Community Psychiatry
The Principles

Community Psychiatry
The Principles

Edited by

Douglas H. Bennett MD FRCPsych
Emeritus Physician, Bethlem Royal and Maudsley Hospitals, London, UK

Hugh L. Freeman MSc MA DM FRCPsych FFCM
Honorary Professor, University of Salford;
Honorary Consultant Psychiatrist, Salford Health Authority, UK;
Editor, British Journal of Psychiatry.

CHURCHILL LIVINGSTONE
EDINBURGH LONDON MELBOURNE NEW YORK AND TOKYO 1991

CHURCHILL LIVINGSTONE
Medical Division of Longman Group UK Limited

First published 1991

ISBN 0-443-03308-0

British Library Cataloguing in Publication Data
Community psychiatry.
  1. Medicine Psychiatry
  I. Bennett, Douglas H.   II. Freeman, Hugh 616.89

Library of Congress Cataloging in Publication Data
Community psychiatry : the scientific background / edited by
Douglas H. Bennett, Hugh L. Freeman.
     p.   cm.
  Includes bibliographical references.
  Includes index.
  ISBN 0-443-03308-0
  1. Community psychiatry.   I. Bennett, Douglas H.
II.Freeman, Hugh L. (Hugh Lionel)
  [DNLM: 1. Community Psychiatry. WM 30.6 C73435]
RC455.C6175 1991
616.89--dc20
DNLM/DLC
for Library of Congress   90-2528
                                              CIP

Produced by Longman Singapore Publishers (Pte) Ltd.
Printed in Singapore.

Contributors

Boris M. Astrachan MD
Professor and Head, Department of Psychiatry, University of Illinois at Chicago, Illinois, USA

Leona L. Bachrach PhD
Research Professor of Psychiatry, Maryland Psychiatric Research Center, University of Maryland School of Medicine, Catonsville, Maryland, USA

Douglas H. Bennett MD FRCPsych
Emeritus Physician, Bethlem Royal and Maudsley Hospitals, London, UK

J.L.T. Birley FRCP FRCPsych
Emeritus Consultant Psychiatrist, Bethlem Royal and Maudsley Hospitals, London, UK

A.P. Boardman BSc PhD MB BS MRCPsych
Senior Registrar, Division of Psychiatry, United Medical and Dental Schools, Guy's Hospital, London, UK

Alexander C. Brown MD FRCPsych
Consultant Senior Lecturer, Department of Mental Health, University of Bristol, Bristol, UK

G.W. Brown
Professor of Social Policy and Social Sciences, Royal Holloway and Bedford New College, University of London, UK

Traloach S. Brugha MD MRCPsych
Senior Lecturer, Department of Psychiatry, University of Leicester; Honorary Consultant Psychiatrist, Leicestershire Health Authority, Leicester, UK

John E. Cooper BM FRCP FRCPsych
Professor of Psychiatry, University of Nottingham Medical School, Nottingham, UK

T.K.J. Craig MB BS MRCPsych
Senior Lecturer, Division of Psychiatry, United Medical and Dental Schools, Guy's Hospital, London; Director, Research and Development for Psychiatry, London, UK

Hugh L. Freeman MSc MA DM FRCPsych FFCM
Honorary Professor, University of Salford; Honorary Consultant
Psychiatrist, Salford Health Authority, UK; Editor, British Journal of
Psychiatry.

David Goldberg DM FRCP FRCPsych
Professor of Psychiatry, University of Manchester; Director, Mental
Illness Research Unit, Manchester, UK

Peter Huxley BA MSc PhD
Professor of Psychiatric Social Work; Director, Mental Health Social
Work Research Unit, University of Manchester, UK

David Jolley BSc MB BS FRCPsych
Consultant Old Age Psychiatrist, Withington Hospital, Manchester;
Honorary Lecturer, Manchester University, UK

Susan Jolley MB ChB MRCPsych
Consultant Old Age Psychiatrist, Withington Hospital, Manchester;
Honorary Lecturer, Manchester University, UK

Heinz Katschnig MD
Professor of Psychiatry, Psychiatric Clinic, University of Vienna, Austria

Julian Leff BSc MD FRCPsych MRCP
Director, MRC Social and Community Psychiatry Unit, Institute of
Psychiatry, London; Professor of Social & Cultural Psychiatry, University
of London, UK

David L. Marshall MB BS MRCPsych
Consultant Psychiatrist, Somerset Health Authority, Wells, UK

Richard F. Mollica MD MAR
Assistant Professor of Psychiatry, Harvard Medical School; Director,
Harvard Program in Refugee Trauma, Harvard School of Public Health;
Clinical Director, Indochinese Psychiatry Clinic, St Elizabeth's Hospital,
Boston, Massachusetts, USA

Isobel Morris MSc
District Clinical Psychologist, Lewisham and North Southwark Health
Authority, London, UK

Jennifer Newton PhD
Prevention Research Officer, National Association of Mental Health
(MIND), London, UK

Edna H. Oppenheimer MA
Senior Lecturer, Addiction Research Unit, Institute of Psychiatry,
London, UK

Jim Orford MA PhD
Reader in Clinical and Community Psychology, University of Exeter;
Top Grade Psychologist, Exeter Health Authority, Exeter, UK

E.S. Paykel MD FRCP FRCPsych
Professor of Psychiatry, Addenbrooke's Hospital, University of
Cambridge, UK

James Raftery MA
Lecturer in Health Economics, Department of Clinical Epidemiology &
Social Medicine, St George's Hospital Medical School, London, UK

John W. Rawlinson RGN RMN DipN CertEd
Tutor, Avon College of Nursing and Midwifery, Bristol, UK

Geoff Shepherd BSc MPhil PhD
Consultant Clinical Psychologist, Head of Psychology Department,
Fulbourn Hospital, Cambridge, UK

Digby Tantam BA MA MPH PhD MRCPsych
Professor of Psychotherapy, Department of Psychology & School of
Postgraduate Medical Education, University of Warwick, UK

Contents

Introduction

We have called this book *Community Psychiatry: The Principles*, because it is our intention to present the subject as essentially a branch of medicine. This does not mean that it has been written entirely by doctors: as will be seen in the list of contributors, a significant number of them are in fact non-medical scientists. However, what they all share is the principle that community psychiatry should be approached from the standpoint of scientific investigation, rather than from an ideological or idealistic one. In the present state of knowledge, fragmentary as it is in many respects, much of this subject must inevitably rest for the time being more on well-informed subjective judgements than on established facts. But this is very different from making the available data fit a pre-determined framework that may be essentially political — which, regrettably, is the way that community psychiatry has often been approached up to now. In this Introduction, we will deal with several topics that have not been considered at length in other parts of the book.

Definition

We see community psychiatry as motivated, first and foremost, by the humanitarian goals of medicine in general, and not by a wish to take part in the imposition of any particular vision of human society. It is ironical, in fact, that those who persistently denounce psychiatry for being 'coercive',' manipulative', or 'repressive' are often the most anxious to make people conform to their own ideological blueprint of how life should be organised.

We have also tried to separate 'community psychiatry', as we understand it, from the very different concept of 'community mental health'. Endless tedious argument has gone on over many years about the definitions of these and other related terms, and it seems unlikely there will ever be universal agreement about them. Very simply, we do not see 'community mental health' as an offshoot of medical science, in the way that 'community psychiatry' is. In so far as there is any consensus about the meaning of 'community mental health', it refers to a concern with the perceived moral and psychological welfare of a society, rather than to levels of psychiatric morbidity; correspondingly, any action that it may involve would not be primarily through medicine or related professions. To complicate the situation further, though, the phrase 'community mental health service' is often used to mean one which undertakes the care *for* a particular community. Instead, we have preferred to talk of a 'community-based' or 'district' psychiatric service, and so far as possible, these terms have been used throughout the book.

With very few exceptions, existing books on this subject have originated in the United States and have been strongly coloured by experience and prevailing ideas there. In contrast this work comes from Great Britain, though three of the contributors are American and one is from Continental Europe. It follows the consensual British view that community psychiatry is an eclectic, non-ideological, and largely atheoretical discipline, but one which is open to and capable of absorbing ideas or data from any school, provided that these are found pragmatically to be capable of reducing disease, distress, or disability. Whatever is shown empirically to be effective can be drawn into the model, and none need be excluded on dogmatic grounds alone; although this understanding of community psychiatry owes more to the biological model than to any other single one, it is equally open to psychodynamic concepts or to such sociological ones as social support and social networks.

As a psychologist, Whitehead (1988) sees community psychiatry as 'pulling the focus finally away from a largely biologically based illness model to one where social and psychological factors in causation, maintenance and alleviation are given full weight.' To what extent the structure of services needs to be changed by this conceptual shift, or whether it could be done largely by altered work practices and retraining of staff within existing arrangements, is a question on which there is little agreement.

Those principles of district-related service organisation which originated mainly in the United Kingdom in the 1950s and 1960s have since been influential in many parts of the world, but particularly in Northern and Western Europe. In doing so, they seem to be more durable than the American Comprehensive Community Mental Health Center model, which, while it seemed to be all-powerful in the 1960s, has failed to deliver what it promised — as was surely inevitable, given the grandiose and imprecise nature of its goals, combined with the modest resources actually applied. Another wave of uncritical enthusiasm was aroused by the Italian reform of 1980, but this time with a strong underpinning of political ideology; ever since then, a number of local services in Italy — unrepresentative even of that country — have been put up by enthusiasts as the model to which every mental health service ought to conform. The Italian reform has promoted some useful improvements (some of which had already started before it was implemented), but these have little to do with the political or philosophical rhetoric that accompanied it. Franco

Bassaglia may indeed have provided the inspiration for it all, yet there is no evidence that either the political mobilisation of society or the transformation of societal attitudes that he predicted has occurred to any meaningful extent (Papeschi 1985). Where services have improved in Italy — and this has been mainly confined to the northern half — the changes have been very largely along lines already familiar elsewhere, while the gaps and deficiencies remain as egregious as in most countries. A national survey of the evaluative research that had actually been done (Crepet 1988) did not record a single well-designed study, including a control group, to investigate the effectiveness of the new model of care. Up to 1990, improved psychiatric services in Italy appear to be comparable with those in some other European countries, including the UK, but not significantly better.

The underlying theme of this book is in fact one of transition from the mental hospital — a process occurring today in almost all industrialised countries though accompanied by hardly any systematic evaluation. In the rest of the world, though, non-indigenous services never reached more than a small fraction of the population, so that the development of modern community psychiatry there must follow a different path, which is likely to be closely linked with primarily medical care. The Western European and North American mental hospital was essentially a construction of the early nineteenth century, but one strongly influenced by the principles of the Enlightenment and, in Britain, by evangelical religion. At the mid-period of that century, it had become established as one of the most important of public services, but why such relatively enormous sums of both capital and revenue should have been given over to the care of mental illness by states which in general avoided intervention in the lives of their subjects — except to maintain law and order — is a question that still remains largely unanswered. The view derived from Marx via Foucault is that this was basically a mechanism of social control, with the specific purpose of removing unproductive or disruptive members of the adult population from the arena of work. However attractive this might be to some as a theory, it finds little or no support in the increasing volume of detailed historical research which is now reaching fruition. Even historians who start with a conspiratorial view of the asylum find, on examining its detailed records, that in almost all cases, those admitted were severely disturbed through mental illness or retardation; they came in when their families could no longer cope, or because they had no families (Walton 1988). They were not heroes or heroines of the class struggle.

The other persisting question is why the asylums, which began with great optimism and high discharge rates, should over time have become so overwhelmed by the increasing chronicity of their patients that they had to be constantly enlarged and supplemented by new institutions. Views on this, however, must be influenced not only by history, but by increasingly sophisticated psychiatric or social–psychiatric knowledge. It has been suggested that the incidence of schizophrenia may have risen during the 19th century, but in trying to explain the steady rise in asylum populations, this view perhaps pays insufficient attention to the influence of culturally different patterns of life on the outcome of the illness, in countries with or without traditions of custodial care. There were also the effects of the severely restricted asylum setting on people confined as pauper–lunatics without the kind of relief from symptoms that comes from present-day medication. A significant proportion of those affected by schizophrenia at that time and since suffered severe, permanent disability of a kind now described as 'negative syndromes'. In the early asylums, as with any service that is set up to deal with whole populations, such patients will have presented little problem in terms of numbers at first, but as time went on, the original hopes of treating the treatable were dissipated by the accumulation of increasing numbers of chronic patients. Their chronicity was the product of the inherent handicaps of the illness, combined with the effects of institutionalism.

However, the explanation of chronicity does not relate only to schizophrenia. Many of the asylum patients also had serious physical disease, particularly tuberculosis, syphilis, or epilepsy, which would have made their discharge even more difficult. Some were too mentally retarded to manage in society outside, and no special institutions yet existed for them. Some had a mixture of medical and social handicaps, none of which singly would have required long stay in an institution, but which when combined, kept people in the asylum because there was no other facility that was able or willing to accept them. This historical excursus is critical to understanding the processes through which mental hospitals could now be replaced by a more appropriate pattern of services, two centuries after they evolved in a recognisably modern form. Unless the lessons of the Victorian asylum are fully learned, though, it is possible that the same cycle might occur, where naive optimism is followed by disillusion, but this time within the ambit of 'community psychiatry'. For all its faults, the classical mental hospital had in its time a utility in its resources of space and staffing, which enabled it to cope with cases affected by multiple and undifferentiated problems and to offer continuity of care over many years, if often at a considerable cost in the development of secondary disabilities. Furthermore, it nearly always had a place available when there was an emergency, and did not charge for its services. It would be ironical if concern about those patients within mental hospitals suffering from chronic mental illness — which was one of the main motivating forces behind the community psychiatry movement — should in the end result in that same group of people suffering from lack of adequate care, but this time outside any hospital.

Community psychiatry has demonstrated that it has replaced many but not all of these functions of the mental hospital. A relatively small number of people with challenging behaviour or severe disabilities will still require 24-hour residential care, whether willingly sought or legally enforced, and whether in a hospital, a nursing home, or a residential unit in the general community. Smaller hospital units will be relatively more expensive per case than psychiatric hospitals, though needed for significantly fewer patients, who will be severely ill or disabled and requiring more intensive care than most in-patients did in the past. Nevertheless, the total cost of in-patient care is likely to be reduced. What ought to be a pragmatic question, though, of how the community can cope best with the needs of relatively small numbers of people who have severe disabilities tends to be converted into an ideological issue, whereby all care within a hospital by professional staff is labelled as 'oppressive'. Similarly, the need to protect the community from the very few individuals showing intractable and dangerous behaviour is often denied by those responsible for planning or managing services, mainly because the facilities required to deal adequately with this problem are expensive, particularly in staff time. Community psychiatry must also recognise that there is a need for the provision of services in the community which offer continuing care for chronic patients over the years, with the easy availability of 24-hour emergency services that will offer immediate help when problems arise acutely. If such high-dependency care for limited numbers of chronic patients is not available outside hospital, community psychiatry will not be adequate to serve the mental health needs of whole populations in the 1990s.

Psychiatric training

One of the most unsatisfactory aspects of psychiatry in many countries, at least until the 1980s, was the low standard of its specialist training, associated with a generally poor quality of medical recruits; similar problems affected the other mental health professions. (This chapter will not discuss the training of non-medical mental health workers.) In Britain, outside the two main postgraduate centres (at London and Edinburgh), psychiatric training occurred mostly in mental hospitals on an apprenticeship basis, and was not assessed by any higher examination comparable to those in general medicine or surgery. In 1971, though, the new Royal College of Psychiatrists introduced both rigorous require-ments for training schemes and a specialty examination with high clinical and academic standards. Combined with the increasing numbers of medical graduates (many of whom were now women), these changes dramatically raised the quality of doctors coming into British psychiatry, but their training was essentially hospital-based — like that of every other medical speciality, as well as that of nurses and other health professionals. Somewhat similar developments occurred in Northern Europe and Commonwealth countries, but in the USA most teaching centres remained dominated by psychoanalysis until the strong re-emergence of biological psychiatry in the 1980s.

However, just as this newly devised British system was settling down and beginning to produce well-trained specialists, the national trend towards community psychiatry required it to be fundamentally rethought. One possibility would have been to separate off a sub-speciality of community psychiatry, with its own training requirements comparable to those, for example, of forensic psychiatry, but this option was not supported (Freeman 1985). Instead, community psychiatry has generally been viewed as 'a way of working with patients which...will demand an extended range of expertise from all psychiatrists' (Royal College of Psychiatrists 1989). This means integrating experience of community-orientated developments into the existing training programme, but without loss of any of the core skills of psychiatry, such as the management of disturbed patients or familiarity with the whole range of abnormal mental phenomena. If patients are to be able to continue receiving skilled medical treatment, when that is the required option, psychiatrists should neither retreat into a narrow medical role nor 'make a virtue of feeling deskilled by adopting the generic role of 'mental health worker'' (Peet 1986).

Though there is no consensus about the range of expertise needed for community-orientated psychiatry, the College's report saw essential differences from hospital-based practice in the variety of settings where patients are seen, more explicit liaison with other health care workers, greater consideration of local conditions, and fewer grade-specific tasks. Since some of the required skills should be expected of other members of a multi-disciplinary team, the question arose whether such training might also be shared with these professions? The possible advantages of such sharing, including better cohesiveness of teams, had to be balanced, though, against a risk of eroding the special roles and skills which each profession brings to the multi-disciplinary management of patients (see Ch. 1). Full-time hospital work, at least for the first year, still seems the most effective way for a doctor to become skilled in the essential tasks of history-taking, examination of the mental state, clinical investigation, and case-presentation. On the other hand, this report advocated at least a year's experience of community-orientated psychiatry, with work in primary care, day facilities, domiciliary assessment, crisis intervention, and consultation to other agencies. To avoid loss of the experience of managing chronically ill psychotic patients, trainees might follow cases in the community for a year or more.

Such a dispersal of the training experience of psychiatrists, though, ought not to involve the break-up of well organised schemes with high academic standards: to do so might risk returning to something like the old mental hospital apprenticeship. Not only is there still a need for the collective wisdom and facilities of large teaching centres, but also for the support and mutual learning that comes from trainees' shared experience. At the same time, many established clinicians will need some retraining for a modified style of working, as well as continuing medical education to maintain their core professional skills. However, all these activities have to be paid for, and doctors who do not earn their living from private practice, like members of other professions involved, cannot reasonably pay the cost themselves. In Britain, a National Health Service in the grip of ideological upheaval does not seem well placed to meet these new demands, yet if it does not, the quality of service must inevitably fall and 'community psychiatry' cannot properly succeed. In most other countries also, insufficient attention had been given to the systematic training of psychiatrists for community-based work.

Compulsory treatment in the community?

Because of the sometimes damaging effects of psychosis on the perception of reality, and because of the dangers to the patient or others which may result from this, nearly every country has legal provisions whereby such people can be compulsorily admitted to a hospital and be given treatment there. However, these laws mostly originated in a time when the classical mental hospital was the only place where patients with severe psychiatric disorder could be managed, and in many countries the laws have become seriously obsolete. Even when updated, as in the English Mental Health Act of 1983, it is rare for them to acknowledge the fact that with current psychiatric treatments and patterns of services, the place of residence of the patient has become much less important than the care being received. These considerations apply particularly to services which strongly emphasise management within the home whenever possible, though they are relevant to all with a community orientation.

A 'Community Treatment Order' (CTO) is a mechanism which might answer the dilemma of separating compulsory treatment from unnecessary residence in a hospital, but it remains a highly controversial option. Some states of the USA use it as a 'least restrictive alternative' to compulsory admission, though it may then be applied more through legal negotiations similar to plea-bargaining, rather than as a matter of clinical judgement (American Psychiatric Association 1987). It is sometimes known there as 'out-patient commitment'. In England, however, the use of extended leave to ensure continued medication, while the patient remains subject to a compulsory admission order, was ruled to be illegal (R v. Hallstrom 1985). As a result, the only policy that services can follow, if consent to treatment is persistently refused, is to wait until the patient has deteriorated sufficiently to become liable for compulsory readmission. In Victoria, Australia, CTOs have had legal effect since 1986: so far, staff there have not attempted to treat patients against their will outside hospital. However, the Orders seemed to have improved compliance in some cases, as well as committing the treating agencies to a firm plan of management in the community (Dedman, 1990).

In any population, the number of people likely to require a CTO would be very small indeed, but nearly all would be suffering from schizophrenia or another major psychosis. Usually, the case is one of the 'revolving door' type, in which improvement in hospital is invariably followed by the patient stopping treatment after discharge and then suffering relapse. Each relapse is not only distressing to the patient and relatives, but is likely to cause progressive erosion of the network of social support, with possible loss of job, home, and friendships.

It would clearly be very undesirable for any such measure to be used mainly as a way of covering up deficiencies in a psychiatric service; the CTO would in fact work best in places where the service is well-organised and financed, so that cases requiring an Order would be very few. For a CTO to be appropriate, the patient should have had a previous period of severe mental illness which had responded to the proposed treatment, and ready access should be available to be a second opinion and to a legal Tribunal. It is likely that most patients placed on a CTO would then agree to receive treatment, but community psychiatric nurses in Britain have been understandably concerned about the situation they might face if any patient did not do so. Probably, admission to hospital would then be more appropriate than the compulsory administration of treatment in a community setting, but this should not result in such delay that the patient deteriorates to a serious extent. Alternatively, if the English law and many others could be altered so that admission was to a 'service' rather than to a hospital, many of these major problems would not occur. Certainly, their number can be reduced by mental health staff keeping in close touch with relatives or other concerned individuals and by coordinating their own work in relation to any particular patient. Using a retrospective examination of case records and other information, Sensky et al (1990) showed that a group of psychiatrists at a London hospital were consistent and selective in their criteria for recommending patients for hypothetical compulsory community treatment.

Asylum

By an unfortunate semantic change, of the kind described by Hoggart (1988) as 'the cultural accretions of language', the word 'asylum', which should indicate a secure place of shelter, became largely restricted in meaning to a 'total institution' (Goffman 1961) — one usually pictured as huge, remote, parsimonious, and authoritarian. On the other hand, 'community' was increasingly equated with cohesive and caring neighbourhoods, so that 'by a process of tautology, being "in the community" becomes an administrative goal in itself' (Wing 1990). Since the genuine function of asylum was forgotten in this, a deconstruction of terms is now needed to identify the essential elements of that function and to see whether or not they have been incorporated into the network of a community psychiatric service. In Britain, the Short Report (1985) emphasised that 'the concept of asylum has nothing inherently to do with large or isolated institutions.' Nor is there necessarily anything custodial about it: the protection of vulnerable people does not include that of society, except from the embarrassment of witnessing odd behaviour. Wing (1990) suggests that shelter from cruelty, exploitation, pauperism, and social isolation on the one hand should be balanced by 'reparation', which consists of identifying the causes of social disablement, treating any physical or mental disorders, and providing the means of rehabilitation and resettlement, where possible. This group are to be distinguished from the very small number who need constant nursing care on a long-term basis, for whom the hospital–hostel is likely to be the most acceptable solution (Hyde et al 1987).

Within the spectrum of psychiatric illness, those needing asylum rather than the high-dependency regime of a hospital unit or 'hospital–hostel' are predominantly suffering from chronic psychoses. 'Typically, they are middle-aged and single or divorced; they have few visitors and are unemployable within the hospital. Many have failed at integration into the community and some roam the hospital grounds resisting all further attempts at rehabilitation... A few have behavioural characteristics that would attract attention (outside)' (Fottrell 1990). Some still remain as long-stay in-patients, avoiding efforts to resettle them, but many more are 'in the community', in the sense that they are cared for by relatives, live isolated in bedsits or lodgings, are in charitable shelters, on remand in prison, or sleeping rough. Because most are no longer in psychiatric beds, calculating their number becomes more and more difficult, but Robertson (1981) estimated these as about 50 per 100 000 population for England, or about 150 in an average Health District, many of whom will be aged 65 and over.

The provision of care for this group should follow a clearly defined policy, coordinated between health services, social services, voluntary organisations, etc. In Britain, though, very little attention and virtually no experiments have been devoted to the alternative structures that might serve the function of asylum (Wing 1990); nor has there been any controlled comparison of the possible facilities that might replace the mental hospital in this respect. People with severe chronic disability, particularly if this is psychiatric, have a low priority with health services, worldwide.

Since the 1970s, long-term accommodation provided within the network of community mental health services in most countries has generally been small-scale and in ordinary housing. But many of the chronically disabled need a moderate degree of supervision — in some cases indefinitely — and providing this in many small units involves heavy costs, administrative complexities, and difficulties in monitoring standards. One view is that it would be more economical and effective to provide some facilities for larger groups of residents; these could often be converted from existing buildings, particularly where mental hospitals are sited fairly near the population they serve. But there are difficulties; many patients do not wish to be admitted or to stay in hospital (Johnstone et al 1984) and perhaps cannot be compulsorily committed. The conversion of a former asylum may be extremely costly and planning permission not easily obtained; even then, the stigma associated with the hospital's past may haunt it. People can, of course, be cared for and rehabilitated in new small units; the methods of providing such care without institutionalising them have been described, if not heeded (Garety and Morris 1984). Deinstitutionalisation is still formulated incorrectly as structuring units physically in new ways and in new places, rather than in changing staff attitudes and forming new relationships between patients and staff.

This raises the question of how the effects of a change of accommodation on individuals can be assessed, since once a system of care has fallen into disrepute, as the mental hospital system did after World War II, it tends to be assumed that any change will be for the better. Wing (1990) has proposed four standards by which the function of asylum ought to be evaluated within a community-based mental health service: (1) Are the functions of asylum being carried out at least as successfully as in the best (not the worst) hospital-based services of the past? (2) Are the disadvantages thought to be inherent in the old system being avoided? (3) Are problems being introduced which are specific to the new service? (4) Are new advantages (e.g. extra choice) being derived from increased interaction with families and with the general public? Simply setting out questions of this kind will draw attention to the very inadequate way in which many post-hospital developments have been carried out and to the lack of planning, evaluation, and effective management that is to be found in the development of community-based psychiatric services throughout the world.

Evaluation

Of these generally missing processes, evaluation is perhaps the most critical for the development of a scientifically-based community psychiatry (see also Ch. 1). For both clinicians and administrators in most countries, the facts of life in the 1990s are that no significant increase in real resources for mental health care is to be expected, so that changes must result only from the reallocation of existing funds, staff, or buildings. Any new service, e.g. community mental health centres or psychiatrists' sessions in primary care, will eventually be at the expense of some existing one, and this makes it essential to evaluate both the process of change and the outcome of the new service (Strathdee 1990). Hafner & An der Heiden (1989) define three levels at which evaluation should be done: (1) the mental health sector of a national system of health and social services; (2) the psychiatric service in a defined catchment area; and (3) individual facilities and programmes within a district. The usefulness of the evaluation will depend mainly on the nature and quality of the information being collected; for instance, the number of discharges from in-patient care, although easy to record reliably, conveys nothing about the outcome of these individuals' stays in hospital.

The information required is of two main kinds. Firstly, that relating to patients' psychopathology, social functioning, quality of life, and any other types of handicap all need to be measured by reliable and valid techniques such as the Present State Examination. Secondly, information relating to the services received: because packages of care are complex, the use of all services within the network should be recorded in relation to individual patients, ideally through a cumulative case register (e.g. Wooff et al 1983). However, if the packages are poorly defined, as they have been in many comparisons of extramural with institutional care, it will not be possible to obtain results that have external validity, i.e. that are generalisable to other settings (Bachrach 1982). Ultimately, it cannot be shown that the objective of a mental health service (minimising the morbidity of individuals with psychiatric disorders) is being achieved, unless there is detailed evidence that such outcomes are related to processes within the system of mental health care. If an individual is exposed to the system, it is usually assumed that the outcome is a result of its intervention, particularly if that intervention has been changed, but unless the evaluation has taken account of other possible factors, this does not exclude the possibility that some other factor was responsible for that outcome. Existing studies have rarely done so, however. Since conditions change constantly, the functioning of the mental health care system at the district level needs to be evaluated continuously, and the cumulative case register is the most effective way of doing so (Wing 1989). Most regrettably, the British case registers have largely ceased to exist, due to the withdrawal of official funding, whilst that in Mannheim was closed down through political action; however, some registers continue to function in Europe (Ten Horn et al 1986).

Although the run-down of psychiatric hospitals is a fact in most countries, and many of the hospitals will be closed sooner or later, there is virtually no evidence about the effectiveness of this policy, particularly in relation to the cost of community alternatives (O'Donnell 1990). Both Weisbrod et al (1990) in Wisconsin and Hoult et al (1984) in Sydney found that a community-based system was more efficient than an institutional one for patients with a wide range of psychiatric diagnoses, but this alternative care needed to be comprehensive in nature, continuous over long periods, and assertive rather than merely reactive. O'Donnell points out that in model programmes such as these, there is usually a degree of enthusiasm and high morale which would not necessarily be found everywhere; just as psychiatric hospitals varied greatly in their quality, so inevitably will community-based alternatives. There is no evidence that in-patient care can be completely replaced without very adverse consequences, since all comparative studies have included the admission to hospital of some patients who had been originally allocated to community care. Furthermore, the effectiveness of community mental health centres, psychiatric work in primary care, crisis intervention teams, case management, and various kinds of residential settings all remain largely unknown in any scientific sense.

When the question is faced of how to evaluate mental health services in terms of money values, difficulties become even more formidable. In the first place, many of the phenomena with which these services are concerned are scarcely expressible in financial terms: the cost of absence from work, for instance, can be calculated, but hardly the relief of distress that results from successfully treating depression. Weisbrod et al (1980), who made one of the most sophisticated financial comparisons of two contrasting types of psychiatric care, pointed out that what appears to be a cheaper service may in fact be merely one that has shifted part of its costs into forms whose costs cannot be calculated, e.g. the stress and poorer quality of life experienced by informal carers. Their own method was to measure in monetary terms all costs that were measurable, but also to identify explicitly all other relevant costs. This rigorous approach has not often been equalled.

Another complication arises from the fact that in the process of deinstitutionalisation, the less handicapped will almost invariably leave hospital first. This usually results in an over-optimistic view being taken by administrators and planners of what the total cost will eventually be of resettling the entire hospital population. Yet, 'because of this selective process, it can't be assumed that today's money will also buy the same services for tomorrow's clientele' (Knapp 1990); the packages of care which the most dependent patients will need are more expensive than their care in hospital would have been. There has also been much confusion from calculations of the costs of services which are based on the average for large numbers of patients, with very varying characteristics; this does not provide a reliable basis for planning. In Britain, the TAPS project in London has approached these financial questions in a highly sophisticated way, but even a wealth of data relating to the closure of two mental hospitals will not provide definitive answers for an entire country on the costs and efficiency of a new pattern of services. So far as other countries are concerned, the generalisability of such findings for them must inevitably be much less.

Another approach to the needs of evaluation is the construction of 'standards of care', arising from the work on Quality Assurance (QA) in Australian mental health services (Rosen et al 1989). The QA process requires that information on the service is continuously fed back to all service-providers concerned, and that there is a mechanism to ensure that improvement in quality is maintained. However, if standards of care are laid down, the management of the service should be able both to ascertain that effective use is being made of existing resources and to identify any extra resources that are needed. Rosen et al propose that the standards should meet most of the following requirements of a district mental health service: (1) in applying to both community and hospital facilities, to all professions, and to all phases of care; (2) in involving both users and providers in providing standards for their local conditions; (3) in being linked to desirable outcomes, rather than being focused only on structures and processes. All standards would also be specific to mental health care. The main phases of care to be evaluated would be: initial contact and assessment, acute management, ongoing management and rehabilitation, and long-term follow-up. This work is as yet in its early stages; one fundamental question, though, which remains problematic for all forms of evaluation is — what is to happen when the needs which are identified cannot be met with the resources made available (from whatever source)? Theoretically, a population which 'wills the ends' must also 'will the means', through whatever machinery exists, whether public, private, or mixed. In practice, though, such a logical result rarely emerges, since people tend to decide that they should both have their cake and eat it.

The UK Department of Health has emphasized that indicators of outcome are needed not only by planners, policy-makers and health authorities, but also by clinicians, if they are to evaluate the effectiveness of their work and identify areas for improvement (Jenkins 1990). For mental health, outcome consists of changes in patients' functionings, morbidity, and mortality, but because of their complexity, any indicators used are likely to be only indirect or partial measures. Since psychiatric in-patients represent only 1–2% of the total of psychiatric morbidity in most countries, indicators which refer primarily to them will clearly be of only very limited value. Jenkins has proposed a preliminary series of indicators of health care input, process and outcome for nine diagnostic categories of psychiatric disorder. In the case of schizophrenia, for example, the suggested outcome indicators are: local prevalence figures (with grading levels of disability), hospital first-admission and readmission rates, and rates of employment, suicide, standardized mortality, and homelessness in local patients. Up to now, most available information on mental health services has been related to input or process, but this is ultimately only a preliminary stage to the construction of valid, reliable, and sensitive measures of outcome in individual patients. Without these, there can never be reasonable certainty about the value of developments in community psychiatry. Unfortunately, the division of health activities, such as medical treatment, from social care, including performance in daily living activities, makes assessment of the outcome of some vulnerable groups even more difficult, since inputs in one system may have to be measured as outcome in the other.

The role of consumers

Although not strictly a part of the scientific approach to community psychiatry, the ex-patients' movement requires mention here. Earlier attempts had in fact been made to give the patient a greater say in his/her treatment; for instance, the therapeutic community movement adopted the democratic ideals of the post-war period and sought to provide 'opportunities for patients to take an active part in the affairs of the institution' (Rapoport 1960). Rapoport, however, did not feel that these aims were wholly compatible with the satisfactory adjustment of ex-patients to life outside hospital. Later 'patient government' became popular in the United States, although at Yale Psychiatric Institute, it was felt to be 'an anemic institution with sporadic existence'. Power-sharing was tried and though playing a part in liberalising psychiatric hospital life, did not generally satisfy patients, who are pursuing other aims today (Rubenstein & Lasswell 1966).

In 1985, the House of Commons Social Services Committee said that members had had difficulty 'in hearing the authentic voice of the ultimate consumer of community care...Services are still mainly designed by providers, whether families or clients, and in response to blueprints rather than in answer to demand' (Short Report 1985). The current movement is usually described by psychiatrists and by some others (Chamberlin 1978) as the 'ex-patients' movement'. However, the terms used by and the ideals of its proponents in America, Canada, The Netherlands, Britain, Australia, and New Zealand vary widely. For some it is 'advocacy', for others 'empowerment', patients' rights, user participation, liberation, or consumer networks, while the most extreme proponents are against 'psychiatric oppression', or see themselves as 'survivors' from mishandling in institutions. American practice, drawing on experience from the black, women's, and gay movements, strongly resists the inclusion of non-patients in their movement and sees dangers in allowing professionals to set goals for it. In this sense, they are separatists and maintain an independence of and opposition to psychiatric ideology (Chamberlin 1987). Others, though, take a more conciliatory stance and work with the mental health system.

These divisions are exacerbated by the problems of funding which face every one of these groups, while another difficulty lies in the nature of consumerism. Material consumers are advised which goods to buy on the basis of information about their efficacy and cost; they are not involved in the manufacture or sale of these goods. The consumers of a treatment service, on the other hand, wish to be involved in the planning, development and evaluation of the service, as well as to be consulted about care, support, and treatment programmes which they will receive (WHO 1989). There is an understandable need for consumers to get their views and needs taken seriously and to receive better care by enabling more equal and more intelligent transactions to take place between such persons, their representatives, and health care personnel. However, the situation is viewed in differing ways by the general public, the patients, their families, and professionals respectively. The general public's interest and fears are aroused by the occasional dramatic episode of violence which shatters the framework of publicly predictable behaviour, while families are tied by the burden of caring for relatives or by fears for their safety, if they refuse care. Professionals are motivated by anxieties about their responsibility for giving safely correct care, lest they come under attack from relatives, the public, or the law. Even public attitudes as expressed respectively by MIND and the National Schizophrenia Fellowship (NSF) in Britain or the National Alliance for the Mentally Ill in the USA, differ in their attitudes to treatment and hospital care, although the involvement of ex-patients with both *Mindlink* and the NSF's *Voices*, for instance, is encouraged.

Even so, growth of the movement has been slow in the United Kingdom. Efforts to secure advocacy for those with learning difficulties (or mental retardation) by the Advocacy Alliance, a consortium of five nationally known voluntary organisations (Sang & O'Brien 1984), has only involved three hospitals and formed 30 long-term relationships in six years. In America too, Chamberlin (1981) concludes that while millions have been in the physchiatric system at some time in their lives, the movement has reached only a small fraction of them.

The ex-patients' movement has clearly been most concerned with the needs of in-patient users (Barker & Peck 1987), but difficulties are or will be present in the future community management of people with psychiatric disorders. Anxieties about Community Treatment Orders are voiced by one 'users'' spokeswoman as giving the psychiatric profession the right 'to drug citizens compulsorily in their own homes' (Lindow 1990). The same author feels that the government's White Paper *Caring for People* (Department of Health 1989) also threatens users with stigma by suggesting that district health authorities should 'keep appropriate registers'. One unresolved question, though, is how to assess the legitimacy of claims by individuals that they 'represent' the users of the mental health care system. Since the latter number several million in the United Kingdom (if all levels of psychiatric disorder are included), it is difficult to see in what way their views and wishes in general have been sought.

The UK Department of Health's discussion paper on planning district mental health services (Department of Health 1990) gives priority both to improving the quality of services and to making these more responsive to the views of their users. District Health Authorities are advised to identify the main users and to find out which activities *they* regard as key indicators of good performance. Each agency providing services is also to have an effective system to obtain these views, which will vary according to the groups concerned: patients may be surveyed through questionnaires or interviews, GPs through surveys on the pattern and quality of services, and surveys of the community may examine overall perceptions of the adequacy of the priorities of its mental health service.

The concept of an ex-patients' movement perhaps expresses too many ideas at the same time and tries to embrace too many different forms of action. Even so, without considering this development, community psychiatry could be portrayed as the transfer from caretaking in large old institutions to caretaking in smaller, newer institutions. Great advances have been made for the physically handicapped in recent years by giving them *physical access* to buildings through structural, architectural modification; they can get access with the use of ramps and lifts to hotels, churches, theatres, and even buses. But those who have been mentally ill still need *social access*. This is more difficult to achieve, for it requires that those who are not psychiatrically disabled have to change their attitudes. Full acceptance of the psychiatrically disabled would mean that they require access to the law and to employment, to have a wage, income maintenance, or adequate insurance, to be able to vote wherever they live, and not to be socially excluded. This seems as far off, perhaps, as physical access was 25 years ago, but some groups are being consulted and are participating in the planning and management of services (Renshaw 1988). It is difficult to say how the movement will develop or whether, as in the United States, it will go in a number of directions. There is no doubt, though, that in one form or another, it will continue to grow.

London and   H.L.F.
Oxford, 1991   D.H.B.

ACKNOWLEDGEMENT

Some material in Chapter 2 previously appeared in the chapter by HL Freeman in 'Mental Illness, Changes & Trends', edited by Philip Bean (1983). This appears by kind permission of John Wiley & Sons.

REFERENCES

American Psychiatric Association 1987 Involuntary commitment to outpatient treatment: report of the Task Force on Involuntary Outpatient Commitment. American Psychiatric Association, Washington

Bachrach L L 1982 Assessment of outcomes in community support systems: results, problems and limitations. Schizophrenia Bulletin 8: 39–61

Barker I, Peck E (eds) 1987 Power in strange places: user empowerment in mental health services. Good Practices in Mental Health, London

Chamberlin J 1981 On our own: patient-controlled alternatives to the mental health system. McGraw Hill, New York

Chamberlin J 1987 The case for separatism: ex-patient organising in the United States. In: Barker I, Peck, E (eds) Power in strange places. GPMH, London

Dedman P 1990 Community treament orders in Victoria, Australia. Psychiatric Bulletin 14: 462–464

Department of Health 1990 Developing districts. HMSO, London

Department of Health & Social Security 1989 Caring for people: community care in the next decade and beyond. Cmd 849, HMSO, London

Fottrell E 1990 Asylum for psychiatric patients in the 1990s (letter) British Medical Journal 300: 468

Freeman H L 1985 Training for community psychiatry. Bulletin of the Royal College of Psychiatrists 9: 29–32

Garety P A, Morris I 1984 A new unit for long-stay psychiatric patients: organisation, attitudes and quality of care. Psychological Medicine 14: 183–192

Goffman E 1961 Asylums. Penguin, Harmondsworth

Häfner H, An der Heiden W 1989 Evaluation of care for the disabled mentally ill: theoretical issues. European Archives of Psychiatry & Neurological Sciences 238: 179–184

Hoggart R 1988 A local habitation. Chatto & Windus, London

Hoult J, Rosen A, Reynolds I 1984 Community-orientated treatment compared to psychiatric hospital-orientated treatment. Social Science & Medicine 18: 1005–1010

Hyde C, Bridges K, Goldberg D, Lawson K, Sterling C, Faragher B 1987 The evaluation of a hostel ward: a controlled study using modified cost benefit analysis. British Journal of Psychiatry 151: 805–812

Jenkins R 1990 Towards a system of outcome indicators for mental health care. British Journal of Psychiatry 157: in press

Johnstone E C, Owens D G C, Gold A, Crow T J, Macmillan J F 1984 Schizophrenic patients discharged from hospital: a follow-up study. British Journal of Psychiatry 145: 586–590

Knapp M 1990 The direct costs of community care of chronically mentally ill people. In: Henderson J H (ed) Comprehensive Mental Health Care. Gaskell, London (forthcoming)

Lindow V 1990 Participation and power. Open Mind 44: 10–11

O'Donnell O 1990 Cost effectiveness of community care for the chronic mentally ill. In: Henderson J H (ed) Comprehensive Mental Health Care. Gaskell, London (forthcoming)

Papeschi R 1985 Denial of the institution: a critical review of Franco Bassaglia's writings. British Journal of Psychiatry 146: 247–254

Peet M 1986 Network community mental health care in north-west Derbyshire. Bulletin of the Royal College of Psychiatrists 10: 262–265

Rapoport R N 1960 Community as doctor: new perspectives on a therapeutic community. Tavistock, London

Regina v Hallstrom 1985 Judgement of Mr. Justice McCullough in the High Court of Justice, Queen's Bench Division, Royal Courts of Justice, 20 December

Renshaw J 1987 Preface In: Barker I, Peck E (eds) Power in strange places. GPMH, London

Robertson G 1981 The provision of inpatient facilities for the mentally ill: a paper to assist NHS planners. DHSS, London (unpublished)

Rosen A, Miller V, Parker G 1989 Standards of care for area mental health services. Australian & New Zealand Journal of Psychiatry 23: 379–395

Royal College of Psychiatrists 1989 Report of the working group on the training implications of the move towards community orientated treatment. London

Rubenstein R, Lasswell H D 1966 The sharing of power in a psychiatric hospital. Yale University Press, New Haven

Sang R, O'Brien J 1984 Advocacy: the UK and American experiences. Project paper No. 51. King Edward's Fund for London, London

Sensky T, Hughes T, Hirsch S 1990 Compulsory treatment of psychiatric patients in the community. British Journal of Psychiatry (in press)

Short Report 1984 House of Commons Social Services Committee Report on community care with special reference to the adult mentally ill and mentally handicapped. HMSO, London

Strathdee G 1990 Delivery of psychiatric care. Journal of the Royal Society of Medicine 83: 222–225

Ten Horn G H M, Giel R, Gulbinat W H, Henderson J H 1986 Psychiatric case registers in public health. Elsevier, Amsterdam

Walton J K 1986 Casting out and bring back in Victorian England: pauper lunatics. In: Bynum W F, Porter R, Shepherd M (eds), The Anatomy of Madness, Volume 2. Tavistock, London

Weisbrod B A, Test M J, Stein L I 1980 An alternative to mental hospital treatment II: economic benefit–cost analysis. Archives of General Psychiatry 37: 400–405

Whitehead A 1988 Bringing science to community care. British Journal of Clinical Psychology 27: 199–200

WHO 1989 Consumer involvement in mental health and rehabilitation services. Division of Mental Health, WHO, Geneva

Wing J K (ed) 1989 Contributions to mental health planning & research. Gaskell, London.

Wing J K 1990 The functions of asylum. British Journal of Psychiatry (in press)

Wooff K, Freeman H L, Fryers T 1983 Psychiatric service use in Salford: a comparison of point–prevalence ratios 1968 and 1978. British Journal of Psychiatry 142: 588–594

1. Principles and prospect

D. H. Bennett   H. L. Freeman

Community, according to Le Bon (quoted by Dennis 1958), is one of those words which are 'uttered with solemnity, and as soon as they are pronounced an expression of respect is visible on every countenance and all heads are bowed'. Some have also felt that the concept has a moral imperative (Hawks 1975), while yet others see it as a popular device to conceal various confusions and contradictions (Pinker 1982) or as a code word to embrace all good work. Titmuss (1963) expressed a similar view, seeing the 'statutory magic and comforting appellation' of community care as pulling the wool over our own and other people's eyes. Though it is difficult to determine the origin of the use of 'community care' in psychiatry, the Annual Report of the Board of Control for 1930 is said to have included the term (Hunter & McAlpine 1974); in 1946, Blacker used it to distinguish between a 'closed hospital psychiatry' for mentally retarded and psychotic patients, and psychiatry 'in the outside world', concerned with the treatment of neurotics and with child guidance. But it only came into more general use in Britain in 1957, when the Royal Commission on the law relating to mental illness and mental deficiency referred to it as 'treatment and training without bringing people into hospital, or discharging them from hospital sooner than in the past' (Royal Commission 1957). Even so, the subsequent 1959 Mental Health Act made no legislative requirement for such a policy to be followed (see Ch. 2).

'Community' has also been employed to refer to the 'community mental hospital', which would not only provide inpatient facilities but develop outpatient services within the community it served (WHO 1953), as well as to the 'therapeutic community', consisting of a 'dynamic', non-institutional form of psychiatric care (Hinshelwood & Manning 1979). Limitation of the term 'in the community' to mean psychiatric services outside the hospital was regarded as unfortunate by the British Seebohm Report, which saw both hospitals and residential homes as part of the community (Report of the Committee on Social Services 1968). Endless argument has in fact occurred over the precise meaning of this and related phrases, such as 'community mental health'. However, a usefully pragmatic view of the question was that of Rehin & Martin (1963), who regarded a community mental health service as any scheme 'directed to providing extramural care and treatment ... to facilitating the early detection of psychiatric illness or relapse and its treatment on an informal basis, and to providing some social work service in the community for support or follow-up'. The trend towards community care combined the new practices of psychiatrists, who were pragmatically doing what they believed to be right, with some general anti-institutional feelings in public opinion. Parker (1971) stated that 'community care' had 'attained a currency reached by few other slogans in the history of social policy in Britain... was easy to comprehend and offered clear-cut guidelines for policy and action'. However, whose responsibility it was to follow these guidelines was then by no means clear.

Though 'community psychiatry' had begun in Britain as an attempt to provide treatment for psychiatric patients outside mental hospitals, its meaning later changed when it was used to describe a national plan for district-based services (Bennett 1978). To be effective, such a practice would need to be grounded in social psychiatry, i.e. the relationship of social factors to psychiatric illness and of that illness to society: it involved the aim of caring, not just for the identified patient, but for a whole population over a significant period of time. Wing (1979) regards this model — sometimes called 'secondary community care' — as most suitable for people who would formerly have been at risk of becoming long-stay mental hospital patients, but not for individuals who were unlikely to have been inpatients for long, and still less for those who would never have seen a psychiatrist at all formerly. However, this view seems to discount the extra benefit which the moderately ill would gain from improving the availability of psychiatric treatment to the population as a whole: in fact, both Freeman (1963) and Bennett saw service to a broadened clientele as one of the primary aims of a community orientation.

Freudenberg (1976), who was influential in the development of British mental health policy, stated that community psychiatry 'assumes that people with psychiatric disorders can be most effectively helped when links with family, friends, workmates, and society generally are maintained, and aims to provide preventive, treatment, and rehabilitative services for a district, which means that therapeutic measures go beyond the individual patient'. That statement clearly expressed the pragmatic, common-sense, and atheoretical basis on which British policy proceeded, but as Freudenberg said, it was largely an assumption, which had not been confirmed by empirical evaluation — as is still largely the case.

An American view by Serban (1977) described community psychiatry as having three aspects — firstly, a social movement; secondly, a service delivery strategy, emphasising the accessibility of services and acceptance of responsibility of the mental health needs of a total population; and thirdly, a means of provision of the best possible clinical care, with emphasis on the major psychiatric disorders and on treatment outside total institutions. Most British developments could be regarded as a combination of the second and third of these aspects. Granted the prevailing complex of values, beliefs, and norms in the country, such a reorientation of psychiatric services towards a more community-based structure was probably inevitable in the 1960s and 1970s, though this did not necessarily imply any change in the types of treatment or care employed. However, a 'community' includes institutions, which in turn include hospitals, and to some extent mental hospitals; it is the mode of use of these institutions which is critical. They can either be closed systems in themselves, drawing in a selected group of clients and treating them by separation from their social contexts, or alternatively, can be part of a service network which extends in various ways into the population served — sometimes called a 'dispersed institution'. Moving the inpatient facilities of a psychiatric service from a large mental hospital to the general hospital serving that sector of population is the most conservative step in changing the overall pattern of care.

Finally, there was a very useful definition of community psychiatry by Sabshin (1966) — 'the utilization of the techniques, methods and theories of social psychiatry and other behavioral sciences to investigate and meet the mental health needs of a functionally or geographically defined population over a significant period of time, and the feeding back of information to modify the central body of social psychiatric and other behavioral science knowledge'. This was contrasted with the public health model, particularly as advocated by Caplan (1964), which saw community psychiatry as being primarily concerned with applying techniques of prevention, at different levels, and with achieving such vague aims as 'positive mental health'. In the USA, the development of comprehensive community mental health centres was strongly influenced by Caplan's views, and started with the assumption that these facilities could prevent psychiatric illness, promote mental health, and improve the general quality of life. Such ambitious aims were not achieved, though; most outpatient care continued to be provided by private practitioners, while the centres made a disappointing contribution to the major problems of chronic psychosis and dementia (see Ch. 19). This model, in fact, had little to say about making clinical care available to those who are currently ill, and its effectiveness remains entirely unproven.

Mechanic (1981) commented on Caplan's proposals that 'some of the concepts implicit in preventive psychiatry are unfortunate not only because they are grandiose, naive, and an obvious projection of political values, but also because they continue to divert attention from making remedial efforts which are more consistent with existing knowledge and expertise'. Examples of these efforts, which are still inadequate in almost every country, include ante-natal and post-natal care, family planning services, and community facilities for those with chronic mental illness.

Mechanic goes on the ask 'by what values do we divert attention from these needs to pursue illusory goals? The greatest weakness of preventive psychiatry in the 1960s was substitution of vague ideals for tangible action and a failure to specify clearly how psychiatric expertise could lead to the laudable goals that were advocated'. It is an unfortunate fact that so little is still known of the aetiology of most major psychiatric disorders that primary prevention is possible to only a very limited extent, and this has provided endless opportunity for the critics of psychiatry to condemn it for 'patching up', instead of preventing the illnesses from occurring. However, until scientific knowledge advances much further, psychiatrists have little alternative in general but to develop as well as they can those measures of secondary and tertiary prevention which are now proved to be effective. Examples of these include the use of depot neuroleptics to prevent or delay relapses of schizophrenia, and the similar role of lithium in recurrent affective disorder (see Ch. 17).

To return to the meaning of 'community', it has never been easy to define this in sociological terms although certain themes are constantly repeated. These include: locality, the interaction of people, their common bonds, and their combined actions. Such themes represent aspects of the individual's social situation, his relationship to his sickness, and his means of coping with it — all of which have to be studied empirically. However, there is yet another meaning. Most long-term psychiatric patients want to get back into society, but they can only truly live there if they have some responsibility (perhaps with help) for their own lives and for making their own decisions. The quality of their lives is not significantly changed by improving living conditions in the psychiatric hospital, where decisions are not their own but are made by staff. In hospital, the quality of *care* can certainly be increased: doctors and hospital staff are preoccupied, as they should be, by the nature of the regimes and treatments which they prescribe. However, in the general community, since there has to be a compromise between treatment and living, a balance must be struck between the patient's way of life, the family's needs (where relevant), and medical treatment, which often has to be rearranged to take account of the demands of daily life. Strauss (1984) points out that while health personnel have a part to play in this scheme, this is a secondary role, since it is the patient who has to carry on, day by day, in the face of his disorder. Professionals have much to learn about how to help families and patients in their actual life situations, which, for the professions, are new places of work.

'Community' is therefore a term which can be attached to treatment outside hospital walls, to treatment in the hospital itself, to the work of clinicians outside the hospital, to the public health approach and to prevention (Acheson 1985). At the present time, it seems to have most meaning as a way of working in which professionals, patients, and their families or other supporters form new partnerships and use those services which everyone uses. In spite of these observations, the reader may still find the word used loosely and in different ways throughout this book; 'community psychiatry' and 'community mental health' are examples of terms in such common use that they cannot now be changed, although of course they refer to different concepts. The best we can hope to do is to avoid narrow definitions, and try to explain what we mean by the terms we use.

COMMUNITY MENTAL HEALTH

For William Alanson White (1917), 'mental hygiene' was the last word in preventive medicine. Since the asylum, the poor house, and the prison housed the results of failure, a split had developed between mental hygiene on the one hand, seeking the prevention of mental disorder and the promotion of 'positive' mental health, and traditional psychiatry on the other, which cared for the mentally ill, including those who did not recover. According to Kingsley Davis (1937), the adherents of mental hygiene hid their middle-class social values and mores, but in fact behaved not as scientists, but as practising moralists. Later, the word 'hygiene' was dropped, because of its medical connotations, and its successor 'mental health' embraced the belief that society, not merely the ways of individuals, also needed to be changed. This concept of mental health led to an extension of the category of people who should be defined as deviant from this point of view, moving well beyond the traditional focus on psychopathology; the new pattern of community mental health system was said to offer 'help to anyone and everyone (who has) problems of failure or maladaptation' (Dinitz & Beran 1971). Those who accepted such views rejected concepts of 'illness' and 'mental', and regarded themselves, irrespective of any lack of training, as having the right to treat, so that it was 'difficult to distinguish between clinical expertise and faith healing'.

It was in the early 1960s that the 'community' label became fixed to mental health, but 'community mental health extends far beyond the medical model. Psychiatrists may be involved in it as may other professionals, politicians, columnists, citizens of all kinds and consumers of mental health services who see it as an area of legitimate concern' (Schwartz 1972). This growth of public and political interest, seen by many psychiatrists as involvement by outsiders in what had been their particular world, also meant that services were increasingly influenced by shifts in government policy and by the confusions of a rapidly changing society (Levine 1981). The differences between this movement and traditional psychiatry were illustrated by the comment that running a community health programme was no longer a function of clinical skill, but one of adapting to and sometimes even changing the local political, social, and economic environment, and in becoming deeply involved in the life of that community (Levenson & Brown 1968). Thus, in community mental health, the limits of those to be treated, those able to treat, and the means of treating them were greatly expanded to include, for instance, the problems of ethnic minorities, the women's movement, peace on the planet, as well as other political and social issues for which psychiatry has in fact no answers and no related expertise. This assault on conventional models led — at certain times and places — to the effective dissolution of all boundaries: of concepts, criteria, roles, facilities, and organisational structures.

The rise of this movement in the USA is well illustrated by comparing the composition of the Joint Commission on Mental Illness in 1961 and that of the President's Commission on Mental Health in 1978. On the Joint Commission, there were 26 doctors and 20 others — many of whom represented professional organisations. The smaller President's Commission had a total of 20 and these included only three psychiatrists (President's Commission 1978); its members were selected to achieve a balance of representation, as well as the advocacy of special minority interest groups. It failed, however, to provide any critical analysis of the relevant issues based on adequate data or careful reasoning (Levine 1981). Community mental health thinking provides no firm theoretical basis for the provision of services adequate to care, for instance, for the elderly confused or those chronically sick and disabled from psychosis. Using the model of prevention tends to provide consultation services operating through a variety of local agencies; these include crisis intervention, and provision for those with social problems which are not necessarily causing them any serious psychological distress (Freeman 1983, Goldberg 1971).

NON-SPECIALIST COMMUNITY PSYCHIATRY

Epidemiological findings since the 1960s have indicated that psychiatric symptomatology is much more extensive in the community than was previously recognised (Hill 1969), and so a decision has to be made as to who, in future, will be part of the psychiatrist's constituency. Although the trend to community psychiatry in a general sense has been proceeding slowly for more than 50 and perhaps 100 years (see Ch. 2), it does not reduce the need for specialised psychiatric services to be maintained, and for the limited professional skills that are available to be concentrated and applied where they can be most effective. In their analysis of the literature, Goldberg & Huxley (1980), showed that out of a population of 1000, 250 people each year experience symptoms which may be regarded as psychiatric or psychological in nature; in Britain, 230 of these refer themselves to general practitioners (GPs), but of these, only 17 are referred to psychiatrists and only 6 admitted to hospital. Thus, there are three types of patients — a group who would perhaps be best helped by general medical intervention, those who are seeking non-specialised psychiatric help, and finally those who require specialist psychiatric care.

Whilst little is known about the quality of work of GPs in dealing with mental health problems, their activities are often buttressed (in Britain at least) by the contributions of social workers (Cooper et al 1975), psychologists (Griffiths 1985), nurse therapists, (Marks 1985), and those psychiatrists (Mitchell 1983, Strathdee & Williams 1984) who have formed close working liaisons with the primary care group. It is thought by many that the high prevalence of minor psychiatric symptomatology reinforces this need for better non-specialised care services, rather than for the recruitment of more specialist psychiatrists (e.g. Brook & Cooper 1975). The importance of such generalist care is that (when done well), it can provide more continuity, avoid unnecessary labelling or stigma, and see the presenting symptoms in relation to other aspects of the individual's physical and mental condition. Thus, it can bridge the specialities, prevent fragmentation of care, and protect the patient from the possible therapeutic excesses or narrow-mindedness of a specialist technocracy (Titmuss 1965, WHO 1973). It is difficult to draw the line, though, between generalist and specialist care (Sturt & Waters 1985), and some community crisis-intervention services or mental health advice centres may have added to the confusion by treating only a similar body of patients to those of primary care (Bouras et al 1986, Gleisner 1982). This may reflect not only a failure to define the goals of the specialist service adequately, but also a realisation that patients with difficult neurotic problems may not receive adequate help from their particular GPs.

However, those whose illness causes them difficulty in performing social roles, whose behaviour stresses the tolerance of their social network, or who need intensive medical and nursing care at times may well require periods of hospital care (Leff 1986). Since the vulnerability of such patients to the stimulus of life events means that their periods of social failure are liable to recur, they are likely to need a specialist community service, based on a centre linked to a general hospital psychiatric unit, which is always available. On the other hand, those who suffer less severely usually require care from a generalist service system, which in Britain and some other countries is based on general practice. There seems no reason why nurses, psychologists, occupational therapists, social workers, and doctors should not operate in either service (Reed & Lomas 1984), but the nature of the work should be different in the two settings; insisting that primary care teams — still a limited feature of general practice — are the cornerstone of community psychiatry (Shepherd 1989) does not provide a model that is widely relevant. An examination of the influence of one pioneering psychiatric intervention service which offered open access to the public showed that it only reduced the admission of those patients with non-psychotic diagnoses (Boardman et al 1987). However, Williams & Balestrieri (1989) found that close involvement of psychiatrists with the primary care team particularly reduced admission rates and bed usage among patients suffering from affective and personality disorders. Neither study, though, demonstrated direct benefits to patients, in terms of reduced morbidity.

Ferguson et al (1990) have described the evolution of outpatient work into a primary care setting, with the purpose of offering combined care — through more effective liaison and regular contact between GPs and the psychiatric team — in an environment with which patients are already familiar. This was augmented by a day hospital, drop-in centre, and other facilities situated within the sector of population served — an inner-city area of Nottingham. The team operated on an inter-disciplinary basis; patients were seen either at the GP's surgery or in their own homes, but were offered in-patient or day-patient admission if this was thought necessary. At the end of five years, a cohort of patients treated by this service was compared with a matched cohort, treated by a more conventional service in the same city. In terms of diagnosis, there was no difference between the two cohorts; acceptance by patients of both services was good, but those who received most of their care in the community were less troubled by feelings of stigmatisation. It was concluded that the reductions in admission rates and bed usage by the community service had not been at the expense of increased symptomatology or social dysfunction, and that the sustained contact with patients negated suggestions of 'neglect' by community-based services in general. Perhaps the main questions raised by these results are whether the *élan* of such an innovative service can be maintained indefinitely and if so, whether it will have the resources to keep regular contact with a steadily increasing number of patients who have chronic or recurrent illnesses. The more conventional, hospital-based service returned a much higher proportion of its patients to the care of their GPs after an episode of specialist treatment, and this is the way that at least a proportion of primary practitioners prefer to operate, since the close liaison required by the community service may not be acceptable to them.

Strathdee & Williams (1984) found that the modes of involvement of British psychiatrists in primary care could be divided into three main groups. The most common was the 'shifted outpatient model', where the psychiatrist still undertakes both assessment and treatment, as in a hospital outpatient clinic, but this activity is moved to a general practice setting. Next most frequent was the 'consultation model', where the psychiatrist helps the GP in assessing the patient and advises on management; in the case of psychotherapy, the patient may not actually be seen in this process. Finally, in the 'liaison attachment model', a few psychiatrists were undertaking supervision and training of social workers, community psychiatric nurses, or other primary care professionals, without necessarily seeing any of their patients. These British models, however, depend strongly on the capitation-fee arrangements of NHS general practice, and have little application to the many countries where the fee-for-service system is used; there, either transferring the care of less severely ill patients to specialists or spending time in consultation with them would result in significant loss of income for GPs. Also, senior British psychiatrists receive extra payments for certain domiciliary visits to patients, when the GP may also be present, and this incentive to collaboration is absent in most other countries, where such visits are unusual. Finally, the question has been raised (Fahy 1989) whether increased involvement by psychiatrists in the 'vast burden of covert and badly managed morbidity in primary care' may be at the expense of more important tasks, such as responding to emergency cases and providing high-quality care to the chronically ill. The same principles might be applied to other branches of medicine, but these specialists have not so far been drawn to any large extent into direct involvement with their patients at the primary-care level.

SPECIALIST COMMUNITY PSYCHIATRY

While community mental health may be seen as a reaching out to try and change or rehabilitate a sick society, the aims of specialist community psychiatry are more modest. Stated most simply, this is the psychiatry practised by those doctors working in the community who take into account the fact that patients are members of varying social systems (Schwartz 1972). It is a form of clinical practice, not a tool of social reform — the scientifically based art of treating psychiatric disorder and emotional disturbance (Loeb 1966). Therefore it is, or should be based on empirical research, for it is interested in differentiating the phenomena of psychiatric disorder and seeking standard terms to characterise them: only thus can the serious be distinguished from the trivial, or the long-lasting from the evanescent. If both social and clinical phenomena can also be defined and measured, it is possible to study systematically that interaction of clinical and social events which is the substance of social psychiatry (Wing 1971). Unlike Viola Bernard (1964), who believed that the terms 'community psychiatry' and 'social psychiatry' could be used interchangeably, Sabshin (1966) rejected definitions influenced by the public health model which stressed prevention. His view of responsibility for a defined population means that the hospital psychiatric service cannot select the people for whom it will care, but has to deal with the relevant morbidity of the whole population, members of which may put the sick individual at risk, but may also be put at risk by him. Community psychiatry has often emphasised *where* psychiatry should be practised, and for whom and by whom, but Sabshin's model provides a theoretical base for *how* it is done, using social psychiatric studies of clinical phenomena which are being influenced by social events (Bennett 1978). However, 'mental health needs' have to be seen in terms of reasonably definable boundaries: in the case of personality disorders, for instance, the points where these merge into variations of normal personality traits may not be universally agreed.

At the same time, there is no doubt in the minds of many, that the 'where' of community psychiatry is also important. Particularly in its beginnings, it led, in ill-considered instances, to the premature discharge from hospital of poorly prepared and inadequately supported patients. Patients were then 'in' but not 'of' the community: the situation described in Germany as *gemeindenahe* or *near the community*. Thus, the community was seen from the vantage point of the mental hospital — it was 'out there' for a person who moved into a hostel or nursing home from the institution. On the other hand, for one who is capable of living in his/her own dwelling, an old people's home is not 'in the community'; for such a person, community cannot be seen as merely meaning non-hospital. The assumption that if you are in hospital you are dependent, and if you are out of hospital you are independent, means that where the 'community' is will depend on your capacity to deal with it. Whereas for the Royal Commission (1957), the community was outside the hospital, for the Seebohm Committee (1968), the hospital was in the community. But making the site of treatment more local is certainly important in itself: it offers decentralised treatment, which can be more individual, since it is able to take into account both the patient's clinical condition and the nature of his/her behaviour and habits, which can then be considered in their context, i.e. in relation to the family and social environment. It may then be possible to mobilise local social services and to incorporate support given by employment, education, social welfare, and housing authorities, together with that provided by the churches and other voluntary bodies; such a service is much less stigmatising and less handicapping, insofar as it facilitates the use of culturally approved forms of care. It should also be less likely to miss unobtrusive morbidity, such as that of chronically handicapped psychotic patients, if it has a detailed knowledge of its sector of population. Goffman (1961) emphasised the importance of ensuring that where one lives, where one works, and where one spends one's leisure time are not directed by the same authority; if that is not the case, there is less risk of institutionalisation and desocialisation.

Out of hospital, the patient has to achieve some kind of balance between living on the one hand and coping with the limitations of illness or disability on the other: he/she may have to cope with poverty, limitations of choice, lack of support, and stigma, together with the problems caused by the symptoms of the disorder (Strauss 1984). In a system of community psychiatry, staff should help the individual to cope with the experience of illness and disability since quality of life is not governed primarily by living in the general community rather than in hospital, but by how he/she lives with the illness. In this situation, it is important how both professionals and others help the patient, his/her family, and friends to manage the isolation, marital discord, transformation of domestic roles, and other difficulties that may inevitably arise. Staff tend to be anxious about this, and have every reason to be so if the patient is seen as living in a situation where there are no 'agents' to help and no adequate helping strategy is being constructed professionally. While health personnel have an important part to play in this scheme, they are far from being the only important figures in the patient's daily life, for in this new situation, he is in *his* community and not in *their* hospital (Hoult 1986).

So far as services in Britain are concerned, district psychiatry can be seen to have remained so far fairly closely within the conventional models of medicine, nursing, and social work, but to have primarily extended outwards from institutions. Its theoretical basis is an eclectic, but fundamentally biological form of psychiatry. To complement this, the work of voluntary bodies and of non-professional individuals or organisations within the population, although difficult to quantify, is making an increasing contribution, stressing in particular the right of the consumer to have a say in the nature of services required. Even so, the bulk of care is still provided by public services, financed by national and local taxation, and as such, is still to some extent paternalistic. Describing the rise of professional society in England during the past century, Perkin (1989) states that its animating spirit has been 'the professional social ideal which defends and justifies their collective self-interest in terms of the service performed... by each hierarchy ... and the principle of social justice it upholds'. The claims of professionalism were thus a reformulation of *noblesse oblige* — meeting the obligation owed by those with status and resources to those who have little or none, in a way which would contribute to social cohesion. It is not surprising that, following the principle of functional utility, this should have been done paternalistically, and in such a way as to preserve the corporate autonomy of the professions — particularly medicine.

THE MULTIDISCIPLINARY TEAM

Another important aspect of community psychiatry is that much of the conventional dyadic relationship between patient and doctor has been replaced by one with a multidisciplinary professional team (MDT). This has occurred primarily because of the heterogeneous nature of the clinical service in psychiatry, especially when practised outside hospital or the private consulting room, and the multidimensional disabilities of long-term patients; close and structured collaboration is believed necessary to ensure co-ordination of the special skills of each discipline involved (Soni et al 1989). It is also assumed that this will result in a more equitable division of labour, the development of comprehensive therapeutic plans for patients, and a stimulating and supportive work environment, though in practice, all these are rarely achieved (Øvretveit 1986). On the other hand, MDTs may remove legitimate options from both clients and members, and maintaining the cohesiveness of the team itself can take time away from the direct care of patients.

Øvretveit described four types of team organisation, according to whether or not there is a formal leader and the degree of authority and accountability assumed by that member. Soni et al state that MDTs should not be established unless the managers concerned have accepted the training needs of the different professions involved for this kind of work and have allocated the money required, and unless a formal statement of policy and procedures has been agreed. They add that members of MDTs come from different levels in the hierarchies of their respective professions, and therefore have varying abilities to participate in the decision-making process; in Britain, only the consultant psychiatrist is independent of any structure of line management. So far as clinical decisions are concerned, team members should be responsible either to its leader or collectively to their colleagues in the MDT, but the boundary with non-clinical matters is often uncertain, so that divided loyalties may cause conflicts and so harm the quality of service. The more directly an individual member is controlled by his/her own professional hierarchy, the more likely it is that such difficulties will arise, for instance, over the recruitment of new staff. Theoretically, a team that was wholly independent in management and budgetary terms would be relatively free of such problems, but it would then be involved in constant negotiations and bargaining with other bodies, e.g. for access to hospital beds, so that the end-result would most likely be no better.

As part of the development of MDTs, the traditional primacy and leadership role of doctors among the health professions have been strongly challenged in many countries. Whereas it had been usual for clinical decisions to be a medical prerogative — though after consultation with the members of any other professions involved in the case — MDTs often work through collective decision-making, in which the doctor is only one voice. If there is a team leader, this may well be a non-medical member. Arrangements of this kind resonate with current trends towards egalitarianism and with the anti-medical and anti-psychiatric tendencies that emerged in the 1960s, but their implications for health care have generally been poorly thought out (Sims 1989).

In the first place, in Britain and other countries, the clinical responsibility of the psychiatrist has a legal basis which cannot be abdicated, particularly in the case of patients who are compulsorily admitted to hospital or those who afterwards engage in litigation. Secondly, one of us (DHB) pointed out some years ago that true blurring of roles between the professions in psychiatric care could not happen without the blurring of salaries, but in Western countries, there has so far been no trend in that direction. Therefore, the much higher remuneration of the psychiatrist needs to be reflected in a greater degree of responsibility. Thirdly, as the only team member free of management hierarchies, the consultant psychiatrist is in the strongest position to act as advocate for the patient and to promote innovations. Fourthly, the extensive training and experience of the psychiatrist give him a sapiential authority which should perhaps be reflected in his influence within the team. Fifthly, senior doctors are likely to remain longer in any particular post, as the members of the other professions will largely move out of direct contact with patients if they are promoted. Finally, there is still a strong expectation amongst patients and amongst other organisations, such as the police, that the doctor is in charge and is the person who will make major decisions about treatment and care; such expectations should not be ignored, since the resulting uncertainty may be strongly anti-therapeutic (Sims 1989).

Yet a clear model of work for psychiatrists outside the hospital or consulting room has not yet emerged; this is not altogether surprising, since the time has been relatively short since community psychiatry began to evolve in its present sense. Construction of such a model will require the clear definition of those tasks within the overall care of psychiatric patients (whether in or out of hospital) which require the specific skills of a specialist doctor. Whether or not this will generally include the function of inter-professional leadership remains to be seen, but if it does, then such leadership should be neither authoritarian nor weak, but should respect the professional skills and autonomy of other members of the care team.

In this connection, the concept of the 'key worker' was an important development of the 1980s and has emerged as an essential aspect of the activities of MDTs. It represents a departure from conventional medical practice, where *all* responsibility for the patient was assumed to reside ultimately in the senior doctor, though other professions (such as nursing) would have responsibility limited to their specific tasks. In the MDT, each profession is acknowledged to possess certain special skills, which the others do not possess to the same extent; therefore, the appropriate member (or members) will be called on whenever the patient is in need of that particular skill (or skills). So far as prescription of medication is concerned, for instance, *only* the doctor has the legal authority to do that, and must therefore be involved whenever this form of treatment becomes an issue. The key worker concept does not challenge or deny the particular functions of any profession, or of any other group of workers in the mental health field who have a clearly identified function. It has nothing to do with the 'deprofessionalisation' which was a prominent aspect of 1960s community mental health and anti-psychiatry, and which re-emerged 20 years later, mainly as a way of reducing staff costs. When a key worker is identified, that person takes responsibility for maintaining continued contact with the patient and for providing general monitoring and counselling, as well as keeping the other members of the team informed of the case and seeking their views on it when necessary. The key worker will be concerned about whether the patient is receiving any relevant benefits or services that are available and in addition, will contribute his/her particular professional skills, calling on other members of the MDT when their own are needed. Which member will be chosen as the key worker for any individual case may depend primarily on what the particular needs of that patient are, but may also be influenced by the size of members' case loads or other responsibilities that they have outside the work of the MDT. In principle, though, there should be no bar to any member of a team — psychiatrist (senior or junior), hospital nurse, social worker, psychologist, occupational therapist, or the GP — becoming the key worker for any case. What is most important is that a key worker should be identified, particularly in the case of long-term or recurrent disorders; however, the role of a key worker is not the same as that of a case manager (see below).

ALTERNATIVE APPROACHES

Though the results of experiments to provide treatment on a totally different foundation from the national model have so far been unconvincing, local services which depart substantially from the average have certainly been developed within Britain and other industrialised countries. These have mostly emphasised crisis intervention, making a multidisciplinary team available to patients in their homes, sometimes on a 24-hour and 7-days-a-week basis. The best known is that operated from Napsbury Hospital to the London Borough of Barnet (Scott 1980); this aims to involve family and neighbours in the intervention process, and to identify psychosocial transitions which may have led to the crisis situation. After the service began operating, the hospital first admission rate dropped by over 30% — though it was previously well above the national average. This service generates strong loyalties, but also antagonisms; it involves long hours of work for the staff, with possible stresses in their personal lives, and heavy travel costs. Hospital and financial data, though, tell nothing of the experience or outcome of patients, nor of the feelings of relatives, GPs, or others in the community about the service they receive. These matters have still to be fully assessed.

Dingleton Hospital in Scotland, has an even longer experience of a community crisis intervention service, but for a very different, largely rural population. It undoubtedly benefits from a particularly high standard of general practice and from a close-knit society in the small

Border communities (Jones 1987). However, in industrialised countries as a whole and especially in city areas, there may be significant numbers of people suffering from psychiatric disorders who are not part of any meaningful social network; in these cases, crisis intervention may have much less to offer. Though the work of Langsley et al (1969) has often been cited in support of the 'preventive' approach, evidence is lacking that such arrangements remain effective in the long term. There is also the problem that the personal and interpersonal crises which occur in any population are so many that it would be quite impossible to intervene professionally in most of them. Leighton (1982) has described this as 'like trying to drink the ocean'. Nor has it been proved that such intervention would have the positive results that have been claimed for it. Mechanic (1981) states that crisis intervention theory is based on a vague conceptualisation that environmental trauma and lack of coping ability cause mental illness, but that the evidence for this is incomplete and far from secure. Neither is there much evidence that the advocated type of troubleshooting, although perhaps valuable in reducing distress, has any impact on the rate at which formal psychiatric illness occurs, or that it would necessarily be directed at those who are likely to become ill if untreated (see Ch..5). However, a distinction needs to be made between, on the one hand, managing acute illnesses by crisis intervention and on the other, responding rapidly to the acute needs of chronic patients (Hoult & Reynolds 1984), which ought to be achieved by every psychiatric service.

Crisis intervention services in Britain are of three main types: those operating alongside conventional referral systems; those which are an integral part of a local mental health service, screening all its referrals; and thirdly, selective services which target a particular kind of client, e.g. those attempting suicide (Renshaw 1989). A service which is immediately available, in an informal setting, is likely to be popular with many users, as well as providing a satisfying style of work for some staff. However, the pressures to set up such a service may result from problems — e.g. inadequate screening of cases before admission, poor communication between professions, or geographical separation of a hospital from the community service — which could have been dealt with more directly. Other relevant factors are that some patients prefer the security of the hospital when they are ill, staff with other duties may not be able to commit the necessary time to crisis work, and inexperienced junior doctors may have to carry the burden of making decisions. The aims and priorities of crisis services have not always been well enough defined, and they are likely to achieve little in themselves, unless the team has access to a wide range of mental health facilities in the area its covers.

In Tameside, Greater Manchester, a mental health centre where intervention followed mainly non-clinical lines was developed in a converted house (Gleisner 1982). Professional role differences there have been minimised, patients have access to their case notes, and no medication is administered; however, conventional treatment and care are also available within the district service, and it might well be that the two kinds of facilities deal with different kinds of patients. A similar service operates in one sector of the London Borough of Lewisham (Bouras 1982). Since these reports, community mental health centres have shown an extraordinary growth in Britain as a base for the delivery of psychiatric care. In the U.S.A. such facilities, designed to increase accessibility to psychiatric help, have been criticised for their basic philosophy that mental illness could be prevented by simple counselling and social intervention: less than half of the proposed 2000 centres were in fact opened and their numbers were already declining in the 1980s (Mollica 1980). In England, these centres, often enthusiastic for preventive work and the promotion of 'positive' mental health, grew from 22 in 1980 to over 82 in 1988 (Sayce 1989). At the same time, however, a study of the Lewisham centre by Boardman et al (1987) showed that it had done nothing to reduce the admission of patients to the local mental hospital, there being no district general hospital psychiatric unit; this was because patients with severe and long-lasting disabilities were not being seen and perhaps also because the centre was not operating a 24-hour service. Sayce claimed that these centres provide a local and swiftly accessible service, though unless they can close the gap between rhetoric and reality, they will not serve the needs of the seriously ill, but only look after the 'worried well' — which should be the task of the primary care services. These unconventional facilities, then, hover on the line separating non-specialist and specialist community psychiatry, and since their funding comes from both health and social services budgets this may well lead, in Britain, to conflict about the nature of the population served. (Developments of this kind are also discussed in Ch. 12.)

DISTRICT PSYCHIATRY

Psychiatry, which ought to concern itself with whole communities rather than with individual patients alone, therefore needs to be aware of the social structures of these communities and with their environments (Freeman 1985). Those psychiatrists who have a district responsibility will have the opportunity to become very familiar with living conditions in their territory, and may well wish to intervene when overcrowding or high-rise accommodation, for instance, seem to be affecting people adversely, though there have been few instances of this happening in practice. Within each community, the pattern of social networks — a factor first clearly analysed by Bott (1957) — seems to be relevant to much psychiatric disorder, particularly non-psychotic conditions. Deficiencies in the social environment are a well established consequence of being mentally ill, while some of the increased prevalence of neurotic morbidity observed, e.g. in the lowest social class may be partly explained by deficiencies of social bonds (Henderson 1980). However, determining which of these elements is primary, or whether a third leads to both, is a problem on which research still continues. The relationship of psychiatric disorder to social factors is extremely complex and not only may different social factors be important in different diseases, but the same social factors may operate differently in separate conditions (see Brown, Ch. 3). Jones (1988) has pointed out the illogicality whereby 'society' is blamed for being at the root of psychiatric disorders, yet when redefined as 'the community', is supposed to be the healing matrix within which these problems are best managed. Furthermore, the virtues of communities were being discovered just around the time when social and cultural changes were causing them to break up and lose their cohesion in many cases — for instance, the long established working-class communities of the north of England, which were mostly bulldozed out of existence around the 1960s.

District psychiatry in Britain, though, is a concept which has not developed on a theoretical basis such as that of social networks or psychodynamics, but rather through pragmatic action, and it has been mainly studied from the viewpoint of social administration. Among the professional staff involved, it has required psychiatrists particularly to step out of their traditional clinical role in certain respects, and to intervene in some social situations, as well as in the process of developing services: 'the professional in the community care context is a facilitator, co-ordinator, and integrator' (Mechanic 1989). The character of district psychiatry has been strongly influenced up until now by the relationship between primary medical care and specialist services within the NHS; overall, the most common reason for referral by a GP to a psychiatrist in Britain is failure of the patient to respond to the GP's initial treatment — which is usually medication. One of the commonest forms of activity developed by psychiatrists in district services is that of regular visits to primary health centres, where consultations can be held with the care team and patients be seen nearer to their homes. In some cases, but by no means all, a useful dialogue develops between specialist and primary care staff as a result of this regular contact (Strathdee & Williams 1984) (see above and Ch. 12). However, since the most common pathway to specialist psychiatric care in Britain up to now has been referral by a GP to a psychiatrist for a *medical* consultation, the trend to multidisciplinary teamwork in mental health services — where initial contact might be with a member of one of several professions — will require some rethinking of these accustomed methods.

Wing (1979) has summarised the essential characteristics of a mental health service for a community as that it should be responsible, comprehensive, and integrated. This is an appropriate goal to which the further evolution of district psychiatry could aim, though the limitations of public spending in Britain make the achievement of plans for it seem fairly distant. Various methods have been used to transfer funds from the hospital to the community sector (DHSS 1981), but if total resources are too restricted, such measures cannot improve things much overall. For instance, although the number of very old people in the population is continuing to increase rapidly, places in local authority residential homes in England actually fell by 9000 from an already inadequate level between 1976 and 1981 (Grundy & Arie 1982); the government response to the Griffiths report on community care (DOH 1989) envisaged the replacement of much of this service by the purchase of care in private or voluntary homes by social services. The 1983 Mental Health Act for England & Wales laid a duty on both health authorities and local authority social services to provide aftercare for people who have been treated for psychiatric disorder. This requirement, though, remained inoperative for several years, not least because most social services departments were unable to provide even a minimum complement of approved social workers, with the qualifications specified in the Act; some were still not providing a 24-hour service for mental health emergencies in 1990.

Two other important aspects of district psychiatry are establishing priorities and maintaining continuity. If a service aims to deal with all the mentally disordered in a population, it is reasonable to maintain that this can only be done by focussing limited resources primarily on those groups who have the greatest need of them. To some extent, this will require a reversal of articulated demands, which are likely to come most strongly from those of higher social status, with less severe neurotic and personality disorders. Where psychiatry is mainly practised privately, clients of this kind are likely to take up most of the resources available. On the other hand, it can be argued that in terms of human needs, the three groups which most require these resources are those suffering from the most severe and long-term disorders — schizophrenia, dementia, and mental retardation. All are predominantly chronic conditions, difficult to treat by curative medicine, and needing prolonged care by relatives or public services; since few demands come from the patients themselves, there must be positive discrimination in their favour, if they are not to be neglected. So far as psychotherapy for less severe conditions is concerned, it might be necessary for the specialist services in a district to follow a policy of 'benign neglect'. In other words, responsibility for it might have to remain at the level of primary care, but with the offer of training and consultation for those professional staff involved. This view does not minimise the distress and disability caused by neurotic disorders, but unless specialist mental health services could be very greatly expanded — which probably could only be at the cost of reductions in other areas of the public services — the best approach to these problems is probably through strengthening the capability of primary care.

Continuity is one of the most important aspects of psychiatric care, and at the same time one of the most difficult to achieve; in a condition like schizophrenia, where episodes of illness may occur over most of a lifetime, it may make all the difference between success and failure. Mechanic (1989) warns that 'community care experiments... have yet to demonstrate that these programs can maintain their early momentum over long periods of time or communicate their enthusiasm to others. Yet the conditions they treat are chronic and difficult... often intractable, and require effective and aggressive services over the long range... Despite much rhetoric there is continuing difficulty in maintaining a supportive network of mental health services'. In a district service, individuals will come and go, but the commitment to its task should always be carried on within the professional team, and over the course of years, their collective knowledge of the community and its people may well be an asset of steadily increasing value. This policy does, however, demand an integrated structure of adequate services within which it can be deployed, yet developments in the NHS since 1988, such as the proposals for self-governing hospitals with 'competition', represent a serious threat to whatever degree of integration had been achieved in Britain during the previous 40 years. The roles of purchaser and provider of health care services are to be separated — as they are to be with social care services — and purchasers are to specify the quality of services purchased, as well as their volume; how 'quality' is to be defined, let alone measured, remains so far unknown, but some of the problems of evaluation are referred to below and in the Introduction. Continuity of care, though, is unlikely to be achieved without the development of systematic information systems for any population which, in industrialised countries, are now likely to be computerised. On the scale of a sector or district, such systems are relatively easy to introduce, but maintaining the consistent input and high quality of data needs constant attention. If clinical staff receive regular reports from the system, in a form that is useful to them, and if the required data come from a clearly defined group of patients, they are more likely to co-operate reliably with the information system. Incorporating ratings of the mental state or social behaviour can also provide material for clinical audit or other attempts at evaluation (Taylor & Bhumgara 1989).

THE EFFECTIVENESS OF COMMUNITY TREATMENT

Developments towards community psychiatry have proceeded up to now mainly on an ideological basis, yet choices of that kind ought to be made from evidence about the relative effectiveness of alternative systems. Proving effectiveness, however, is a problem with most changes in psychiatric care (or indeed, with medical care in general), evaluation being usually restricted to the level of monitoring processes, or of the utilisation of resources. It therefore consists mostly of empirical studies, dependent on a shared ideology or common-sense view of what is desirable, and would more accurately be described as recording. Yet the actual objective of the service activities is an improved outcome in individual clients or those around them, in such terms as reduced symptoms or better performance of social roles; without knowledge of this, one cannot be sure that the effectiveness of treatment programmes is really being increased, e.g. by more staff or facilities. Rehin & Martin (1963) emphasised that 'to demonstrate the efficiency of community care... it will not be enough to point to declining first admission rates... we shall need to know if the patient's illness has been fully and more lastingly remitted, if his family are socially more capable of living a satisfactory life'. But in fact, objective evaluation of all professional activities is immensely difficult — 'clinicians... are convinced of the benefits accruing from clinical autonomy, improved channels of communication and the close liaison with community services... but such benefits... may be extremely difficult to measure and to demonstrate, partly because they concern intangibles' (Cooper & Morgan 1973).

These authors add that evaluation of community services is even more difficult than that of hospital services because of the problems of monitoring clinical change in that setting, and of identifying all the variables by which it may be influenced. An exhaustive investigation which followed the introduction of a sectorised service for part of Stockholm (Lindholm 1983) was unable to find any difference between the outcome of former mental hospital patients discharged to that area and that of patients remaining under the care of the conventional service. In Mannheim, Häfner & Klug (1982) examined changes in the utilisation of psychiatric services, following the change from a hospital-centred to an integrated, community-based structure; the workload of all services increased, particularly outpatients and crisis intervention, and particularly for depression and alcohol-related disorders. The more extensive availability of care was found to be covering some needs that had been previously unmet. There are no British studies which look critically at the effectiveness of community care or treatment as a alternative to that given in hospital. However, as Bennett (1978) has pointed out, the mental hospital was never properly evaluated either, and always dealt only with a selected group of clients, leaving the rest to manage as well as they could outside. Very often, evaluative studies make use of criteria such as 'reducing admissions' or 'closing hospitals', which are easy to measure but in themselves convey no useful information about changes in the morbidity of patients or in the experience of carers, unless other parameters have been clearly described. The aims of mental health services need to be more clearly conceptualised, but this requires identification of clients' needs, specification of standards of care, and monitoring the provision of services, as well as meaningful evaluation of outcomes.

One American review of outcome studies (Braun et al 1981) suggested that when individuals were placed in the community with adequate support, social therapy, and extensive planning, the results were much more successful in terms of readmission, independence, and developing self-esteem than when such help had not been provided; those individuals fared no less well than residents in traditional mental hospitals. Avison & Speechley (1987) found that there had been few theoretical or methodological advances in the past 20 years in relation to the factors supposed to measure community adjustment: undue reliance continued to be placed on readmission, employment, and community tenure. Another study — of a small service in Canada which took a very positive view of community-based treatment — acknowledged that ex-patients are able to undertake some of their responsibilities at work and at home, 'even while in considerable distress' (Fenton et al 1982). However, evaluation of community psychiatric services cannot take place in isolation; every element has connections with other services, both public and private, e.g. social security, housing, child care, penal, or general medicine. Comprehensive evaluation needs to take account also of changes in the demand on these services which result from changes within the mental health sector.

CURRENT CONCERNS IN BRITAIN

Dissatisfaction with the old custodial Poor Law asylums stretches back more than 100 years: that we have had community care 'for centuries' (Murphy 1987) is true in the sense that people were managed in the community — though often very badly — before asylums were built. The decline in the bed occupancy of mental hospitals in the London health regions since the mid-1950s has been at a remarkable rate — about 3000 beds per annum in England as a whole — and showed no sign of leveling off in recent years (Fig. 1.1); 'the convergence of the individual graphs is striking but unexplained' (Leff 1986). This rundown is so uniform between the different hospitals that it cannot be accounted for by the discharge policies of doctors, by administrative changes, or by the decisions of patients or their relatives. Because of criticisms that mental hospitals have dumped large numbers of unprepared patients in the community, Miller, one-time director of mental health services in New York State, examined the changes that occurred in the State's hospital populations over a 16-year period. In March 1965, there were 85 000 people residing in the State's psychiatric hospitals; between that date and March 1981, 39 500 of these residents (nearly a half) died in hospital without ever having been discharged, while 31 200 were discharged (but most of these had been admitted to hospital less than a year before their discharge), and of these, 21 000 had so far never been readmitted within New York State. In March 1981, there were 25 000 residents still in

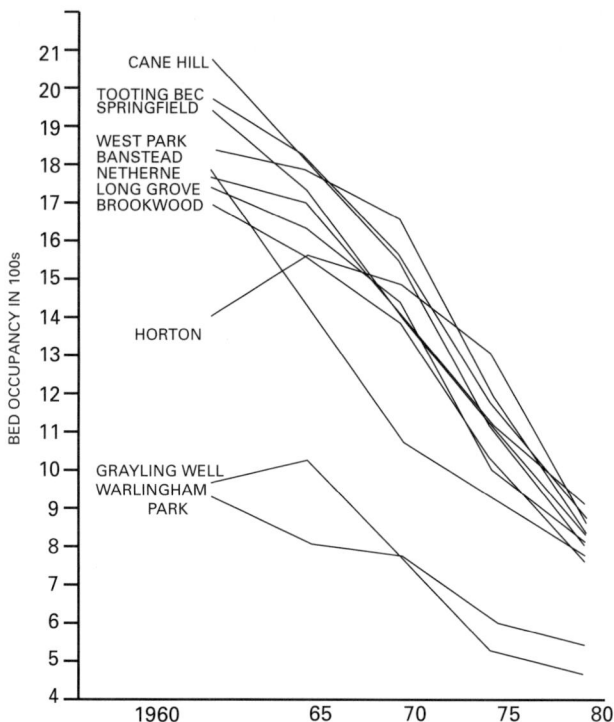

Fig. 1.1   Bed occupancy of mental hospitals in London health regions since the mid-1950s.

hospital who had been there in March 1965, though the average length of stay had, of course, become much shorter over that period. Whilst there must be some uncertainties about these figures, Miller concluded that the greatest contributors to the reduction of the hospital populations had been death and the discharge of long-stay patients, who had been replaced by patients with shorter stays (Miller 1985). Whether or not those long-stay patients were in general prepared for discharge and whether or not they went to suitable extramural situations were not questions that could be answered by the study, however.

The DHSS Statistical Bulletin (1988), reviewing the reduction in the number of long-stay residents of mental hospitals in England and Wales during the period 1976–1986, reported similar findings: twice as many had died in hospital as were discharged. In 1976, 46% had been in hospital for 5 years or more and this proportion had reduced to 33% in 1986; approximately 12 000 patients had died in hospital, while 6000 had been discharged during the decade. Only one British commentator has taken Miller's view, saying that in addition to those discharged, 'more patients have been dying in hospital than have been admitted for long-term care' (Mahoney 1988). Weller (1985), examining where patients have gone from one London psychiatric hospital (Friern), did not consider deaths, although these may have some relevance to the relatively small number of residential and day places provided in relation to the larger diminution of hospital populations in Britain (Murphy 1987). Within the UK, Scotland has followed a much more conservative policy than England, and the level of bed provision has remained at about 50% higher in the former country.

A general move away from institutional care since World War II in industrialised countries has been seen in the disappearance of orphanages and large children's or old people's homes, although prisons so far remain unaffected. The diminution of mental hospital population has been referred to as 'deinstitutionalisation' in the United States, but Gruenberg (1977) regarded this as a 'slogan which confuses issues', like community care: a reduction in the population of mental hospitals, with rising readmission rates, is rather an *indicator* (his italics). To call a policy 'deinstitutionalisation' substitutes this indicator for a more accurate measure of the development of extramural care which would measure changes in individuals' morbidity — 'something like a child trying to push the speedometer needle to make the car go faster'. Paradoxically, a high proportion of those who have become long-stay patients in mental hospitals are now capable of functioning in a non-hospital setting, while many of those in the community, who have similar problems, actually need sheltered accommodation and a greater degree of support — short of 24-hour attendance but with the 24-hour availability of help.

Nevertheless, as mentioned above, some hospital-type accommodation has to be provided for those with acute or profound needs: this should not be given in a former Poor Law institution, restyled as a hospital, but in a facility such as a local general hospital psychiatric ward, which is acceptable to the population and appropriate to present-day circum-stances (Freeman 1963). For a few long-stay patients, a 'ward in a house' solution has proved both acceptable and effective in several parts of Britain, and has been more extensively evaluated than many innovations (Bennett 1980, Wing 1982, Goldberg et al 1985, Gibbons 1986). Therefore, a person needing full-time residential psychiatric care in a high-dependency environment, with 24-hour cover, does not have to reside in a conventional hospital, since the same can be provided in a small, informal setting, provided that an adequate number of trained staff are permanently available. Although staff expenses appear high in such hospital-hostels, capital costs are low and the involvement of residents in catering and domestic duties makes support services relatively cheap.

But how many hospital beds will in fact be needed? In Barclay's view (1988), this question cannot be answered in terms of any fixed ratio, since there are so many variables involved — economics, social policy, the attitudes of psychiatrists, employment conditions, and the value of social welfare benefits, as well as the cost of residential accommodation and public housing. Barclay adds that over the past 40 years, no fixed bed-to-population ratio has proved reliable, but that 'the number required has constantly become less'. No one knows when the irreducible minimum will be reached, though it seems likely that the move of patients from residence in psychiatric hospitals will continue in most developed countries. The main change at the end of the 1980s is that the concept of community psychiatry has been extended almost imperceptibly, as innovations have been tried in many countries; meanwhile, institutions in the process of running down undergo the risks of demoralisation, and health authorities in Britain have made plans for the widespread closure of mental hospitals. The point has been reached where it is being proposed by some health and social service authorities that even the most seriously disabled psychiatric patients will now be cared for in their own homes or in some non-hospital form of residential facility (Murphy 1988).

It has also been suggested (Turner 1988) that there can be no real community care if hospital admission remains part of the legal basis for treating those who are most persistently and severely ill. However, even if they accept that our former asylums may have no place in today's service, few experienced professionals deny a continuing need for psychiatric beds in general hospitals and for small autonomous units to provide more secure long-term care and rehabilitation for some patients. Criticisms are heard that discharging psychotic patients leads to increased vagrancy, a larger prison population, more suicides, isolation in bedsitting rooms, and homelessness (Bassuk et al 1984, Weller et al 1989); some of those claims, however, are difficult to evaluate. Both the numbers of the homeless and the prison population continue to rise in Britain and both will certainly include a number of psychotic or post-psychotic, rootless wanderers, some of them determined to avoid treatment, others to avoid admission, who travel as a 'stage army' between prison, doss-house, and mental hospital — where such a hospital still exists. However, homeless mentally ill and mentally disordered offenders in significant numbers 'long antedate community care policies' in Britain (House of Commons Committee 1985). A report on the homeless in London (Canter et al 1989) showed that the number of men living rough on the streets had risen from 247, counted by the National Assistance Board in 1966, to 753 in April 1989: this suggests an increase of 500, although the survey — by Salvation Army personnel — may not have included men sleeping rough in buildings. The number of mentally ill sleeping rough has increased to some extent and there are grounds for anxiety about homeless, indigent men wandering the streets of London and, to some extent, other large cities; such problems are worse in all cities than elsewhere, since socially withdrawn and paranoid individuals tend to drift into them. Weller et al (1989) found that 41% of groups of destitute people, examined at successive Christmases between 1985 and 1988, had either current or past evidence of psychosis; 90% originated from outside London. Timms & Fry (1989) reviewed studies of the homeless, which estimated that 20–50% currently suffered from schizophrenia or other serious mental illnesses; most were not then receiving any psychiatric treatment, though they had typically been in contact with psychiatric services in the past and had dropped out of contact. No doubt this problem should not be separated from the wider need for affordable rented accommodation in cities, particularly for single persons.

In 1978, Gunn et al surveyed the prison population in the south-east of England. While a third of sentenced prisoners could be regarded as 'psychiatric cases', it was clear from analysis of the interviews that the proportion of patients who were actively psychotic was probably as low as 1%, which would have meant something like 350 psychotic prisoners in the whole system in England and Wales: however, the number may well have risen somewhat since that time (Gunn personal communication). Bowden (1990) also maintains that there is little evidence to support the view that appreciable numbers of people are in prison who should be inpatients in psychiatric beds. Fowles (1990) provides numerical evidence to prove that former mental hospital patients are not in prison in any significant numbers. There may be mentally ill young men coming into prison who have never been in mental hospitals, since some of the newer psychiatric units are less willing than the older institutions to admit difficult patients with long-term problems (Coid 1988). In Sydney, Australia, 200 ex-long-stay hospital patients who had been most recently discharged were followed-up 3 to 40 months later; this survey revealed only one homeless individual, two former patients who gave serious problems to the police, and six others who were petty nuisances (Andrews et al 1989). Claims that suicides have increased since community care became more common do not seem so far to have been substantiated (Roy 1982, Sturt 1983, Wilkinson 1982).

One aspect of the run-down of psychiatric hospitals which rarely receives sufficient attention is that in the discharge of long-stay patients, the least handicapped will almost invariably leave hospital first. As a result, experience gained in the early stages of the deinstitutionalisation process tends to give a misleading impression of the ease with which hospital residents can be resettled outside. However, as the process goes on, groups with more and more severe levels of disability are reached, and these will require progressively greater amounts of care and support — often permanently — when they leave hospital. What planners and administrators usually fail to understand, though it is clear to most clinicians, is that the run-down of inpatients results in the average level of disability steadily rising, *both* among the remaining hospital residents and among those resettled outside. Furthermore, care in both settings becomes steadily more expensive over the course of time, in terms of annual expenditure per patient (Häfner & Heiden 1989).

Of course, mental illness involves a burden on relatives, which is often dutifully or even cheerfully borne. Much depends on the family circumstances, its size, and the age of caring relatives, as well as on the nature of the individual temperaments and family relationships. Even so, neither treatment in hospital nor in the home seems to relieve some burdens completely or to relieve others at all (Fenton et al 1982). In the well-known comparative study undertaken in Chichester and Salisbury, some burden was lessened by the hospital service, although severe problems were relieved equally by hospital and community treatment (Grad & Sainsbury 1968). However, in Fenton's Canadian study, admission to hospital did not relieve any aspect of burden more effectively than did home treatment. Much, of course, depends on the way burden is measured. Hoenig & Hamilton (1969) differentiated between 'subjective' and 'objective' forms, and showed that the fact of patients being out of hospital increased neither so far as relatives were concerned, although this finding may have been influenced by the fact that the social services often took action to modify problems that became too much for families to bear. Interestingly, they found more complaints of subjective burden in households in social classes I and II, although the objective burden there appeared to be smaller than in families from classes III to V.

Nevertheless, in countries where mental hospitals are being closed, families are worried about difficulties in getting help for themselves and, as they see it, lack of necessary hospital care for their patient members, though Creer & Wing's findings (1974) that the groups of relatives they studied wanted more help from the extramural services, rather than more mental hospital care, seem typical. A study of patients discharged from an English mental hospital showed that in spite of severe burden on relatives and the poor living conditions of some patients, less than a handful wished to return to hospital and equally small numbers of relatives wished them to do so (Johnstone et al 1986). In another study of 50 long-term mental hospital patients and 100 elderly confused patients resettled in York, it was found that the former long-stay patients were well supported in their residential settings, but that the resettlement of the elderly confused was less successful; their care was both episodic and fragmented, and a heavy burden fell on elderly relatives (Jones 1985). Even if there was more effective extramural support, doubts about the fitness or advisability of community alternatives to hospital admission linger in the minds of many, in particular for those patients who suffer from forms of organic brain disease or trauma and are aged under 65, since there is no accepted pattern of care for them in Britain. The Worcester Development Project (Hall & Brockington 1990) has suggested that about 7 places per 100 000 population are needed for long-term care and supervision, mainly for people suffering from organic brain disorders. However, this is for a district consisting of small towns and rural areas; in inner-city populations, the rate could well be several times higher.

The process of change from the centralised, medically or professionally dominated institution to a decentralised, diffuse system, involving a wide range of agencies, people, and facilities, has many aspects. It is still often assumed that mental hospitals were excellently run and highly therapeutic for the mentally ill, though at the same time recorded that they were 'grossly overcrowded and seriously lacking any therapeutic facilities or therapeutic programmes' (Cumming & Cumming 1957). Society tends to deny the presence of mental illness for as long as possible, but when this can no longer be done, it then rationalises isolation of the patient with the belief that hospital care is ideal. Lyth (1988) suggested that hospitals are organised primarily as a defence against public and nursing anxiety, and that to some extent, change is inevitably an excursion into the unknown: it implies a commitment to future events that are not entirely predictable and to their consequences, thereby provoking doubt and anxiety. Since any significant change within a social system implies changes in existing relationships and in the social structure, there are important psychological reasons why people are reluctant to contemplate changes which remove the insulation of mental illness or undermine well established institutional defences against deeper anxieties (Parker 1985). On a more pedestrian level, there may be resistance to closure of institutions from trade unions and from local businessmen and shopkeepers, who equate maintenance of a local hospital with their personal interests — financial or otherwise (Greenblatt 1976). Much of the literature, though, refers to North American hospitals, whose size and degree of institutionalism were on a much greater scale than those known elsewhere.

There have also, of course, been difficulties not only in running down psychiatric hospitals but in the provision of new services: in Britain, these derive to some extent from the problems of unifying the management and funding of the new facilities, and of transferring money from hospitals to local authority social services. The health and social service sectors have generally found it difficult to co-operate effectively, so that for instance, an increase in child care demands has led to a decrease in mental health work by social services (Fisher et al 1984), while the conflicting memberships, methods of financing, and responsibilities of the two bodies, as well as the pressure of the increasing numbers of people who are old and frail, all challenge central government's desire to secure an overall reduction in local authorities' spending. The difficulties of achieving integrated planning between the local authority, the health service, and social security also highlight the barriers to change. Attempts at joint funding have not been enthusiastically received, since local authorities feel that such commitments may force them into later

financial difficulties (Chant 1986). However, from 1991, health authorities will act as agents of central government in paying a specific grant to
local authorities for the social care of psychiatric patients on the basis of
assessments of individual need (DOH 1989), and will have the
responsibility of monitoring this service: in this way, it is hoped that many
patients who would otherwise have had to spend significant periods in
hospital may receive appropriate care outside.

SOME MODEL SERVICES

Dane County, Wisconsin operates a system, repeated in some other parts
of that State, where the county pays for both the hospital and the
community service. The money is transferable, so that if there is more
use of the hospital services in Mendota State Hospital, there is less
money for the district services and thus the risk of job losses for
community staff who have difficult chronic cases admitted to hospital. In
this way, the dollar follows the patient (Stein & Ganser 1983). There are
other interesting aspects of the service, including an assertive approach by
staff, who do not wait for the patient to contact them, but seek him/her
out, though PACT — the Programme for Assertive Community
Treatment — is said to be 'non-intrusive'. A crisis intervention team offer
24-hour help, while a mobile community team offer case management
and organise money and medication for about 180 chronic patients with
schizophrenia who, supported in this way, can take responsibility for
much of their lives (Muijen & McNamee 1989). The staff also work with
families, giving education and support to them and to other helpers
(Stein & Test 1978, 1980). This comprehensive system of community
care has been carefully evaluated, and it has been shown that the
programme is an effective way of helping chronically mentally ill people,
decreasing the hospital admissions and symptoms of the experimental
patients, while improving their employment and socialisation, when
compared with control patients. It provided a model for services in New
South Wales.

In that Australian state, about 1 million of the 3 million inhabitants of
Sydney are served by well organised community services, which after
some hesitation are being extended. Part of the service has been carefully
evaluated (Hoult & Reynolds 1984, Hoult 1986) and no extravagant
claims have been made, since 40% of the experimental patients were still
admitted to hospital, although the average length of stay was reduced to
8.4 days for the experimental group, compared to 53.5 days for the
controls. Hoult refers to the importance of forming a therapeutic alliance
with the patient and his family and of reducing their mutual burden:
equally important is the willingness to involve both patient and relatives
or care-givers actively and to provide them, where appropriate, with
information, support, guidance, and counselling. Such a service needs

sufficient multidisciplinary staff, and each team has about 10 members, who are available through the 24 hours. They offer case management in which a designated professional has responsibility for checking that the needs of a small number of disabled former patients are being met by those services which should be providing varied aspects of care. They are nevertheless more accessible than most psychiatric services — with many long-distance pagers and available telephones, and are more mobile — each team has about six cars — as well as more assertive, not being time-limited in their interventions. Two areas also have mobile treatment teams, on the Madison model, for the management of long-term patients. About eight areas with populations of 100–150 000 people have their own group homes, hostels, living skills centres, day centres, and respite houses, while two have 'ward in a house' schemes. Another important difference from most British services is that this one is intentionally health-led and health-funded; as there are no local authority social services for the mentally ill, social workers are employed by the health authority.

One British service that has replaced the mental hospital (which has been demolished) with a comprehensive community service is in the Torbay district of South Devon. This too is a health-led, health-financed service, although the staff work closely with local authority social services, who co-operated in its development. Contrary to the views of the Audit Commission (1986) and to the Griffiths' report (1988) it demonstrates the possibility of changing things and transferring funds in the NHS where there is the will and a specific programme for doing so (Boswell 1988). Change from the old mental hospital-based service to the new community service was accomplished without staff redundancies; all were offered comparable jobs, some non-nursing staff being employed as assistant nurses, and others as 'service assistants'. There are altogether 400 mental health staff, looking after the Torbay population of 240 000; five local mental health centres have been provided, as well as an inpatient unit in the district general hospital. For an initial period, transport, housing, and removal costs were supplemented by the health authority responsible for the whole of Devon, so that the South Devon experience was probably made possible by the release of funds from closing high-cost mental hospitals (Mahoney 1988). However, it would be premature to claim that arrangements such as this represent a successful model for the future until results of systematic evaluation are available, including measures of morbidity in different categories of patients.

DEALING WITH LONG-TERM PROBLEMS

One of the inescapable facts of psychiatric disorder is that its severe forms tend to run a chronic or recurrent course, whether the individuals concerned are resident in or out of hospital. If community psychiatry is to provide comprehensive care to whole populations, it will have to structure its services so that they can respond to these long-term needs in a sensitive and effective way. This will not happen, however, unless the services' objectives are clearly identified and their performances monitored. Moving services away from psychiatric hospitals, which generally could not escape the duty of managing the most difficult and disabled patients, carries the risk that these groups may then be neglected — however inadequate hospital care may have been for them in the past. This is because both clients and facilities become dispersed into situations where there are competing demands from people with less severe morbidity. The fall-back function of the mental hospital therefore has to be re-established, but within a comprehensive community-based service.

In the past, services have often failed to be effective because the acute model has been applied uncritically to long-term problems. The objectives of the service and its plans (if any) for meeting these have never been clearly formulated, patients have received no help with their problems of everyday living, the responsibilities of different professionals have not been made clear, liaison between them has been unsatisfactory, and neither patients nor relatives have been involved in the care plans. Acute episodes are often referred to as if they usually represent individuals who were previously unknown to the mental health services, but in fact, a high proportion of these people will have a previous psychiatric history, which may well be extensive. In many cases, such an episode will be merely the rapid worsening of a state of chronic illness or disability, and largely through migration patterns, problems of this kind occur at relatively high levels in certain environments, e.g. inner-city areas with declining populations (Freeman 1985). There is no general agreement on the best pattern of care for these people, and services must vary a good deal according to local circumstances. However, a number of special initiatives — particularly in England — have aimed to ensure that community-orientated services do not neglect long-term problems in the populations for which they are responsible.

Dean & Gadd (1989) restructured the psychiatric service for an inner-city area of Birmingham where there had been a high use of inpatient care, with many compulsory admissions; two-thirds of the population of 25 000 was born outside the UK. The multidisciplinary team based themselves in a local resource centre, where organised activities and social support are provided for the chronically ill, together with a service for acute patients who are being managed mainly at home. Urgent referrals are seen on the same day by a doctor and nurse; if necessary a patient can be admitted to hospital at any time, and those unable to attend the centre are visited regularly. The very compact nature of the area makes it easy both for patients to attend the centre and for staff to visit them; also, the high proportion of Asian patients, with their extended families, probably allows home care to be successful more often than would be likely in other populations.

In a similar area of London, from which 60% of admissions to acute psychiatric beds had previously been the readmissions of patients with long-term problems, a new MDT, additional to the existing sector teams, was established at a community base (McClean & Leibowitz 1990). Between inpatient episodes, little support had been available to people of this kind from the community nursing service or nearest day hospital, but this team has emphasised the continuity of the key worker role, and patients are seen mostly at home or at their GP's surgery. Social support is focused through weekly groups, mostly open-ended and held jointly with non-psychiatric agencies, aiming to re-attach patients to normal activities within the community. All known cases are reviewed at least every three months, and about 100 had been listed for permanent care at the end of two years. Those who refuse all care are monitored through relatives or neighbours. The nature of such work is summed up in the authors' statement that 'every patient contact is a draining contact', so that the risk of staff 'burn-out' may well be great.

In the past, the role of the professional in mental health services has needed to include not only the application of clinical skills but also an administrative function, as seen for instance when a psychiatrist writes about a patient's progress to a GP, asks the community nurse to monitor the use of medication, informs the social worker of a problem in the patient's housing, and arranges to see the patient again. Without attention to these organisational aspects, clinical care is unlikely to be successful in the long term. Where the key worker concept is used, that professional usually takes administrative responsibility in addition to his/her professional duties for the patient concerned. Yet the skills required for administrative and co-ordinating work differ from those required for direct care of patients. An alternative model is that of case management, where the administrative duties for a number of patients are separated from the clinical and are assumed by another worker, who does not have any therapeutic function. On the other hand, this person may have budgetary responsibility, involving the purchase and monitoring of the best possible package of care for those patients with the funds available. It seems reasonable to relieve highly trained professional staff of largely routine functions, which do not require their specific skills and which to some extent may now be computerised. However, little reliable information has so far been produced as to how well this system works in practice — particularly over long periods. Anecdotal evidence suggests that case managers on the whole may not have sufficient status to direct the activities of professionals, though their work will be appreciated insofar as it reduces the non-clinical tasks of therapeutic staff.

An early attempt in this direction was by Freeman et al (1979), who set up a central office for a health district, where records were kept on every schizophrenic patient, the basic data coming from a case register. However, funding was not available for long enough to evaluate the system, e.g. by comparing the outcome of patients on it with that of similar patients elsewhere; it might have a particularly useful application in countries where staff costs are relatively low.

A further project in the same area (Salford) tested a case management system for long-term schizophrenic patients (Wolff & Whitehead 1988). With the help of an administrator and clerk, using a personal computer, a team of psychiatrists, community psychiatric nurses, and occupational therapists, with representatives from psychology and social work, met monthly. Reviews and care plans were completed for 25 patients in one year; written plans were drawn up in consultation with patients and relatives, so far as possible, but only two patients actually attended review meetings. As part of the care plan, a key worker was appointed for each case; the writing down of medical and social assessments and of the plan itself assisted staff to keep their objectives and strategies more clearly in mind. At the end of the project, though, it was clear that systematic working together of this kind was unlikely to continue in the absence of a team co-ordinator. Unless staffing levels are such that care-givers have no difficulty in meeting their patients' needs — a situation which is unlikely to be common — administrative tasks of this kind tend to be neglected. However, employing administrative staff for case management involves extra expenditure, which managers and politicians usually find very unwelcome.

In England, health authorities have each been required to set up a Care Programme to provide co-ordinated care for people disabled by chronic mental illness who are living mainly in the community, from 1991 (DOH 1990). This acknowledges that some such patients can only be maintained out of hospital satisfactorily if they receive appropriate social care, in forms such as meals, physical comfort, and human contact. The programme is painstaking but requires training and a change in attitude and further evaluation. What is not made clear is whether or not extra money will be provided to develop these services, in the transitional period before mental hospitals are closed; this is the financial 'double-bind' that has delayed the development of extramural services in Britain and some other countries for many years.

Wing & Furlong (1986) argued that services for the chronically disabled should be planned on the basis of these people's identified needs, analysed as being due to either intrinsic impairment, social disadvantage, or personal distress. The problems which are defined in this way should then be met by specific forms of care, which include medical treatment, rehabilitation, shelter, etc. When the relevant individuals from a population have been identified epidemiologically, the aggregation of their total needs should form the basis for planning long-term services. A variety of options will be needed, so that individual packages of care can be designed and then modified over time, but the system has to be managed in such a way that integration and continuity are always preserved. Wing & Furlong state that disability has three main aspects — occupational, residential and recreational — and that individuals may have varying degrees of handicap within these dimensions. They also identify five factors that may well limit the degree of possible independence, and that may need special attention from the services. These are: risk of harm to self or others; unpredictability of behaviour and liability to relapse; poor motivation or capacity for self-management; lack of insight; and low public acceptability. Use of this kind of sophisticated analysis by well trained staff could lead to an enormous improvement in the quality of life of chronically disabled people, most of whom are likely to be living outside hospital in the future. However, such progress would depend on enough resources being available in each district to provide the required treatment and care options for those patients' needs. Many of the people with long-term psychiatric disorders also have problems of physical health, such as epilepsy, chronic bronchitis, or the sequelae of alcohol abuse; their package of care will have to be capable of responding to these needs. Up to now, little reliable information has emerged in any country about the efficiency of treating patients of this kind on a community basis as a general policy; what one can reasonably say is that to be efficient, a community service will have to have a comprehensive range of facilities and staff.

CONCLUSION

One cannot doubt that many mental hospitals have no future — at the beginning of 1990, 55 in the UK were scheduled for definite and 22 for probable closure — but if there is not enough money for community services, there will certainly not be enough to spend also on the maintenance of decaying institutions. Over 30 years ago, a well known medical superintendent said that we should ask ourselves seriously whether the interests of the mentally ill are best served by providing more psychiatric beds or building bigger and better mental hospitals — 'perhaps we should concentrate our efforts on treating the patients within the community of which they form a part' (Rees 1957). Different areas of Britain and other countries not only require a differing number of beds on account of their socio-economic and environmental conditions (Hirsch 1988), but have staff with diverse traditions and outlooks, offering varying patterns of service: the hospital facilities may be of various kinds, social services may be highly or poorly involved, managers may be lively or unimaginative, psychiatrists may be innovative or change-resisting, while voluntary effort may be excellent or almost non-existent.

Above all, when former institutional patients are living in the community and the mental hospitals are closed, that is only the beginning, or rather, a step in the process of the change. Some believe that these old lunatic asylums should be preserved, their buildings and ground converted, but this has not been supported (Burrell 1985). One possible future problem for Britain and other countries was described by Pepper et al (1982) in the USA — young patients who have never been admitted to hospital but are dissatisfied with existing treatment programmes, and reject both them and aftercare, at the same time as abusing alcohol and other drugs. In the UK, as in many other countries with very competitive political agendas, housing departments, social work services, social security, employment services, and even the medical services do not give the mentally ill and especially the chronically ill, high priority. People in general are ambivalent about the question; in California, while many people 'do not support community care, all seem strongly opposed to institutional care' (Elpers 1987). There is danger that through preoccupation with the abolition of outmoded institutions, loss of asylum for the chronically handicapped, the civil rights of the mentally ill, the burden on families, or the costs and organisation of community services, the reasons for the changes in psychiatric care will be forgotten.

This discussion recalls the views of Davey (1867), who was anxious to *develop hospital treatment not asylum care* and to secure the relief and cure of the disordered mind (see Ch. 2). The community approach, through its concern with each person's adaptive capacity and with the risks of desocialisation, as well as with the organisation of appropriate support and if necessary shelter, should help to limit disease, disability, and if possible distress, not only in those who suffer, but in their families and others. The variations are endless; they greatly influence the pace of change which is described in the various chapters of this book. But progress requires professional staff to accept — as many certainly do — that the treatment of psychiatric disorders is significantly influenced by the way in which they are defined and the way in which they are managed. What can be achieved does not depend on manpower or capital investment alone; those are needed, but we are travelling slowly along the path of change and Utopia is a challenging vision, rather than a promise. It is better, therefore, if people accept 'that which you cannot turn to good so to order it that it be not very bad. For it is not possible for all things to be well unless all men were good, which I think will not be yet this good many years' (More 1516).

REFERENCES

Acheson E D 1985 That over-used word "community"! Health Trends 17: 3

Andrews G, Teeson M, Stewart G, Hoult J 1989 Community placement of the chronic mentally ill. Hospital and Community Psychiatry (in press)

Audit Commission 1986 Making a reality of community care. Her Majesty's Stationary Office, London

Avison W R, Speechley K N 1987 The discharged psychiatric patient: a review of social, social-psychological and psychiatric correlates of outcome. American Journal of Psychiatry 144: 10-18

Barclay W A 1988 Report to the Minister of Health N.S.W. from the Ministerial Implementation Committee on Mental Health and Developmental Disability (chairman Barclay W A). Volume I Government Printer New South Wales

Bassuk E L, Rulin L, Lauriat T 1984 Is homelessness a mental health problem? American Journal of Psychiatry 141: 1546-1550

Bennett D H 1978 Community psychiatry. British Journal of Psychiatry 132: 209-220

Bennett D H 1980 The chronic psychiatric patient today. Journal of the Royal Society of Medicine 73: 301-303

Bernard V W 1964 Education for community psychiatry in a university medical centre. In: Bellak L (ed) Handbook of community psychiatry and community mental health. Grune and Stratton, New York

Blacker C P 1946 Neurosis in the mental health services. Oxford University Press, London

Boardman A P, Bouras N, Cundy J 1987 The mental health advice centre in Lewisham Service usage: trends from 1978 to 1984. NUPRD, London

Boswell D 1988 Care in the community: a comprehensive local mental health service in South Devon. BBC Broadcast Notes 16644: 3 The Open University Milton Keynes

Bott E 1957 Family & social network. Tavistock, London

Bouras N 1982 Mental health advice centre: 3 years of experience. Research Report No 1 Lewisham Health District, London

Bouras N, Tufnel G, Brough D I, Watson J P 1986 Model for the integration of community psychiatry and primary care. Journal of the Royal College of General Practitioners 283: 62-66

Bowden P 1990 New directions for service provision: a personal view. Institute of Criminology, Cambridge. (20th Cropwood Conference). (In press)

Braun P, Kochansky G, Shapiro R et al 1981 Overview: deinstitutionalization of psychiatric patients, a critical review of outcome studies. American Journal of Psychiatry 138: 736-749

Brook P, Cooper B 1975 Community mental health care: primary team and specialist services. Journal of the Royal College of General Practitioners 25: 93-110

Burrell J 1985 A sane environment. Building Design 18 October: 8-10

Canter D, Drake M, Littler T, Moore J, Stockley D, Ball J 1989 The faces of homelessness in London: interim report to the Salvation Army. Department of Psychology, University of Surrey, Guildford

Caplan G 1964 Principles of preventive psychiatry. Tavistock, London

Chant J 1986 Making ends meet in a continuum of care. In: Wilkinson G, Freeman H (eds) The provision of mental health services in Britain: the way ahead. Gaskell, London

Coid J 1988 Mentally abnormal prisoners on remand. I. Rejected or accepted by the NHS. British Medical Journal 296: 1779-1782

Cooper B, Morgan H G 1973 Epidemiological psychiatry. Charles C. Thomas, Springfield, Ill

Cooper B, Harwin B G, Depla C, Shepherd M 1975 Mental health care in the community: an evaluative study. Psychological Medicine 5: 372-380

Creer C, Wing J K 1974 Schizophrenia at home. National Schizophrenia Fellowship, Surbiton

Cumming E, Cumming J 1957 Closed ranks: an experiment in mental health education. Harvard University Press, Cambridge, Mass

Davey J G 1867 On the insane poor in Middlesex and the asylums of Hanwell and Colney Hatch. Journal of Mental Science 13: 314-319

Davis K 1937 Mental hygiene and the class structure. Psychiatry 1: 55-65

Dean C, Gadd E 1989 An inner city home treatment service. Psychiatric Bulletin 13: 667-669

Dennis N 1958 The popularity of the neighbourhood community idea. Sociological Review 6: 191-206

Department of Health & Social Security 1981 Care in the community: a constructive document on moving resources for care in England. HC 81: 9 DHSS, London

Department of Health & Social Security 1983 Health service development: care in the community and joint finance. DHSS, London

Department of Health & Social Security 1988 Statistical Bulletin: Results of mental health enquiry 1986. Government Statistical Service, London

Department of Health 1989 Secretary of State's statement to Parliament on community care. DOH, London

Department of Health 1990. Services for people with a mental illness. DOH, London

Dinitz S, Beran N 1971 Community mental health as a boundaryless and boundary-busting system. Journal of Health & Social Behaviour 12: 99-108

Elpers J R 1987 Are we legislating reinstitutionalization? American Journal of Orthopsychiatry 57: 441-446

Fahy T 1989 Comments on psychiatry in primary care. In: Henderson J H (ed) Comprehensive Mental Health Care (in press) Gaskell, London

Fenton F R, Tessier L, Struening E L, Smith F A, Benoit C 1982 Home and hospital psychiatric treatment. Croom Helm, London

Ferguson B, Cooper S, Brothwell J, Markantonakis A, Tyrer P 1990 The clinical evaluation of a new community psychiatric service based on general-practice psychiatric clinics. (Submitted for publication)

Fisher M, Newton C, Sainsbury E 1984 Mental health social work observed. Allen & Unwin, London

Fowles A J 1990 The mentally abnormal offender in the era of community care. Institute of Criminology, Cambridge (20th Cropwood Conference). (In press)

Freeman H L 1963 Community mental health services: some general and practical considerations. Comprehensive Psychiatry 4: 417-425

Freeman H L 1983 Concepts of community psychiatry. British Journal of Hospital Medicine 30: 90-96

Freeman H L 1985 Mental health and the environment. Churchill Livingstone, London

Freeman H L, Cheadle A J, Korer J R 1979 A method for monitoring the care of schizophrenic patients in the community. British Journal of Psychiatry 134: 412-416

Freudenberg R K 1976 Psychiatric care. British Journal of Hospital Medicine 19: 585-592

Gibbons J S 1986 Care of 'new' long-stay patients in a district general hospital unit. The first two years of a hospital hostel. Acta Psychiatrica Scandinavica 73: 582-588

Gleisner J 1982 A community mental health centre. British Journal of Clinical & Social Psychiatry 1: 71-73

Goffman E 1961 Asylums: essays on the social situation of mental patients and other inmates. Doubleday, New York

Goldberg D 1971 The scope and limits of community psychiatry. In: Shagass C (ed) The role of drugs in community psychiatry. Modern problems of pharmacopsychiatry 6. Karger, Basel

Goldberg D, Huxley P 1980 Mental illness in the community: the pathway to psychiatric care. Tavistock, London

Goldberg D P, Bridges K, Cooper W, Hyde C, Sterling C, Wyatt R 1985 Douglas house: a new type of hostel ward for chronic psychotic patients. British Journal of Psychiatry 147: 383-388

Grad J, Sainsbury P 1968 The effects that patients have on their families in a community care and control service: a two year follow up. British Journal of Psychiatry 114: 268-278

Greenblatt M 1976 Historical factors affecting the closure of state hospitals. In: Ahmed P, Plogg S G (eds) State mental hospitals: what happens when they close. Plenum, New York

Griffiths R 1988 Community care: agenda for action. Her Majesty's Stationary Office, London

Griffiths T A 1985 Clinical psychology in primary health care. In: Watts F N (ed) New developments in clinical psychology. Wiley, Chichester

Gruenberg E M 1977 Community care is not "deinstitutionalization". In: Serban G (ed) New trends of psychiatry in the community. Ballinger, Cambridge, Mass

Grundy E, Arie T 1982 Falling rate of provision of residential care for the elderly. British Medical Journal 284: 799-802

Gunn J, Robertson G, Dell S, Way C 1978 Psychiatric aspects of imprisonment. Academic Press, London

Häfner H, Klug P 1982 The impact of an expanding community mental health service on patterns of bed usage. Evaluation of a four year period of implementation. Psychological Medicine 12: 177-190

Häfner H, Heiden W 1989 Effectiveness and cost of community care for schizophrenic patients. Hospital & Community Psychiatry 40: 59-63

Hall P, Brockington I F 1990 The closure of mental hospitals. Gaskell, London

Hawks D 1975 Community care: an analysis of assumptions. British Journal of Psychiatry 127: 276-285

Henderson S 1980 A development in social psychiatry. The systematic study of social bonds. Journal of Nervous & Mental Diseases 168: 63-69

Hill D 1969 Psychiatry in medicine. Nuffield Provincial Hospitals Trust, London

Hinshelwood R D, Manning N (eds) 1979 Therapeutic communities: reflections and progress. Routledge & Kegan Paul, London

Hirsch S R 1988 Psychiatric beds and resources: factors influencing bed use and service planning. Gaskell, London

Hoenig J, Hamilton M W 1969 The desegregation of the mentally ill. Routledge & Kegan Paul, London

Hoult J 1986 Community care of the acutely mentally ill. British Journal of Psychiatry 149: 137-144

Hoult J, Reynolds I 1984 Schizophrenia: a comparative trial of community orientated and hospital orientated psychiatric care. Acta Psychiatrica Scandinavica 69: 359-372

House of Commons Social Service Committee 1985 Community care with special reference to the adult mentally ill and mentally handicapped people. Her Majesty's Stationary Office, London

Hunter R, McAlpine I 1974 Psychiatry for the poor. Dawsons, London

Johnstone E C, Owens D G C, Gold A, Crow T J, Macmillan J F 1986 Schizophrenic patients discharged from hospital: a follow-up study. British Journal of Psychiatry 145: 586-590

Jones D 1987 Community psychiatry in the borders. In: Drucker N (ed) Creating community mental health services in Scotland. Scottish Association for Mental Health, Edinburgh

Jones K 1985 After hospital: a study of long term psychiatic patients in York. Department of Social Policy & Social Work University of York, York

Jones K 1988 Experience in mental health: community care and social policy. Sage, London

Langsley D G, Flowenhaft K, Machoptha P 1969 Follow-up evaluation of family crisis therapy. American Journal of Orthopsychiatry 39: 753-758

Leff J 1986 Planning a community psychiatric service: from theory to practice. In: Wilkinson G, Freeman H (eds) The provision of mental health services in Britain: the way ahead. Gaskell, London

Leighton A H 1982 Caring for mentally ill people. Cambridge University Press, London

Levenson A I, Brown B S 1968 Social implications of the community mental health center concepts. Proceedings of the American Psychopathological Association 57: 117-127

Levine M 1981 The history and politics of community mental health. Oxford University Press, Oxford

Lindholm H 1983 Sectorised psychiatry. Acta Psychiatrica Scandinavica 67; Supplement 304

Loeb M B 1966 Community psychiatry. What it is and what it is not. In: Roberts L M, Halleck S L, Loeb M B (eds) Community Psychiatry. University of Wisconsin Press, Madison

Lyth I M 1988 Containing anxiety in institutions. Free Association Books, London

Mahoney J 1988 Finance and government policy. In: Lavender A, Holloway F (eds) Community care in practice. Wiley, Chichester

Marks I 1985 Nurse therapy in primary care. Royal College of Nursing, London

McClean E K, Leibouitz J 1990 A Community mental health team to serve revolving door patients. (Submitted for publication)

Mechanic D 1981 In: Bloch S, Chodoff P (eds) Psychiatric ethics. Oxford University Press, Oxford

Mechanic D 1989 Painful choices. Transaction, New Brunswick, NJ

Miller A D 1985 Deinstitutionalization in retrospect. Psychiatric Quarterly 57: 160-172

Mitchell A R K 1983 Liaison psychiatry in general practice. British Journal of Hospital Medicine 30: 100-106

Mollica R F 1980 Community mental health centres: an American response to Kathleen Jones. Journal of the Royal Society of Medicine 73: 863-869

More T 1516 Utopia. Dent, London

Muijen M, McNamee G 1989 A visitor's view of Madisons' program for assertive community treatment (PACT). Psychiatric Bulletin 13: 352-355

Murphy E 1987 Community care I: problems. British Medical Journal 295: 1505-1508

Murphy E 1988 Community care II: possible solutions. British Medical Journal 296: 6-8

National Assistance Board 1966 Homeless single persons. Her Majesty's Stationary Office, London

Øvretveit J 1986 Organisation of multi-disciplinary community teams. Health Services Centre, Brunel University, Uxbridge

Parker R 1971 In: Proceedings of the 1971 annual conference of the National Association for Mental Health. NAMH, London

Pepper B, Ryglewicz H, Kirshner M C 1982 The uninstitutionalised generation: a new breed of psychiatric patient. In: Pepper B, Ryglewicz H (eds) The young adult chronic patient. New Directions for Mental Health Service No 14 Jossey Bass, San Francisco

Perkin H 1989 The rise of professional society. Routledge, London

Pinker R 1982 The Barclay Committee on Social Workers. Their role and tasks. In : Appendix B. Bedford Square Press, London

President's Commission on Mental Health 1978 Volume I U.S. Government Printing Office, Washington

Reed J, Lomas G (eds) 1984 Psychiatric services in the community. Croom Helm, London

Rees T P 1957 Some observations on the psychiatric patient, the mental hospital and the community. In: Greenblatt M, Levinson D J, Williams R H (eds) Free Press, Glencoe

Rehin G F, Martin F M 1963 Some problems for research in community care. In: Freeman H L, Farndale J (eds) Trends in the mental health service. Pergamon, Oxford

Renshaw J 1989 Crisis intervention services information pack. Good Practices in Mental Health, London

Report of the Committee on Local Authority and Allied Personal Social Services 1968 The Seebohm report. Command 3703 Her Majesty's Stationary Office, London

Roy A 1982 Suicide in chronic schizophrenia. British Journal of Psychiatry 141: 171-177

Royal Commission on the Law Relating to Mental Illness and Mental Deficiency 1954-1957 1957 Command 169. Her Majesty's Stationary Office, London

Sabshin M 1966 Theoretical models in community and social psychiatry. In: Roberts L M, Halleck S L, Loeb M B (eds) Community psychiatry. University of Wisconsin Press, Madison

Sayce L 1989 Community mental health centre: rhetoric and reality. In: Bracx A, Grimshaw C (eds) Mental health care in crisis. Pluto Press, London

Schwartz D A 1972 Community mental health in 1972: an assessment. In: Barten H H, Bellak L (eds) Progress in community mental health Vol II. Grune & Stratton, New York

Scott R D 1980 A family orientated psychiatric service to the London Borough of Barnet. Health Trends 12: 65-68.

Serban G 1977 In: Serban G (ed) New trends of psychiatry in the community. Ballinger, Cambridge, Mass

Shepherd M 1989 Primary care of patients with mental disorder in the community. British Medical Journal 299: 666-669

Sims A C P 1989 Paper given to Social & Community Section Meeting. Royal College of Psychiatrists, Stratford-upon-Avon

Soni S D, Steers L, Warne T, Sang W H 1989 Multi-disciplinary teams and line management. Psychiatric Bulletin 13: 657-661

Stein L I, Ganser L J 1983 Wisconsin's system for funding mental health services. In: Talbott J A (ed) Unified health systems: utopia unrealised. New directions for mental health services No 18. Jossey Bass, San Francisco

Stein L I, Test M A (eds) 1978 Alternatives to mental hospital treatment. Plenum, New York

Stein L I, Test M A 1980 An alternative to mental hospital treatment I conceptual model, treatment program and clinical evaluation. Archives of General Psychiatry 37: 392-397

Strathdee G, Williams P 1984 A survey of psychiatrists in primary care: the silent growth of a new service. Journal of Royal College of General Practitioners 34: 618-625

Strauss A L 1984 Chronic illness and quality of life. Mosby, St Louis

Sturt E 1983 Mortality in a cohort. Psychological Medicine 13: 441-446

Sturt J, Waters H 1985 Role of the psychiatrist in community-based mental health care. Lancet i: 507-508

Taylor J, Bhuumgara K 1989 The safety net project. Psychiatric Bulletin 13: 667-679

Timms P, Fry A 1989 Homelessness and mental illness. Health Trends 21: 70-71

Titmuss R M 1963 Community care — fact or fiction? In: Freeman H L, Farndale J (eds) Trends in the mental health service. Pergamon, Oxford

Titmuss R 1965 Role of the family doctor in the context of Britain's social services. Lancet i: 1-4

Turner T 1988 Community care. British Journal of Psychiatry 152: 1-3

Weller M P I 1985 Friern hospital: where have all the patients gone? Lancet i: 569-570

Weller M P I, Tobiansky R I, Hollander D, Ibrahimi S 1989 Psychosis and destitution at Christmas 1985-88. Lancet ii: 1509-1511

White W A 1917 Underlying concepts in mental hygiene. Mental Hygiene 1: 14

Wilkinson G 1982 The suicide rate in schizophrenia. British Journal of Psychiatry 140: 138-141

Williams P, Balestrieri M 1989 Psychiatric clinics in general practice: do they reduce admissions? British Journal of Psychiatry 154: 67-71

Wing J K 1971 Social psychiatry. British Journal of Hospital Medicine 5: 53-56

Wing J K 1979 In: Meacher (ed) New methods of mental health care. Pergamon, Oxford

Wing J K (ed) 1982 Long-term community care: experience in a London borough. Psychological Medicine Monograph Supplement 2

Wing J K, Furlong R 1986 A Haven for the severely disabled. British Journal of Psychiatry 149: 449-451

WHO 1953 Third report of the expert committee on mental health. Technical Report Series No 73 WHO Geneva

WHO Regional Office for Europe 1973 Psychiatry and primary medical care. EURO 5427, Copenhagen

Wooff K, Whitehead C 1988 Working together for the chronically mentally disabled. World Health Forum 9: 420-425

2. Origins and development

H.L. Freeman   D.H. Bennett

Though mental and physical health are closely related, facilities for the mentally ill throughout the world have been segregated into a separate category for as long as they have existed. This category has always been an inferior one in respect of status, resources, and the stigmatisation of its patients, whatever may be the advantages of specialisation of experience or of the more extensive space of mental compared with general hospitals. Psychiatric services everywhere have mostly been ill-coordinated with the overall pattern of medical and social care, and often fragmented within themselves so that, for instance, the staffs of mental hospitals have no responsibility for patients outside — a situation still to be found in many parts of Europe. One further factor that has usually distinguished psychiatric from general hospitals is some form of geographically defined responsibility, resulting from mental hospitals being provided by a level of government which did not accept any financial responsibilities outside its political boundaries. But since the geographical area has usually been large — e.g. that of the former London County Council (LCC) or a State of the USA — it was rarely possible for a meaningful working relationship to develop between any hospital and a particular community.

In the first half of the nineteenth century, both in the United States and Britain, it came to be generally accepted that if the mentally ill were admitted to an asylum, they would be less neglected or even abused, and would have a better chance of recovery than if they remained outside. This was the era of 'Moral Treatment' and in 1845, an Act of Parliament required every county in England to provide an asylum. Before long, though, these ideas about the curability of mental illness were questioned: industrialisation and urbanisation in England, and massive immigration and financial stringency in the United States led to asylums becoming increasingly overcrowded. Thus, the proportion of incurable patients grew, the chances of providing successful moral treatment were reduced, and discharge rates dropped. As early as 1830, John Conolly had proposed, in *An Inquiry Concerning the Indications of Insanity*, that not all deluded patients needed hospital treatment, unless their behaviour was dangerous; for puerperal patients, he regarded it as even contraindicated, since they were morbidly susceptible to new impressions, which would be bad in the asylum. Such cases would have a better chance of recovery if nursed at home. Connolly suggested that if anyone became insane, he/she should be visited by a medical officer from the county asylum, which should also send a nurse, if required. A register of all insane persons should be set up for each county, and a doctor should visit acute cases at least once a week (even once a day, if he was the sole attendant). Small houses adjacent to the asylum were also proposed to house small numbers of patients whose relatives did not want them to be admitted. Later, Connolly abandoned these revolutionary ideas, accepting the essential role of the asylum in mental illness (Haw 1989). In 1867, James Davey, a former superintendent of both Hanwell and Colney Hatch asylums, stated that such institutions were 'not adapted by their magnitude and arrangement to the *cure* of mental disorders'. He proposed that a hospital of not more than 250 beds — 'otherwise it can be no hospital but simply an asylum' — should be built in the neighbourhood of London, with 'all those means and appliances held essential, either directly or remotely *to the relief and cure of the disordered mind*' (Davey 1867). At the same meeting of the Medico-Psychological Association, Dr Belgrave suggested that 'incipient' cases would be best treated as outpatients (Belgrave 1867). The suggestion was not well received, however, in part because it was not properly understood, and both these proposals for moving treatment of the 'curable' patient from the asylum languished. The first recorded outpatient centres were not opened until 1890, and although Dr Davey's proposal was considered by the LCC in 1889, it was abandoned through lack of funds (Walk 1962, 1976). Then, in 1909, Dr Henry Maudsley gave the LCC £30 000 to build a hospital in Central London whose aim was to provide early treatment for mental patients admitted without any form of legal constraint.

The Reverend Hawkins, a clergyman also working at Colney Hatch, had become concerned about the difficulties which discharged female patients had in establishing themselves in society; with Lord Shaftsbury, he established the Mental After Care Association (Hawkins 1871). The propaganda of this small society was very discrete, its work in community care proceeding patiently in the early years of the twentieth century (Rooff 1957) and remaining confined to the Greater London area. It did, however, offer a possible form of care that was not 'institutional' in the accepted sense.

In the United States, things took a rather different turn. In the 1860s and 1870s, neurologists had developed private practices for the care of people who would now be called psycho-neurotic. They believed that in this work, they were more scientific than were the asylum superintendents, although in fact no more scientific justification existed for their interventions than for moral treatment. A number of these neurologists combined in 1880 to found the National Association for the Protection of the Insane and the Prevention of Insanity; its aim was humanitarian reform, the use of science, and the prevention of mental illness, but disagreements led to the break-up of the organisation after only four years (Leighton 1982).

A further example of this desire of change, together with conflicts over the means to be adopted, was seen in the Connecticut Society for Mental Hygiene. Adolph Meyer, a distinguished neuropathologist of Swiss origin, established this Association with Clifford Beers, a former patient who wanted to bring about reform in the States mental hospitals. Meyer was the founder of the school of 'psychobiology' and saw psychiatry as a field of scientific research and practice, while Beers was a layman who had written an autobiographical book, 'A Mind that Found Itself'. Their co-operation broke down in 1910 when Meyer could not continue to agree with Beers' crusading and propagandist approach and was anxious to institute programmes which could test the value of aftercare and of giving help to the ex-patient (Leighton 1982).

Thus, at this stage, on both sides of the Atlantic, there was dissatisfaction with the asylum, a desire to separate the curable patient from the incurable, and faith in the preventive possibilities of early treatment. The American movement, however, was less medical, and had wider lay participation, as well as a strong belief in the possibilities of prevention. While the mental hygiene movement only lasted 30 years, in their approach to the need for change, Meyer and Beers represented two attitudes which are replicated today respectively in the form of community psychiatry and the community mental health movement. Meyer represented the cautious, questioning, research-minded doctor, and Beers the enthusiastic reformer, certain about what should be done and impatient for political and administrative action.

Change was slow, however; in Britain in the 1920s, the opening of the Maudsley hospital to non-certified patients and the growth of the Mental Aftercare Association were important developments (Jones 1960). Malarial therapy for GPI, the first specific medical technique in psychiatry, reinforced hopes of effective treatment and also of social change in the experience that the mentally ill might expect. Asylum patients suffering from this disease who needed laboratory examination and medical treatment were often transferred to general hospitals, where legal controls did not apply, and this led to a realisation that such controls might be less necessary than had been thought. There was also continuing public unease about the ways in which the mentally ill were treated in the asylums: it was widely thought that some sane persons were being detained as insane, that the whole system of lunacy administration was wrong, and that widespread cruelty existed. Evidence of poor standards and of abuses at Prestwich Hospital, Manchester appeared in 1922 in a book by Dr Montagu Lomax, who had worked there as an assistant medical officer, but the medical establishment and asylum authorities closed ranks to discredit it (Harding 1990). A Royal Commission on Lunacy and Mental Disorder was established in 1924, and when it reported two years later, voluntary treatment, i.e. without legal commitment, was recommended whenever possible. The report stressed both psychiatry's relationship to general medicine and the need for the aftercare of discharged hospital patients in the community; it was also recommended that the connection with the Poor Law should be abandoned (Royal Commission on Lunacy 1926). This set a pattern which has been followed and further developed in subsequent legislation. Although the Poor Law was not finally abolished until 1948, the Mental Treatment Act of 1930 introduced voluntary treatment, permitted money to be spent on outpatient services by local authorities, and made the whole system more humane in a number of ways: for instance by replacing the word 'asylum' with 'mental hospital'.

During the 1920s, the new alternatives to mental hospital treatment which evolved were: general hospital psychiatry (at first only for outpatients and at certain teaching hospitals); psychotherapy based on Freudian theory — almost all in private practice; child guidance clinics; and, after 1930, outpatient clinics operated by the staff of mental hospitals. In terms of numbers, their impact for some time was very small, but they had a greater importance in demonstrating that the mental hospital was not the only possible focus of care, particularly for such a wide spectrum of conditions as that of psychiatric disorder.

However, World War II then caused a delay of almost a decade before any major change could be seen in the delivery of British psychiatric services; the only significant exception was a pioneering integrated arrangement in Portsmouth, developed by Dr Thomas Beaton. A desire to avoid the admission of patients who were not certifiable led him to develop outpatient services and relationships with local general practitioners and with the public. For the first time, these facilities were available to both psychotic and neurotic clients, and a unified inpatient and outpatient service was provided by the mental hospital staff which was, however, little emulated and soon forgotten; it was conceptually too far ahead of its time (Freeman 1962). As Newton (1988) points out, 'existing services have long-established operational procedures, professionals are trained to think and work in particular ways, and professional boundaries are commonly understood and observed. A new programme which requires changes to firmly held traditions will run into all kinds of practical problems'. But one should not overlook the fact that even then, mental hospitals admitted only a small proportion of those in the community with even serious psychiatric morbidity; the main precipitants of admission were that they caused unusual disruption or lacked supporting relatives (Mills 1959).

In a study at Napsbury Hospital, Bott (1976) found that there had been a change in the pattern of admissions in the mid-1930s: 'a new population started coming into the hospital, [one] which left more readily as well as coming in more readily'. Her interpretation of this is that general practitioners had communicated to patients and relatives a belief that madness might now be curable. An attitude of hopefulness, together with a feeling of social responsibility towards the helpless, was even more evident in Britain during and after World War II; there was then a general social and political consensus about the responsibility of the State for those who had suffered war's rigours and dangers. It became accepted by all leading politicians that it was the proper function of government to ward off severe stress, not only among the poor but in all classes of society. In the late 1940s, Beveridge's plan for a Welfare State was realised in a series of enactments which aimed to secure freedom for all from want and disease. Its egalitarian philosophy of 'bread for all before cake for anybody', which included the implementation of the National Health Service, had a profound effect on the care of the mentally ill.

Similar changes had taken place somewhat earlier in the United States, where, during the Depression, the realisation that not only the lazy and unmotivated, but respectable friends and neighbours could be unemployed and on Relief, led to some change in the philosophy of welfare. In the 'New Deal', Americans became rather more willing to accept the idea that economic subsistence was a right and not a privilege, and this was manifested in some concern for disadvantaged groups, including the mentally ill in State Hospitals.

During World War II, there had been concern among senior psychiatrists in Britain that problems of neurotic illness might have increased in the civilian population, whilst the medical services to treat them had been curtailed. In the interests of the war effort, a national survey was organised by Dr C P Blacker, to examine whether there had been such an increase as to require new facilities. From the epidemiological point of view, the exercise was not very successful — which is not surprising, considering that it had no reliable baseline for comparison — but it did provide a detailed picture of the services then available for non-psychotic patients: in these terms, the favoured London region was said to be 'in a class by itself'. Compared with the outpatient clinics run by mental hospital staff, those organised by the voluntary hospitals themselves were found to be, on average, longer established, holding more sessions, better staffed, and seeing more neurotic patients and new cases, although these differences were tending to become less marked. At that time, 71% of clinics were being held in voluntary hospitals, and the rest in a variety of settings.

In 1946, Blacker saw that in the previous 20 years, psychiatrists had developed new growing points, located in what for institutional psychiatrists was the 'outside world'. Like Hill (1969) he feared a schism between a restrictive and 'closed' psychiatry in the large mental hospitals,

limited to the care of those suffering from psychosis and mental retardation, and an 'extramural' psychiatry — often known as 'psychological
medicine' or 'medical psychology' in the teaching hospitals — concerned
mainly with neurotic patients, child guidance, industrial psychiatry, and
prevention. Blacker felt that this schism had been overcome in the
Portsmouth service, but not much elsewhere.

By the early 1950s, there had been another very significant development — the discovery in France of the neuroleptics — although opinions
still vary about the relative importance of the pharmacological action of
these drugs, compared with social and psychological measures. Both
Ødegard (1964) and Shepherd et al (1961) maintained that the introduction of neuroleptics into more traditional hospitals acted merely as a
catalyst, facilitating the shift towards a new pattern of care, rather than
being the cause of that new approach, while Bennett (1967) emphasised
that their effectiveness was related to social and psychological as well as
to chemical effects. But it cannot be disputed that the neuroleptics did
allow the acute disturbances of psychosis to be controlled in most cases,
without putting the patient to sleep. For the first time, therefore, it was
possible to manage many seriously ill psychotic patients outside mental
hospitals — in general hospitals, in their homes, and in the new types of
facilities that were being developed, such as day hospitals. Certainly, it
was remarkable that in both Britain and the USA, an apparently inexor-
able rise in the resident populations of mental hospitals suddenly reversed
in 1954 — shortly after the introduction of neuroleptics — and has
continued downwards ever since, post hoc if not entirely propter hoc.
However, the same pattern was not seen in some other countries, such as
France and West Germany (Mangen 1985) and there seems to have been
no simple relationship between these falls in resident numbers on the one
hand and use of medication, economic or political circumstances, or
professional practices on the other; any connections between these must
have been very complex.

Though large numbers of mentally disturbed people have always
remained in the general community, this was often at a terrible cost to
their relatives. What was new in the 1950s was that many people with
serious psychiatric illness who would previously have been admitted to
mental hospitals were not being admitted, because a genuine alternative
now existed. At this same time, the more extensive use of ECT —
particularly for outpatients — brought quick relief to many people with
severe affective disorders who might previously have had to spend long
periods in a mental hospital. However, Brill (1980) suggests that the
radical developments of the 1950s in mental health services were part of a
broader trend in public affairs. Although it had long been known that the
social environment is an important influence on psychiatric disorders,
World War II led to a greatly increased sensitivity to social issues, as well
as to a greater confidence in the ability of governments to overcome such
problems by social engineering.

THE WHO REPORT OF 1953

One of the most influential documents of the early post-war period on mental health services was a Report of WHO's Expert Committee on Mental Health — *The Community Mental Hospital* (WHO 1953). Its initial proposition was that every society needs a certain provision of beds for those people who are mentally ill and as a consequence, either constitute a danger to or otherwise create grave social problems in the community; the minimum ratio for this kind of emergency care was seen as 0.1 beds per 1000 population. Having reached that target, authorities were recommended to then concentrate on employing qualified staff for outpatient consultation and treatment, as well as for activities in the community such as public education. The most favourable setting for this extramural work would be the principal general hospital serving the community concerned. The service could then hope to develop specialised offshoots, e.g. for child psychiatry, psychotherapy, epilepsy, alcoholism, and post-discharge support. Day hospitals — of which very few then existed — were advised particularly for 'people suffering from severe psychoneuroses for whom the help of individual or group psychotherapy is not sufficient'.

The core of the report was its advice on inpatient services: 'The most important single factor in the efficacy of the treatment given [is] an intangible element which can only be described as its atmosphere'. That appropriate atmosphere was said to be one of a 'therapeutic community' which depended mainly on interpersonal relationships, starting with those between the medical director and his psychiatric staff, and cascading down to those between patients themselves. Purposeful activities were seen as one of the most important characteristics of the therapeutic community, and their planning as an important task of the hospital psychiatrist, but there should be a gradual transition, helped by social work, therapeutic clubs, pre-discharge employment, sheltered workshops, and night hostels.

There was said to be much confusion about the role of the psychiatric nurse, because this was in many respects different from that of the nurse in a general hospital; as a result, patients who did not need general nursing might be left to the care of untrained attendants. However, the UK, Holland, and Switzerland had established full training within mental hospitals for psychiatric nurses, which was parallel to that of general nursing. The therapeutic community was said to demand from the psychiatric nurse 'an understanding of her relationship with individuals and with groups, which becomes her most important nursing skill', but 'if the hospital is to become a therapeutic community...it must model its architecture and its plan on that of a community'. Therefore, new psychiatric hospitals should never have more that 1000 beds, and the optimum size was somewhere between that and 300; where population density was small, the lower limit would be preferable, as it would be where there were shortages of trained staff. The hospitals should be composed of small buildings — 'take the village as its model' — and allow most patients to live in small groups; it should also be very near the community served.

The report commended boarding-out (both for chronic patients and as a transition to discharge), accepted residential institutions for the elderly demented, and was sceptical of special hospitals for particularly difficult groups of patients. The overall culture and interests of general hospitals was said to be generally unsuitable for psychiatric patients — concern was expressed that if the general hospital creamed off the most treatable cases, 'there is no more certain way of turning the community mental hospital into a 'madhouse' and depriving it of its role of a therapeutic community'. Considering the condition of most mental hospitals at that time — particularly outside North-West Europe — the report was remarkably progressive and forward-looking. However, in taking the 'therapeutic community' as its guiding principle, it did not acknowledge the extent to which this was attenuated from the original formulation by Main (1946) and by Maxwell Jones (1952): 'therapeutic atmosphere' would in fact have been a phrase more true to the Report's opening analysis. The Committee was also rather illogical in focusing on the individual authority of the medical director, whilst at the same time urging a principle which required that power resided in the institutional community as a whole.

The conclusion was that psychiatric services could be regarded from two different viewpoints: (a) the 'classical', where the psychiatric hospital extends into the community via its extramural activities; and (b) the 'modern', where the medico-social team is responsible for all the mental health problems of the community, and considers the psychiatric hospital as one of its tools. If it was appropriate to the social organisation of a particular country, the latter was seen to be generally preferable. In retrospect, though, it seems doubtful whether there is in fact any meaningful difference between the two: (a) could be regarded as one means of achieving (b) which is suitable for countries with an established system of psychiatric hospitals.

GENERAL HOSPITAL PSYCHIATRY IN BRITAIN

The first general hospital psychiatric unit in Britain was opened at Guy's Hospital, London in 1728, and with the spread of voluntary, subscription-based hospitals, others during that century at Edinburgh, Manchester, Liverpool, and Leicester; however, the Manchester Lunatic House, next to the Infirmary, was remarkable in having over 100 beds by 1800. Had that pattern continued, the whole subsequent British history of the care of mental disorder might have been totally different, but in fact, both private madhouses and the new county asylums caused increasing competition, so that by the 1840s, the Manchester unit was much under-occupied, later moving out to the country as a private hospital. The same story occurred eventually at the other voluntary hospitals, and it then became the usual practice for any patient in them who was found to have overt mental illness to be removed to an asylum (Mayou 1989). In the marginal area of psychoneurotic and 'functional' disorders, though, patients often came under the care of physicians and neurologists — at least until psychiatric services were more generally established.

The other main root from which British general hospitals of today originated was the infirmary accommodation of the Poor Law Institutions, in which both physical and mental disorders and patients of all ages were at first mixed up, usually in dreadful conditions. From the mid-1860s, though, separate units were provided for the infirm, either within existing workhouses or often in new buildings, and after the Poor Law reforms of 1929, these became municipal hospitals.

Following the 1890 Lunacy Act, almost all of them had included a mental observation ward, to which disturbed patients were admitted and then transferred to an asylum, unless they recovered quickly. In some hospitals, however, there were much larger units ('mental blocks'), where psychiatric patients might remain for a considerable time; their history is poorly documented, but after they were taken over by the NHS in 1948, the unit populations were usually found to consist of an ill-defined mixture of chronic psychotics, epileptics, the mentally retarded, and cases of senile dementia. Most observation wards developed into active psychiatric units during the 1950s, but the particular problems of services in London resulted in the six wards there continuing for a decade or so longer (Eilenberg et al 1962).

The tradition of general hospital care, which effectively died out in the mid-nineteenth century, was slowly and falteringly re-established after World War I, but mainly confined to outpatients. In this process, the wartime experience of 'shell shock' (which would now be called Post-traumatic Stress Disorder) and the problems of chronic disability which often followed this condition, provided an important impetus. In practice, a small élite of 'physicians in psychological medicine', working mainly in voluntary teaching hospitals, offered minor psychotherapy and some rudimentary medication, but did not attempt to deal with psychotic patients. This situation, though, was changed by the Mental Treatment Act of 1930, which permitted local authorities to pay for their staff to undertake outpatient services, but usually in other premises, such as voluntary hospitals, since most mental hospitals were not easily accessible. Their clientele was rather different from that of the teaching hospitals, including more psychotic patients and many seen before or after admission to a mental hospital.

The Board of Control — the regulatory body for England and Wales —

did its utmost to encourage the development of outpatient work by mental hospitals in the 1930s, but this proved an uphill task. In 1934, a survey by the Board showed that 120 clinics were operating, compared with 29 just before the passage of the Mental Treatment Act; 92 of them were being held in general hospitals. During 1933, there had been some 45 000 attendances by almost 10 000 patients (of whom 44% went to London County Council clinics). Fourteen hospitals (12 of them voluntary) were said to have 'beds available for mental patients'; however, at Hitchin, this did not seem to be very meaningful, since the survey records that, 'Dr Fuller only attends...when asked to do so by the hospital staff, and only one [out-] patient was treated in 1933' (PRO, MH 5/250). Social workers were said to be attached to 39 clinics. In 1936, the Minister of Health stated that there were 143 outpatient clinics associated with public mental hospitals (Hansard 7 April 1936). Clinics were usually conducted by the medical superintendents or their senior assistant medical officers, and though the Board of Control meticulously analysed the information it received, very little is known as to what actually went on in them. In 1935, there were still two London teaching hospitals which lacked even an outpatient clinic for psychiatry, and the rest had only minimal facilities. In 1938, local authorities in England and Wales were caring for 131 000 inpatients in mental hospitals (Webster 1988).

EVOLUTION OF THE DISTRICT CONCEPT

It is difficult to say at what point the 'District Psychiatry' model fully emerged, or just how it came to be adopted in Britain as a national policy, though there are indications of this in the Annual Reports of the Chief Medical Officer, Ministry of Health in the mid-1950s, particularly 1958, where a definite change of attitude away from the mental hospitals can be seen. Ministry planning was greatly influenced by the example of tuberculosis, where a very large demand for hospital beds diminished almost overnight, following the discovery of effective drugs in the late 1940s. It seemed not unreasonable then to expect a similar change with schizophrenia, and when the neuroleptics were discovered, that millennium had apparently arrived, though the experience of a few more years showed that this was a more complex situation than with tuberculosis. In fact, there seems to have been a slow evolution of the 'District Psychiatry' concept over some time, which represented the final common path of a number of influences; in terms of the WHO Expert Committee's dichotomy (1953), it mainly represented the 'classical' model. These influences were as follows:

The Amsterdam Home Treatment Service

This was started by Querido in the 1930s as an expedient to deal with the shortage of mental hospital beds in the city, caused by financial stringency; it became widely known internationally in the 1950s, and was then one of the most influential models in social psychiatry for some two decades. Starting with the practical necessity to minimise hospital care for financial reasons, it went on to promote treatment of psychiatric disorder in the general community as a primary goal, and to work out theoretical formulations as a basis for this work. Priority was given to the re-establishment of equilibrium in the patient's pattern of human relations — a process that was generally thought to take place better in the community itself. Providing a city-wide, 24-hour emergency service was shown to result in a lower level of admissions than before, but the services' administrative independence, in a separate category from both mental hospitals and private practitioners who undertook most of the outpatient care, was not a feature that was widely copied (Querido 1968) (see Ch. 22).

The Thirteenth Arondissement Service

During the 1950s, Paumelle started a unit where treatment and occupational therapy were available to psychiatric patients in a working-class area of Paris. Developing from that, an association was established with support from both official and voluntary funds, which became responsible for all psychiatric care in that administrative area of about 200 000 people. The district was then divided into seven sectors, for each of which there was a multidisciplinary team, which visited patients at home and remained responsible for them in all facilities, including the psychiatric hospital; hence the term *politique du secteur*. The orientation was strongly psychoanalytical, though in 1964, only 10% of patients received individual psychotherapy. A small psychiatric hospital, day hospital, workshop, social clubs, child psychiatry service, and various community organisations were developed for the area (Chick 1967). This model, however, was not widely followed within France itself, except in limited respects (see Ch. 22).

Day hospitals

The first day hospitals (apart from some forerunners in Russia) were established in London and Montreal, respectively, in the late 1940s. They demonstrated that many psychiatric patients could benefit from a category intermediate between inpatient and outpatient status, thus introducing the principle of part-time hospital care, which added a new element of flexibility to services. Later, it was clear that a large proportion of those needing psychiatric care *could* be dealt with primarily as day patients, though not necessarily that this was the best means of treating them. Arrangements for day care spread rapidly in Britain, and to a lesser extent in other developed countries; one of the reasons was a wish to save money, compared with inpatient treatment, though good-quality day care proved to be expensive in staff time, and many of its clients might never actually have been admitted as inpatients (Farndale 1963). In other words, there was a broadening of the psychiatric clientele to include a group with a lesser degree of morbidity than in people who would previously have been admitted to mental hospitals (see Ch. 13).

General hospital units in Lancashire

Industrial Lancashire, in the north-west of England, was noteworthy for a relatively large number of county boroughs, i.e. medium-sized towns which provided all their own services and were answerable only to the national level of Government, until the local government reorganisation of 1974. Each had a former municipal hospital with a large psychiatric observation unit, from which patients would usually be sent on to a mental hospital if they needed more than a brief stay. When the NHS began, the Manchester Hospital Region found itself with only one mental hospital per million people; these hospitals were all overcrowded, neglected, and short-staffed. It was decided to use the very modest extra resources that became available to develop local psychiatric services in the observation units at general hospitals in several of the county boroughs (Smith 1961). Although the evolution of this process is not well documented, it seems clear that a few influential doctors were largely responsible for it.

Originally, it was assumed that links would be preserved with the nearest mental hospital, particularly for long-stay beds. However, the psychiatrists appointed to run these units soon preferred to 'consume their own smoke', i.e. to use only the beds within their own units, though they did not take over the care of those chronic patients from their populations who had previously been admitted to mental hospitals and remained there. Considering that they were largely setting off into uncharted territory, the enterprise and apparent success of these psychiatrists in such places as Oldham, Bolton, Burnley, Blackburn and Blackpool was remarkable, though they may have sometimes overstated their case, since the overall poverty of resources probably restricted referrals. The claim that these units dealt with *all* cases of psychiatric disorder in the catchment area requiring specialist attention raised questions about the boundaries of psychiatric responsibility that were never adequately faced. Nevertheless, their experience eventually came to the attention of those responsible for the development of the NHS, and the example was a potent influence; Godber (1988), who played a key role in national policy at this time, has stated that the Manchester Region experience did more to gain acceptance of the general hospital unit than anything else.

However, the generalisability of this model could be questioned. In Kathleen Jones' view (1979), 'Each of the success stories in hospital/local authority co-ordination was based on a double accident: an adminstrative solution where hospital and local authorities were roughly coterminous... and an accident of personality which provided them with psychiatrists willing to reach out into the community and to experiment with a community-based service'. That individual personalities are often of critical importance is at present a rather unfashionable view, though an historical study of the service in Salford supported it (Freeman 1984). Experimentation, however, always has to start somewhere and, as Muir Gray (1979) has commented on the early Public Health movement. 'Essential for change to occur are *changeurs*, those individuals and groups who have the commitment and ability to realise the potential energy for change.' Without such examples, little new would happen, yet unless they are able to achieve lasting changes in administrative systems, the achievements of these agents are unlikely to survive their departures, as Beaton's experience in Portsmouth showed.

Extension of the mental hospital service

It was also shown that a very similar model could be developed from a mental hospital, when this was situated actually within its catchment area — usually a county borough; in most cases, the medical staff had been employed by the local authority until the inception of the NHS in 1948. During the late 1950s, developments in York, Croydon (May & Wright 1967), and Nottingham attracted much interest; co-operation was made easier by the hospital's catchment area being substantially coterminous with the borough's boundaries. In fact, the difference between a large general hospital unit such as that at Oldham (Freeman 1960) and a medium-sized local mental hospital that had shed much of its chronic population was scarcely significant. Bennett (1978) criticised these arrangements on the grounds that they offered 'only specialised, segregated care for the mentally ill, who often retained their sick role', but breaking down mental hospitals' previous isolation was a considerable achievement. The relationship between the hospital and the local authority varied, but usually did not go far beyond discussions on the admission of disturbed patients, requests for the aftercare of discharged cases, or help in finding employment or accommodation for them (May & Gregory 1963). In Croydon, community care was not seen as an alternative to hospital treatment, but rather as part of a district psychiatry which provided various forms of clinical and social help.

BRITISH MENTAL HEALTH POLICY, 1948–1960

The early years of the NHS were preoccupied with setting up an administrative structure, repairing some of the wartime neglect, and establishing uniform conditions for staff; even though most of these were miserably paid, the cost of the service soared far beyond the unrealistic financial predictions on which it had been founded (Webster 1988). The fact that very little new hospital building occurred for over 15 years at least had the effect of preventing any additional mental hospitals coming into being — something that seemed likely to happen in the early 1950s. In general, psychiatric services were still little different from the 1930s. However, even relative to the NHS in general, the rate of increase in services was particularly small in psychiatry, which carried very little weight within the medical establishment. In addition to this lack of resources, the tripartite administrative division of the NHS — into hospitals, family doctor, and local health authority services — made development of comprehensive services very difficult. Though the Macmillan Royal Commission had concluded in 1926 that mental disorder should be 'dealt with on modern public health lines', there was still very little sign of this happening. For instance, in some regions, a psychiatric patient requiring admission might still be taken into any mental hospital which had a vacancy, however far this was from his home; if he had several readmissions, each might be to a different hospital, so that no continuity of care was possible. The same situation was not unusual in other industrialised countries at that time.

Outside hospital, there was virtually no provision for the mentally ill except a more widely available service of family doctors — though hardly any of these had had much teaching or experience in psychiatry. (The role of the GP is the subject of Ch. 12.) In 1948, with the ending of the Poor Law, local health authorities were given the duty of providing officers (DAOs) who would undertake compulsory admissions to mental hospitals, but there was no requirement for them to have any knowledge of mental illness, and some very curious individuals undertook the job at times, in the smaller authorities — a situation that remained unchanged with the inception of the 1959 Mental Health Act, except that they were given the new title of Mental Welfare Officer. In a general sense, these were community mental health workers, but they were administratively subject to the Medical Officer of Health, though not normally able to expect any professional guidance from him or his medical colleagues. Very few doctors indeed in public health had any special training in psychiatry, and the rigid bureaucracy of local government had virtually no experience of employing professional staff with a caring function, who would expect to make their own decisions on the basis of their professional skill. A few qualified psychiatric social workers (PSWs) were employed in more progressive local authorities, although there were only eight such staff nationally in 1951. However, their position was usually a difficult one, and they tended to retreat into isolated corners of professionalism, viewed with suspicion or hostility by the rest of their colleagues, who were mostly untrained. In 1962, a study of 100 schizophrenic patients discharged from mental hospitals in the London area found only four who had been visited by a social worker in the follow-up year (Parkes et al 1962). This was the unpromising social work basis on which 'community care' had to be established.

As mentioned earlier, the total resident population of British mental hospitals began to fall after 1954, in spite of the fact that admissions were continuing to increase steadily — a trend encouraged by progressive psychiatrists, believing that more could be done therapeutically for patients who came in at an early stage of illness. In fact, substantial changes were brewing within the mental health services, even though little was yet to be seen on the surface; almost certainly, one reason for them was the recruitment into the Armed Forces of many psychiatric doctors of high quality during World War II. Afterwards, most of these joined the NHS as consultants, and they provided a marked contrast with the rather poor quality of medical staff that had usually been found in mental hospitals up to then. Amongst other things, they were generally intolerant of the traditional system of hierarchical authority under a medical superintendent, which was incompatible with their status in the NHS, and which contributed much to the institutionalism of mental hospitals. Very likely, their 'oedipal' rebellion against this system, which eventually resulted in the abolition of superintendents (except in Scotland), was a positive factor for change. Another was the therapeutic community concept, developed within wartime psychiatry by Main and Maxwell Jones; although often honoured more in the breach than the observance, this was a potent ideological force, which caused many old habits to be questioned and added psychological and social dimensions to the more organically based regimes in psychiatry. Paradoxically perhaps, the WHO Expert Committee (1953) saw 'the creation of the milieu of a therapeutic community and the fostering of the relationships and activities which compose it' as 'the therapeutic task of the medical director', adding that this 'can never be created under the direction of a lay administrator; it is... a technical psychiatric task'. In historical terms, this was an almost exact repetition of the situation in early nineteenth-century asylums, where the necessity for medical direction of 'Moral Treatment' was equally stressed.

Yet another influential concept was the 'Open Door', pioneered particularly in the late 1940s by Dr George Bell of Dingleton Hospital in the Scottish Borders. Though the history of psychiatry already contained many examples of institutions that had been operated without locked doors for certain lengths of time, the old norm had always re-established itself eventually, except for a favoured élite of patients. The rationale for this policy of locking up was never examined objectively — any more than was the 'certified' status of most chronic mental hospital residents, who had no wish to leave in any case. However, Bell's example (achieved before neuroleptics were widely available) had a more permanent effect on this occasion, and ward doors were progressively unlocked in Britain throughout the 1950s and 1960s, contributing to a more therapeutic atmosphere and to a greater acceptability of the hospitals to prospective patients. The same process was much slower to occur in Europe and the USA (Gruenberg 1972). A few years later, though, when mental hospitals had taken on a major new function of psychogeriatric care, the problem of the senile wanderer caused some doors to be re-locked — but this was for different reasons.

Mention has already been made of the first day hospitals, which brought a new kind of flexibility into psychiatric facilities, contrasting with the rigid administrative procedures of the mental hospital system. Outpatient care also grew rapidly, from the early years of the NHS, and became even more important with the introduction of neuroleptics, anti-depressants, and tranquillisers, since these could often be used extra-murally. Industrial therapy, with a rehabilitative aim, began to replace the unpaid labour of a minority of mental hospital patients in their ancillary departments; it found its most intensive development in the Industrial Therapy Organisation at Bristol (Early 1960). Therapeutic social clubs and hostels were set up in some areas, e.g. Salford (Freeman & Mountney 1967) and small numbers of psychiatric beds became available in several general hospitals, though only for highly selected patients. In its best Wakleyan tradition, *The Lancet* published a series with the title *In the Mental Hospital*, which focused on the changes that were stirring in that previously torpid scene, and these in turn stimulated professional staff in psychiatry to attempt further new developments. One of these was the fostering of links between a psychiatric hospital and the population it served, particularly through the local authority health department. However, when one county (Lancashire) contained 17 semi-autonomous health divisions and 17 independent county boroughs, collaboration between all these and the mental hospitals was unlikely to be close.

Such changes resulted in a widespread feeling among psychiatrists and allied professions that progress was being seriously impeded by obsolete provisions of the law. Apart from the amendments of the 1930 Mental Treatment Act, these were still embodied in the 1890 Lunacy Act which, as Jones (1972) pointed out, was preoccupied overwhelmingly with the need to set up safeguards against possible illegal detention, rather than with providing care to those who needed it. Its effect was to impose a rigidity on the whole system that made innovation, early treatment, and flexible use of resources extremely difficult. These legal operations were supervised by the Board of Control, a surprisingly progressive body, which in the 1930s had — largely unsuccessfully — tried to persuade local authorities to run their mental hospitals in a more enlightened manner. In the early 1950s, it found a way round some of the more irksome provisions of the law by allowing admission of patients to mental hospitals on a 'non-statutory' basis, to 'de-designated' wards. (Patients could only be admitted under the Lunacy Act to accommodation that was legally designated for that purpose.) By this new means, psychiatric patients had the same legal status as medical patients in a general hospital; in practice, the arrangement clearly worked well, and provided the example for a fundamental reform of the law governing mental disorder.

As a result of these currents of opinion, a Royal Commission was set up in 1954; it reported three years later and recommended sweeping changes in the relevant law. The usual fate of such reports is to gather dust in some Whitehall pigeon-hole, but the government of the day found itself short of new legislation, and embodied virtually all the Commission's recommendations in the 1959 Mental Health Act. Both the report and the Act were founded on the beliefs that as a medical discipline, psychiatry did not need detailed legal control of its activities, and that the focus of its operations should shift, as far as possible, from institutions to the communities served by them. However, there has been a widely prevalent misunderstanding ever since that the Act legislated for a policy of 'community care'. It certainly removed any possible legal barriers to the implementation of such a policy, and spelled out the responsibilities of local authorities to provide extramural services, specifically mentioning hostels among these. But the only positive duty for the authorities was the same as before — to provide officers who would undertake compulsory admissions. Furthermore, both that particular government and every successive one refused to 'earmark' for mental health purposes any of the money which local authorities received from them, as part of the general policy of 'block grants'. However, from 1991, local authority social services are to receive specific grants to encourage them to contribute to the services needed by mentally ill people living in the community.

As Macmillan (1965) pointed out, the greatest weakness of British national policy, in connection with implementation of the 1959 Act's objectives, was its dependence on local initiatives and on voluntary action by local authorities for the development of integrated services. Within the budget of each authority, though, mental health had to compete with all other demands, and it was rare for it to get any significant share. Probably no more than lip-service was ever paid generally to the policy of setting up a network of community-based services as an alternative to mental hospitals, since the scale of resources that would have been required for this task never existed in the local authority financial system. Most authorities did very little, and a significant number did nothing at all; many years after the Act was passed, the differences between the best and worst authorities remained as wide as ever.

The Joint Commission on Mental Illness and Health in the United States was established later; reporting in 1961, it said that 'the objective of modern treatment of persons with major mental illnesses is to enable the patient to maintain himself in the community in a normal manner'.

To do so it is necessary: to save the patient from the debilitating effects of institutionalisation; if the patient requires hospital admission, to return him to home and community life as soon as possible; and thereafter to maintain him in the community as long as possible. The Commissions in both countries sought the avoidance or at least substantial reduction of hospitalisation. At first, the discussion of deinstitutionalisation and community care was little more than a recognition by psychiatrists that hospital populations were continuing to decrease, in spite of rising admission rates, but before long, a substantial change was beginning to take place. For some 90 years, some psychiatrists had been expressing dissatisfaction with the mental hospital and had been trying to move patients into environments which offered better chances for the treatment of 'recoverable' patients. In a subtle way, this view now widened to include all psychiatric patients, no doubt representing the effect of the liberalisation of admission procedures and hospital policies, as well as public feelings of therapeutic optimism, generated by the apparent success of chemotherapy and by more general improvements in medical treatment. Patients who at one time might have been forced to enter hospital and stay there were now free both to come in and to leave; they could decide to have treatment or no treatment at all, if they were not a danger to themselves or to others.

There was growing dissatisfaction at this time with institutional life, not only for the mentally ill but for other groups in society. It was a period of relative economic affluence and the provision of social security in Britain made it easy for patients who might, through poverty, have been forced into institutional care, to survive in society and for their families to maintain them at home. In respect of other European countries, Mangen (1985) stated that 'only when insurance liability was extended could extra-mural services develop rationally'. Even so, as the US Joint Commission (1961) noted, while people feel sorry for the mentally ill, 'they do not feel as sorry as they do relief to have out of the way, persons whose behaviour disturbs and offends other people'. These various views and changes contributed to the combined phenomenon of rising admission rates and declining resident populations in mental hospitals. There seemed to be a growing feeling, though rarely explicitly stated, that discharge to the community was not merely a move to a more satisfactory setting for treatment or care, but that the community setting was itself therapeutic (Hawks 1975, Jones M 1952). Discharge to the community appeared to become, for some patients at least, morally and therapeutically desirable and defensible, without involving any need to provide functional equivalents to hospital care.

DEVELOPMENTS IN THE 1960s

In 1961, Tooth & Brooke published an analysis of the fall in numbers of residents of mental hospitals in England and Wales which had occurred during the previous five years, and they unwisely (in statistical terms) continued this projection down to zero for long-stay patients in 1975. This simplistic use of a trend whose causes were largely unknown seems to have influenced Enoch Powell, as Minister of Health, to proclaim, in a characteristically apocalyptic speech, the forthcoming end of British mental hospitals (1961), though much later (1989), he stated that he had actually foreseen the mental hospital sector being reduced to about half of its then size. Instead, inpatient accommodation for psychiatric patients was to be provided in district general hospitals (DGHs) and only at half the existing rate, in relation to population. The first national 'Hospital Plan' for these hospitals was published in the following year, though the actual role of psychiatry in them remained ill-defined for some time: in fact, the plan was largely the aggregation of unco-ordinated ideas and hopes from different authorities, without definite provision either for the capital to construct the new buildings or the revenue to operate them. Considering the penny-pinching way in which the NHS had actually operated from its beginning, this lack of financial realism was surprising. However, as the first attempt ever to assemble information on a national basis of the building plans of the Regional Hospital Boards, it was an important development. At the time, there was no organisation below the national level with the responsibility for planning *health* services as a whole; the consequence was that hospital authorities had to fill the vacuum as well as they could (Webster 1988).

In 1963, the Ministry of Health published a 'National Plan' for community care; like the 'Hospital Plan' (with which it was completely unco-ordinated), it was merely an assembly of proposals by individual local authorities, without any obligation on them to provide these services, or any guarantee that the proposals would actually be carried out. However, it was at least an official acknowledgement, for the first time, that provision for psychiatric patients ought to be considered in the general context of community health and social services. In the following year, the Ministry issued a circular to hospital authorities on '*Improving the Effectiveness of Psychiatric Hospitals*'; it recommended changes of the kind that have been described above, and particularly urged hospital – local authority collaboration. However, as no extra funds were provided, its effect was limited. This circular was the only specific government advice on mental health services issued in the 1950s and 1960s, though official approval was clearly given to such integrative arrangements as those in Nottingham.

The situation at this time in Britain was administratively an unusually fluid one, so that where a group of like-minded professional staff came together, they could strike out in a new direction, provided that their ideas did not require spending much extra money. In this, the clinical autonomy of NHS consultants and their position outside administrative hierarchies was particularly important. There was a strong feeling of optimism abroad — communicated particularly at the Annual Conferences of the National Association for Mental Health — and those involved felt that the problems of mental disorder could be largely conquered on the basis of their professional skills, if the resources could be obtained to do it. This feeling was not shared, however, by Titmuss (1961) who emphasised the enormous scale of the needs to be met in community care, compared with the puny efforts so far directed at them, which had not increased in real terms during the previous decade. The current optimism was remarkably similar to prevailing feelings in the early nineteenth century, when the newly established asylums were seen as a definitive answer to the problems of severe mental illness. Ironically, though, that had largely been a reaction to the 'community care' of workhouses, small private madhouses, and families. At both periods, there was strong and confident medical leadership. It was also significant, though, that by the later 1960s, there had been more Parliamentary interest, and more items in newspapers, radio, and television than ever before, indicating 'a significant heightening of the salience of mental illness in terms of both overt political activity and broader social awareness' (Martin 1984).

During the 1960s, several different models of services for defined communities were developed in England through local initiatives:

(a) In Salford, extramural services were begun by the local authority; a new consultant had access to all facilities serving the population, and obstacles to their integration were removed. The social workers became active partners in policy-making and training (Freeman & Mountney 1967). The fact that the Medical Officer of Health devolved his administrative control over the activities of the local authority mental health services down to specialist social workers and doctors (mainly from the NHS) was of crucial importance and was then almost unique.

(b) In Nottingham, the local authority handed over direction of its social workers to the medical superintendent of the mental hospital, but did not otherwise contribute to the organisation or facilities of mental health services (MacMillan 1956).

(c) In West Ham, a consultant without hospital attachments developed a community service centred on local authority child guidance clinics; hospital services for adult psychiatry remained unchanged (Kahn 1967).

(d) In Worthing, the mental hospital pursued an extramural policy of its own, unco-ordinated with the local authority (Carse et al 1958). Its success was claimed primarily on the basis of a substantial reduction in admissions, yet this was not long since a high admission rate had generally been thought to indicate a successful mental hospital. This doubtful criterion illustrates the problems of evaluation, described above.

(e) In York, the mental hospital and local authority co-operated closely through a joint committee and personal relationships, but their services were otherwise unchanged (Freeman 1963).

(f) In Lancashire, consultants based in general hospital units developed integrated services, in which the local authorities co-operated, but provided few initiatives of their own (see above).

(g) In Scotland, Wales, and Northern Ireland, little change occurred in psychiatric services during this period, except for the arrangements initiated by Maxwell Jones at Dingleton Hospital (see Ch. 1).

At this time, though, the majority of patients residing and treated in the community were not discussed in terms of 'community psychiatry'; that term was reserved for the ones who were being resettled in society after a mental hospital stay. There was increasing awareness of the needs of the elderly mentally infirm, the emotionally disturbed adolescent, the drug addict, the chronic alcoholic, and the psychopathic offender, as well as those who were socially adrift in society without employment, home, or family ties and who constituted a burden on the economy and on the public conscience (Hill 1969). Thus, community psychiatry was changing its constituency: it was no longer to be thought of merely as an extension of the mental hospital. Even so, the hospital remained an essential theme in all discussions of the subject, in the sense that community psychiatry was seen as being the opposite of the kind practised within mental hospitals, while the movement of care and treatment away from those hospitals remained a central preoccupation of government.

However all these arrangements were thrown into a state of upheaval by the reorganisation of social services in England & Wales, which absorbed mental health social workers into a unified department for each local authority in the period 1971–1974. Mental Health specialism came into disfavour because of the generic ideology of the new social services departments, who believed that human needs could not be neatly divided into sections, but the new methods were only superficially conceptualised by the time they were introduced. The Seebohm Committee which advised the reorganisation had in fact devoted relatively little attention to mental health, and it seems that the special needs of this group were not adequately considered (Seebohm 1989). Next, in the 1974 NHS reorganisation, mental health services were taken from local authority health departments and absorbed into their social services. Opinions remain divided as to the overall value of this exercise, but nearly all psychiatrists regarded it as a disaster (Society of Clinical Psychiatrists 1977). Though admittedly most districts did not have a mental health social work service of high quality before the changes, those which had devoted resources to creating one found it disappearing before their eyes, as staff were shuffled and reassigned. Jones (1979) has pointed out that 'integration' of social work meant loss of the common understanding of professionals working in mental health, and thus an actual *dis*integration from their point of view, which was particularly unfortunate since medical and social needs are often inseparable. An official view (Brothwood 1973) was that 'many more social workers are now involved in helping the mentally ill' and that 'the area teams will provide the continuity of care', but reality since then has rarely corresponded to that.

DISTRICT PSYCHIATRY IN THE 1970s

The early 1970s was a period in which managerialism was thought to be the key to solving the major problems of society, and in addition to the Seebohm reorganisation, it saw those of the NHS and of local government. The NHS changes of 1974 had objectives which were broadly right, but made the fundamental mistake of introducing one tier of management too many; the 'health district' was a concept which only emerged at a fairly late stage of the planning. However, the subsequent 1982 reorganisation made the district the basic unit of management, and this contributed usefully to the development of locally-based psychiatric services. Mental hospitals had lost their separate management committees (HMCs) in 1974, and though this may have resulted in some drainage of resources to other specialities, the record of most such bodies had generally been a dismal one. As a result of local government reorganisation, though, towns as large as Bristol or Blackpool which formerly provided their own social services (reorganised only three years earlier) now found themselves part of a large county for that purpose, and the results of this change seem to have been generally unfortunate for the development of mental health services because of the unwieldy bureaucratic structures that were created.

A contemporary assault on familiar values was signalled in many European countries by the 1968 students' revolt against university and other authorities; this process was relatively muted in Britain, but the same social impulses were abroad there too, challenging what was seen as the oppressive forces of established order, together with moral and medical orthodoxy. Around this period, psychiatry ceased to be solely a professional concern, but 'went public'; it was not only psychiatrists, nurses, and social workers, but an increasing number of laymen who judged psychiatric illness and its management to be legitimate matters of public as well as professional interest (Martin 1984). Citizens of the western democracies, who expected to involve themselves in discussions and to judge between complicated courses of action, felt both obliged and willing to make their views known on these matters (Robb 1961) and to challenge the specialised knowledge of practitioners. Attracted and persuaded by simplistic notions derived from a kind of sociology which embraced Existentialism and Marxist philosophy, some sought to overturn long established distinctions between sanity and insanity, and to put the blame for psychiatric disorder on a disordered society. As a result, the chronicity of some mental illness came to be under-estimated, as the willingness and ability of society to care for its mentally ill members was exaggerated. (Leighton 1982).

Contemporary mental health policy in Britain, though, really dates from the publication of *Hospital Services for the Mentally Ill* by the Department of Health & Social Security (DHSS) in 1971. It outlined 'the essential elements of a comprehensive integrated hospital and community service based on a department in a district general hospital': in this, 'the inpatient, day patient, outpatient, general practitioner and local authority services jointly form a comprehensive service for patients in an area, to be used as flexibly as possible, in which the emphasis is on rehabilitation, on the preservation of continuity of the patient's personal relationships and of his contacts with the local community'. It was said to be important that the DGH psychiatric department should be supported by psychogeriatric assessment facilities and by a well developed geriatric department. Even more important was 'the provision of adequate community services by local authorities... Without this, an effective comprehensive service cannot be provided'. Generally speaking, each area of about 60 000 population was to be served by a multidisciplinary therapeutic team, including a consultant psychiatrist, which had its facilities in a division of the hospital. Referral of long-stay patients from DGH units to mental hospitals was to be avoided and mental hospitals were expected to run down towards closure; this process might be accelerated by transferring the residue to other mental hospitals or to small 'community hospitals'. However, 'It should be the responsibility of the local authority social services department, where necessary, to find suitable residential accommodation for patients discharged from hospital'. Norms of provision were: 0.5 beds and 0.65 day places per 1000 population for general psychiatry; 10–20 beds per 250 000 for psychogeriatric assessment; at least six general psychiatric outpatient sessions per 100 000 per week; and small numbers of beds for children and adolescents. Sainsbury (1973) pointed out, however, that the precise objectives of the new pattern were not stated, and that the main proposals had not been the subject of research specifically to assess their effects.

This was a clearly formulated policy, which in its general objectives was consistent with current thinking in British psychiatry. However, its advice was over-rigid ('only in exceptional circumstances should a division admit a patient from outside its district'); it ignored the need for specialised services such as psychotherapy; it denied the possibility of new long-stay patients accumulating; its reliance on social service provision was completely at variance with reality; and it provided no reliable data on which its norms might have been based. Also, since the number of general hospital units was then still quite small, it should have been made clear that the process of providing them throughout the country was bound to be a very long one indeed. In 1968, a pilot project had started in the Worcester area with the objective of providing a community-based service and closing the mental hospital (Hassall 1976), but calculating the cost of this development on a nationwide basis might have resulted in a rethink of policy, particularly as the Department of Health & Social Security (DHSS) had to augment the local social work service in Worcestershire by paying for four additional salaries over a number of years. The process of closure was finally completed only in 1989 (Hall & Brockington 1990).

In a symposium on this national policy (Cawley & McLachlan 1973), Brothwood emphasised the official view that the hospital function was to provide medical and nursing care for those in whom this was the primary need, whereas there was no justification for making the chronically handicapped into long-stay hospital residents. However, long-term provision of beds and day places for the aged with severe dementia was added — though not necessarily in the DGH — as well as medium-security beds, which were to be on a regional basis. Sectorisation was said to improve communication between staff members, ensure continuity of treatment, and foster co-operation with the area team of social workers; furthermore, somebody had to have the final responsibility for treating patients such as chronic schizophrenics whom no one else would willingly accept. It was also advised that the staff of a DGH unit should constitute a single entity with that of the related division of the local mental hospital. In 1970, 94 DGH psychiatric units were operational in England & Wales, though varying greatly in size, but they accounted for only 15.5% of all hospital admissions of the mentally ill; in more recent years, NHS statistics have not distinguished between DGH and mental hospital activities.

Wing (1973) pointed out that since the problems of chronically handicapped people are both medical and social, these two aspects of the service must be integrated to be effective — 'An active supervisory service... for chronic schizophrenic patients must form an essential part of any community care system' — and continuity of contact must be maintained. It was likely that a locally-based comprehensive service would in fact attract an increased clientele, thus demanding more resources, while research on emergency referrals (Gleisner et al 1972) showed that these were often handled by inexperienced staff, whereas an experienced multidisciplinary team should be generally available, if unnecessary hospital admission was to be avoided. Account had not really been taken of these needs, nor of the build-up of new long-stay patients that was already occurring.

As far as sectorisation was concerned, most British psychiatrists expressed their concern that this should be interpreted flexibly, in view of the special interests of individual consultants, the legitimate preferences of GPs or patients, and varied local conditions, e.g. of population density. There was also the danger of professional isolation where consultants worked single-handedly, without sufficient contact with their peers. Birley (1973) estimated that in 1970, for each 60 000 of the population, there was an average of just over two psychiatric doctors in post, one of whom was a consultant; this figure included child psychiatry. In view of the huge number of people in the population suffering disabilities from neuroses, personality disorders, and interpersonal problems, it seemed most unlikely that most of these could ever be dealt with by experienced specialist staff. There were also the many people with chronic disabilities from psychoses or organic brain syndromes, who had complex needs. In terms of staff numbers and quality, therefore, it appeared that only a rudimentary service could be provided for much of the country — a point which drew attention once more to the gross disparities of resources in Britain from place to place. Furthermore, though much responsibility was now being shifted on to local authorities to replace functions of the mental hospitals, central Government could do little to influence local situations, whilst experience up to then allowed no confidence that a reasonable level of community-based mental health services would be provided everywhere by the social services.

Government policy was finally promulgated in the White Paper *Better Services for the Mentally Ill* (DHSS 1975a). This acknowledged that adequate supporting facilities in the community were not generally available, and laid down four main objectives: expansion of social services provision; relocation locally of specialist services; establishment of suit-able organisational links within the service; and increase in staffing levels. The new pattern of staffing was to consist of: (a) Primary Care Team — GPs, health visitors, home nurses, social workers; (b) Specialist Therapeutic Team — psychiatrists, nurses, social workers, occupational therapists, and psychologists; (c) Social Services (non-specialist); and (d) Volunteers. The DGH psychiatric unit was to be seen 'not simply as an inpatient department but as a centre providing facilities for treatment on both a day and inpatient basis and as the base from which the Specialist Therapeutic Team provides advice and consultation'.

It was acknowledged that there were many old long-stay patients who could not realistically be discharged, and that new long-stay patients were accumulating, some of whom would have to remain in hospital accom-modation. The Government's aim was said to be 'not to close or run down the mental illness hospitals but to replace them with a local and better range of facilities'; where a mental hospital served more than one Health District, it should be split into divisions, each serving a district and integrated with the staff and facilities there. There was to be a radical change in the balance of resources, decreasing those for inpatient care and increasing those for outpatient, day, and residential care within the community. This represented a much more sophisticated approach, but although drawing attention to the financial aspects, it said very little as to how these were to be met: in fact, within any reasonable time-scale, there was still no possibility of the necessary amounts of capital being available to build all the required DGH units. Nor was the likelihood any greater of all local authorities providing the level of community services that were needed to make up for reduced hospital accommodation and to improve standards. Early & Nicholas (1981) reported that the resident population of a Bristol mental hospital had fallen by 59% over the period 1960–1980 and that 23% of the remaining patients needed sheltered accommodation outside, yet the county Social Services had just closed their one hostel, and were spending only 0.7% of their budget on adult psychiatric services. The White Paper gave no indication either of how effective Primary Care Teams were to be formed, equipped with the necessary skills, or encouraged to work together (Jones 1988).

A year after its appearance, Freudenberg gave a semi-official restatement of the policy of 'District Psychiatry' (Freudenberg 1976), acknowledging the view that psychiatric intervention 'should be intimately related to processes which occur in social contexts in the community' (Grinker 1975). One of the main determinants of a community-based policy had been recognition of the detrimental effects that large, often isolated institutions had on patients, particularly schizophrenics; the number of occupied psychiatric beds in Britain had fallen by 60 000 in the previous 20 years, and it was hoped that hospital care would be further reduced by screening patients before every admission and by maximum use of outpatient and day care. The network of facilities in a district was seen as consisting of a number of small manageable components, all within easy reach of the community they serve. However, in view of national economic difficulties, a low-cost policy was advised, with less specialised facilities being established first; the same approach has been proposed by Freeman (1979).

In Freudenberg's view, if responsibility was clearly related to a defined, manageable population area, the psychiatrist and multi-professional team would develop a thorough knowledge of psychiatric disorder there, and would be more closely linked to the primary care team. They should become more aware of patients' social circumstances and networks and of the general characteristics of the community, including its agencies and representatives — 'Without such reorientation the development of community psychiatry is not possible. In turn, the community eventually also demands a much greater say in the way services are run'. Freudenberg went on to suggest that prevention should then become more feasible, though acknowledging that much of these activities went far beyond the responsibility of psychiatry. Of such preventive measures, crisis intervention seemed to be the most directly relevant, but its effects were unevaluated — as they still are. Nor was there any indication of how 'the community' was to influence the operations of the National Health Service locally: in fact, that would have run counter to the managerialism which was increasingly evident in the NHS, while American experience of local control of community mental health centres had been far from encouraging on the whole.

As far as the social service contribution to district services was concerned, day centres were being planned on the basis of 0.6 places per 1000 population, but at the projected rate of progress in 1976, it would have taken 25 years to provide this for the whole country. Day centres provide shelter, occupation, and social activity; they relieve the strain on caring families, give help with personal relationships, and encourage participation in work or community activities. Sheltered longer-stay accommodation was being recommended on the basis of 0.15 places per 1000 population, of which about half should be in staffed homes; the same prolonged time-scale was envisaged as for day care.

For new long-stay patients (i.e. under age 65, and in hospital between one and three years), a DHSS study (1975a) had projected a need of 0.17 hospital places per 1000 population, which might be provided in 'hospital hostels', from which patients could attend a day hospital or centre, though the Camberwell case register had indicated a larger need than this. The basic flaw in national policy which Macmillan had pointed out a decade earlier — that it depended on local authorities who were often poor or unwilling — thus remained unchanged, though some modest improvement had come from the system of joint financing with health authorities. However, the progressive restriction of public spending from 1976 onwards meant that the time-scales forecast by Freudenberg were no longer relevant; in fact, some local authority services were actually being reduced. Bewley et al (1981) pointed out that 'new' long-stay patients have in fact often had a long psychiatric career in other hospitals previously; in their 5-year follow-up of 1467 mental hospital patients, only 17 of the 81 'new' chronic patients reviewed had not earlier been in other psychiatric hospitals. Since 1980, though, national political pressure in Britain for the rapid closure of mental hospitals has intensified, in spite of the fact that alternative services in most areas remain far from comprehensive, and there is widespread anxiety — amongst both professional staff and relatives — about the future care of patients with long-term illnesses.

During the period 1970–1975, psychiatric doctors and nurses employed by the NHS increased in numbers by 31% and clinical psychologists by 64%; outpatient attendances increased by 11.5% and day patient attendances by 55%, but the total number of inpatient admissions did not change much overall (first admissions actually decreased by 10%). There seemed to have been some shift, therefore, from inpatient to day care, and an increase in the amount of professional time available per patient — though teaching, research, and administration would also make demands on this (Williams & Clare 1981). To some extent, therefore, the objectives of national policy were then being met, though little or nothing was yet known of the effect of this on patients. By 1986, there were about 52 000 occupied psychiatric beds in England & Wales, compared with 150 000, 25 years earlier; excluding accommodation for inpatients, NHS units offered nearly 20 000 day-care places, whilst a further 10 000 were provided by social services and voluntary organisations. Residential places for the mentally ill in local authority, private, or voluntary homes numbered over 10 000 (Audit Commission 1986).

During the 1980s, there was more action in determining priorities, as well as in financing and managing services, by a government anxious to reduce expenditure, but no change in direction, and 'undramatic progress along lines already well established' (Martin 1984) continued. Two policy documents were *Care in Action* (DHSS 1981a) — an indication of a policy for closing mental hospitals — and *Care in the Community* (DHSS 1981b), which sought views on specific ways of transferring money from the NHS to local authorities. This led to the attachment of grants to identified persons moving from hospital to local care and was designed to facilitate the rundown of mental hospitals, as set out in *Care in the Community & Joint Finances* (DHSS 1983). The health service unions and voluntary organisations also produced reports (MIND 1983, Richmond Fellowship 1983, COHSE 1984) on these developments: MIND was particularly concerned with the values and principles on which mental health services should be based and on respecting the client as a full citizen with appropriate rights and responsibilities. Finally, a new Mental Health Act 1983 for England & Wales, replaced that of 1959, which had successfully reduced the previous legal impediments to treatment, but incurred some allegations of infringing the civil liberties of a minority of committed patients, while leaving the rights of those who needed protection to the discretion of psychiatrists alone. This Act was perhaps an uneasy compromise between the affirmation of civil rights and what could be achieved by law, but affecting less than 10% of mental hospital patients and not touching the needs of the mentally disordered in the community (Jones 1988). In this, its followed an earlier trend in the USA, where increased activity by lawyers resulted in many patients leaving mental hospitals, but without evidence that this had benefited them in terms of reduced morbidity or handicaps. It laid a duty on both health authorities and local authority social services to provide aftercare for people who have been treated for psychiatric disorder. This requirement, though, remained inoperative for several years as described above.

In 1986, the independent Audit Commission reviewed the progress that occurred in the previous decade towards meeting the targets set out in *Better Services for the Mentally Ill* for England. Its conclusions were on the whole very gloomy, particularly as reduction in hospital facilities was found to have proceeded much more rapidly than the development of community services which were supposed to replace them. One of the main reasons for this was the lack of bridging finance to cover the transition period between the old pattern of services and the new, but other problems identified were marked disparities in standards from place to place, organisational confusion, and the division of responsibility between various agencies. However, the Commission also noted features which they had found to be associated with successful progress towards community-based care and which included: committed local agents of charge, focus on action rather than machinery, integration of services across agency boundaries, a multidisciplinary approach, and partnership between statutory and voluntary agencies. The conclusion was that a way out of the impasse would require either a separate agency for community care receiving contributions from both health and social services, or else full responsibility being assumed by the NHS which would obtain care from social services on a contract basis. However, the subsequent Griffiths Report (1988) chose an arrangement which differed from both of these.

Thus the end of an historical view of changes in the mental health services, which from the beginning had been designed to facilitate an improvement of treatment for patients, sees a forceful attack on the use of the treatment ethic as a justification for compulsory intervention. This attack may be taken, perhaps, as an example of a 'community mental health' activity rather than one of community psychiatry; the similarities and differences between these two kinds of activity were discussed in Chapter 1, while developments since 1980 are considered in more detail in Chapter 21. Changes similar to those in the United Kingdom following World War II occurred to varying extents in some other countries, and are described in Chapter 22.

REFERENCES

Audit Commission 1986 Making a Reality of Community Care, HMSO, London
Becker A, Murphy N M, Greenblatt M 1965 Recent advances in community psychiatry. New England Journal of Medicine 272: 621-626
Belgrave T B 1867 Discussion on Dr Davey's paper. Journal of Mental Science 13: 399-400
Bennett D H 1967 Social therapy and drug treatment in schizophrenics: a review. In: Freeman H, Farndale J (eds) New aspects of the mental health services. Pergamon, Oxford
Bennett D H 1978 Community psychiatry. British Journal of Psychiatry 132: 209-220
Bewley T H, Bland M, Mechan D, Walsh E 1981 New chronic patients. British Medical Journal 283:1161-1164
Birley J L T 1973. In: Cawley R, McLachlan G (eds) Policy for action. Oxford University Press, London
Blacker C P 1946 Neurosis & the mental health service. Oxford University Press, London
Bott E 1976 Hospital and society. British Journal of Medical Psychology 49:97-140
Brill H 1980 Notes on the history of social psychiatry. Comprehensive Psychiatry 21:492-499
Brothwood J 1973 In: Cawley R, McLachlan G (eds) Policy for action. Oxford University Press, London
Carse I, Panton N E, Watt A 1958 A district mental health service: The Worthing experiment. Lancet i:39-41
Cawley R, McLachlan G 1973 Policy for action. Oxford University Press, London

Chick J 1967 in: Freeman H L, Farndale J (eds) New aspects of the mental health services. Pergamon, Oxford

COHSE 1984 The future of psychiatric services: The Mallison Report. COHSE, Berstead, Surrey

Davey J G 1867 On the insane poor in Middlesex and the asylums of Hanwell and Colney Hatch. Journal of Mental Science 13:314-319

Department of Health & Social Security 1971 Hospital services for the mentally ill. HMSO, London

Department of Health & Social Security 1975a Better services for the mentally ill Cmnd 623. HMSO, London

Department of Health & Social Security 1975b Statistical Report Series, No 12. HMSO, London

Department of Health & Social Security 1981a Care in action: a handbook of political and priorities for the health & social services in England. HMSO, London

Department of Health & Social Security 1981b Care in the community Discussion document. London

Department of Health & Social Security 1983 Health service development: care in the community and joint finance. DHSS, London

Early D F 1960 The industrial therapy organization (Bristol). Lancet ii: 754-757

Early D F, Nicholas M 1981 Two decades of change: Glenside hospital population surveys 1960-80. British Medical Journal 282: 1446-1449

Eilenberg M D, Pritchard M J, Whatmore P B 1962 A 12 month survey of observation ward practice. British Journal of Preventive & Social Medicine 16: 22-27

Farndale J 1963 In: Freeman H L, Farndale J (eds) Trends in the mental health services. Pergamon, Oxford

Freeman H L 1960 Oldham and district psychiatric service. Lancet i: 218-221

Freeman H L 1962 The Portsmouth mental health service 1926-52. The Medical Officer 107: 149-151

Freeman H L 1963 In: Freeman H L, Farndale J (eds) Trends in the mental health services. Pergamon, Oxford

Freeman H L 1979 In: Meacher M (ed) New methods of health care. Pergamon, Oxford

Freeman H L 1984 Mental health services in an English county borough before 1974. Medical History 28: 111-128

Freeman H L, Mountney G H 1967 In: Freeman H L, Farndale J (eds) Trends in the mental health service. Pergamon, Oxford

Freudenberg R K 1976 Psychiatric care. British Journal of Hospital Medicine 19: 585-592

Gleisner J, Hewett S, Mann S 1972 In: Wing J K, Hailey A M (eds) Evaluating a community psychiatric services. Oxford University Press, London

Godber G E 1988 In conversation with Hugh Freeman. Psychiatric Bulletin 12: 513-520

Griffith S R 1988 Community care — agenda for action. HMSO, London

Grinker R R 1975 In: Hamburg D A, Brodie K H (eds) American handbook of psychiatry Vol 6. Basic Books, New York

Gruenberg E M 1972 Obstacles to optimal psychiatric service delivery systems. Psychiatric Quarterly 46:483-496

Hall P, Brockington I F 1990 The closure of mental hospitals. Gaskell, London

Harding T 1990 'Not worth powder and shot'. A reappraisal of Montagu Lomax's contribution to mental health reform, British Journal of Psychiatry 156: 180-187

Hassall C 1976 The Worcester development project. International Journal of Mental Health 5: 44-50

Haw C M 1989 John Connolly and the treatment of mental illness in early Victorian England. Psychiatric Bulletin 13:440-444

Hawkins H 1871 A plea for convalescent homes in connection with asylums for the insane poor. Journal of Mental Science 17:107-116

Hawks D 1975 Community care: an analysis of assumptions. British Journal of Psychiatry 127:276-285

Hill D 1969 Psychiatry in medicine. Nuffield Provincial Hospitals Trust, London

Joint Commission on Mental Illness and Health 1961 Action for mental health. Basic Books, New York

Jones K 1960 Mental health & social policy. Routledge & Kegan Paul, London

Jones K 1979 In: Meacher M (ed) New methods of mental health care. Pergamon, Oxford

Jones K 1988 Experience in mental health: community care and social policy. Sage, London
Jones M 1952 Social psychiatry. Tavistock, London
Kahn J H 1967 In: Freeman H L, Farndale J (eds) Trends in the mental health services. Pergamon, Oxford
Leighton A H 1982 Caring for mentally ill people. Cambridge University Press, New York
MacMillan D 1956 An integrated mental health service. Lancet ii: 1094-1095
MacMillan D 1965 In: Freeman H L (ed) Psychiatric hospital care. Baillière, London
Mangen S P 1985 Psychiatric policies: developments and constraints In: Mangen S P (ed) Mental health care in the European Community. Croom Helm, London
Main T F 1946 The hospital as a therapeutic institution. Bulletin of the Menninger Clinic 10: 66-70
Martin F M 1984 Between the acts: community mental health services 1959-1983. Nuffield Provincial Hospitals Trust, London
May A R, Gregory E 1963 An experiment in district psychiatry. Public Health 78:19-25
May A R, Wright S L 1967 In: Freeman H L, Farndale J (eds) New aspects of the mental health services. Pergamon, Oxford
Mayou R 1989 The history of general hospital psychiatry British Journal of Psychiatry 155: 764-776
Mills E 1959 Living with mental illness. Routledge & Kegan Paul, London
MIND 1983 Common concern. Mind publications, London
Muir Gray J 1979 Men against disease. Oxford University Press, Oxford
Newton J 1988 Preventing mental illness. Routledge, London
Ødegard O 1964 Pattern of discharge from Norwegian psychiatric hospitals before and after the introduction of the psychotropic drugs. American Journal of Psychiatry 120: 772-778
Parkes C M, Brown G W, Monck E M 1962 The general practitioner and the schizophrenic patient. British Medical Journal i:972-976
Powell J E 1961 In: Proceedings of the 1961 Annual Conference of the National Association for Mental Health. NAMH, London
Powell J E 1989 In conversation with Hugh Freeman. Psychiatric Bulletin 12:402-406
Querido A 1968 The development of socio-medical care in the Netherlands. Routledge & Kegan Paul, London
Richmond Fellowship 1983 Mental health and the community. Richmond Fellowship Press, London
Robb J H 1961 Decentralisation and the citizen In: Roberts J L (ed) Decentralisation in New Zealand Government Administration. Oxford University Press, London
Rooff M 1957 Voluntary societies and social policy. Routledge & Kegan Paul, London
Royal Commission on Lunacy & Mental Disorder 1926 Report. HMSO, London
Sainsbury P 1973 In: Cawley R, McLachlan G (eds) Policy for action. Oxford University Press, London
Seebohm Lord 1989 In conversation with Hugh Freeman. Psychiatric Bulletin 13:465-470
Shepherd M, Goodman S, Watt D C 1961 The application of hospital statistics in the evaluation of pharmacotherapy in a psychiatric population. Comprehensive Psychiatry 2:1-9
Slater E 1981 Interview. Bulletin of the Royal College of Psychiatrists 5:178-181
Smith S 1961 Psychiatry in general hospitals. Lancet i:1158-1159
Society of Clinical Psychiatrists 1977 Psychiatry & the Social Worker
Titmuss R 1961 In: Proceedings of the 1961 Annual Conference of the National Association for Mental Health. NAMH, London
Tooth G C, Brooke E M 1961 Trends in the mental hospital population and their effect on future planning. Lancet i: 710-713
Walk A 1962 Mental hospitals. In: Poynter F N L (ed) The evolution of hospitals in Britain. Pitman, London
Walk A 1976 Medico-psychology, Maudsley and the Maudsley. British Journal of Psychiatry 128:19-30
Webster C 1988 The health services since the War, Vol I. Problems of health care. The National Health Service before 1957. HMSO, London
WHO 1953 Third Report of the Expert Committee on Mental Health. HMSO, London
Williams P, Clare A 1981 Changing patterns of psychiatric care. British Medical Journal 282:375-377
Wing J K 1973 In: Cawley R, McLachlan G (eds) Policy for action. Oxford University Press, London

3. A psychosocial view of depression

G. W. Brown

A comprehensive review of the role of social and psychological factors in the aetiology and course of depression is beyond the scope of a single chapter. Instead, I will attempt to integrate the findings of one research programme comprising a number of general population studies of depression in Britain. However, as some fellow scientists remain sceptical about how much the depression within such samples is of relevance to that found within specialist psychiatric practice, it may be useful to open with a discussion of the comparability of these two groups of depressed people.

'DISTRESS' VERSUS 'DISEASE'

Environmental changes play an essential role in the generation of emotion, and the interplay between plans and events determines a good deal of such experience — one feels more sadness on the death of one's own than a neighbour's dog. Emotions do at times emerge for no apparent reason, and may therefore have a purely biological origin, although outside influences should probably never be entirely ruled out since they may operate unobtrusively through a prevailing social situation or some accumulation of incidents (Frijda 1986). While this is beyond serious dispute, a common view in psychiatry reverses this position for clinical depression. It is claimed that the depressive conditions seen by psychiatrists are of a different order from those in the general population and, at least by implication, that this is because one concerns 'disease' and the other 'distress'. For example, in *The Reality of Mental Illness*, Roth & Kroll (1986) assert that 'the persons going to psychiatric clinics *differ* from those with the milder type of disorder one discovers in the community. There are of course people in the community in distress. But although there is some overlap they are generally not the people who attend psychiatric clinics and hospitals.' In support of this view, a report of the MRC Social Psychiatry Research Unit is cited, which concluded that 'most disorders seen in the community are essentially transient distress reactions which are very different in nature from classical depressive illness' (Bebbington et al 1980, 1981a, Tennant et al 1981a). Roth &

Kroll go on to add that 'even the conditions which resemble depressions are much less severe than those that bring people to psychiatrists'. In short, there is little overlap between community and patient populations and 'real' depressions are effectively channelled into psychiatric care. While there can be no doubt that *some* psychiatric patients are much more severely mentally ill than most non-patients in the general population, current evidence suggests that the rest of this argument is generally misleading.

In the first place, it is necessary to take into account the well-established finding that there are major differences in the behaviour of general practitioners (GPs) when dealing with affective disorder, some referring few or no patients to psychiatrists and others referring many (Goldberg & Huxley 1980). There is no reason to believe that the populations served by GPs who refer patients contain disorders of a different order of severity to those who do not. It follows that many possible patients never see a psychiatrist, and in this sense alone, claims made for a more or less comprehensive coverage are unpersuasive. Furthermore, epidemiological data are usually presented in a misleading fashion, overlooking the fact that conclusions will be greatly influenced by what threshold is taken by investigators to define a depressive condition. If this is kept low, so that quite mild disorders are included as depressed, then those identified as depressed in the general population will be bound to be, as a group, much less seriously disturbed. In a nutshell, the argument is as follows: those treated by psychiatrists for depression will, by and large, reach a certain minimal threshold of severity. If, as has usually occurred, a lower threshold is taken to define who is depressed, relatively more of the depressed in the general population will fall near this threshold and, therefore, as a group, it will be bound to contain a smaller proportion of severe cases. But if the threshold is raised, this proportion will begin to approach that of the patient series.

This can be illustrated with a hypothetical, although by no means unrealistic example, using three levels of severity of depression: A — cases of marked severity; B — cases of moderate severity; and C — borderline cases, not meeting minimal requirements for caseness. To be compatible with Roth & Krolls' position, I will define 'caseness' (i.e. A+B) as the level of symptomatic disturbance usually reached by patients referred to psychiatric services. (Later, a more systematic definition will be given.) Assume that during a single year, 20 women are referred to psychiatrists from a particular local population, with 6, 12, and 2 women falling into categories A, B and C respectively, and that from the same population, 100 women develop depression over the same period, with 10, 30 and 60 in these same three categories. Clearly, as the data are presented, the disease-versus-distress perspective has some credibility; patients are a good deal more disturbed, with 90% of those referred belonging to the two worse categories (18/20), compared with only 40%

(40/100) of those depressed in the general population. Moreover, this difference is greatest for the most severe A category. While this is the kind of argument used by Kroll & Roth, the picture changes if we concern ourselves with the relative severity of the two categories of *caseness* of depression. With a new denominator A + B instead of A + B + C, there is hardly any difference between the proportions in category A — 33% for patients, and 25% for the general population (and, of course, in the remaining category B — 67% versus 75%).

In fact, such claims and counter-claims are largely irrelevant and detract attention from the real issue which is the number of clinically depressed people from the same local population who are receiving or not receiving psychiatric care. In the present example, there are double the number of cases in the general population than in the patient series — 40 and 18 — and this ratio is probably conservative where actual rates are concerned. There is now reasonably convincing evidence that many who are clinically depressed are not seen by psychiatrists (e.g. Goldberg & Huxley 1980, Myers et al 1984, Helzer et al 1985) and at any one time, half of these will have been depressed for at least one year. There is, in fact, reason to believe that even with a quite strict criterion of caseness, only a minority of such disorders are channelled into psychiatric care in Britain, whether they are chronic or not (Brown et al 1985). What appears to be reflected by claims for comprehensive coverage by some psychiatric services is the wish to convey the view that depressive conditions can exhibit symptoms of such a severe and psychotic nature as to place them outside any continuum with ordinary emotions of distress and sadness, however, this might be extended. (Roth & Kroll also wish to distance psychiatry from the more extravagant and misleading claims of the not fully defunct anti-psychiatry movement.) While there can be no doubt that this view is correct, it is not, however, usually made clear that the majority of depressives seen by psychiatrists do not have these extreme features. In order to represent such conditions, it would probably be necessary to create a still more severely disturbed category A, containing, for example, 15% of depressed patients but hardly any from the general population. However, most of the depressive conditions seen in psychiatrists' patients consist of constellations of more everyday signs or symptoms of depression, i.e. lack of concentration, feelings of hopelessness, lethargy, loss of weight, etc.

There is no epidemiological evidence that would contradict this less conservative view; one recent study has shown that only half of the patients treated by (GPs) with antidepressant drugs meet the criteria for major depression (Sireling et al 1985a & b). On the other hand, the study also confirmed that major depression was more often unrecognised than recognised by GPs. This is not, however, a contradiction, and it indicates that GPs treat many patients with antidepressants who fall below the threshold of severity of depression that is generally seen in outpatient psychiatry. This is quite consistent with there being many more cases of clinically relevant depression in the general population than in psychiatric settings.

But it is not only over the issue of severity that such radical claims have been made. It has also often been suggested that depressive disorders can be neatly pigeonholed as 'psychogenic' or 'biological', and this may include a hint that only phenomena primarily brought about by physiological, constitutional or organic factors should be of concern to psychiatry. Again, one response must be that there can be no doubt about the existence of 'endogenous' depressive conditions that have no link with environmental stressors; a better term would be 'endogenomorphic' (Klein 1974, Wilner 1985) but current evidence, again, suggests that patients of this kind are a minority (Brown & Harris 1978, Brown et al 1985). It would probably be more realistic to start seeing the development of clinical depression in terms of some complication of despair, with the attendant sense of pointlessness and lack of energy, and then to seek reasons, both psychosocial and biological, why some instances referred to psychiatrists meet no more than the minimal criteria needed to define clinical depression, while others display a more extreme picture. Whilst such a basic environmental view might be seen as a radical departure from much current psychiatric thinking, it may gain more acceptance if three riders are borne in mind.

First, depression is certainly not a unity, in either a clinical or an aetiological sense. For example, a recent study of women admitted to a Psychiatric Mother and Baby Unit suggests that there is an important biological component among those developing clinical depression shortly after the birth where relatively few women had experienced anything untoward in social terms. This did not hold among those women with an onset during their pregnancy, the majority of whom had at least one major social problem (Martin et al 1989), but despite these apparent aetiological differences, the two groups showed no obvious differences in symptomatology.

Secondly, I will not be dealing with the relatively rare bipolar conditions that undoubtedly have an important genetic component, and may well be far more independent of psychosocial influences. Thirdly, while a major loss or disappointment frequently precedes the onset of a depressive disorder, this is rarely enough to be pathogenic in itself; some additional vulnerability is usually necessary for the condition to emerge.

POPULATION STUDIES OF DEPRESSION

Research on depression cannot afford to rely solely on the study of identified patients because of the very real danger of bias arising from the way in which individuals are selected into psychiatric care. For example, those coming to see a psychiatrist may more often think that they require medical care than others with comparable conditions in the same population from which patients are drawn (Ginsberg & Brown 1982). Only material from the general population will allow us to distinguish inherent characteristics of depressive disorders from those that reflect the way patients are filtered into the psychiatric services.

So far, most surveys have been carried out with women. Women have usually been shown to have about double the rate of depression than men, although this does not hold for the comparatively rare bipolar conditions (Nolen-Hoeksema 1987, Weissman & Klermann, 1977).* Recent surveys have sought to define 'caseness' of depression in terms of the kind of characteristic bodily and psychological symptoms that are met in outpatient practice (Sashidharan, 1985). In the Bedford College Diagnostic Scheme, utilising a shortened version of the Present State Examination (PSE), a person has to suffer from depressed mood and at least four of the following ten symptoms of depression: hopelessness, suicidal ideas or actions, weight loss, early waking, delayed sleep, poor concentration, neglect due to brooding, loss of interest, self-depreciation, and anergia (Finlay-Jones et al 1980). (The PSE has quite a high threshold of severity for including individual symptoms — e.g. for 'suicidal ideas' some plan of action has to have been entertained (Wing et al 1974). Using this, or a similar definition of caseness, depression has been found to be common; in urban areas of the UK, as many as 15% of women over the age of 18 can be expected to suffer from depression of caseness severity within the compass of any year (Brown & Harris 1978, Bebbington et al 1981a & b, 1984, Surtees et al 1983). A number of these episodes may be fairly short-lived, but about half will have lasted for at least one year. A number of non-depressive symptoms are always present; the average number of total symptoms rated for cases of depression in a recent survey, using the shortened version of the PSE, was 19.1 (Brown et al 1985). There also appear to be considerable social-class differences in prevalence; this was shown in a survey in Camberwell in the early 1970s and there has been support for this in subsequent surveys (e.g. Brown & Harris 1978, Bebbington et al 1984, Surtees et al 1983, Surtees 1986). In a survey in Islington in 1981 of working-class women with a child at home, 22% had experienced a caseness condition during the prior year, the great majority of these involving depression (Brown et al 1985). Moreover, these estimates do not include sub-clinical depressive conditions; if those with less severe states, but still involving characteristic symptoms (e.g. borderline cases in the Bedford College Diagnostic Scheme) are included, such rates are roughly doubled (Brown

---

*Studies of students are among the few that have failed to show differences (Jenkins & Clare 1985). However, the overall results in relation to sex may be misleading; depressed men may more often have been missed because they refuse to be seen, are more often found in institutional contexts such as prison, or are defined in terms of an associated condition such as alcoholism.

& Harris 1978, Brown et al 1985, see also Bebbington 1986, Craig et al 1987).

The issue of vulnerability is so central to this argument that a preliminary discussion of prior research and ideas may be useful; the basic notion is that those who are vulnerable will only develop depression once a relevant life event has occurred. Inadequate social support from core ties appears to be particularly critical for women, but less is known about men in this respect; it is possible that in their case, vulnerability only emerges with greater limitations in bonds of intimacy (e.g. Murphy 1982, Bolton & Oatley 1987, Eales 1988).

However, the matter is complicated by the fact that vulnerability may not remain constant and may well change once an event has occurred; for example, at the death of her mother, a woman may receive support from her husband of a kind she has not known for years. If, however, the notion of vulnerability is restricted to the pre-event situation, it is possible to avoid the tricky task of trying in some way to amalgamate such differing patterns of support; in the present example, this would allow an empirical test of whether such improvement is able to lessen the impact of long-term neglect. The distinction between the pre- and post-event situation is therefore a device to help us keep track of what is happening. One possible reason why long-term situations, such as chronic neglect on the part of a husband, can induce vulnerability is that they work through a person's sense of self, especially via feelings of low self-worth. Furthermore, such feelings are important because they increase the likelihood of general hopelessness, once a major loss or disappointment has occurred — the feeling that nothing can be done about restoring what has been lost, replacing what has gone, or emerging from a deprived situation in which one is trapped (Beck 1971, Brown & Harris 1978, Oatley & Bolton 1985). If this view is correct, then although prevailing inner states such as low self-esteem may play a contributory role, it is the final experience of general hopelessness that is critical.

Little has so far been done to test this idea, since in epidemiological-type research, such feelings are easily confused with signs of the depressive disorder itself. However, the theoretical perspective remains important, since it is potentially able to explain how highly disparate experiences, relating to provoking events and various vulnerability factors, can combine to produce clinical depression. The perspective is also a genuinely psychosocial one, in which the development of hopelessness depends on the interplay of the outer world (e.g. lack of support) and the inner world (e.g. lack of self-worth). Therefore, whether a husband's last-minute support will be able to stave off feelings on the part of his wife about her life as a whole may well ultimately depend on whether there appears to be any likelihood of a radical long-term change in his behaviour; without such hope, her feelings of low self-esteem resulting from his long-term neglect may well dominate her response.

Since there are formidable difficulties in measuring inner states close to the point of onset of depression, research has so far understandably concentrated on establishing the relevant behaviour by detailed questioning, e.g. what the husband did before and after an event. However, recent longitudinal studies, to be reviewed below, have allowed valid estimates of one inner state — self-esteem — to be made prior to the occurrence of the event, and the possible development of hopelessness, or depression; this was something which had been impossible in the cross-sectional studies that have so far made up the bulk of research enquiries. In the pre-event period, two processes need to be distinguished; the first is the ongoing *vulnerability*, while in the second, these same factors, or quite different ones, may increase the chances of an event occurring — a question of *event-production*. Matters are complicated by the fact that the two processes may overlap. To take an example: while the break-up of a marriage will not necessarily lead to clinical depression, the resulting isolation and lack of support may well, in time, lead to vulnerability, or in the form of feelings of low self-worth. Such feelings may in turn be event-producing, e.g. if a person embarks on risky sexual adventures in an effort to deal with them. A dual effect of this kind will typically take place over time, i.e. low self-worth may first play a role in event-production, and then act as a vulnerability factor to increase the risk, in the context of any resulting event.

CONTEXTUAL MEASURES OF LIFE EVENTS

I will refer here particularly to the results of two of the population surveys already mentioned. That carried out in Camberwell, South London, in the early 1970s, saw 458 women between 18 and 65; details of their lives and psychiatric history were discussed with them and systematically rated (Brown & Harris 1978). Although it was predominantly a working-class inner-city area, a middle-class population to the south of the borough was included. The second, more ambitious longitudinal study was subsequently carried out in Islington, an inner-city area in North London. This aimed to contact women before any onset of a depressive disorder of clinical severity, in order to provide a better test of the theoretical ideas emerging from earlier cross-sectional studies. Working-class women with a child at home were selected, since the earlier research had suggested that they were most likely to develop depression. In addition, all single mothers were included, regardless of occupational or social-class criteria, as they were also probably at a higher risk. There were two main phases, approximately one year apart. In the first, quality of personal ties, support received, and measures of self such as self-esteem, self-acceptance, and self-definition were rated, together with any psychiatric disorder — either at interview or in the preceding 12 months. A second phase comprised details of any psychiatric disorder and of life events and difficulties occurring during the follow-up year, together with actual social support received during any important crisis, as well as the woman's response to it (Brown et al 1985, 1986a). There was also another contact for most of the women, a further year later, which was important for studying the long-term course of the disorders. Between the studies in Camberwell and Islington, a rural population in the Outer Hebrides was examined (Brown & Prudo 1981, Prudo et al 1981), and there was a special enquiry in Walthamstow to explore the aetiological role of early loss of mother (Harris et al 1986).

These and other recent enquiries in the UK have placed central emphasis on the study of life events; most have utilised the Bedford College Life Event and Difficulty Schedule (LEDS), based on interviewing and consensus ratings which were designed to eliminate bias (see Brown & Harris 1986b, 1989b). Only events with severe long-term threat have proved to be important for depression, and these in turn have provided the basis for a more detailed exploration of aetiological processes: for such threat to be defined, it had still to be present some 10 days after the occurrence of the event. Also associated with onset were *major difficulties*, i.e. those with a high level of threat, lasting at least two years and *not* involving purely health difficulties. The results of the original survey in Camberwell concerning the role of severe events have been replicated on at least 10 occasions (Table 3.1, Column 2); when such events and difficulties are taken into account, their impact is considerable. An epidemiological measure of population-attributable-risk that gives the proportion of onsets related to a prior event or difficulty, and that allows for their juxtaposition by chance, was 73%; for severe events alone, the average was 54%. In the latest survey, carried out in Islington, these were 81% and 88%, respectively.

Although findings concerning difficulties have been less consistent than those for events, major difficulties have often made an important additional contribution to risk (Table 3.1, Columns 2, 3 and 4), and the term *provoking agent* is used to cover the presence of either a severe event or a major difficulty. It is possible that some populations, particularly in the inner city, more often have severe events arising from such difficulties, thereby reducing the number of onsets with a major difficulty alone. Additionally, there must be some uncertainty about the exact role played by these difficulties, particularly in relation to vulnerability. In this respect, there are several possibilities. First, rather than having a direct effect, the difficulties may serve as a methodological safety net, in the sense of indicating the presence of an unrecorded severe event, perhaps because it was not mentioned, or it fell outside the period studied (typically about six months), or because it was erroneously characterised as non-severe. Alternatively, there is also evidence that a less threatening event can at times serve to bring home to a person the full implications of

Table 3.1 Summary of population studies using LEDS of women in the 18 to 65 age range giving relationship of severe events and major difficulties to onset of caseness of depression (chronic cases of depression excluded)

		Onset cases			Non-cases
Studies (random sample unless stated)	Length period studied	Severe events	Major difficulty	Severe event or major difficulty	Severe event or major difficulty
		% with at least one event/difficulty			
		%	%	%	%
Brown & Harris (1978) Camberwell.	38/52	25/37 68	18/37 49	33/37 89	115/382 30
Brown & Prudo (1981) Lewis, Outer Hebrides.	1 year	11/16 69	6/16 38	13/16 81	42/171 25
Costello (1982) Calgary Alberta.	1 year	18/38 47	20/38 53	-	-
Campbell et al (1983) Oxford (working-class with child).	1 year*	6/11 55	6/11 55	10/11 91	21/60 35
		5/12 42	5/12 42	9/12 75	17/52 33
Cooper & Sylph (1973) London (general practice)	3/12	16/34 47	-	-	-
Finley-Jones & Brown (1981) London (general practice).	1 year	27/32 84	6/32 19	27/32 84	32/119 27
Martin et al (1989) Manchester (pregnant women).	1 year	13/14 93	4/14 29	13/14 93	25/64 39
Brown et al (1986) Islington (working-class with child).	6/12*	29/32 91	15/32 47	30/32 94	92/271 34
		25/33 76	14/33 42	28/33 85	107/323 33
Parry & Shapiro (1986) Sheffield (working-class with child).	1 year	12/20 60	3/20 15	14/20 70	62/172 36
Bebbington et al (1984) Camberwell.	10/12	-	-	13/21 62	45/131 34
Total		212/312 68	107/279 38	218/261 84	558/1745 32

*Sample seen on 2 occasions 12 months apart
Average population attributable risk = 73.1%

an ongoing difficulty (Brown & Harris 1978). In order to simplify this review, severe events will, for the most part, be cited as aetiological agents.

Most studies of life events have used a checklist of possible events which are added together to arrive at an estimate of overall adversity or strain. This approach has not been seriously interested in placing events in a biographical setting; the same 'score' is given to, say, birth of a child, whether it involved a single mother living in deprived circumstances or a newly married couple eager to have a child. The placing together of experiences in this way has a long history; there are parallels, for example, with utilitarianism, where all kinds of pleasure and enjoyment were summed to define 'happiness' in terms of a single formula or concept of utility. J S Mill was only the most illustrious of its followers to eventually find this inadequate. To deal with events in terms of standard scores to be added (and perhaps subtracted) ignores the fact that they occur in settings, and because of this, are usually an integral part of our lives and concerns. 'A setting has a history, a history within which the histories of individual agents not only are, but have to be, situated, just because without the setting and its changes through time, the history of the individual agent and his changes through time will be unintelligible' (MacIntyre 1981). Our sense of self largely derives from such settings, together with the roles and purposes associated with them and the activity that has gone before (Oatley & Bolton 1985). It is possible, since plans and fantasies about the future can also be involved, for a sense of self to go beyond this and for new identities to be visualised and created, but even here, the current setting will almost certainly provide an essential background for their study.

There are, of course, problems in translating this into effective measurement, but the LEDS has made an attempt, albeit still crude, to do so. The threat ratings are 'contextual', in the sense of attempting to take account of an event's relevance for ongoing plans when assessing its likely meaning, although the idea of 'plan' (or some similar notion such as motive, purpose, or goal) is not ideal, since it conveys striving or awareness of some desirable future state. The more neutral term 'concern' is perhaps preferable, as it suggests that the motivational background can be largely silent until the event has occurred (Frijda 1986, Klinger 1977). It is in so far as life events generate personal meaning in this way that they are important for understanding clinical depression.

The LEDS has attempted to translate some of these ideas by basing measurement on the ability of the investigator to use empathic understanding of the social situations of others to assess the likely meaning of events (Brown & Harris 1989a,b). It is based on the view that people often cannot tell what something means for them until they can relate it to their plans and concerns, and on the assumption that these can be estimated if we have sufficient knowledge of the person in biographical terms. Because of the way the LEDS is structured, the interviewer has to find out a good deal about the person, and it is therefore possible to make a reasonable estimate of how most people would react to an event, given a particular set of current and biographical circumstances. Furthermore, it is possible to make such an assessment while ignoring what the person said he or she had actually *felt* about the event (See Brown & Harris 1989, Chapter 1 for a justification of this approach).

LOSS AND DEPRESSION

There has been a general agreement about the critical importance for depression of loss (e.g. Bibring 1953, Beck 1967, Paykel 1974, Finlay-Jones & Brown 1981, Miller & Ingham 1983, Dohrenwend et al 1986). In the Islington study, the majority of severe events occurring in the six months before the onset involved the experience of loss, disappointment, or failure (see Brown et al 1987, Brown 1989), and most had occurred within a few weeks of the onset itself. Twenty-nine of the 32 women developing depression at a caseness level in the follow-up year had at least one associated severe event. For 12 of the 29, it presented a threat to their identity as a wife or mother about which they could do very little — at least in the immediate future — and for most of them, it was part of a long history of failure and disappointment in one or both of these roles.

Mrs Jones is typical. She was 38 years old when we saw her; she had come to London from Jamaica 20 years before, and lived with three children in a comfortable flat, rented from the local authority. One son had left home in the previous year after a quarrel, and she had had no contact with him since then; this separation had in fact led to an episode of depression, from which she had largely recovered. A second episode occurred in the follow-up year when she learned that her son had got into trouble with the police and faced a criminal charge. She occasionally saw him in the street, but they did not speak. She conveyed a sense of loss and disappointment when talking of him: 'That they should turn out like that. I think I made a mistake. It is the result of my actions... There is no way I can help him now'. She dwelt on the effects of her divorce, 10 years before, and the difficulty she had had to obtain custody of the children. She also conveyed some sense of a double failure, as her attempts to obtain further qualifications for her job by studying full-time had run into difficulties during the previous year.

The second set of eight women had a more diverse set of experiences, but all appeared to feel imprisoned in a non-rewarding and deprived setting, with the event itself underlining how little they could do about extracting themselves. Any way forward appeared to be blocked. Five of the eight had events concerning poor housing, or debt, or both. However, there were usually wider ramifications; for example, one woman, a single mother, lived with an extremely hyperactive child, and another, again a single mother, was pregnant by a man who had let her down when her flat had been set on fire (the severe event), so that she had been left homeless. Of the remaining three events, two concerned severe physical handicap — one involving a husband and one the woman herself. The eighth woman was unusual in the sense that the circumstances leading to the event were not blatantly distressing; when we first saw her, she reported feeling trapped in a dull and unrewarding marriage, and the subsequent event was a love affair going badly wrong. These eight women were distinguished from the first 12 because they appeared to be trapped — the event itself brought this home to them. However, some also felt a failure in some aspect of their core identity, and doubtless, some at least of the first group saw themselves as trapped. The distinctions so far are ones of degree, the dominant theme for both groups remaining one of loss, failure and disappointment.

The final nine women had all lost a core person they had known for some time; for some it appeared to be no more than a break in the contact, but the women had good grounds to feel rejected. Six, in fact, continue the same theme of failure and disappointment. One woman, for instance, had lived alone except for her son (born six years before) and had originally conveyed how she disliked her unmarried status, how she found it too much responsibility, and was lonely and wished to marry. During the following year she became close to a man for the first time in six years; the severe event was finding out that he was going out with another woman. Another had a similar experience, a further two cases involved having trouble and breaking contact with a sister to whom they felt close. Another involved a husband leaving home, and another the death of a child in circumstances that might convey some element of failure on the woman's part. The remaining three women experienced a death (mother, husband and friend, respectively), but there was no obvious reason for them to feel in any way responsible, or for that matter rejected. For one of these women (and possibly one other), there appeared to be an element of 'over-reaction'; she had an excellent marriage and a wide circle of friends. But overall, there does not seem to be much doubt about the message; the events presented, for the most part, an integral threat to core aspects of the sense of identity and self-worth of the women.

FURTHER REFINEMENTS OF SEVERE EVENTS

Some have sought to play down the significance of such results because only about one in five women experiencing severe events go on to develop depression at a caseness level: this is usually expressed in terms of the small amount of variance explained (r^2). Andrews & Tennant (1978) go so far as to suggest that because of this, life events are unlikely to have clinical or preventive importance. But they fail to point out that this situation is the same for almost all aetiological agents in medicine- for instance, the factor of heavy smoking explains a good deal less than 1% of the variance of lung cancer (Cooke 1987). This is not to deny that it is necessary to go further — in search of factors that potentiate risk — but most instances of depression still appear to be brought about by a severe event, just as in an analogous way, most instances of lung cancer are associated with heavy smoking. It is difficult not to see this as a fact of clinical and preventive significance.

Having established the role of severe events, the most important way forward has been to consider why, for one reason or another, people are more or less vulnerable to their effects. But there is another, more obvious possibility that also needs to be examined; just as some types of tobacco lead to a greater risk of lung cancer, so certain severe events may lead more often to depression.

In the Islington research, the strength of the aetiological link was increased when the classification of events was refined in a number of ways. The first is of particular interest, given the somewhat uncertain status of long-term difficulties. For each severe event occurring in the follow-up period, a judgement was made about whether there was a 'link' between it and any ongoing marked difficulty present at the time of the first interview. For example, the threat of eviction because of rent arrears experienced by one woman, matched the ongoing difficulty she had had concerning such payments. Ongoing difficulties were often the source of such matching 'D-events' (D standing for difficulty). However, although this kind of link with a marked difficulty was much the most common reason for defining a D-event, a *causal* relationship between the two was not essential. For example, an event could be so considered if it had been rated severe because of the presence of the difficulty. Thus, a pregnancy rated severely threatening because of poor housing would be considered linked to the difficulty and therefore a D-event. Such events were, however, usually related to the difficulty; in a straightforward way, e.g. a husband leaving home in the context of marital disputes over his heavy drinking and violence, or a difficulty with a child (say misbehaviour at school) culminating in an event with the same child (say referral to a Child Guidance Clinic). Almost a quarter of the women with a severe event had at least one such D-event, i.e. where it was linked with a preceding ongoing difficulty; and there was a three-fold greater risk of depression among them than among the rest of the women with a severe event (Table 3.2, Part A). Eales (1988), in a study of unemployed men, found an apparently similar effect; unemployment was far more likely to lead to depression among men who had had a history of financial or employment difficulties for some time.

A special analysis, involving the re-rating of all severe events on a more fully graded threat scale, suggested that something more than severity of threat of the D-events is needed to explain this greatly increased risk (see Brown 1989). The issue is unsettled,but there is some suggestion that following a D-event, women were more likely than those with other severe events to respond with profound feelings of hopelessness, which

Table 3.2   Onset among 130 Islington women with a severe event in Islington by whether it 'matched' certain first interview measures

---

A. Severe event matching prior difficulty of 6/12 or more (D-event)

		% onset
	Yes	46 (16/35)
	No	14 (13/95)
	p < 0.001	22 (29/130)

B. Severe event matching prior commitment (C-event)

		% onset
	Yes	40 (16/40)
	No	14 (13/90)
	p < 0.01	22 (29/130)

C. Either severe event matching prior difficulty or prior commitment (i.e. D-event or C-event)

		% onset
	Yes	37 (24/65)
	No	8 (5/65)
	p < 0.001	22 (29/130)

---

has been proposed as commonly forming a key link in the development of depressive disorders (vide supra). When questioned in detail, only about a fifth of the women reported that they responded with a more or less complete lack of hope to a severe event, but 38% said they did so in response to a D-event, compared with only 9% to all other severe events. This suggests that a woman is more likely to feel profound hopelessness following the arrest of her son if it has been part of a history of troubles than if it comes more or less out of the blue. Since the rating of hopelessness is based on material collected after any onset of depression, it is open to inaccuracy and bias, and the result must be seen as no more than suggestive. The result, however, is made more plausible by the fact that the association held for those *not* developing depression as well as for those who did (Brown et al 1987).

It is also possible to characterise severe events in terms of the fact that they matched prior role conflict. Such conflict, often arising from diverging obligations, such as that between domestic and external spheres, was fairly common. Events that matched the area of conflict were called 'R-events' — R standing for role conflict. Such conflict at the time of the first interview commonly covered conflicting demands of work and domestic responsibilities; for example, a woman's worry at first interview about work demands and care of her child would match the subsequent event of the child being found stealing. Since risk is also increased by R-events and there is a great deal of overlap with D-events, a combined 'D/R-event' category will be used in the final overview of the Islington material.

A third way of matching severe events proved to be quite independent of the first two. We discussed with the women, at some length, various domains of their lives — children, marriage, housework, employment, as well as other activities, and social contacts outside the home — and each woman's degree of commitment (behavioural as well as subjective) to each domain was rated. In making the rating, we kept in mind that it was possible to be highly dissatisfied with, say, a particular marital situation and yet be highly committed to the *idea* of marriage. All but 18% of the women had at least one marked commitment in one of the six areas considered, with an average for the sample as a whole of 1.52.

Severe events matching high commitment were termed 'C-events' (C standing for commitment), and women with a C-event were also much more likely to develop depression (Table 3.2, Part B). Measurement was straightforward — all severe events, for example, concerning a child would automatically match if a woman was high on commitment to motherhood. Their greater risk appears to reflect the fact that marked commitment increases the saliency of a loss or disappointment. The result, incidentally, confirms the emphasis that has been placed on relevant plans and concerns in rating the long-term threat of events.

However, despite the welcome increase in ability to predict depression that is provided by such a classification of events, it is still necessary to consider how far ongoing vulnerability helps in the understanding of who will develop depression, given the occurrence of a loss or disappointment.

VULNERABILITY

Various vulnerability factors were isolated in the original Camberwell enquiry, and it was speculated that low self-esteem might provide a common underlying explanation. One purpose of the longitudinal study was to make a direct test of this, and it now appears that low self-esteem does play such a role; it was judged on the basis of the extensiveness and severity of negative comments that a woman made about herself at the time she was first seen. (In other publications, the term 'negative evaluation of self' has been used.) Once a severe event had occurred, the chances of the onset of depression were doubled if low self-esteem had

Table 3.3 Low self-esteem at first interview and onset depression among 303 Islington women

| | Severe event | |
Low self-esteem	Yes % onset	No % onset
Yes	*34* (17/50)	*6* (2/31)
No	*15* (12/80)	*1* (1/142)
	p < .02	ns

been present. It met the definition of a vulnerability effect, since risk was low unless there was both a severe event and low self-esteem (see Table 3.3).

The result can probably be taken seriously, since self-esteem was measured before the follow-up period, and furthermore, the Edinburgh MRC Unit for Epidemiological Studies in Psychiatry reached somewhat similar conclusions (Ingham et al 1986, 1987, Miller et al 1989). However, it still remains to settle the exact role of low self-esteem, and this cannot be done without at the same time taking into account its correlation with the quality of social support. I will concentrate on support from core relationships, as research has so far failed to reveal any protective effect from less central ties. (Core ties are defined as those with husband, lover, or anyone described as 'very close', in response to direct questioning at the time of our first interview.)

SOCIAL SUPPORT

In recent research, the notion of support has been closely linked with the concept of vulnerability. In our Camberwell study, lack of confiding and intimacy with a husband or lover was the most important vulnerability factor, and this has now been documented on many occasions (Brown & Harris 1986b). However, the intimacy measure used in those studies contains an important ambiguity; it takes account of both confiding behaviour in general and also that behaviour during the aftermath of any critical event occurring before the onset of depression, thus confusing pre-event and post-event periods. This means that any difference between the two has to be amalgamated in the one rating, although where there is a discrepancy, most weight is typically given to behaviour at the time of the crisis.

More extended examples may be helpful. A woman's lack of confiding and intimacy with a husband or lover has been the most commonly studied vulnerability factor, but there are various possible permutations of support. The most obvious involves long-term lack of support from a core tie, especially a husband. One way this may act is to decrease self-esteem and, through this, to increase the risk of depression once a crisis occurs. However, more fortunate women are not necessarily protected. To be part of any close relationship is to place oneself in jeopardy; any satisfactory relationship opens up the possibility of betrayal and rejection. A second possibility, therefore, is that a woman with apparently effective support, initially, may receive none once a crisis has occurred, and that being so 'let down' serves to increase her risk of depression, despite (or perhaps because of) earlier support. A third possibility is that a woman who has been without support from her husband for some time receives, once the event has occurred, effective help from someone else — say a close female friend — and in this way is rendered less at risk. The first possibility concerns the pre-event situation and the last two the post-event situation. The second, concerning being 'let down', will, if anything, act to suppress the effect of positive features of the social environment prior to the event, and the third, concerning alternative support will, if anything, act to suppress the effect of negative features prior to the event.

Since the Islington survey was based on a longitudinal design, it was easier to contrast measures of support in the pre-event and post-event periods and, as discussed earlier, to deal with only the first in terms of vulnerability. The description of support once an event had occurred was therefore kept quite distinct; this was discussed in terms of 'crisis support' i.e. confiding about the event, receiving at least 'moderate' active emotional support from the same person, and not receiving a negative reaction on the person's part at some point in the crisis (Brown et al 1986a). It turned out that if pre-event and post-event situations differed, it was the latter that predicted the onset of depression. Therefore, in what follows, it is necessary to take account of both the pre-event measures of support and what transpired once the event had occurred. While the full results are complex, Table 3.4, dealing with married women with a severe event, illustrates the basic findings. Cell 'd' shows those who received no support from their husband on either occasion; as expected, they have a high rate of depression. Cell 'b' shows women who did confide in their husband at the earlier point, but who failed to obtain crisis support from him; they were, in other words, 'let down', and had a particularly high rate of depression. It is only those in cell 'a', who received support on both occasions, that were at a low risk. (There were few in cell 'c' in Table 3.4 receiving support with the event from their husband, which was unexpected in terms of the earlier situation, when there was no confiding; the risk of depression for these women was still high.)

One further point about the table is of interest. The marginal totals on the right-hand side show that lack of confiding in a husband, as recorded at first interview, although predicting depression, fell well short of statistical significance. However, it would be highly misleading to see this

Table 3.4 Confiding in husband at first interview, crisis support during the follow-up year and onset of depression among those with a severe event(98 married Islington women)

Confiding in husband at first interview	Crisis support from husband during follow-up		
	Yes % onset	No % onset	Total % onset
Yes	4 (1/23) 'a'	40 (6/15) 'b'	18 (7/38)
No	29 (2/7) 'c'	26 (10/38) 'd'	27 (12/45)

(Crisis support not known for 3).

in terms of the absence of a link between early support and subsequent risk of depression. In practice, a basic association has been suppressed by the high rate of depression among those who were 'let down'. Once these women are omitted, as just seen, cell 'a' of Table 3.4 shows the expected result. A further important point is not shown about cell 'd', i.e. women who received no support on either occasion from their husband. Among these, there was a complete absence of depression for 17 who received crisis support from someone named earlier as very close, usually a woman. But this only occurred for those in cell 'd', i.e. as long as a woman had not been let down by her husband. The three distinct effects discussed earlier have therefore been isolated, but only those in cells 'c' and 'd', involving absence of confiding at first contact, can be said to represent a vulnerability effect.

The full data show that married women were particularly prone to be let down, either by a husband or someone whom they had named as 'very close'. By contrast, single mothers who had been confiding in someone 'very close' practically always received support in the crisis from at least one such person. Their high risk of depression was related less to being let down than to lacking support in the first place (Brown et al 1986a).

PRIOR PSYCHIATRIC SYMPTOMATOLOGY

Critics of a psychosocial view of depression have cited as contrary evidence the predictive importance of prior depressive symptoms (see Akiskal 1985), and it is necessary, therefore, to consider whether ongoing psychiatric symptomatology plays a role in the processes so far outlined. In Islington, chronic sub-clinical symptomatology was an important predictor of caseness of depression (Brown et al 1986b). For inclusion, symptoms had to be present at the time of the first contact with the woman and to have lasted for at least one year; the conditions were almost always borderline cases of anxiety or depression, although a few non-depressive conditions at a caseness level were included. In interpreting this result, it needs to be borne in mind that such chronic symptoms, as much as low self-esteem, may reflect the quality of a woman's core relationships. Indeed, it is just such a link that appears to explain the result; such symptoms showed no tendency to predict subsequent depression *unless they were accompanied by a marked social difficulty*. Furthermore, this link was entirely the result of the occurrence of later D-events (i.e. severe events linked to ongoing difficulties), such as a husband leaving home, in the context of a long-term marital difficulty. The original report should be consulted for a full discussion of alternative interpretations, but its final conclusion was that there was nothing to suggest that sub-clinical symptoms raise risk, except in the presence of ongoing difficulties, which presumably had often played a role in their perpetuation (and perhaps onset) in the first place.

I know of no published evidence which suggests that the inclusion of subjects with chronic sub-clinical conditions before the onset of a frank depressive disorder is a threat to the psychosocial perspective so far outlined. Indeed, given the documented role of ongoing difficulties in the aetiological process, results are just what would be expected. At the same time, there is an obvious need to replicate this result, and current evidence is certainly insufficient to rule out the possibility of an independent biological effect.

RECOVERY FROM DEPRESSION

One of the most significant public health problems presented by depression is that, at any one time, half of those suffering from it at a caseness level are chronic, i.e. the episode has lasted for at least one year and usually a good deal longer. It is therefore important to establish whether or not psychosocial factors play a role in its perpetuation or recovery.

Material collected over a three-year period in Islington has confirmed findings from the Camberwell research that ongoing difficulties do play a role in perpetuating depression at a caseness level. However, equally important is a new finding that recovery from chronic depression (including any major improvement) is related either to a reduction in ongoing difficulties or to the occurrence of a 'fresh start event' (see Table 3.5). The latter is a new concept, involving the idea of starting again. While this often goes with a reduction in difficulties, the two indicators of positive change by no means always go together, and furthermore, fresh start events appear to make a distinct contribution. Perhaps surprisingly, the events often involve a significant degree of threat (a quarter were rated severe events). The important quality appears to be that they convey some hope that things could be better, such as reconciliation with a son and daughter-in-law after the birth of a second grandchild, starting divorce proceedings by taking out an injunction against a husband, the husband getting a job that relieves considerable financial difficulties and tension at home, or an extremely violent husband being sent to prison for several years because of his attack on the woman and her mother (Brown et al 1988).

Table 3.5 Recovery or improvement among 48 Islington women with chronic depression in terms of a fresh-start event or difficulty-reduction

| | Fresh-Start event or difficulty-reduction | |
| | Yes | No |
Initial difficulty score	% recovered or improved	
0–2 (low)	100 (6/6)	63 (5/8)
3–6	71 (5/7) ⎫ 60	50 (2/4) ⎫ 21
7+ (high)	54 (7/13) ⎭	10 (1/10) ⎭
Totals	62 (18/26)	36 (8/22)

The majority of women in Islington recovering from chronic depression had either experienced difficulty-reduction or a fresh-start event, and in this sense, the general importance of a cognitive-affective approach to depression is underlined, i.e. the changes either involved relief from ongoing adversity or state of deprivation, or the hope of this. Among women who recovered without either of these experiences were a number whose depression had been brought about by the death of a husband or child, and there may well be a small group of chronic depressions following a bereavement that only dissipate with time.

There was also a hint that under certain circumstances, the level of social support played a role. There have been other suggestive studies (Surtees & Ingham 1980, Tennant et al 1981a,b, Parker et al 1985, Miller et al 1987), and it is possible to make a provisional case that the process of recovery is often the mirror-image of the psychosocial processes leading to onset.

EARLY LOSS OF MOTHER AND PAST ADVERSITY

So far, I have dealt chiefly with the year before the development of a depressive disorder, but the aetiological model of the original Camberwell enquiry included, as a vulnerability factor, loss of mother before the age of 11, due either to death or a separation of at least one year. Such loss was associated with a much raised incidence of depression once a provoking agent had occurred, and along with this went a greater overall prevalence of depression at a caseness level (Brown et al 1977).

There has been a good deal of controversy about this finding (Brown & Harris 1986a, Harris & Brown 1985, Crook & Eliot 1980, Tennant et al 1980, Harris et al 1986), but its significance is underlined by its replication in two further population studies. An enquiry in Walthamstow screened 3000 women to provide all instances of early loss of parents; those with an early loss of mother before the age of 11 had a much higher rate of current depression, and this also held for losses between the ages of 11 and 17. Differences for loss of father did not reach statistical significance, although there was some suggestion that his loss by separation may have been associated with an increased risk (Brown et al 1986c, Harris et al 1986, 1987). In the Islington survey, a high rate of depression again occurred among those losing a mother between 11 and 17, suggesting that the original Camberwell cut-off at age 11 may have been rather too hastily adopted (Bifulco et al 1987).

The aetiological processes involved are undoubtedly complex, and recent research suggests that more important than the early loss of the mother itself was the quality of replacement parental care (Harris et al 1986, 1987, Bifulco et al 1987). If this was inadequate (in terms of an index of parental indifference and lax control, termed 'lack of care'), the risk of current depression was doubled. In order to learn more about this link, it is necessary to go on to trace a person's history through a series of

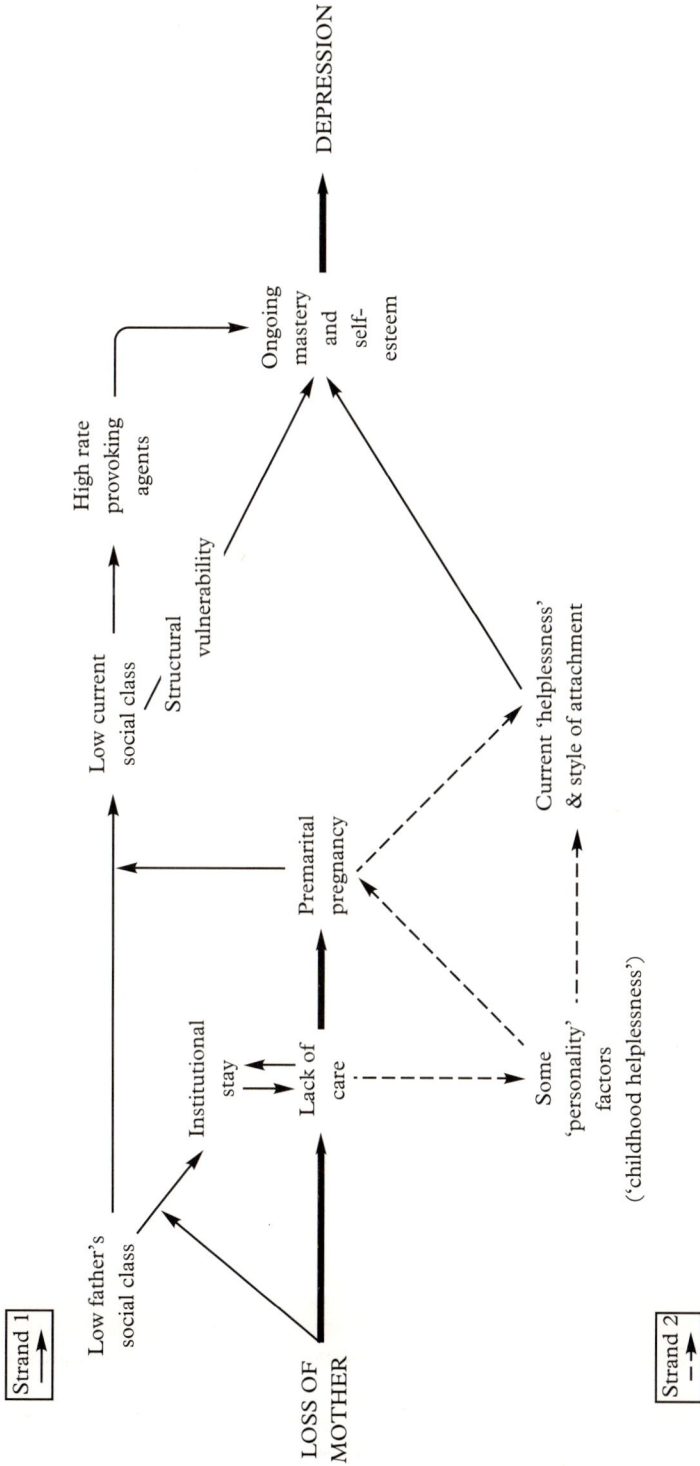

Fig 3.1 Causal model showing main lines of impact of loss of mother.

possible experiences from the early loss itself to later depression, i.e. to gain some sense of a person's life trajectory after the loss and its immediate aftermath. But such an exercise should not be approached in a spirit of determinism; it is now quite clear that intervening experiences can serve to reduce as well as increase the risk of depression in adult life (Quinton & Rutter 1984a,b, Rutter et al 1983, Rutter 1988). In attempting to chart this chain of circumstances, it became clear that certain subsequent experiences in adolescence and early adulthood were particularly associated with the development of vulnerability and with the experience of provoking agents (Harris et al 1986, 1987).

Premarital pregnancy played a particularly critical mediating role and, like lack of care itself, was associated with later risk factors (Brown 1988). What seemed to be crucial about such pregnancies was that they trapped women in relationships which they might well not otherwise have chosen and which then became a source of severely threatening events and major difficulties, e.g. housing and financial problems consequent upon a couple starting a family too young to have built up adequate savings, or marital difficulties with undependable partners. The women also emerged as less upwardly mobile, in terms of social class, than their peers without such pregnancies. In interpreting this complex of experiences, a conveyor belt of adversities was outlined on which some women were moved from one crisis to another, starting with lack of care in childhood and passing via premarital pregnancy to current working-class status, lack of social support, and high rates of provoking agents (see Strand 1 in Fig. 3.1). However, to attribute this chain of circumstances solely to environmental factors might prove short-sighted. Although it was often hard to see from the women's accounts of their lives how they could have left this conveyor belt once their childhood had located them on it, a more personal element could almost certainly have played a role (Strand 2 in Fig. 3.1). There can be little doubt that at any point in time personality attributes such as helplessness and low self-esteem, that are part of the second strand, can influence how the external environment represented in the first strand is interpreted and dealt with, and the consequences of this can in turn powerfully influence future Strand 1 experiences. It should also be kept in mind that the experience of premarital pregnancy among women in the 1980s may be different from the cases studied in the Walthamstow enquiry. This experience is certainly more common, and the measure may in future need to be refined if it is to serve as a useful predictor of the same chain of adverse experiences.

The notion of life structure is a complex one, and other results could still be added. For example, full-time employment among Islington women was associated with a particularly high risk of depression. In such instances, full-time work was usually linked with either evidence of strain or role conflict, and the risk itself appeared to be a direct result of the way subsequent crises, particularly concerning core ties, resonated with the meaning of the work for the women. However, those in part-time work had a lower risk than non-workers, and this appeared to relate to a configuration of factors involving greater shortcomings in non-workers' marriages and the fact that they were looking after younger children. Nonetheless, some direct protective effect of part-time work may have been present, since such workers felt more secure about their marriages even when objective sources of insecurity were controlled (Brown & Bifulco 1989). However, this kind of further result can be seen as an elaboration of the points already developed, and it is therefore now possible to attempt some kind of overall view.

AN OVERALL VIEW — INTRODUCING THE CONJOINT INDEX

This summary of findings provides pieces from which a more synoptic view of depression can be built. Since suitable pre-onset biological measures are as yet scarce (REM latency is perhaps the only serious candidate) and the necessary collaborative research has not yet been carried out, this overview has to be restricted to the role of psychosocial factors.* The task of synthesis is nonetheless a difficult one, given that a number of the factors so far outlined are highly inter-related. I have therefore kept the final overview as simple as possible and have aimed to present a picture that is full enough to be informative, despite a certain crudeness in detail.

It may be useful to start by summarising what has emerged so far concerning (i) time order, and (ii) the factors of the aetiological model itself, contrasted with the more speculative mechanisms or processes used to interpret them:

	Pre-event	Event	Post-event	Outcome
Factors	Lack of confiding in husband, Low self-esteem, etc.	D/R-event, etc.	Husband's lack of crisis support, 'Let down' by husband. Other crisis support, etc.	Onset of depression.
Processes or Mechanisms.	Vulnerability, Event-production.	Experience of loss/ disappoint-ment.	? Drop in self-esteem.	? General hopelessness.

*See Cartwright (1983) for an innovative attempt to relate biological (REM latency) and social measures (divorce).

It will be recalled that one factor (e.g. low self-esteem) may be involved in more than one process (e.g. vulnerability and event-production), and that there may be important changes in the factors over time (e.g. pre-event confiding in a husband being replaced in the post-event period by the experience of being 'let down').

A large proportion of episodes of depression in the general population follow fairly closely in time on an important loss or disappointment. If an episode does not follow fairly soon, most people appear safe, at least from developing depression at a caseness level, until the occurrence of another critical loss or disappointment. For example, Eales (1988) concluded in his study of unemployed men that depression usually occurs soon after the loss of job, and failing this, it will not occur without a new crisis, which may or may not arise from the unemployment as such. However, even if depression does not follow a loss or disappointment, a person may be subject to increased risk in terms of event-production. For example, the original event (e.g. the husband's stroke) may result in a serious ongoing difficulty (e.g. subject needs to give up her job to be with him), and this increases the risk of depression via a subsequent severe D-event matching the difficulty (e.g. a more debilitating stroke some months later). A second avenue, also via event-production, is that severe events will increase in number as a result of the person trying to cope with feelings of distress by risk-taking behaviour.

The example also suggests how key aetiological factors will generally have their roots in the prior 'life structure' — a term used by Levinson (1978) to deal with the way the internal and external worlds meet in an individual. It is a useful term because it emphasises that there will usually be some structure and regularity in a person's life; Levinson includes not only behaviour, but also unexpressed longings, moods, regrets, and attitudes about life, as well as anything in the external world relevant to them (Sloan 1987). In the Islington enquiry, a good deal of energy was expended in recording this structure (O'Connor & Brown 1984). The resulting instrument — the Self Evaluation and Social Support Schedule (SESS) — deals with external manifestations of current life structure in areas such as marriage and motherhood, and with how activities are internally represented in terms of feelings of self-worth, security, mean-ing, satisfaction and dissatisfaction, sense of control, etc.

However, this distinction between what I will henceforth refer to as 'environmental' and 'psychological' is a matter of degree. Our material about any one person was collected from that subject only and, although we went to considerable effort to obtain examples of behaviour in order to rate environmental measures such as amount of confiding with husband and quality of his emotional support, the accounts are clearly liable to reflect the woman's feelings to some degree. Moreover, although we certainly do not claim that the environmental is uninfluenced by the psychological and vice versa, the two sets of measures were not equivalent; they aimed to measure a distinct phenomenon and there is evidence that they managed this reasonably well. For instance, while an assessment of confiding in your husband (based on detailed questions about what actually occurred) related to the subsequent risk of depression, a straightforward rating of a woman's belief in the amount of confiding differed a good deal and was quite unrelated to the risk of depression. Even more significant, the exercise was certainly justified in the empirical sense that (as will be reported) as far as predicting depression is concerned, knowledge of both aspects proved to be far more informative than knowledge of just one, and this is the basic rationale for a Conjoint Index incorporating both.

In order to see how low self-esteem relates to outward imperfections in relationships or roles, the 70 measures of SESS dealing with environmental aspects of a woman's life, such as the frequency of quarrels in the home, quantity and quality of interaction at work, undependability of husband, and security of job, housing, and social network were considered; measures were then selected (by multiple regression) that were most highly associated with low self-esteem. For married women, the final items in the resulting index (Negative Elements in Close Relationships) were negative interaction with children, negative interaction with husband, lack of primary quality in the relationship with the husband, and the security-diminishing characteristics of her housewife role (a measure largely reflecting shortcomings in the practical and financial help provided by her husband). For single mothers, the selected items were negative interaction with children, strife within the home, and lack of a 'true', very close relationship (someone named as 'very close' with whom there was confiding and frequent contact). In addition, women were included in both versions of the index if at the first interview they had an ongoing marked difficulty that had lasted for at least six months and that involved someone in the home (or occasionally a lover, or husband in contact but living away).

Once this index had been taken into account, only low self-esteem and the presence of chronic sub-clinical symptoms added to the prediction of depression in the following year. Given a severe event, it was the combination of the environmental measure and one or other of the two psychological states that predicted onset (Table 3.6). Once this was taken into account, none of the component measures related to onset of depression, but given their joint occurrence and a severe event, the risk was considerable — 48% (24/50) compared with 6% (5/80).

The Negative Elements of Close Relationships Index is an empirically rather than theoretically based measure; it was developed by finding what correlated with low self-esteem, which means that it is still necessary to settle just what it entails. In addition to describing obviously distressing behaviour, it can at times reflect dissatisfaction and irritability on a woman's part, attempts to downplay a situation of potential difficulty, as well as a fairly sensitive device for picking up the early signs of serious trouble in core relationships. Its present importance probably lies in the

Table 3.6   Negative elements in close relationships and discomfiture at first interview and later onset depression among 130 Islington women with a severe event

Negative elements in close relationships	Low self-esteem *and* chronic subclinical symptoms % onset	Low self-esteem % onset	Chronic Subclinical Symptoms % onset	Nil % onset
Yes	(7/18) 39	(10/23) 43	(7/9) 78	(3/27) 11
		48 (24/50)		
No	(0/2) 0	(0/7) 0	(1/6) 13	(1/38) 3
		7 (1/15)		

fact that it confirms the fact that some intimation of what was to occur later was present at the time of first interview. This is reflected in the first component of the model — the process of event-production already discussed in general terms.

The negative elements in the Close Relationships Index also reflected, at times, quite subtle shortcomings in the quality of relationships, and it was just such features that predicted some major problems in the follow-up year. For example, one woman was included in the index because of a 'moderate' rating on 'negativity of interaction' with husband, despite a high rating on the parallel positive scale, many other favourable ratings, and no other negative rating as part of the index itself. The one 'moderate' rating was based on the woman's comments that there could 'be tension when we go out together and he's in one of his moods', that 'He sometimes gets on my nerves when we are home together and I want to get on with work' (he was unemployed), and that 'He's very quick-tempered'. During the follow-up year, he became highly disturbed as part of a paranoid disorder, and it turned out that she had underplayed the difficulty his selfish and unreasonable behaviour had brought to the marriage in a crisis more than a year before first interview. The term 'discomfiture' will be used to describe the presence of one or the other of the two psychological states of low self-esteem or chronic sub-clinical symptoms; it conveys something of their reactive quality to the environment, and reflects the fact that the negative feelings and chronic symptoms might be far from overwhelming, at times coexisting with a good deal that was positive. In order to simplify this presentation, a woman will be said to be positive on the *Conjoint Index* if there is a presence of discomfiture and negative elements in close relationships, i.e. a woman has to be positive on the environmental index of negative elements in close relationships and positive on one or other of the psychological measures of low self-esteem or chronic sub-clinical symptoms. The term conjoint is used to reflect the fact that environmental and psychological had both to be present.

Women positive on the Conjoint Index were far more likely to have a later matching D/R-event (i.e. a severe event arising out of an ongoing difficulty or role conflict), but no more likely to experience any other kind of event. Thirty-nine per cent (31/80) of those positive on the Conjoint Index experienced a D/R-event compared with 5% (12/223) of other women. The first component of the model is therefore:

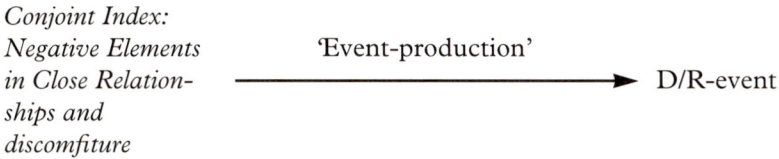

Conjoint Index:
Negative Elements   'Event-production'
in Close Relation- ————————————————————▶ D/R-event
ships and
discomfiture

This association of the Conjoint Index is hardly surprising, given that the D/R-events must be linked with a prior difficulty or source of conflict, but more surprising perhaps is its complete failure to predict any other kind of event. Because of this clear-cut result, the 43 women with a D/R-event will be dealt with separately below. The occurrence of a D/R-event, as such, did not contribute very much to a raised risk of depression; it was when the woman was also positive on the Conjoint Index that there was a greatly increased risk. This, of course, is just what would be expected if the Conjoint Index acted as a vulnerability factor.* The index acts to increase risk by 'producing' D/R-events and then by acting as a vulnerability factor, once such an event has occurred:–

Onset among women with D/R-events (N = 43)

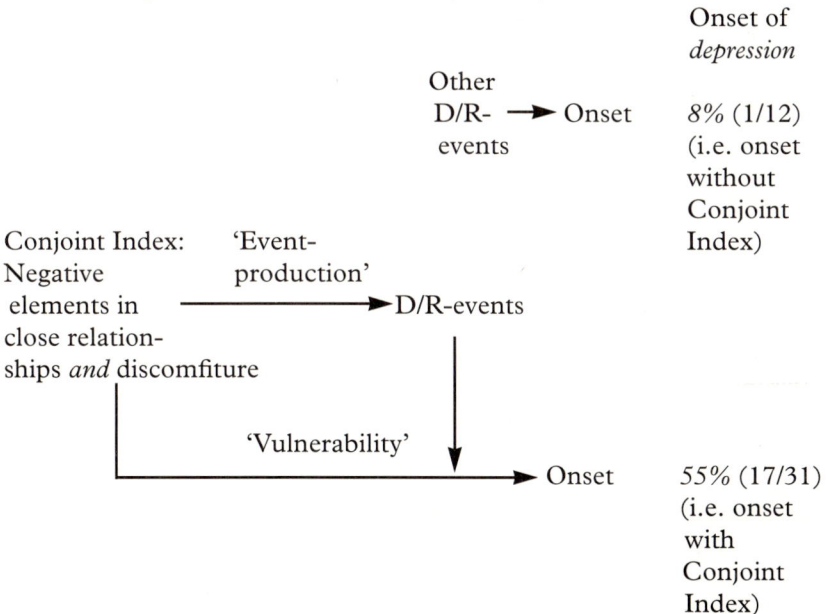

Onset of
depression

Other
D/R- ——▶ Onset   8% (1/12)
events   (i.e. onset
without
Conjoint

Conjoint Index: 'Event-   Index)
Negative   production'
elements in   ————————▶ D/R-events
close relation-
ships *and* discomfiture

'Vulnerability'

▶ Onset   55% (17/31)
(i.e. onset
with
Conjoint
Index)

---

*It is possible to conclude that the Conjoint Index acts as a vulnerability factor, since without a severe event, it is rarely associated with onset (see Appendix 1).

Therefore, in this first model, it is necessary to keep in mind both the event-production and vulnerability functions of the Conjoint Index, and the fact that it was the coming together of the two that was highly related to the onset of depression.

A second model, without event-production, is sufficient to deal with the rest of the women experiencing a severe event, but here again most of the onsets were a consequence of the Conjoint Index acting as a vulnerability factor; it was again the occurrence of a severe event (but not a D/R-event) and the Conjoint Index in the same woman that led to a greatly increased risk of depression:–

Onset among women with severe events other than
D/R-events (N = 87)   Onset of
                                                                        depression

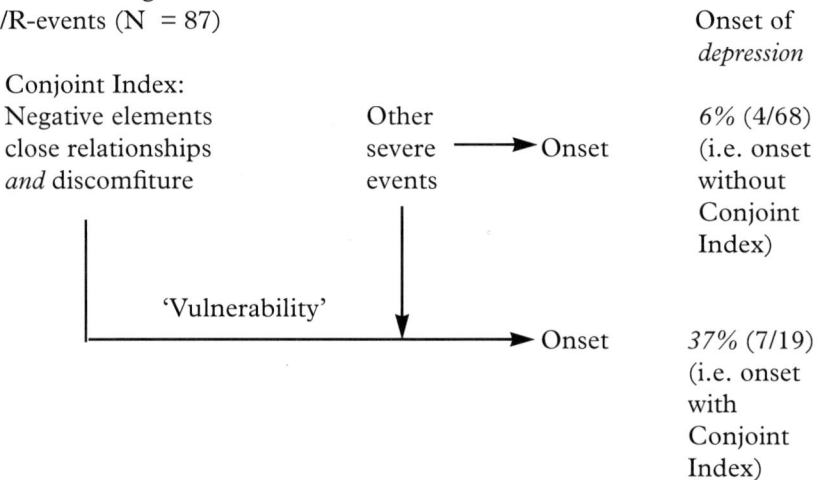

Conjoint Index:
Negative elements   Other   6% (4/68)
close relationships   severe ──────► Onset   (i.e. onset
and discomfiture   events   without
                                                            Conjoint
                           │   Index)
      ┌────────────────────┤
      │ 'Vulnerability'   │
      │   ▼
      └──────────────────────────► Onset   *37% (7/19)*
                                                            (i.e. onset
                                                            with
                                                            Conjoint
                                                            Index)

The effect of current life structure and its correlates, as reflected by the Conjoint Index, is so overriding in these two models that it is associated with most cases of depression in the Islington sample. However, there are still two issues that need to be incorporated in any overview — adequacy of support in a crisis, and early experience as exemplified by lack of care.

THE CONJOINT INDEX AND SUPPORT

Following the earlier discussion, inadequacy of support will be defined here as either lack of crisis support *or* being 'let down', and in this way restricted to events in the follow-up year. Not unexpectedly, it is highly correlated with all three pre-event factors of the Conjoint Index — negative elements in close relationships, low self-esteem, and chronic sub-clinical symptoms. In this sense, its central role in the development of depression is to complement the tightness of the links already discussed — an overlap which is consistent with the emerging picture of depression as grounded in shortcomings within close relationships.

Inadequacy of support is best seen as a mediating factor, linking the components of the Conjoint Index with onset of depression. It follows that the situation at the time of first interview often presaged subsequent inadequate support and the occurrence of D/R-events (e.g. learning of a husband's affair when he had been unpredictable and unsupportive for some time), although the signs of this could, at times, be quite subtle.

Therefore we have:

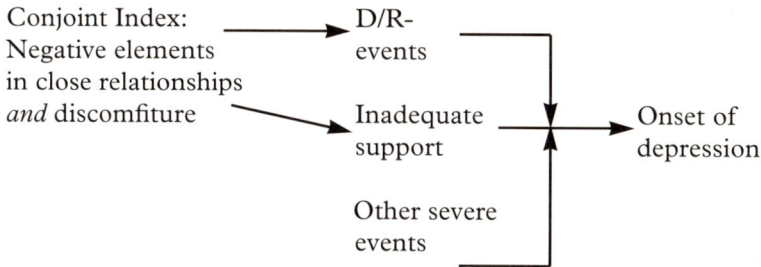

Conjoint Index: ⟶ D/R-events

Negative elements in close relationships *and* discomfiture ⟶ Inadequate support ⟶ Onset of depression

Other severe events

Since the association between inadequate support and the Conjoint Index is high, actual changes in the patterning of results brought about by the inclusion of inadequate support in the model are relatively modest (details are given in Appendix 2). The correlation between the Conjoint Index and depression changes very little in numerical terms when such inadequacy of support is taken into account. But in the light of this and the earlier result (see Table 3.4), inadequacy of support appears to be a particularly critical intervening link between the Conjoint Index and the onset of depression. Crisis support is post-event and cannot be seen as a vulnerability factor; yet despite the fact that women could be 'let down', there was a great deal of continuity between pre-event and post-event situations; indeed, the Conjoint Index, in practice, even predicted reasonably well those who were to be 'let down'. In terms of actual results, there is yet another strong interactive or synergistic effect. It is the occurrence of *both* the Conjoint Index and later inadequate support that is linked to a high risk of depression (Table 3.7); of those who experienced a severe event, as many as 59% (22/37) of those with both

Table 3.7 Conjoint Index (negative elements in close relationships and discomfiture) at first interview, inadequacy of support among 130 Islington women with a severe event and onset depression

Conjoint Index: negative elements in close relationships *and* discomfiture	Inadequate support in crisis		
	Yes % onset	No % onset	
Yes	59 (22/37)	17 (2/12)	(1 nk)
No	18 (4/22)	2 (1/55)	(3 nk)

the Conjoint Index and later inadequate support developed depression, compared with 18% (4/22) of those with only poor support, and 4% (3/67) of the remaining women.

Life structure at one point in time therefore appears to be implicated in the development of a good deal of depression, at least in the context of life in an inner city. Furthermore, those at a high risk formed a surprisingly small proportion of the population. In Islington, most of the onsets (26/32) occurred among the quarter (80/303) of the women who were positive on the Conjoint Index. However, this picture needs to be seen in dynamic terms. During the follow-up year some women were added to this high-risk group because of life events and lack of support, while others were removed by improvements in life structure, often via fresh-start events or reduction of a difficulty.

THE CONJOINT INDEX AND LOW SELF-ESTEEM

The tight interrelationship of the factors makes it difficult to interpret the exact role that low self-esteem plays in the model. However, it is easier to consider the possibilities if we break from the conservative assumptions about time order made so far. It is likely that the environmental component of the Conjoint Index plays a critical role in determining the psychological component (in the form of discomfiture), rather than vice versa. Let us therefore assume that 'negative elements in close relationships' is by and large an antecedant factor that is highly predictive of most of the remaining factors in the model. The components of the model as a whole are so highly related that it is still possible to exclude it, in the sense of treating it as an antecedent factor, and yet for the following factors in the model to show an equally powerful link with onset. A woman's discomfiture in the presence of either a D/R-event or inadequate support is critical — 51% (24/47) of such women developed depression, compared with only 6% (5/79) among those remaining, with a severe event.

Table 3.8   Low self-esteem and chronic subclinical conditions, and onset among the 130 women with a severe event in terms of two immediate risk factors

		D/R-event and/or inadequate support in crisis				
Low self-esteem	Chronic sub-clinical condition	Both	D/R-event Alone	Inadequate Support	Neither	Total
			% onset			% onset
Yes	Yes	60 (6/10)	0 (0/2)	33 (1/3)	0(0/5)	35 (7/20)
Yes	No	50 (4/8)	0 (0/3)	50 (6/12)	0 (0/6)	34 (10/29)
No	Yes	83 (5/6)	67 (2/3)	-	17 (1/6)	53 (8/15)
No	No	33 (1/3)	0 (0/6)	18 (3/17)	0 (0/36)	6 (4/62)
			(4 nk support)			

Low self-esteem has much the same order of effect as chronic sub-clinical symptoms (see right-hand column, Table 3.8). However, Table 3.8 makes it clear that low self-esteem is unrelated to onset without the presence of one of the immediate risk factors, i.e. a D/R-event or inadequate support. But here it needs to be added that neither of these two immediate risk factors is related to a high risk without discomfiture, in the form of either low self-esteem or chronic sub-clinical symptoms. It follows that low self-esteem is unlikely to be merely epiphenomenal, since on the whole, a negative psychological state appears to be necessary for depression to occur.

A particularly important possibility is that *adequate* support may be sufficient to neutralise the harmful effect of low self-esteem. Unfortunately, because of the inter-relationship of the factors in the model with low self-esteem, of those subjects experiencing a severe event, only 16 had both adequate support and low self-esteem (5 of them also had a D/R-event). Nonetheless, the fact that none of these 16 developed depression suggests that effective support in a crisis may be enough to suppress any link between low self-esteem and depression, even in the presence of a severe event. (Logistic regression shows the difference to be statistically significant.) Despite the intricacies of the data, it is difficult to think of a more plausible explanation.

Moreover, this argument deals only with the effect of low self-esteem once a severe event has occurred, but there are other possible effects. Self-esteem might play a role in event-production, and furthermore, it might be further reduced after the occurrence of a severe event, although this cannot be tested with the present design. Nor would it be surprising if such a fall was of particular importance following being 'let down'. Self-esteem certainly appears to fall about the time of onset of a depressive disorder (e.g. Lewinsohn et al 1981). Therefore, although I have emphasised the possibility of low self-esteem leading to feelings of general hopelessness, once a severe event has occurred, it may prove to play a role at a number of points in the aetiological process. (A more detailed discussion can be found in Brown et al 1990a, b & c.)

THE CONJOINT INDEX AND EARLY EXPERIENCE

An *Index of Early Inadequate Parenting*, based on the experience of lack of care from a key carer or the presence of marked antipathy from such a carer, has been used as a means of incorporating early experience into this overall picture. (The results were similar if only the lack of care measure was used.) Such early inadequate parenting is reasonably highly related to the Conjoint Index. However, in terms of the link between past experience and severe events, it was the current situation that was critical; for example, the past was entirely unassociated with the occurrence of a D/R-event (so heavily implicated in onset) unless there was also the relevant event-producing life structure. Such results suggest that the current environment provides the essential intervening link between inadequate parenting and depression.

In terms of the second key aetiological factor — inadequate support — there was a small and statistically non-significant link with early inadequate parenting that was independent of the Conjoint Index,* as well as some hint that a personality characteristic stemming from early experience might be involved. Women with inadequate parenting were more likely than others to turn to unsuitable or inappropriate people for support, once a crisis had occurred (Andrews & Brown 1988); those who did so also tended to romanticise close relationships and to deny any incipient problems. It often seemed that the women wanted to believe, in spite of clear contrary evidence, that those they had named as closest to them were reliable, helpful, and supportive. While this exploratory analysis suggests that some personality factor may play a role, this does not mean that it is necessarily outside the confines of the model that has been outlined. Indeed, it is not unlikely that its importance for depression stems only from the fact that it leads in some way to inadequate support.

BORDERLINE CASE CONDITION

Mild depressive disorders — borderline case conditions in the Bedford College terms — are also common in the general population, and are frequently seen by GPs and in medical outpatient clinics. They play a role in the development of physical disorders (e.g. Murphy & Brown 1980, Creed 1989, Craig 1989), and when present in mothers, also appear to raise the risk of serious accidents to their children (Brown & Davidson 1978). They overlap to a certain degree with depressive conditions defined by other diagnostic schemes such as the SADS/RDC and PSE/CATEGO, but probably form less than half of those classified as 'cases' by such schemes (see Dean et al 1983). Finally, they can be included in the models that have been outlined. They are also often provoked; in Islington, two-thirds (17/27) of the depressive conditions were preceded by a severe event (21/27). However, several studies have now suggested that vulnerability effects are on the whole absent. For example, of those with a severe event, 10% (5/50) who were positive on the Conjoint Index developed a borderline case condition, compared

---

*Findings for those with a severe event were:

Early inadequate parenting	Conjoint Index		Total
	Yes	No	
	% inadequate support		
Yes	83 (19/23)	44 (7/16)	67 (26/39)
No	69 (18/26)	25 (15/61)	38 (33/87)

(Of those with early inadequate parenting, 49% (35/72) were positive on the Conjoint Index compared with 19% (45/231) of the remaining women.)

with 15% (12/80) of those not positive, a difference well below significance. The most likely explanation is that women who are well-supported are not protected from depression altogether, but in response to a major loss or disappointment, are more likely to develop a borderline case than a disorder of caseness severity.

SOME FINAL COMMENTS

Systematic research on the role of psychosocial factors in the aetiology and course of depressive disorder has been largely confined to the last 20 years. The research has not been uncontroversial and because of this, I have presented certain results in some depth, rather than a summary of work in the field as a whole — a review that would inevitably make it more difficult for the reader to assess the evidence supporting this perspective. In so far as a psychosocial view is relevant, the present review has conveyed that depression is about loss, disappointment and rejection from which there is no obvious way forward. But there will need to be commitment, and usually a sense of self, staked in what has been lost; it is probably also necessary for there to be a sense that the stake was legitimate and possession deserved. Kluckholm & Strodtbeck (1961) distinguish between the 'desirable' (in terms of cultural norms) and the 'desired' (in terms of personal preference): depression may well be most likely to occur where the two converge. A woman may develop depression when the lover with whom she has been living returns to his home abroad, despite the fact she knew all along that he would have to return, due to his national status. In a strict sense, her sense of possession here is illegitimate. But her depression would not spring from the loss of the person (that would be a matter of grief and pining) so much as from her sense that at her age she should have a reliable man to care for her children, and her chances have been that much more reduced by the time they have spent together and by the need to mourn his loss. Moreover, loss of what is felt to be deserved is likely to be experienced in terms of a lowering of self-worth; the greater the sense of being in the right, the greater this worthlessness. It is therefore particularly the loss of a legitimately desired resource, the realistic assessment of shockingly poor chances of renewal or replacement, and a sense of general hopelessness about moving forward that seem most relevant (see Freden 1982 and his discussion of Becker 1964, 1971 for a similar emphasis). Current cognitive theories of depression emphasis the unrealistic pessimism of the depressed patient about the future. This would clearly make such hopelessness even more likely; sadly, among working-class women, in inner-city areas at least, assessments are often all too realistic.

These factors are not necessarily sufficient to bring about a depressive disorder. Various other influences have been discussed, most notably those stemming from childhood and from emotional support around the time of the onset of depression itself. Moreover, the tendency has been emphasised for the various influences to be interrelated, as has the need, if depression is to occur, for a number of them to be present. Because of this, it would be highly misleading to give undue weight to any one factor (or even two) in the final model. For example, we have seen that there is very high risk of depression (approaching 50%) when a number of risk factors occur together. But despite the fact that a matching D/R-event and inadequate support in a crisis are of central importance, they were insufficient, even when occurring together, to produce such a high risk without the presence of one of the background psychological factors of low self-esteem and chronic sub-clinical symptoms. Some of the reasons for this may be related to issues of measurement, but on the whole, it probably reflects a real effect. By and large, the necessary psychosocial conditions for the development of clinical depression appear to have some kind of history. They do not emerge out of the blue, and some trace of harbingering conditions can usually be documented in both the environment and psychological state of the person. Perhaps the essential insight is that the general hopelessness which has been posited as the most likely common final pathway to depression is unlikely to develop following an important loss without earlier intimations of hopelessness into which the loss can feed.

Given the continued (and if anything increasing) allegiance of psychiatry to an essentially biological view of the major psychiatric disorders, such an approach will inevitably be controversial. While I believe that the response of some — to argue in terms of a contrast between 'distress' and 'disease' — is unnecessarily divisive, that response has been useful in bringing the issue of diagnostic classification to the fore. For instance, the need to distinguish between 'cases' and 'borderline cases' of depression is now well recognised. Some aspects of the controversy appear to have abated; there is now, for example, fairly wide agreement that cases of depression in the general population are of significance for psychiatry, although not necessarily best dealt with by psychiatric services. There can also be little doubt that the same aetiological factors play a role in depressive conditions treated by psychiatrists, as first documented in the early work by Paykel and his New Haven colleagues, who emphasised the importance of 'exit' events for depressed inpatients (Paykel 1973). However, a satisfactory evaluation of such research would need to cover highly complex issues concerning factors determining diagnosis, treatment effects, and who receives care; available space is not sufficient to review these here. It seems reasonable, though, to conclude that the part played by psychosocial factors in cases of depression treated by psychiatrists may only be somewhat less than that in respect of depression in the general population (see Brown & Harris 1986a, for a summary).

This review has been narrow in a second sense. In choosing to deal with issues in depth, I have inevitably failed to cite a good deal of important research. About the central role of life events, however, there does not seem to be much dispute; only a handful of clearly negative reports exist, and these may well be the result of methodological differences (Finlay-Jones 1981, Brown & Harris 1988b, 1989). There must be more uncertainty, though, about the areas of vulnerability and support, but even here, the results of recent research broadly support the view I have outlined (Alloway & Bebbington 1987). So far, the main source of doubt about the critical role of support derives from a study by a group in Canberra (Henderson et al 1981), and there is reason to believe that its essentially negative findings are not a threat to the position I have outlined (Henderson & Brown 1988) (See also Ch. 4).

However, the formidable nature of the problems faced in the study of support in relation to depression is clear from the research reviewed. While, for example, the notion of being 'let down' makes a good deal of theoretical sense, there is the real possibility that a woman's response to a crisis (and perhaps her incipient depression) may at times have contributed to this rejection — her 'over-emotional' response to the severe event, for instance, alienating would-be supporters. There has also been some suggestion in the Islington material that personality factors influence the kind of support received. Under these circumstances, there is no room for dogmatism, and in the end, fully convincing evidence may only emerge with experimental research. However, no research programme can expect, at present, to do more than produce plausible evidence for or against a particular aetiological viewpoint; from this rather less stringent view of scientific activity, findings are reasonably convincing. Here, it is useful to bear in mind that the Conjoint Index, based on material collected at first contact with the women in Islington (involving negative elements in close relationships and discomfiture) correlated with the subsequent onset of depression almost as well as the measures concerning support in a crisis in the follow-up year, that were collected retrospectively. Even if I have placed too much weight on the role of support in the crisis itself, there does not appear to be much doubt that measures of interpersonal relationships can be highly effective in predicting who will become depressed.

The role of major difficulties also requires further elucidation. Their exclusion, as provoking agents, from the review of the Islington survey created no problem, since only one onset, occurred among the 30 women with such a difficulty and no severe event. However, they have contributed a good deal more in other enquiries, and it is important to learn more about their role. We have seen that they can be of consider-able importance in providing the necessary background for D-events — one of the most potent aetiological agents among Islington women. There is also interesting evidence that the impact of major difficulties can, at times, be mediated by quite minor events that appear to force a reassessment of the ongoing life structure, e.g. the engagement of a woman's sister, when she herself is in a difficult marriage (Brown & Harris 1978).

The research concerning early experience has created, if anything, more controversy than that on support. However, even here, some consensus appears to be emerging, particularly about the importance of the quality of the relationship with parents in childhood after the loss itself (e.g. Munro 1966, Abrahams & Whitlock 1969, Jacobson et al 1975, Crook et al 1981). Parker (1979, 1983), investigating the relationship with parents in childhood among depressed neurotic patients, has produced evidence for this view, but the assessment of 'parental bonding' by a questionnaire is open to the limitations of this type of measure.

There are also some essentially negative findings on early experience, but recent studies have tended to support the importance of the quality of early care, if not that of loss (e.g. Birtchnell 1980, Birtchnell & Kennard 1981). Indeed, the basic findings concerning early loss now seem reasonably well established, and research begins to turn more to the question of the mechanisms involved. One of the central questions must be how far early experience leads to cognitive sets such as helplessness, that in turn lead to increased risk (i.e. the personal, Strand 2) independently of developments in the environment (i.e. the environmental, Strand 1). Given the close link between various factors in the model, this will technically be difficult to tackle. But these close links are, of course, a part of reality, and their theoretical and practical implications need to be faced.

The big omission from this review has been the burgeoning field of biological research. Here, there must be disappointment that in spite of recent advances, collaborative research has been rare. This situation will be bound to change, once biological markers of risk are more firmly established. (Calloway et al 1984 and Dolan et al 1985 provide interesting examples of collaborative research based on measures of biological function while patients are depressed.) It is only necessary to record that there is no problem, in principle, in incorporating such factors into the kind of models that have been outlined. No inherent conflict exists between the two traditions, and one of the exciting possibilities of the next decade is that they will move more closely together, as biological researchers become more involved in questions of aetiology. Gilbert (1984, 1989) has given stimulating accounts of some of the lines that this might take. So far, almost the entire effort of biological workers in psychiatry has been expended on establishing correlates of depression and in seeking to unravel the neurochemical effects of drug treatment. Some biological mechanisms can be expected to parallel the kind of processes outlined above, but others may make a separate contribution, although not necessarily entirely independently of psychosocial factors.

Finally, I have said nothing about the implications of the research for psychiatric services. Knowledge about the aetiology and course of disorders does not necessarily translate easily into effective practice. Indeed, as far as social factors are concerned, their major impact may at first be through pressure to rethink established ideas. Nonetheless, there appear to be a number of strategic points for intervention (Newton 1988). In terms of prevention, the work on early loss and quality of early care points in a number of directions; in particular, the crucial role of decisions about life plans such as marriage, motherhood and employment has been implicated. There can, of course, be no universal prescription outlining advice to a young woman who has become pregnant out of wedlock, but discussion with a counsellor of the kind of issues dealt with in this review may help towards a more informed decision about the future. However, it needs to be recalled that only some one-third of those developing depression were reported to be at a high risk because of adverse early experience(though, of course, more sophisticated research may well increase this proportion). In any case, in so far as the past was important, it usually appeared to be mediated by current circumstances. In terms of any effort at prevention, one of the most important implications of the work is that it should be possible to make a more refined assessment of women at risk, i.e. not just women who have experienced a certain kind of loss, but in addition, those with particular characteristics. Especially critical here are those women with children who are at a high risk because of both environmental factors (negative elements in core relationships) and psychological factors (low self-esteem or chronic sub-clinical symptoms). We saw also that the importance of these factors appeared to be largely mediated by the quality of support in the face of major losses and disappointments; the critical fact is that only a quarter of the women seen in Islington were at risk in this way. This is particularly important when resources are considered.

It has been argued that in prior work on intervention, one mistake has been made through targeting one risk factor (e.g. a major loss), when it would have been possible to narrow down the large target group and thereby use the time far more productively. Those, for instance, who already have good confiding relationships will be likely to find 'outside' support of less value than those without significant core support. Such work also promises to enable more informed decisions to be made about the type of support likely to be helpful; one obvious point is that in providing support (say for an elderly or handicapped person) which, by doing things increases a sense of dependency, may be deleterious as far as the risk of depression is concerned (Rodin 1983, 1985, Newton 1988). However, the findings on high-risk women have other practical implications. One obvious need is to carry out collaborative work with exponents of cognitive therapy; it is dispiriting that so little is known about parallel changes in the patient's social milieu in this apparently successful therapy (Teasdale 1988), or for that matter in drug treatment. The importance in terms of prevention of the wider economic and cultural context is too obvious to need comment.

The size of the problem, even if only a quarter of inner-city working-class women with children are at a high risk, is considerable. The obvious strategic point of entry are the women who are suffering from chronic depressive conditions. The fact alone that at any one time half of the depressive disorders are of this kind represents a major public health problem. It will also be necessary to keep in mind that depression is often accompanied by other psychiatric conditions (particularly anxiety) and by physical complaints. The latter are particularly common among the elderly, where events concerning physical ill-health play a greater role in onset and in course (Murphy 1982, 1983). The study of chronic depressive conditions has also suggested the presence of powerful social effects. Here, it is possible to speculate about a range of interventions, from social work with women with marital problems (e.g. Corney 1987), befriending schemes using the volunteer help of local women (e.g. Pound & Mills 1985), to various kinds of intervention by GPs (e.g. Goldberg 1982). During the next decade, we will learn a good deal more about such schemes. There will also certainly be an increased tendency to develop direct collaboration between psychiatrist and GP in the latter's surgery. While there must be some doubt about the ability of the various kinds of intervention I have listed to make a truly substantial impact without parallel changes in the status of women — particularly in terms of altering the balance of resources channelled into the work of raising children — this is no excuse for not trying. Moreover, as long as some of the efforts are carefully evaluated, and in so far as knowledge about effective intervention accumulates, it could only add to the pressure for more basic changes in society.

Acknowledgements

I should like to thank Tirril Harris, Toni Bifulco and Candida Richards for their invaluable comments on earlier drafts of this chapter: the review in any case reflects to considerable extent the outcome of their labour and that of their colleagues over the last decade.

APPENDIX 1

Vulnerability effect: Conjoint Index, Type of provoking agent and onset in follow-up year (N = 303)

Conjoint Index: Negative elements in close relationships and discomfiture	D/R-event	Other severe event	major difficulty	No provoking agent
	% onset	% onset	% onset	% onset
Yes	55 (17/31)	37 (7/19)	14 (1/7)	4 (1/23)
No	8 (1/12)	6 (4/68)	0 (0/13)	1 (1/130)

APPENDIX 2

Conjoint Index (negative elements in close relationships and discomfiture), type of provoking agent, adequacy of support in follow-up and onset of depression for the 130 with a severe event

Negative elements in close relationships and discomfiture	D/R-event		Other severe event	
	Inadequate support		Adequate support	
	Yes	No	Yes	No
	% onset		% onset	
Yes	65 (15/24)	33(2/6)[1]	54 (7/13)	0 (0/6)
No	25 (1/3)	0 (0/8)[1]	16 (3/19)	2 (1/47)[2]

[1] = 1 not known support.
[2] = 2 not known support.

REFERENCES

Abrahams M J, Whitlock F A 1969 Childhood experience and depression. British Journal of Psychiatry 115: 883–888

Akiskal H S 1985 Interaction of biologic and psychologic factors in the origin of depressive disorders. Acta Scandinavica Supplement 71: 131–139

Alloway R, Bebbington P 1987 The buffer theory of social support — a review of the literature. Psychological Medicine 17: 91–108

Andrews B, Brown G W 1988 Social support, onset of depression and personality: an exploratory analysis. Social Psychiatry 23: 99–108

Andrews G, Tennant C 1978 Being upset and becoming ill: an appraisal of the relation between life events and physical illness. Medical Journal of Australia 1: 324–327

Bebbington P 1986 Depression: distress or disease? British Journal of Psychiatry 149: 479

Bebbington P, Hurry J, Tennant C 1980 Recent advances in the epidemiological study of minor psychiatric disorders. Journal of the Royal Society of Medicine 73: 315–318

Bebbington P, Tennant C, Hurry J 1981a Adversity and the nature of psychiatric disorder in the community. Journal of Affective Disorders 3: 345–366

Bebbington P, Hurry J, Tennant C, Sturt E, Wing J K 1981b Epidemiology of mental disorders in Camberwell. Psychological Medicine 11: 561–579

Bebbington P, Sturt E, Tennant C, Hurry J 1984 Misfortune and resilience: a replication of the work of Brown & Harris. Psychological Medicine 14: 347–363

Beck A T 1967 Depression: clinical, experimental and theoretical aspects. Staples Press, London

Beck A T 1971 Cognition, affect and psychopathology. Archives of General Psychiatry 24: 495–500

Becker E 1964 The revolution in psychiatry. Free Press, Glencoe

Becker E 1971 The birth and death of meaning: an interdisciplinary perspective of the problem of man. Free Press of Glencoe, New York

Bibring E 1953 Mechanisms of depression. In: Greenacre P (ed) Affective disorders: psychoanalytic contributions to their study. International Universities Press, New York

Bifulco A, Brown G W, Harris T O 1987 Childhood loss of parent and adult psychiatric disorder: the Islington study. Journal of Affective Disorders 12: 115–128

Birtchnell J 1980 Women whose mothers died in childhood: an outcome study. Psychological Medicine 10: 699–713

Birtchnell J, Kennard J 1981 Early mother bereaved women who have and have not been psychiatric patients. Social Psychiatry 16: 187–197

Bolton W, Oatley K 1987 A longitudinal study of social support and depression in unemployed men. Psychological Medicine 17: 453–460

Brown G W 1988 Causal paths, chains and strands. In: Rutter M (ed) The power of longitudinal data: studies of risk and protective factors for psychosocial disorders. Cambridge University Press, Cambridge

Brown G W 1989 Depression. In: Brown G W, Harris T O (eds) Life events and illness. Guilford Press, New York, Unwin Hyman, London

Brown G W, Bifulco A 1989 Women, employment and the development of depression: a replication of a finding. British Journal of Psychiatry 156: 169-179.

Brown G W, Davidson S 1978 Social class, psychiatric disorder of mother and accidents to children. Lancet 1: 378–381

Brown G W, Harris T O 1978 Social origins of depression: a study of psychiatric disorder in women. Tavistock Publications London; Free Press, New York

Brown G W, Harris T O 1986a Establishing causal links: the Bedford College studies of depression. In: Katschnig H (ed) Life events and psychiatric disorders: controversial issues. Cambridge University Press, Cambridge

Brown G W, Harris T O 1986b Stressor, vulnerability and depression: a question of replication. Editorial Psychological Medicine 16: 739–744

Brown G W, Harris T O 1989a Life events and illness. Guilford Press, New York, Unwin Hyman, London

Brown G W, Harris T O 1989b Life events and measurement. In: Brown G W, Harris T O (eds) Life events and illness. Guilford Press, New York, Unwin Hyman, London

Brown G W, Prudo R 1981 Psychiatric disorder and physical illness. Journal of Psychosomatic Research 25: 461–473

Brown G W, Harris T O Copeland J R 1977 Depression and Loss. British Journal of Psychiatry 130: 1–18

Brown G W, Craig T K J, Harris T O 1985 Depression: disease or distress? Some epidemiological considerations. British Journal of Psychiatry 147: 612–622

Brown G W, Andrews B, Harris T O, Adler Z, Bridge L 1986a Social support, self-esteem and depression. Psychological Medicine 16: 813–831

Brown G W, Bifulco A, Harris T O, Bridge L 1986b Life stress, chronic psychiatric symptoms and vulnerability to clinical depression. Journal of Affective Disorders 11: 1–19

Brown G W, Harris T O, Bifulco A 1986c Long-term effect of early loss of parent. In: Rutter M, Izard C, Read P (eds) Depression in childhood: developmental perspectives. Guilford Press, New York

Brown G W, Bifulco A, Harris T O 1987 Life events, vulnerability and onset of depression: some refinements. British Journal of Psychiatry 150: 30–42

Brown G W, Adler Z, Bifulco A 1988 Life events, difficulties and recovery from chronic depression. British Journal of Psychiatry 152: 487–498

Brown G W, Andrews B, Bifulco A 1990a Self-esteem and depression 1: Measurement issues and prediction of onset. Social Psychiatry and Psychiatric Epidemiology (in press)

Brown G W, Bifulco A 1990b Self-esteem and depression 2: social correlates of low self-esteem. Social Psychiatry and Psychiatric Epidemiology (in press)

Brown G W, Bifulco A, Andrews B 1990c Self-esteem and depression 3: aetiology issues. Social Psychiatry and Psychiatric Epidemiology (in press)

Brown G W, Bifulco A, Andrews B 1990d Self-esteem and depression 4: effect on course and recovery. Social Psychiatry and Psychiatric Epidemiology (in press)

Calloway S P, Dolan R J, Fonagy P, De Souza V F A, Wakeling A 1984 Endocrine changes and clinical profiles in depression. Psychological Medicine 14: 749–765

Campbell E, Cope S, Teasdale J 1983 Social factors and affective disorders: an investigation of Brown and Harris's model. British Journal of Psychiatry 143: 548–553

Cartwright R D 1983 Rapid eye movement sleep characteristics during and after mood-disturbing events. Archives of General Psychiatry 40: 197–201

Cooke D J 1987 The significance of life events as a cause of psychological and physical disorder. In: Cooper B (ed) Psychiatric epidemiology: progress and prospects. Croom Helm, London

Cooper B, Sylph J 1973 Life events and the onset of neurotic illness: an investigation in general practice. Psychological Medicine 3: 421–435

Corney R 1987 Marital problems and treatment outcome in depressed women: a clinical trial of social work intervention. British Journal of Psychiatry 151: 652–660

Craig T K J 1989 Life stress and psychiatric disorder in the etiology of abdominal pain. In: Brown G W, Harris T O (eds) Life events and illness. Guilford Press, New York, Unwin Hyman, London

Craig T K J, Brown G W, Harris T O 1987 Depression in the general population: comparability of survey results. British Journal of Psychiatry 150: 707–708

Creed F 1989 Life events and appendicectomy. In: Brown G W, Harris T O (eds) Life events and illness. Guilford Press, New York, Unwin Hyman, London

Crook T, Eliot J 1980 Parental death during childhood and adult depression: a critical review of the literature. Psychological Bulletin 87: 252–259

Crook T, Raskin A, Eliot J 1981 Parent-child relationships and adult depression. Child Development 52: 950–957

Dean C, Surtees P G, Sashidharan S P 1983 Comparison of research diagnostic systems in an Edinburgh community sample. British Journal of Psychiatry 142: 247–256

Dohrenwend B, Shrout P, Link B, Martin J, Skodol A 1986 Overview and initial results from a risk-factor study of depression and schizophrenia. Reprinted from Barrett J F, Rose P M (eds) Mental disorders in the community. Guilford Press, New York

Dolan R J, Calloway S P, Fonagy P, De Souza V F A, Wakeling A 1985 Life events, depression and hypothalamic-pituitary-adrenal axis function. British Journal of Psychiatry 147: 429–433

Eales M J 1988 Affective disorders in unemployed men. Psychological Medicine 18: 935–946

Finlay-Jones R A 1981 Showing that life events are a cause of depression — a review. Australian & New Zealand Journal of Psychiatry 15: 229–238

Finlay-Jones R, Brown G W 1981 Types of stressful life event and the onset of anxiety and depressive disorders. Psychological Medicine 11: 803–815

Finlay-Jones R A, Brown G W, Duncan - Jones P, Harris T O, Murphy E, Prudo R 1980 Depression and anxiety in the community: replicating the diagnosis of a case. Psychological Medicine 10: 445–454

Freden L 1982 Psychosocial aspects of depression. Wiley, Chichester

Frijda N H 1986 The Emotions. Cambridge University Press, New York

Gilbert P 1984 Depression: from psychology to brain state. Lawrence Erlbaum and Attolides, London

Gilbert P 1989 Human nature and suffering. Lawrence Erlbaum Associates, Hove

Ginsberg S, Brown G W 1982 No time for depression: a study of help-seeking among mothers of pre-school children. In: Mechanic D (ed) Monographs in psychosocial epidemiology 3: symptoms, illness behaviour and help-seeking. Neale Watson Academic Publications, New York

Goldberg D 1982 The concept of a psychiatric 'case' in general practice. Social Psychiatry 17: 61–65

Goldberg D, Huxley P 1980 Mental illness in the community: the pathway to psychiatric care. Tavistock Publications, London

Hamilton M 1967 Development of a rating scale for primary depressive illness. British Journal of Social & Clinical Psychology 6: 278–296

Harris T O, Brown G W 1985 Interpreting data in aetiological studies of affective disorder: some pitfalls and ambiguities. British Journal of Psychiatry 147: 5–15

Harris T O, Brown G W, Bifulco A 1986 Loss of parent in childhood and adult psychiatric disorder: the role of parental care. Psychological Medicine 16: 641–659

Harris T O, Brown G W, Bifulco A 1987 Loss of parent in childhood and adult psychiatric disorder: the role of social class position and premarital pregnancy. Psychological Medicine 17: 163–183

Helzer J E, Robins L N, McEvoy L T et al 1985 A comparison of clinical and diagnostic interview schedule diagnoses. Physician reexamination of lay-interviewed cases in the general population. Archives of General Psychiatry 42: 657–666

Henderson A S, Brown G W 1988 Social support: the hypothesis and the evidence. In: Burrows G Henderson A S (eds) Handbook of studies on social psychiatry. Elsevier, London

Henderson S, Byrne D G, Duncan-Jones P 1981 Neurosis and the social environment. Academic Press, Sydney

Ingham J G, Kreitman N B, Miller P McC, Sashidharan S P, Surtees P G 1986 Self-esteem vulnerability and psychiatric disorder in the community. British Journal of Psychiatry 148: 375–385

Ingham J G, Kreitman N B, Miller P McC et al 1987 Self-appraisal, anxiety and depression in women: a prospective enquiry. British Journal of Psychiatry 150: 643–651

Jacobson S, Fasman J, Dimascio A 1975 Deprivation in the childhood of depressed women. Journal of Nervous & Mental Disorder 160: 5–14

Jenkins R, Clare A W 1985 Women and mental illness. British Medical Journal 291: 1521–1522

Klein D F 1974 Endogenomorphic depression: a conceptual and terminological revision. Archives of General Psychiatry 31: 447–454

Klinger E 1977 Meaning and void inner experience and the incentives in people's lives. University of Minnesota Press, Minneapolis

Kluckholm F, Strodtbeck F 1961 Variations in value orientations. Row, Peterson and Company, New York

Levinson D 1978 The seasons of a man's life. Knopf, New York

Lewinsohn P M, Steinmetz J L, Larson D W, Franklin J 1981 Depression-related conditions: antecedents or consequences? Journal of Abnormal Psychology 90: 213–219

MacIntyre A 1981 After virtue: a study of moral theory. Duckworth, London

Martin C J, Brown G W, Goldberg D P, Brockington I F 1989 Psycho-social stress and puerperal depression. Journal of Affective Disorders 16: 283–294

Miller P McC, Ingham J G 1983 Dimensions of experience. Psychological Medicine 13: 417–429

Miller P McC, Ingham J G, Kreitman N B et al 1987 Life events and other factors implicated in onset and in remission of psychiatric illness in women. Journal of Affective

Disorders 12: 73–88

Miller P McC, Kreitman N B, Ingham J G, Sashidharan S P 1989 Self-esteem, life stress and psychiatric disorder. Journal of Affective Disorders 17: 65–76

Munro A 1966 Parental deprivation in depressive patients. British Journal of Psychiatry 122: 443–457

Murphy E 1982 Social origins of depression in old age. British Journal of Psychiatry 141: 135–142

Murphy E 1983 The prognosis of depression in old age. British Journal of Psychiatry 142: 111–119

Murphy E, Brown G W 1980 Life events, psychiatric disturbance and physical illness. British Journal of Psychiatry 136: 326–338

Myers J K, Weissman M M, Tischler G L et al 1984 Six-month prevalence of psychiatric disorders in three communities. Archives of General Psychiatry 41: 959–970

Newton J 1988 Preventing Mental Illness. Routledge and Kegan Paul, London

Nolen-Hoeksema S 1987 Sex differences in unipolar depression: evidence and theory. Psychological Bulletin 101: 259–282

Oatley K, Bolton W 1985 A social-cognitive theory of depression in reaction to life events. Psychological Review 92: 372–388

O'Connor P, Brown G W 1984 Supportive relationships: fact or fancy? Journal of Social & Personal Relationships 1: 159–175

Parker G 1979 Parental characteristics in relation to depressive disorders. British Journal of Psychiatry 134: 138–147

Parker G 1983 Parental 'affectionless control' as an antecedent to adult depression. Archives of General Psychiatry 134: 138–147

Parker G, Tennant C, Blignault I 1985 Predicting improvement in patients with non-endogenous depression. British Journal of Psychiatry 146: 132–139

Parry G, Shapiro D A 1986 Social support and life events in working class women. Archives of General Psychiatry 43: 315–323

Paykel E S 1973 Life events and acute depression. In : Scott J P, Senay E C (eds) Separation and depression. Publications 94, American Association for the Advancement of Science, Washington D C

Paykel E S 1974 Recent life events and clinical depression. In : Gunderson I K E, Rahe R D (eds) Life stress and illness. Charles C Thomas, Illinois

Pound A, Mills M 1985 A pilot evaluation of Newpin — home visiting and befriending schemes in south London. ASCP Newsletter 7: No 4

Prudo R, Brown G W, Harris T O, Dowland J 1981 Psychiatric disorder in a rural and an urban population: 2. Sensitivity to loss. Psychological Medicine 11: 601–616

Quinton D, Rutter M 1984a Parents with children in care: 1. Current circumstances and parenting skills. Journal of Child Psychology & Psychiatry 25: 211–229

Quinton D, Rutter M 1984b Parents with children in care: 2. Intergenerational continuities. Journal of Child Psychology & Psychiatry 25: 231–250

Rodin J 1983 Behavioural medicine: beneficial effects of self-control training in aging. International Review of Applied Psychology 32: 153–181

Rodin J 1985 Health, control and aging. In: Baltes M M, Baltes P B (eds) Aging and the psychology of control. New Jersey Lea, Hillsdale

Roth M, Kroll J 1986 The reality of mental illness. Cambridge University Press, Cambridge

Rutter M 1988 Epidemiological approaches to developmental psychopathology. Archives of General Psychiatry 45: 486–500

Rutter M, Quinton D, Liddle C 1983 Parenting in two generations: looking backwards and looking forwards. In: Madge N (ed) Families at risk. Heinemann Educational, London: 66–98

Sashidharan S P 1985 Definitions of psychiatric syndromes — comparison in hospital patients and general population. British Journal of Psychiatry 147: 547–551

Sireling L I, Paykel E S, Freeling P, Rao B M, Patel S P 1985a Depression in general practice: case thresholds and diagnosis. British Journal of Psychiatry 147: 113–119

Sireling L I, Paykel E S, Rao B M 1985b Depression in general practice: clinical features and comparison with out-patients British Journal of Psychiatry 147: 119–126

Sloan T S 1987 Deciding self-deception in life choice. Methuen, New York

Surtees P G 1986 Personal communication

Surtees P G, Ingham J G 1980 Life stress and depressive outcome: application of a dissipation model to life events. Social Psychiatry 15: 21–31

Surtees P G, Dean C, Ingham J G, Kreitman N B, Miller P McC, Sashidharan S P 1983 Psychiatric disorder in women in an Edinburgh community: associations with demographic factors. British Journal of Psychiatry 142: 238–246

Teasdale J 1988 Cognitive vulnerability to persistent depression. Cognition & Emotion 2: 247–274

Tennant C, Bebbington P, Hurry J 1980 Parental death in childhood and risk of adult depressive disorder: a review. Psychological Medicine 10: 289–299

Tennant C, Bebbington P, Hurry J 1981a The natural history of neurotic illness in the community: demographic and clinical predictors of remission. Australian & New Zealand Journal of Psychiatry 15: 111–116

Tennant C, Bebbington P, Hurry J 1981b The short-term outcome of neurotic disorders in the community: the relation of remission to clinical factors and to 'neutralising' events. British Journal of Psychiatry 139: 213–220

Weissman M M, Klerman G L 1977 Sex differences and the epidemiology of depression. Archives of General Psychiatry 34: 98–111

Wilner P 1985 Depression: a psychological synthesis. Wiley, Inter-Science, New York

Wing J K, Cooper J E, Sartorius N 1974 The measurement and classification of psychiatric symptoms: an instruction manual for the present state examination and CATEGO programme. Cambridge University Press, London

4. Support and personal relationships

T.S. Brugha

INTRODUCTION

It would be difficult to dispute the idea that the support that others provide us in our lives is a fundamental component of any notion of 'quality of life'. However, the term 'social support' has also been widely adopted within both medicine and sociology, in a more technical sense, to denote those aspects of relationships that are thought to confer a beneficial effect on physical and psychological health. This subject may therefore have a very wide relevance within the field of medicine, but in a book on community psychiatry, the important question is whether support is also a vital component in the maintenance of psychological health and in the prevention of psychiatric illness. In particular, has it a significant influence on the course of major and long-term psychiatric disturbances?

Discussions of the topic of support can be divided into two somewhat separate arenas within psychiatry. The first of these could be termed the public health field; it is exemplified by the writings of Caplan (1974) and by the American President's Task Panel on Community Support Systems (1978), which asserted that a necessary goal of the community mental health movement should be to 'recognize and strengthen the natural networks to which people belong and on which they depend'. The second arena stems from a more questioning orientation, adopting both theoretical and (in particular) empirical approaches to answer the question with which this chapter began. Research workers in Europe (Brown & Harris 1978, Veiel 1985), North America (Cohen & Wills 1985) and Australasia (Henderson et al 1981) have all contributed to our burgeoning knowledge of social factors in psychiatric disorders, but primarily in the field of the more common, milder affective disorders.

Accordingly, concepts of social support can be divided into both broad and narrow definitions. Broad definitions encompass a wide variety of forms of care that come to individuals through the action of others and that handicapped people, such as the chronically mentally ill, may not be able to provide for themselves, e.g. shelter, nourishment, occupation, clothing (Brugha 1984a). These aids, treatments, and other forms of assistance from others may also be referred to by the rather general term

'Support in the Community'. Narrow definitions, on the other hand, tend to emphasise the specific 'personal' provisions of social relationships and particularly their more subjective components, e.g. confiding, intensity and reciprocity of interaction, or reassurance. Within the field of psychiatry, most research on the latter, more specific aspects of support has been conducted on people with mild, common, affective disorders, who are not in contact with specialist psychiatric services.

This chapter, for the most part, will adhere to the narrower, more specific definitions of support, whilst sometimes also referring to broader approaches. In practice, the 'broader provisions' are provided by social and psychiatric services to those with long-term psychiatric disorders who have need of them; these important issues will not be discussed further here. They consist of forms of care such as assessment procedures, treatments, shelter, welfare, and material aids that people need and do not have the ability to provide for themselves (see Brugha 1984a, Brugha et al 1988). The chapter will begin with a discussion of some conceptual and theoretical issues, followed by a section on methodological aspects. A selective overview of the empirical literature will be followed by a discussion of some of the implications of current work. Management principles that incorporate social network and social support concepts will also be discussed, and the chapter will end with a consideration of the overall implications for public health and social services.

CONCEPTUAL BACKGROUND

The nature of personal relationships

The study of personal relationships by social psychologists and ethologists indicates that much fundamental work on their conceptualisation and measurement has yet to be carried out. Hinde (1978) has made two important general points about personal relationships: the first is that it is necessary to consider not just their behavioural (directly observable), but also their cognitive and affective aspects. The second point is that in order to understand and adequately describe human relationships, it is necessary to take account of the way individuals relate over time. According to Hinde, at a general behavioural level, relationships consist of episodes of *interaction* over time, and the quality, content, and diversity of these interactions should be taken into account. Important cognitive factors that are more specific to human relationships include the nature of exchanges and rewards and how these are perceived by the participants (Hinde 1979); the latter emphasis is particularly relevant to the theme of this chapter.

Attachment theory has had quite a strong influence on notions of support, as for example in the acknowledgement of Henderson (1977) of the importance of the work of Bowlby (1969, 1977). A more general perspective has since emerged that conceives of attachment as being part of an evolved behavioural system that, although more easily observed at the earlier stages of development in the young of many species, may still be a very important influence on the development of adult relationships (West et al 1986) and, in the human case, of neurotic symptoms (Heard & Lake 1986).

The choice of a conceptual model can also reflect professional affiliations. Psychologists have approached the conceptualisation and measurement of personal relationships from both cognitive and behavioural standpoints. On the other hand, epidemiologists and sociologists, concerned with the concept of personal relationships as a (human) social resource, have paid relatively little attention to recent empirical and theoretical work by psychologists, although there is now a growing realisation that personality traits and attitudes may be important in depression (Henderson et al 1981, Brown & Harris 1978, Brugha 1984b, Bebbington 1985).

Until the late 1970s, the social psychiatry literature on the aetiology of non-psychotic disorder was dominated by studies of the role of adversity in depressive conditions, but personal relationships, conceptualised in the form of a positive social resource, have since entered the field. The absence of such resources is sometimes regarded as an independent risk factor, with a direct causal effect on psychiatric disorder (Henderson 1977). However, there is another, perhaps contradictory view of the relationship between support and disorder, in which it is held that the absence of support is unimportant on its own, but that in the presence of stress, it adds significantly to the risk of psychiatric illness (Brown et al 1975, Cassel 1976). In this sense, the presence of support is said to moderate the strength of stress-disorder relationships. This issue will be taken up at several points in this chapter.

Within the social psychiatry literature, there appear to be at least three models of (or ways of conceptualising) social functioning; though these seem to be at odds with each other, all three may be particularly useful to our understanding of social support in the long-term mentally ill.

Firstly, there are those studies that conceive of problems with social functioning as an indirect measure of psychological dysfunction — in other words, as part of the dependent variable. These studies typically describe an individual's social adjustment or social desirability as within the family and place of work (Kreitman et al 1970, Weissman & Paykel 1974, Hurry & Sturt 1981, Waryszak 1982). The second group of studies are appearing in increasing numbers: influenced by social learning theories of adjustment, they are concerned with individuals' coping styles and strategies (Seligman et al 1979, Coyne 1976a & b, Pearlin & Schooler 1978, Firth & Brewin 1982). Athough quite detailed models have been put forward, this kind of approach in general seeks to examine how thoughts (cognitions, attributions, beliefs) or actions affect subsequent health in physical and social environments which are demanding or stressful. The third group of studies, which are the primary focus of this chapter, employ a model in which the subject's social environment is conceived of as a resource, and where the functioning of a single individual can only be understood (and predicted) when consider- ed within the wider context of the behaviour and participation of others. Both 'social support' and 'social network' are terms that appear frequently in this literature. A practical example may help to illustrate these three ways of viewing personal relationships: the complaint — 'Doctor, my marriage isn't working' could be classified as a diagnostic problem (Lipkin & Kupka 1982), as a weakness in personality (a recognition of inadequate interpersonal skills), or as a judgement of a sub-standard spouse who has failed to contribute to the support of the relationship. It is, therefore, particularly important for those working with the social support model to try to consider explanations for their empirical findings by referring also to the other two.

The concept of social support

At an ecological level, a conception of the importance of social support runs through Durkheim's development of his ideas about types of suicide, two of which are termed *egoistic* and *anomic* (Durkheim 1951). These refer to the sense in which, for individual or social reasons, social contact and the influence of norms within a society cease to operate effectively. An example of an important and relevant ecological study is the work of Farris & Dunham (1939) who demonstrated an association between communal social isolation and increased hospital admission rates for schizophrenia in Chicago. The relationship to social support of wider social-class and economic factors and of psychological disorder has continued to be studied during the intervening years (Catalano & Dooley 1977, Liem & Liem 1978). However, it is only recently that the role of social support has been examined at an individual level, partly in response to the widely influential reviews of Caplan (1974) and Cassel (1976).

According to Cassel, social support does not lend itself to precise definition: it appears to consist of both information, in the form of appropriate feedback from others, and also integration within a wider social organisation (although the latter must presumably be taken to be a form of social status that can only be inferred from the verbal and non-verbal behaviour of others). Cobb (1976) also emphasised information — that one is cared for and valued, together with the knowledge that one belongs to a network of communication and obligation. Tolsdorf (1976) included in his definition both action (behaviour) and information (advice and feedback) that assists one in meeting one's goals. Brown & Harris (1978) focused on the importance of a single, close, confiding relationship in which there is trust and a free expression of feelings, usually in the context of an adult sexual relationship. However, others have emphasised both the importance of a wider network of relationships (Schaefer et al 1982, Henderson 1977) and also of tangible, material aid as well as intangible (emotional) support (Schaefer et al 1982, Tolsdorf 1976, Lin & Dean 1984). In his definition of support, Henderson (1977) emphasised its hypothetical status; social support is a commodity received from others during interpersonal transactions, and these transactions are most intense between individuals with strong social bonds. Total time spent together, perceived availability and reciprocity, and the level of attention obtained, are suggested as the more important components of social interaction. Henderson also referred to the literature on primate and human social evolution, human attachment theory, and social network theory; he gave particular credit to the writings of Weiss (1969, 1974) on the functions or provisions of close personal relationships, and to those of Bowlby (1977), who emphasised the importance of trusting relationships.

Weiss (1974) participated in meetings of the Boston chapter of Parents Without Partners, a self-help group, in order to find out why these adults, some of whom had lost their spouses by divorce, had sought out this form of social contact. It was evident that many of them had begun to develop new social relationships through the meetings. Weiss categorised the possible benefits of these social contacts, together with other attachment-providing relationships, in the following way: *Attachment* is provided by relationships such as marriage or a close friendship, and consists of a sense of security, of comfort, and of place; *social integration* 'is provided by relationships in which participants share concerns', together with information, ideas, and 'a shared interpretation of experiences'; *opportunity for nurturance* is provided for by relationships such as those in which an adult gives meaning to his life by taking responsibility for a child; *reassurance of worth* is provided by relationships 'which attest to an individual's competence in a social role'; *a sense of reliable alliance* is provided primarily by kin becuase of their continuing assistance, whether there is mutual affection or not; *the obtaining of guidance* is provided by an authoritative figure who can 'help in formulating and sustaining a line of action'. Particular kinds of information (feedback) from others appear central to Weiss's requirements, but they also refer to the individual subject's own contribution to relationships and not merely to the benefits to be derived from them. Inclusion, by implication, of this reference to the 'providee's' own actions in this theory raises a fundamental question: is it possible to discuss the topic of social support without harking back to the commonsense notion that 'everything you get in life has to be paid for'? Therefore, the usefulness of the term social support might be enhanced by an exclusive emphasis, however narrow and arbitrary, on the supportive aspects of the social behaviour of others, where the term 'supportive' refers both to tangible (material) and intangible provision.

The latter should include problem- or goal-focused information (feedback), as well as qualitative aspects of behaviour (willingness to listen and respond, confidentiality, verbal and non-verbal cues which are accepting rather than rejecting). However, as Hinde (1979) and others have pointed out, the interactional behaviour of any individual involved in a dialogue may be powerfully conditioned by the responses of the other. Therefore, work in this area may yet lead to the unavoidable conclusion that it is neither useful nor feasible to separate theoretical models of personality factors from the study of social support in social relationships. This unresolved issue will also be considered later in this chapter.

Social networks

In advocating the use of social network theory (or perhaps more correctly, the social network method), sociologists have argued that wider social structures may have a major influence on the quality of personal relationships (Wellman 1981). The empirical study of social networks has occurred mainly in the last 30 years (Barnes 1954), although long before this, Cooley (1909) had developed the concept of the 'primary group' to describe those people with whom an individual has 'intimate face-to-face association and cooperation'. According to Mitchell (1969), the social network is 'a specific set of linkages among a defined set of persons, with the property that the characteristics of these linkages as a whole may be used to interpret the social behaviour of the persons involved'. These social networks have both morphological and interactional characteristics. They also have two functions: communication (including, particularly for sociologists, the communication of norms) and instrumentality — or the means whereby people exercise choice to obtain goods and services. There are four morphological characteristics of social networks; *anchorage* refers to the central participant whose behaviour is of concern, sometimes referred to as the ego or centre of a personal network; *reachability* is the extent to which relationships can be used to contact others of impor-tance; *density* is the extent to which the potential links between a defined group of persons do in fact exist; and finally, *range* refers to the number of persons in direct contact with the primary person. The accompanying figure (Figure 4.1) may help to illustrate some of these characteristics. The central participant, EGO, can *reach* D and E through C and possibly through B, via a series of links. However, the density of linkages is low; contacts involving EGO and A can only be direct, and other members of EGO's network cannot facilitate such communication. Furthermore, although D and E might have useful specialised skills that might be helpful to EGO during a crisis, knowledge about these resources would depend on C who could act as a mediator.

The focus of the social network approach on psychiatric disorders can

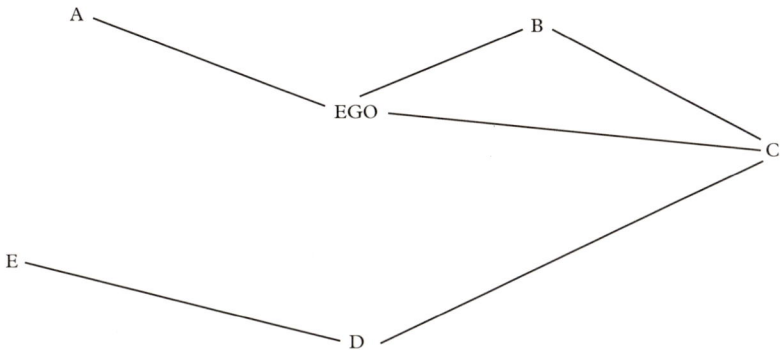

Fig. 4.1 Illustration of social network approach.

be regarded as an extension of sociological interest in it as an important aspect of social behaviour. Tolsdorf (1976) set out to study the social network model 'by utilising it in the study of stress, *support* and coping... to investigate coping and psychopathology using a systems rather than an individual approach'. Another source of interest may have been the popular (although somewhat discredited) view that the nuclear family was replacing more traditional, extended kinship networks. Pattison et al (1975), working in family therapy, attempted to draw on aspects of social network theory for their model of the family, and provided data on the size and density of both normal networks and those of a small selection of neurotics and psychotics. At about the same time, others, including Hammer et al (1978), suggested that the concept of the social network might provide a unifying framework for social research in relation to schizophrenia, while Mueller (1980), in drawing together a wide range of studies, extended the argument to research on psychiatric disorder in general.

Wellman (1981), however, sounded a critical note. He suggested that some workers were using the term 'social network' to describe techniques for measuring social support that made no use of structural concepts such as density and clustering which are specific and, in his view, necessary to the network approach. Density has already been defined as the degree to which persons linked with EGO have links with each other; Figure 4.1 illustrates a small cluster of these individuals (EGO, B and C) *all* of whom know each other, whereas other individuals (A,D,E) are known only to either EGO or to one other member of EGO's network, and do not form part of a visible cluster. Wellman argued for the inclusion of these morphological concepts because they reflect 'large scale social systems'.

However, some social scientists appear to disagree with the idea that social networks substantially reflect the influence of large-scale social systems (e.g. rural and urban systems, villages and housing estates), rather than personal and interpersonal factors such as gender, parenthood, and personality traits or dispositions. Fischer (1982), has reported on a detailed study of both urban and small town social networks, which showed that individual factors such as level of education, income, age, marital status, and gender, were associated with quantitative and qualitative measures of social networks, irrespective of the kind of community in which the person dwelt. Urban and semi-rural social networks did not differ greatly either quantitatively or qualitatively, but they did differ in composition; urban respondents choose to spend more time with friends than with relatives. In his view, personal characteristics and self-selection seemed to explain these differences. Hammer (1980) has argued for a biosocial view, which is not culturally limited, based on data from both western and rural African settings, noting that 'the range of network sizes is surprisingly restricted and fairly consistent'. She has suggested that certain mechanisms may be involved in both the attraction to, and the limitation of, personal connections and that these must be bio-cultural in origin, but also (1981) makes the point that one should analyse 'the properties of the networks around the focal individual, independent of that individual's own behaviour'. Taking both of these views into account, it appears that factors both external and internal to the individual should be considered in attempting to explain, and perhaps even predict, social behaviour. The concept of the social network that is postulated by sociologists and social anthropologists, therefore, embraces not only wider macro-social influences but frequently also factors in the individual, and these might be called personality.

The term 'social network' has often been seen in social psychiatry publications but rarely, as we shall see later in this chapter, with the use of its structural concepts or reliance on the influence of personal factors. The fact that both the individual and the social environment are thought to be influential is not a problem for social network theory; however, it does pose a major question for research on individuals with psychiatric disorder, precisely because such individuals may themselves represent a crucial source of variation in their social network's characteristics. For example, a common psychiatric complaint is that of irritability, in which the person notices an increased tendency to feel like picking a quarrel with others. This tendency, particularly if unexpected, may lead others to withdraw from close contact with such a person, which may in turn lead to much more serious consequences for that individual. Therefore, it seems wise to conclude, at this point, that the structural properties of personal networks might both be influenced by wider socio-economic factors and by the quantity and quality of interpersonal transactions. Returning to the last example, the extent to which unexpected outbursts of irritability are tolerated and accepted is likely to vary considerably, depending on cultural and economic factors, as well as on the individual dispositions of those involved.

Adversity in relation to social support

Research workers interested in the relationship of social support to psychiatric disorder have either sought to study its effects alone (Henderson 1977) or have incorporated it into a multivariate stress-buffering model. Later in this chapter, a series of diagrams will be used to show the different kinds of models that can be used to explain the variety of possible causal relationships.

Dohrenwend & Dohrenwend (1974) advocated the incorporation of a measure of social support, because it may act as an important intervening influence between stressful life events and ill-health. In one multivariate version (the vulnerability model referred to earlier), it is postulated that social support has no independent effect on the risk of disorder, but that it protects against the development of disorder in response to adversity (Brown & Harris 1978).

The stress-buffering model of social support derives some of its inspiration from Cassel's (1976) review of both animal and human studies, in which he developed the hypothesis that the social environment affects host resistance both to biological noxious stimuli such as infectious agents, and to psychological stressors. This model has implications for a range of disorders, in addition to psychiatric disturbances (Berkman & Syme 1979, Welin et al 1985). Although many workers view social support only in relation to its hypothesised effect as a buffer against adversity, others do not agree with this; both Bruhn & Philips (1984) and Surtees (1984) have argued for its importance as a variable in its own right.

The burgeoning use of social support and social network variables in psychiatric epidemiology has also led to theoretical and methodological objections at attempts to examine the buffering effect of social support against adversity (Mueller 1980, Brugha 1981, 1984b, 1986, Thoits 1982, Parry & Shapiro 1986). For example, the observation that many life events may be descriptions of changes in social support leads to the following question: is social support a static resource (rather like savings in the bank), or a fluctuating resource that alters constantly but unpredictably (like stock market shares)? In general, applications of the social support model have made the assumption that social support is a static resource, but in practice, personal relationships may not be like this. A particular case arises in relation to 'exit events' (Paykel et al 1976), which are believed by many to be particularly important in aetiological models of depression; they are not only important adverse experiences (of a particular kind), but can also be indicators of change in social support. Work by Jenkins et al (1981), which places support and adversity at the extremes of a single dimension, also points to the weakness of the theoretical distinction between the two concepts.

This somewhat selective overview of the conceptual background to the literature on personal relationships in psychiatric disorder points to a more general problem — that theoretical distinctions between different conceptual models or constructs (e.g. 'social support', 'coping', 'personality') may be hard to verify empirically, and may need to be radically reviewed in the light of further theoretical as well as empirical work. A number of areas have been suggested in which such overlap may occur, for example, that between exit events and temporal changes in levels of social support, and that between certain psychiatric symptoms and the level of contact and social interaction that a person has with others. It has also been pointed out that in certain populations (e.g. psychiatric patients), the distinction between neurotic symptoms and trait neuroticism may rest more on faith than on empirical data (Katz & McGuffin 1987). Although on face value, the categories of symptoms (and disease categories), personality, and social support and adversity do not appear to overlap in any obvious fashion, there may well be some grounds for concern regarding the tidiness of the apparent boundaries between them. Therefore, in developing empirical research strategies, it is important to construct both instruments and operational definitions of concepts that make specific use of data that can be shown to vary independently of one another, according to the theoretical requirements of a chosen model. It may also be possible to test theoretical models more explicitly, using suitable data, with mathematical techniques such as confirmatory factor analysis (Everitt & Dunn 1983); these research strategies are a vital part of work in the area, and should not be regarded as mere academic curiosities.

METHODOLOGICAL ISSUES

A good study should have a clear aim, relevance to prior scientific literature, and a careful design, as well as information on the estimated power of the study, the source of subjects, response rates, and errors and biases in the data (Alderson 1983). However, of all the standards required of good empirical research, studies of personal relationships and psychiatric disorder are particularly vulnerable to problems of interpretation, arising from the effects of errors in the data, and also from the effects of bias. An additional problem in non-experimental studies is the effect of confounding, which may occur where a variable that the researcher has not considered or measured gives rise to an apparent association between an independent (putative causal) variable and the dependent variable (i.e. a form of psychiatric disorder in most of the studies considered here). This important problem can only be overcome by the use of proper randomisation procedures in experimental studies. An important and relevant example that Henderson et al have studied

(1981) is the suggested influence of prior personality (in this example, neuroticism) on the association between neurotic symptoms and the perceived inadequacy of social support. This will be discussed in more detail below.

In relation to the measurement and classification of psychiatric disorders, reliable methods have been used only in a minority of studies. Whether or not acceptable validity can be achieved in the area of classification, reliability of assessment is central to the success of epidemiological research. In this respect, the PSE-ID-CATEGO system (Wing et al 1974) and the more recent collaborative work of clinicians and epidemiologists in North America using the DIS and DSM III (Robins et al 1981) are important landmarks. Besides the theoretical merits of assessing categories, the onset, duration, and course of disorders should be assessed, but this is done infrequently. Most studies either use only a dimensional score based on a symptom count or, less often, a threshold level on a dimension (Wing & Sturt 1978).

The almost complete absence of data on defined diagnostic categories and sub-categories, and on the course of non-psychotic disorder is a potentially important omission in the literature on social support and psychiatric disorder. This issue has been examined at various times in relation to stress and adversity (Wing & Bebbington 1982, Bebbington 1985, Brugha & Conroy 1985), but hardly any attention has been devoted to it in the context of investigations of personal social relationships, apart from four studies (Brugha et al 1982, Billings & Moos 1984, Hirschfeld et al 1985, Brugha et al 1987b). Nor have reliable measures and classification rules been systematically applied to studies of mixed groups of people with more severe disorders, such as schizophrenia and manic-depressive psychosis (apart from the literature on Expressed Emotion, which is discussed elsewhere in this book).

A number of studies have shown that non-psychotic symptoms, and in particular those of depression, measured both in the general population and in clinical settings, have a significant degree of stability over time (Henderson et al 1981, Keller et al 1982a & b). This finding may be partly, but is unlikely to be entirely due to the kinds of measures used in such studies; clearly, studies that do not separate chronic cases from those of recent onset may produce misleading results. Measures of personal relationships may also be reflecting prolonged depressed mood, with the attendant symptoms of anergia, retardation, and self-depreciation which are seen in many depressed individuals. However, in relation to cases of acute onset, aetiologically important events may go undetected. Both Bebbington et al (1981) and Billings & Moos (1984) have examined these issues in relation to adversity, and both studies encountered technical difficulties. The former judged it inappropriate to compare chronic and acute cases of depression with regard to life events. This is because the three months before onset is thought to be the maximum risk period for short-term adversity in relation to the precipitation of depression, and reliable retrospective accounts of such events could not be obtained over prolonged periods of time from subjects with chronic conditions. Billings & Moos (1984) did not consider the important issue of episode onset, but examined 3, 6 and 12-month periods, prior to the time of data collection for negative life events, in their comparison of newly referred cases of RDC minor and major depression (Spitzer et al 1978) with cases attending psychiatric services for a year. Most of the studies in the literature have based their findings on what a clinician working in hospital would regard as either minor cases of depression or as transient episodes of demoralisation, of relatively little clinical significance. Psychiatrists often label these as cases of 'neurotic' or 'reactive' depression, but many also feel that personality factors may have an important role to play in these minor disorders, and might seriously question the generalisability of the results of such studies to the kinds of clinically severe depressive disorders seen in hospital practice. Patients with anxiety states might also be characterised by differences in measures of social relationships that distinguish them from those who are healthy on the one hand, and those who are depressed on the other.

The same misgivings may be even more crucial in relation to the major psychoses and to long-term, chronic disorders. Much of the descriptive psychopathology of schizophrenia includes items such as 'social withdrawal', or 'delusions of reference and persecution' that are relevant to the manner and degree to which a patient participates in personal relationships with others. Similarly, in the case of those with 'non-schizophrenic' psychoses and more severe personality disorders that also make up a substantial proportion of long-term users of hospital and community psychiatric services (Wing 1982), many of those factors that are regarded as being of importance in the clinical picture are likely to have major implications for a clear examination of personal relationships and what they provide. Examples of these clinical factors include social phobia, lack of drive, and guilty ideas of self-reference. This implies that prospective and experimental studies are required in which these clinical factors are reliably assessed by the investigator.

Although the strongest argument can be marshalled for relating independent variables specifically to the time of onset of a psychiatric disorder, arguments for the assessment of categories do not solely rest on purely theoretical grounds. The empirical validation of categories and hierarchical classification models (Andreason 1982, Sturt 1981), although not without considerable methodological difficulties (Everitt & Dunn 1983), lends further support to the argument for their use in such research.

In contrast to the field of psychiatric nosology, that of personal relationships has rarely been the subject of attempts to validate theoretical models empirically. Weiss's model of the provision of relationships (already referred to) was tested by Duncan-Jones (1981) with confirmatory factor analysis. Using the Interview Schedule of Social Interaction (ISSI) to assess personal relationships in a general population sample (Henderson et al 1981), he concluded that most types of relationships can be broadly accounted for by two major dimensions: 'attachment' and 'social integration'. However, a number of more specific dimensions, corresponding to some of Weiss' categories, could be distinguished within 'social integration'.

Measures of social relationships have been surveyed and critically discussed elsewhere (Brugha 1986, 1988b); however, it is often the case that adequate information about the reliability of such measures is not available and that their face validity may be poor. Data are rarely gathered on, or from, others to whom the focal subject is related, while reporting may be distorted by certain cognitive attributes of the depressed individual, i.e. denial, 'plaintive set' (a tendency to seize any opportunity to describe one's life in its blackest terms), or just plain pessimism. A failure to consider and, if possible, allow for these potential sources of systematic measurement error (or of confounding) may lead to serious errors of inference. Alloway & Bebbington (1987) have discussed problems of inference in relation to research that examines the effects of both life events and social support on psychopathology. In the case of life events, they argue that many of the problems of contamination and of observer and responder bias, as well as the temporal relationship of events to psychiatric disorder have been circumvented by the techniques of Brown & Harris (1978). However, many problems remain for the study of social support, and they suggest that only where two assessments are employed, separated by a period such as six months, will the specific demands of the buffering hypothesis be likely to be overcome; these requirements are rarely adequately met in the scientific literature.

The suggestion above, that personality factors may overlap with other dimensions, requires some further consideration, but personality theory and its assessment cannot be considered fully here. Of all the issues involved, it would be particularly important to demonstrate the long-term stability of personality factors, in contrast to measures of psychiatric disorder, adversity, and social support. Examples of potentially important aspects of personality are: coping capacity and style, patterns of perceiving (e.g. plaintive set or 'polyannaism', of which the latter refers to a uniformly rosy or positive view of the world), and the tendency, now increasingly discussed by cognitive psychologists (Brewin 1985), to attribute the causes of important events in a predictable way. To study the relationship of stable, predictable attributes of individuals, to the other variables under consideration here, aetiological research is needed and is likely to be enhanced by the availability of data gathered in both childhood and adulthood.

EMPIRICAL LITERATURE

The following, selective overview of the empirical literature is based largely on a review completed in 1986. Some recent, important studies are also mentioned, but a more comprehensive update can also be found elsewhere (Brugha 1988a). Both univariate and multivariate, cross-sectional and longitudinal studies will be considered here, but only the last of these categories will be discussed in greater detail. Although multivariate observational studies allow one to explore the relative contribution of different variables (such as the effects of background and demographic variables, e.g. age, sex, and employment status, as well as other theoretically relevant variables such as adversity and personality), the research worker can never be certain that all relevant confounding variables have been considered. On the other hand, there can be much more confidence about causal inferences based on properly randomised experiments in representative population samples. Apart from two discussed below, specific, relevant experimental studies have not yet appeared.

Univariate, cross-sectional studies

Miller & Ingham (1976) interviewed 337 general practice attenders, and asked each to rate nine symptoms, including depressed mood and other (somatic and anxiety) symptoms, on analogue scales. They reported an association between a high depression score and the absence of a personal confidant, and also a lack of more diffuse social relationships with aquaintances. Andrews et al (1978) studied a general population sample of 863 adults in Australia, using the General Health Questionnaire (GHQ) (Goldberg 1972) to measure non-psychotic psychiatric disorders. Using their own measure of 'perceived assistance and support', they also reported a correlation with an elevated ('case' level) score on the GHQ. Further studies in clinical samples (Siberfeld 1978, Henderson et al 1978, Surtees 1980) and in the general population (Billings & Moos 1982, Dalgard 1980, D'Arcy & Siddique 1984, Henderson et al 1981, Leaf et al 1984, Surtees 1984) all report broadly similar findings, in spite of the use of different measures of social support and of psychopathology. Other controlled, observational studies have also reported similar kinds of associations — in pre-pubertal children (Puig-Antich et al 1985) in adolescents (Kandel & Davies 1982), in the elderly (Blazer 1983), in parents of children with cystic fibrosis (Frydman 1981), and in a group of recently divorced women (Wilcox 1981). Apart from Andrews et al (1977), who failed to find an association between social isolation and psychiatric morbidity using the GHQ, no clearly negative cross-sectional studies have been identified. Only one of the studies mentioned above (Henderson et al 1978) has been specifically replicated (Brugha et al 1982).

Very few of the above studies used standardised measures, but

Henderson and his group have developed two detailed measures of qualitative and quantitative aspects of personal relationships and social support — the Social Interaction Schedule (SIS) (Henderson et al 1978) and the Interview Schedule of Social Interaction (ISSI) (Henderson et al 1981). Using the SIS, Henderson et al (1978) found that new cases of non-psychotic psychiatric disorder, who had been referred to a psychiatric outpatient clinic, reported deficiencies in the size of their social networks, as well as increased negative interaction; these patients also perceived their attachment figures as providing insufficient support. In a replication of this study, Brugha et al (1982) confirmed most of these findings.

Although the term 'social network' appears frequently in the social psychiatry literature, hardly any studies have been identified that actually deal with the structural or morphological elements of such a network — the inter-relatedness or inter-connectedness of the members of each subject's primary social group (network density). In a comparison of two sub-groups of 50 divorced women (Wilcox 1981), of whom 25 had made a poor adjustment (judged on the basis of two standardised questionnaire measures of mood and psychological impairment), no major difference in network size or network density could be detected prior to divorce. However, when both groups were followed-up, it was shown that in the poor adjustment group, there was a subsequent significant increase in network density (inter-connectedness) of about 50% and a small reduction in the mean size of their networks (although this finding was not statistically significant). It may be that the use of small sample sizes compromised the statistical power of the comparison. In a small but detailed study, Cohen & Sokolovsky (1978) were unable to find any differences in social network density, when they compared groups of subjects with or without psychotic symptoms, although those with residual symptoms were reported to have significantly fewer relationships than those who had never had psychotic symptoms.

These studies show that psychological dysfunction in a wide variety of people in the general population, as well as some in contact with specialised psychiatric services, is related to their descriptions of the number and quality of their close relationships with others. These findings are sufficiently consistent to justify more substantial studies, in which other possible causal variables are taken into account, but it would be premature to discuss their implications for intervention policies before considering what has been shown by such additional work.

Multivariate, cross-sectional studies

Some methodological issues

In this section, a number of studies will be described in which the relationship between social support and psychiatric disorder is examined in the presence of additional variables, such as adversity. Some readers, who may be unfamiliar with terminology in this area, may find the following explanatory note and diagrams helpful.

The term 'dependent variable' and occasionally, the equivalent term 'outcome variable' will be used to refer to the measure of psychiatric disorder. The term 'independent variable', or occasionally, 'explanatory variable', will be used to refer to an hypothesised causal variable, such as social support, adversity, etc. Figure 4.2 shows the sort of relationship between two variables that was described in the previous section. Those who describe having social support are likely to be well and those who say that support is absent are likely to have an increasing severity of illness.

In the equally fictitious study shown in Figure 4.3, all subjects have also provided information on whether or not they have had a stressful life event during a key period of time; those with adversity are denoted by an asterix, while all the other participants in the study are denoted by a dot. According to Figure 4.3, those who do not experience adversity are, nevertheless, worse off if social support is absent. Those who do experience adversity are worse off than those who do not. The combined effect of absent support and adversity is additive; both of these 'risk factors' are said to be (additive) main effects.

Figures 4.4 and 4.5 show other possible 'causal' relationships when more than one variable is being considered. In the fictitious study shown in Figure 4.4, the combined effect of absent support and adversity is said to be multiplicative; those who have both risk factors (the steeper slope)

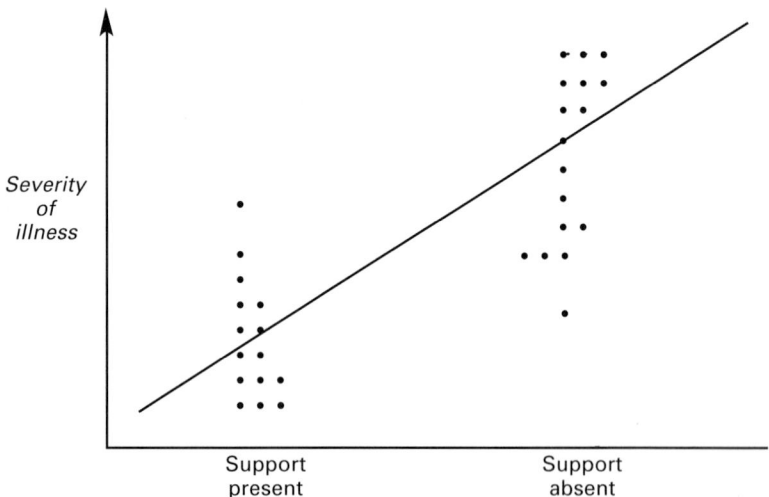

Fig. 4.2 Social support 'appears' to be associated with a lower level of illness; however, no information on exposure to adversity is provided.

are distinctly worse off than those who have only one (the shallower slope). The two effects are said to 'interact' with one another, and in the Figure, one can see that the slopes describing the relationship with illness, of each risk factor, cross over one another (they are not parallel). Figure 4.5 shows an important special case that shares some properties with the study in Figure 4.4. In the study in Figure 4.5, when adversity is taken into account, the association between low social support and illness is found to disappear for low adversity. It is perfectly possible that the study in Figure 4.2 conceals such an effect and leads to the spurious inference that the absence of social support causes illness when, in this hypothetical example, it does not. By taking into account the effect of adversity, we find that there is an interaction between these two variables; adversity is clearly related to illness only in those who do not have support. Those who have support can be said to be buffered or protected from the effects of adversity.

On a final technical point, it should be said that there are mathematical techniques for verifying which of these inter-relationships represents the best explanation of the data gathered in a study. These methods are referred to, nowadays, under the umbrella term of 'generalised linear modelling' (McCullagh and Nelder 1983). But those who are more familiar with terms such as 'analysis of covariance', 'multiple regression analysis', and 'log linear analysis' will find that there is little that is new or unfamiliar here.

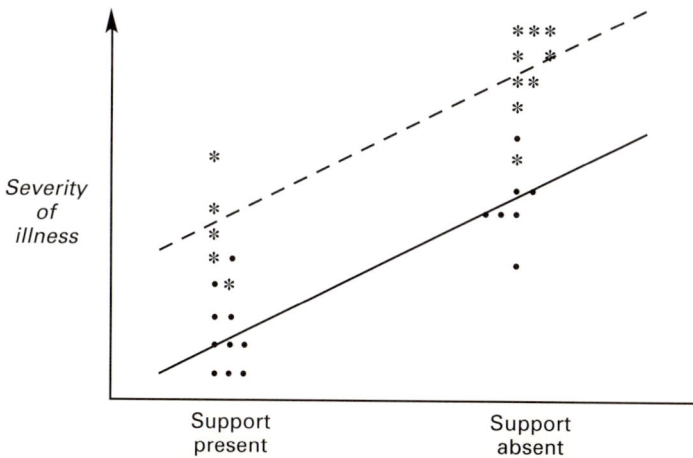

Fig. 4.3 An asterisk (✳) is for a subject with adversity and a dot (•) denotes someone who has not been exposed to adversity. Here we find that social support and adversity are both (independently or additively) associated with a lower level of illness.

Empirical data

Two early studies on the effects of life events on a range of outcome variables, including non-specific indices of psychological distress, also examined the effects of 'psychological assets' (Nuckolls et al 1972) and 'social integration' (Myers et al 1975). Although the methods and results of both were unclear, it would appear that the two explanatory variables were each independently associated with the outcome variable. The study by Andrews et al (1978), mentioned above, clearly showed a main effect, firstly for adversity (using a standardised inventory), secondly for social support, based on a scale of perceived assistance and support that did not specify actual events or points in time, and also for a third explanatory variable — a 'maturity of coping measure'. Step-wise multiple regression analysis of GHQ scores was used on the explanatory variables. To examine the combined effects of these explanatory variables, further mutiple regression analyses were carried out, in which the product of pairs of explanatory variables were also entered into the analysis. The inclusion of multiplicative terms did not account for any additional variation in the dependent variable; the findings suggested that the combined effect of their independent variables was additive, as in the fictional example in Figure 4.3, and that they did not interact significantly with one another.

However, these authors did not state whether or not their data violated

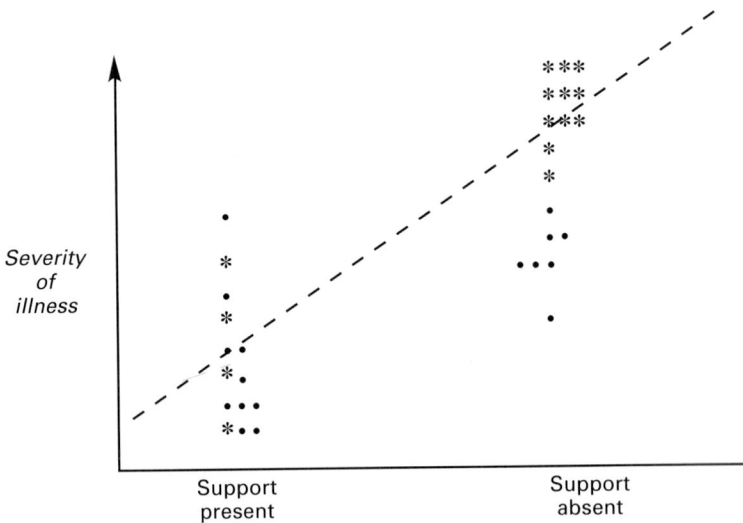

Fig. 4.4   An asterisk (✱) is for a subject with adversity and a dot (•) denotes someone not exposed to adversity. Both low support and adversity are related to illness; but their combined effects are multiplicative: that is, they are significantly more than additive.

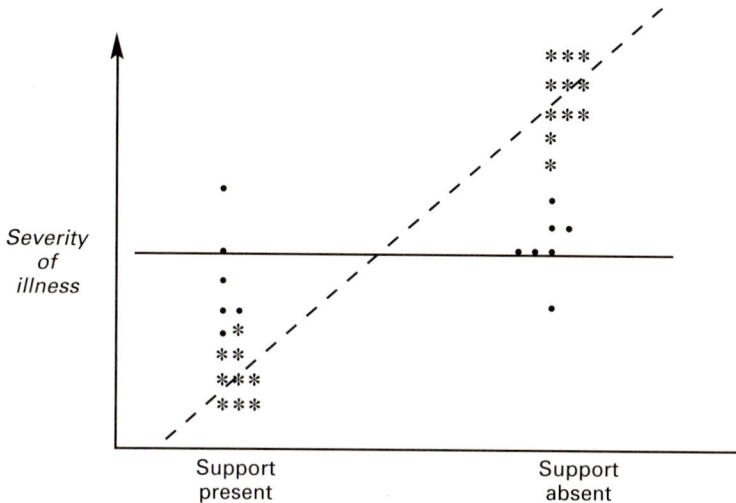

Fig. 4.5   An asterisk (✳) is for a subject with adversity and a dot (•) denotes someone who has not been exposed to adversity. But when exposure to adversity is taken into account in this study, we find that social support is not associated with a lower level of illness; however, those without support are affected by adversity.

the various statistical assumptions required for the use of (least squares) multiple regression analysis, and this omission seems to have been the norm for almost every other study published, since then, in which the technique is used. Nevertheless, studies of random samples of the general population, using similar designs, measures and analyses, have produced comparable findings with respect to adversity, social support and measures of psychological distress (Husaini & Neff 1980, Lin & Ensel 1984, McFarlane et al 1983, Williams et al 1981); three of these studies used the CES-D (Radloff 1977). Samples of more specialised populations have also produced similar results, although rarely using the same measure of social support. Frydman (1981) also claimed to have demonstrated a 'conditional effect', in which low social support only acted in the presence of a life event.

Gore (1978) compared an urban with a rural sample, both studied during a period after the experience of becoming unemployed; a more favourable outcome in the rural group was attributed to a greater amount of social support, compared with that in the urban group. Paykel et al (1980) studied 104 women during their puerperium, using a standardised interview; 24 of them were found to be depressed. Explanatory variables related to depression were: the report of an undesirable life event, a history of psychiatric disorder, 'post-partum blues', marital problems, and age; three social support variables were also related to depression in separate univariate analyses. Turner (1981) drew together four samples from family studies and from a study of mentally ill adults in the community, reporting significant main effects of life event stress and social support on a measure of psychological well-being. Turner & Noh (1983) studied 312 Ontario women during the month after childbirth, in order to examine whether stress and poor social support could explain the relatively worse outcome of women of low socio-economic status; their analysis corroborated this hypothesis.

Although a number of authors infer conditional effects, usually involving measures of social support and stressful life events, very few claim to have demonstrated statistically significant multiplicative interaction effects. D'Arcy & Siddique (1984) used analysis of covariance on data from a postal survey of 417 mothers, all of whom had at least one child. In a sub-group of mothers with pre-school children, a multiple regression model of GHQ score on a measure of support from the spouse and family, and a measure of community support, produced a second-order interaction effect between these two measures. La Rocco et al (1980) used a 'moderated regression analysis' technique in a study of 2010 employed men, and claimed that social support seemed to buffer the effects of job stress on general mental health. Cohen & Haberman (1983), in a study of 70 introductory-course social psychology students, reported perhaps the most clearly presented analysis of all, which demonstrated an interaction effect between the perceived availability of support and negative life events score on the CES-D depression inventory. However, all three studies were carried out on idiosyncratic samples, thus limiting their generalisability.

Many of the multivariate studies described above suffer from a number of technical problems; as pointed out, the use of techniques such as multiple regression analysis requires special care in psychological and social research. Nevertheless, the consistency of the published findings suggests that it would be over-presumptuous to dismiss them completely. However, some studies on representative samples of clinical and general populations have used measures and statistical techniques (such as log-linear analysis (Everitt & Dunn 1983)) in which all the necessary underlying assumptions of the method have been adequately dealt with. For convenience, the results of a number of these studies (all of which provide data in the form of counts which can be set out in $2 \times 2 \times 2$ contingency tables), have been simplified by calculating the relative risk, (or odds ratio) (Alderson 1983) for each of the partial tables. To take a simple example — if the relative risk of developing an episode of depression following a life event is 4, this means that a person's risk of becoming depressed is increased 4 times within a defined period following upon such an event. Therefore, the relative risk provides the reader with a useful indication of the magnitude of the effect of an hypothesised causal agent.

Table 4.1 allows one to examine the relative risk of poor social support and of adversity, as well as that attached to the presence of both factors in a series of studies. Cooke (1987) has discussed this and related techniques with additional examples from the literature. Where the authors themselves supplied the results of a log-linear or a logistic-regression analysis, the finding of a statistically significant main effect for an explanatory variable is indicated by means of a single asterisk in Table 4.1. At this stage, it is worth noting that in none of the quoted studies was evidence provided for a multiplicative interaction effect between the explanatory variables, but some of the authors who had not employed the available statistical tests of probability claim that their data support the 'vulnerability model'. In this model, poor social support has no effect, except in those with adversity (Brown & Harris 1978, Brown & Prudo 1981, Campbell et al 1983, Surtees 1980) (as illustrated earlier in Figure 4.5). None of the studies mentioned in Table 4.1 conform to the rather stringent criteria illustrated in Figure 4.5; the slopes of the lines plotting the effects of the hypothetical causal variables on the measure of psychiatric disorder, in effect, have not been shown to cross one another and the appropriate statistical technique (log-linear analysis), where used, has confirmed that there is no multiplicative interaction effect. If we look at the risk ratios (relative risk levels), in the right-hand three columns of the table, it is apparent that the effect of both risk factors together, is greater than that of a single factor, and in some studies the additional effect is quite substantial. In several, the combined risk exceeds the sum of risks for individual factors, and, in a few (those where individual risks are very small), the combined risk appears to be greater than the product of individual risks. Although some of the studies seem to show that there is no independent risk attached to the absence of support (low intimacy), the effect of adversity (where tested) does not interact with support here either. The data in the table do seem to indicate that the criteria illustrated in Figure 4.5 are almost met in some studies. Perhaps the careful use of more sensitive, continuous measures, rather than of categorical ones, might have detected firmer evidence in favour of the stress buffering model.

The second observation is that the risk ratios vary considerably between studies. This may be partly explained by sampling variation; for example, some of the studies focus on high-risk groups, such as working-class mothers (e.g. Campbell et al 1983), and in addition, measures of variable quality are used. Six studies rely on the PSE-CATEGO-ID system (Wing et al 1974, Wing & Sturt 1978) for assessing psychiatric disorder and on the Bedford College Life Events and Difficulties Scales (LEDS) for assessing adversity and the quality of the subject's relationship with a partner of the opposite sex (Brown & Harris 1978, Brown & Prudo 1981, Murphy 1982, Campbell et al 1983, Bebbington et al 1984, Parry & Shapiro 1986). However, some studies use onset cases only,

Table 4.1   Relative risk of poor social support and of adversity in a series of studies

Source	Sample	N	Explanatory variables Support	Adversity	Risk ratios Low support	Adversity	Combined
Aneshensel & Stone (1982)	Adult general population	998	Having few close relationships	Presence of life event	3.0*	3.5*	5.0
Bebbington et al (1984)	Female general population	147	Low intimacy	Severe event or major difficulty	1.1*	2.1*	3.3
Brown & Harris (1978)	Female general population	419	Low intimacy	Severe event or major difficulty	3.5	14.6	41.6**
Brown & Prudo (1981)	Female general population, rural	187	Low intimacy	Severe event or major difficulty	4.8	16.9	52.0**
Campbell et al (1983)	Working-class mothers	110	Low intimacy	Severe event or major difficulty	5.7	6.45	36.8**
Murphy (1982)	Elderly patients and controls	200	Low intimacy	Severe event or major difficulty	1.0	4.5	19.6**
Parry & Shapiro (1986)	Working-class women	192	Low intimacy	Severe event or major difficulty	2.1*	2.11*	8.26
Salomon & Bromet (1982)	Rural mothers in Pennsylvania	432	Spouse not a confidant	Living near Three Mile Island	1.0	1.5*	2.9
Surtees (1980)	Follow-up of depressed outpatients	71	Available social support	Residual adversity	2.2*	1.9*	3.8

while others use chronic as well as onset cases. Perhaps the most stringent of all was the analysis by Bebbington et al (1984), which used onset cases, ratings of a severe event or major difficulty prior to onset, and a rating of pre-onset intimacy.

Methodological differences can probably account for only some of the differences in the magnitude of the effects revealed in these studies. Nevertheless, there is a degree of consistency in the studies, and particularly in those focusing on groups at higher risk for developing depression in the general population.

A number of cross-sectional multivariate studies have included a measure of coping style or personality. Two have reported a positive association between reports of 'seeking help from close others' and the severity of depression (Husaini et al 1982), or of mental health problems (Warheit et al 1982); both used cross-sectional data. Their findings are in line with the expectation that distressed individuals are more likely to seek help from others. However, any similar findings that emerged from a prospective study which controlled for the severity of initial symptoms would be important, as the amount of support that individuals receive (or report themselves as receiving) may be strongly related to help-seeking. Recent work by Brugha et al (1987b) does not support such a finding — these workers found no association between a measure of help-seeking and subsequent recovery from episodes of clinical depression.

The studies reviewed in this section confirm the importance of social support as a possible causal variable in a wide range of non-psychotic psychological and psychiatric disorders, when other variables have been taken into account. The data set out in Table 4.1 also suggest that the magnitude of the associations found is often quite large; the combined effect of adversity and support, whether additive or multiplicative, has been shown to be quite considerable in a number of studies. As indicated above, when adversity is also taken into account, there is some controversy about the importance of social support. This ranges from the view that support is irrelevant in the absence of adversity, to the view that the effect of adversity on psychological ill-health is not just additive, but is multiplied when support is deficient. However, the importance of these arguments also depends on the realisation that in many respects, adversity is not predictable and preventable, whereas poor social support is relatively more likely to be an ongoing problem that is identifiable and perhaps potentially alterable. As Parry & Shapiro (1986) have pointed out, if poor social support and adversity can be clearly shown to act causally on depression, a major issue for public health policy will arise from the need to devise preventive and treatment strategies for these common, distressing conditions. In the next section, prospective and experimental studies that are designed to answer the crucial question of causality will be discussed.

Prospective and experimental studies

Like experimental studies, prospective studies in which data are gathered from the same subjects at two or more points in time, are costly and technically demanding to carry out properly. Therefore, they can only be justified if prior research, of the kind already described here, lends some support to the suggestion that an important possible cause of an illness has been repeatedly demonstrated. In this section, a selection of such studies will be considered.

Di Mateo & Hays (1981) examined reports of studies in which social interventions were carried out in samples of seriously, physically ill adults; the findings were inconclusive, so that caution was recommended in designing and carrying out further intervention studies. Erickson (1984) has discussed case studies in which family therapy techniques are extended to the wider social network, but again, no specific, conclusive experimental studies are available. Broadhead et al (1983) pointed out that this field of research had not yet produced any notable experimental findings, but emphasised the potential importance of such research for public health policies, suggesting that we could soon expect to see large-scale studies. Since their review was published, two experimental studies have, in fact, been reported.

Parker & Barnett (1987) carried out a controlled, experimental intervention study on highly anxious primiparous mothers. The experimental treatment consisted of either lay or professional assistance, and it was hypothesised that improvement in the treated mothers would be due to the therapeutic ingredient of social support. The intervention cases did show a significant improvement, in contrast to the controls, but there was no evidence that this was due to a change in their reported levels of social support (as assessed by the ISSI). Accordingly, the results were not particularly clear-cut, and could not be said to confirm the social support hypothesis. Dalgard (1986, Dalgard et al 1986) having identified a group of socially isolated middle-aged women at high risk of minor psychiatric morbidity, commenced a long-term intervention experiment; the (randomised) experimental group were invited to take part in various group activities in the community. Long-term psychiatric patients have also been studied, but the results of this are not yet available. So far, the work has shown that the women's social participation and perceived quality of life improved, but the effects on their mental health are not clear; two sub-groups were identified, one much more socially active and the other more passive — the positive effects of increased participation in social activity having been only apparent in the first group (Dalgard et al 1986). This promises to be a very interesting and important piece of work.

In contrast to the lack of experimental work is the growing number of prospective, observational studies; their importance has been emphasised by many workers, in spite of the fact that such studies have neither the power nor precision of controlled, randomised experiments. A particularly important, fully reported study is that of Henderson et al (1981) in Canberra, Australia. This study raises a large number of important theoretical and technical issues, and it is important to give an outline of these.

Their measure of personal relationships — the ISSI — includes many of the elements contained in other less complete social support and social network measures, and as mentioned earlier, its theoretical rationale has received some empirical support (Duncan-Jones 1981). Trained lay interviewers were used to assess a random sample of the adult general population of Canberra. The GHQ (Goldberg 1972) was used in order to generate a probability sample, consisting of all those subjects with symptom scores above a defined, low cut-off point, as well as a sub-sample of individuals with very few or no symptoms. In a second phase of interviews, the Present State Examination (PSE) (Wing et al 1974) was administered to the probability sample. Approximately 170 subjects (representing about one-fifth of the original general population sample) were re-interviewed on three further occasions, over a 1-year period.

Before describing the results of the prospective data analysis, it is necessary to recapitulate the main cross-sectional findings; a multiple regression analysis was carried out on the data, using the Zung depression score as the dependent variable (Henderson et al 1980). Aside from the four dimensions of availability and adequacy of attachment, and of social integration, they also used 'the number of attachments with whom having rows' and an 'objective distress score for adverse experience in the previous 12 months'; this last variable accounted for only 2.2% of explained variance in men and 3.1% in women, once the ISSI variables had been taken into account. The ISSI variables, alone, accounted for a total of 15% of cumulative explained variance in men and 18.3% in women. Their measure of adverse experiences was based on a schedule of life events, previously validated in an Australian population (Tennant & Andrews 1976), and partly derived from the Social Readjustment Rating Scale (Holmes & Rahe 1967). However, it has been argued (Tennant et al 1981) that this method of quantifying life events is inferior to that developed by Brown et al (1975) and Brown & Harris (1978).

The analysis of data collected in this study from the respondents, who were re-interviewed at four-monthly intervals for one year (Henderson et al 1981), showed that in that half of the subjects exposed to the highest levels of adversity in the previous year, deficiencies in social relationships (again using the ISSI) explained 30% of the variance in GHQ scores four months later. However, they explained only 4% of the variance in the half with the lowest levels of adversity.

Similar multiple regression analyses on the four-month follow-up GHQ scores showed that two interaction terms (adversity × adequacy of attachment, adversity × adequacy of social integration) added significantly to the amount of variance accounted for by the adversity and ISSI variables independently (Henderson et al 1981). These analyses were conducted only on subjects who were well at the initial GHQ assessment.

A step-wise multiple regression analysis on the GHQ was administered at the 4-month follow-up interview of 169 subjects, all of whom had been well (non-cases) at the initial interview. A personality measure (the Neuroticism Scale from the EPQ) (Eysenck & Eysenck 1964), had also been administered to them, but unfortunately, only at follow-up and not at the initial interview. Nevertheless, neuroticism accounted for 9.4% of the variance in GHQ score, and the ISSI indices, entered subsequently, also accounted for about 9.4% of the variance. These workers also reported a very high positive correlation between the EPQ extraversion scale and measures of the reported availability of personal relationships.

Use was also made of other measures of 'affiliative tendency' and 'sensitivity to rejection', based on scales developed by Mehrabian (1970). Duncan-Jones (1983) carried out a number of complex, latent variable (multivariate) analyses on the longitudinal data. To reduce measurement error, measures at different points in time were averaged, so that it is more appropriate to regard some of the analyses as being cross-sectional (Henderson et al 1981); path analysis and structural equation modelling (Joreskog & Sorbom 1978) were used. According to the authors, these analyses suggest that the personality measures explain the largest amount of variance in GHQ scores. Stable background social factors, including early life events, also explain a significant, though lesser degree of variance, whereas recent adversity, together with ISSI indices of perceived adequacy and satisfaction with social integration, explain a very small amount of the variance. No other aspects of social relationships, including the availability measures in particular, explain any further variance in GHQ scores (Henderson et al 1981).

It is clear that these workers are aware of many of the study's imperfections (Henderson et al 1981), but one point to which they have paid relatively little attention is the possibility that contamination might exist between some of their independent measures, e.g. the ISSI and the life events measure. Their assumptions that the GHQ is a measure of acute neurotic symptoms and that the EPQ Neuroticism Scale is a measure of an enduring personality trait, also requires particularly critical examination, because of the weight that they have given to their findings which used these two measures. Elsewhere in the work, they report that the 8-month stability of EPQ-N is 0.89 (2 measures), but that of their illness measure (4 4-monthly assessments) is 0.87 — both remarkably stable measures (Table 10.1, Henderson et al 1981). Katz & McGuffin (1987) (already referred to earlier) have argued against the usefulness of EPQ-N in studies conducted on psychiatrically disordered samples, because it largely reflects state variation (symptoms) but trait variation (neuroticism) hardly at all. It remains to be seen whether the latent variable analysis technique can deal adequately with these notable methodological objections. If the EPQ is rejected, however, it appears that the explained variance in illness is accounted for by a combination of adversity, availability of attachment and social integration, affiliative tendency, sensitivity to rejection, and gender (Table 10.5, Henderson et al 1981).

The remarkable stability of the ISSI indices over time is also reported, but Henderson et al do not comment on the significance of the consequent insensitivity of such a measure in a prospective study of this kind. The stability of their measure of personal relationships over time is in itself one of the most interesting findings of their work and appears to be a characteristic of other similar measures (Brugha et al 1987a, Brugha 1988b). It suggests that attention should be given to tracing the developmental origins of these phenomena in early adult life, or even in the social functioning and experiences of childhood.

In spite of these reservations, this work is of importance and significance because of its size, the use of tested, standardised (and mainly interview) measures, and the relative sophistication of the sampling method used. However, it is possible that some of its results may have been over-influential, leading some to conclude (quite prematurely) that the association between deficiencies in social support and neurotic disorders is entirely explained by fixed personality traits in the individuals concerned. A more considered view would be that the conclusion that these workers have reached, concerning the importance of personality factors, raises more questions than it answers.

The importance of this study for social psychiatry relates also to the observation that it broadens the range of aetiological models which can be considered in further research. Furthermore, the criticisms that have followed it may also be of importance in stimulating future research. For example, as a result of the work, the assumption that social support is purely a contingent environmental phenomenon should now be regarded as even more questionable. Henderson et al have also placed on the agenda for future research — and ultimately perhaps for future policy in the health and social services — the need to consider both the individual and his social environment in developing aetiological models of psychiatric disorder. Whereas before, social support was seen as a product of the social environment that bolstered the person's psychological sturdiness, it may now be more appropriate to think of it as a commodity that is exchanged between actors in a continuous process; in this, each person is both provider and recipient, and each has influence on others and through others on himself (Brugha 1984b). The implications for social policy and for clinical practice will be discussed later.

A number of other prospective, observational studies have also appeared since 1980. Reference has already been made to the work of

Surtees (1980), in which 73 psychiatric outpatients were followed-up after approximately seven months (see Table 4.1). Similarly, Mann et al (1981) followed-up 100 attenders at primary health care clinics who had non-psychotic psychiatric disorders; their social support and stress interview (SSSI) scale was found to have contributed, to a small extent, to the one-year outcome score, once severity of initial psychiatric symptoms was controlled for. Williams et al (1981) followed-up 2234 adults in Washington DC; their dependent variable — a 30-item measure of anxiety, depression and positive well being (over the four weeks prior to assessment) — was independently related to each of three explanatory variables: a 9-item index of social contacts and resources, a measure of limitations on physical mobility and a measure of social desirability. Holahan & Moos (1981) carried out a 1-year follow-up of 267 multi-racial couples in San Francisco, using a measure of depression and psychosomatic symptoms. Both negative life change events and family and work relationships (assessing cohesion, expressiveness, involvement and conflict) predicted subsequent symptoms in the expected direction; in addition, when support was controlled for, life change still predicted symptoms.

Schaefer et al (1982) reduced the generalisability of their findings by studying a small sub-group of 100 men and women, aged 45 to 64, derived from a general population sample of 6928 adults, identified some years earlier. At the initial assessment, their own social support interview and questionnaire was used; this assessed informational, tangible, and emotional support from others. Data on guidance and information from the subject's primary social network in the previous month were also obtained, and a 24-item life events questionnaire administered. The Hopkins Symptoms Check List was used at a two-month follow-up interview. Whereas tangible support and contacts with the subject's social network were related to subsequent depression, emotional support and informational support were not. These workers paid special attention to the problems of contamination between exit life events and their social network measures. Their finding that subjective aspects of support (i.e. emotional and informational) were not related to morbidity, whereas social contacts were, is of particular interest because it goes against the argument that the important elements of support are purely subjective and may indeed be a reflection of actual disturbance within the individual, rather than a reflection of important factors in the social environment.

In other prospective studies, Aneshensel & Frederichs (1982) suggested that symptoms of depression and measures of social networks and social support are highly stable over time, while Turner & Noh (1983) found that social support and locus of control explained the increased responsiveness to stress in women of lower socio-economic status. Monroe et al (1983) carried out a 1-year follow-up of 175 college students, and found that depression, assessed by the Beck Depression Inventory (BDI; Beck et al 1961), was predicted by a self-completion life events scale, but was largely unrelated to a variety of social support measures. Husaini & Von Frank (1983) followed-up 235 subjects from an original mixed-race, general population sample of 676, over a 6–18 month period. They found that the CES-D score at follow-up was unrelated to life events (a 52-item list) and only weakly associated with social support, as assessed at the initial interview; they also found a very high correlation between the depression scores obtained at both interviews. In 1091 general population respondents, Lin & Ensel (1984) found a modest independent effect of adversity and social support, assessed at initial interview, on depression (CES-D), at a 1-year follow-up. Ferraro et al (1984) studied 2114 widowed, low-income, elderly community residents and found that those who had been widowed between one and four years before an initial interview went on to increase their friendship networks; however, age was inversely related to friendship and friendship support was more stable than measures of ill-health.

A significant prospective study has been reported from the Bedford College Group in London (O'Connor & Brown 1984, Brown et al 1986); 395 working-class mothers with children were studied, using a new instrument (SESS) measuring self-evaluation and social support, and 353 were followed-up after one year. Of the 32 women who then became depressed (measured on the PSE), 29 had had a provoking agent (a major life event or difficulty) in the six months before onset. Lack of crisis support from the husband and from very close friends (retrospectively assessed) was significantly related to the onset of depression in women with such an event or difficulty. However, in married women, the rating of a confiding relationship, which was assessed prospectively, was not related to the subsequent onset of depression. It was reported that an explanation had been found for the negative findings in married women; those who had confided initially and were subsequently 'let down' (i.e. did not receive crisis support that they expected to receive) were most likely to develop depression (Brown et al 1986). On the other hand, in unmarried women, they did find that the supportive quality of very close relationships was significantly associated with onset of depression.

A particularly interesting series of findings was based on ratings of statements by the mothers — 'Negative Evaluation of Self' (NES) was intended to form part of a measure of self-esteem (O'Connor & Brown 1984). NES was found to be strongly related both to the Time 1 (initial) social support measures and also to the likelihood that a provoking agent would be rated during the following year. The authors noted that NES predicted onset only in the mothers experiencing a provoking agent. The use of new and very detailed investigator-based assessments (SESS) in this prospective study, in conjuction with well established instruments (PSE and LEDS), seems sure to generate many hypotheses about the connections between personal relationships, adversity, self-esteem and depressive disorders.

It is apparent that the studies reviewed in this section are notable for the disparities between their findings. This may be partly due to the fact that different measures have been used on different population samples and, perhaps most important of all, with different lag times between the measurement of dependent and independent variables. Furthermore, it is quite clear from discussion and review of measures of social support (Brugha 1986, 1988b, Brugha et al 1987a) that relatively few workers have given sufficient attention to devising and evaluating such instruments. In this regard, the importance of characteristics of the individual which are termed personality, has been underlined by Henderson et al (1981) and more recently by Brown et al (1986).

In general, the association between deficiencies in social support and subsequent psychological morbidity appears to be stronger than the association between morbidity and previous life events. However, this apparent finding may have to be viewed with scepticism simply because the lag time between 'exposure' and onset of illness may be much more critical in the case of adversity, and studies employing longer lag times (typically greater than three months before onset) may conceal the strength of the association with illness. Brown et al (1986) have also emphasised the point that adversity cannot be adequately assessed without having recourse to retrospectively gathered data; in general, this drawback does not apply to the prospective assessment of support, but it suggests that attempts to examine the 'protective' effect of support against adversity will be equally difficult to achieve, unless a predictable life event like childbirth is made part of the research design.

The present author and colleagues have begun to report a prospective longitudinal study, with repeated measures separated by about four months. Approximately 120 adults from a defined inner-city population, who made contact with hospital-based psychiatric services complaining of depressed mood (Brugha 1986, Brugha et al 1987b, 1990) were studied. Using a new measure of social networks and support (Brugha et al 1987a), subsequent recovery was related to levels of support, when background clinical and socio-demographic factors and follow-up levels of EPQ neuroticism were controlled (Brugha et al 1990).

Thus, the prospective research is encouraging, but the field has become more complicated. Information available from the two experimental studies adds further impetus to the questions raised by the observational studies concerning the relative importance of the individual's own psychological make-up and that of wider inter-personal and social factors. Some of the results appear, on face value, to suggest that there is not a simple causal relationship between support and psychiatric disorder. For example, there may be a further clue in the observation by Dalgard et al (1986) that their sample of lonely middle-aged women appeared to include two distinct sub-groups, of which the second responded poorly to invitations to engage in greater social activity and fared less well in their subsequent pyschological status. This group may consist of women with distinctive personality traits that have contributed both to their psychological distress and to their social isolation; for them, a more appropriate intervention might consist in identifying the nature of these personality characteristics and trying to change them more directly or much earlier in life.

Both the observational and the experimental research suggest that public health strategies, whether remedial or preventive, may have to consider interventions aimed at changing either or both the social environment and the personality characteristics of the individuals at high risk. Primary prevention may even have to be implemented in childhood.

Studies initiated in childhood

Published data on social support, gathered prospectively in childhood with a follow-up assessment of psychiatric disorder in adulthood, appear to be absent. Puig-Antich et al (1985), using a newly developed method with which they claim to be able to measure depression in prepubertal children, have reported on 75 depressed children in whom, compared with 40 normal controls, quantitative and qualitative reductions occurred in social activities with friends, independent of parental marital atmosphere. A follow-up study of 21 of the depressed children showed that most of these deficits cleared up, on recovery from the episode of depression. Rutter & Quinton (1984) compared the adult functioning of 89 women who had been reared in residential children's homes with a group of 41, sampled from the same area, all of whom had previously been studied in childhood by means of standardised questionnaires. The adult outcome of the institution-reared women was substantially worse, but where they were found to be in good psychosocial circumstances in adulthood (supported by a 'good' husband or boyfriend), they functioned as well as the comparison group. Although institution-reared women were more likely to marry men with problems or to be unmarried, their scores in childhood, on a questionnaire measure of deviance, did not predict the quality of their marital relationship status as adults. It is regrettable that the opportunity to assess the adult psychiatric status of these women comprehensively was missed, although criminality and personality disorder were assessed.

Retrospectively gathered data on conduct disturbance in childhood in over 9000 adults in three ECA (Epidemiological Catchment Area Program) centres in the USA were examined in relation to adult psychiatric status (Robins 1985). Although conduct disturbance was much rarer in the childhood of the women, it predicted depressive disorders, anxiety states, and other non-psychotic disorders in adult women, but not in men; conduct disturbance also increased the likelihood of life events in adulthood being reported, particularly in women. The disadvantages of such retrospective data are acknowledged by the author. Similar earlier work from the same group (Helzer et al 1976) showed that both adverse combat experiences and subsequent depression could be predicted, in returned Vietnam veterans, on the basis of similar retrospective behavioural ratings preceding adulthood. The need for prospective studies, using the best possible measures at both life stages, is undeniable.

Studies of categories of non-psychotic psychiatric disorder

The need to consider categories or types of psychiatric disorder has already been mentioned in the section on methodology. Traditionally, in clinical practice, the functional psychiatric disorders have been divided into sub-categories. For example, depressive disorders are often divided into 'neurotic' and 'endogenous' types, the latter applying to cases that feature symptoms such as appetite and weight loss and diurnal variation in depressed mood. Cases of depression that include the presence of hallucinations and delusions are either subsumed within the endogenous category or are considered separately as part of a third 'psychotic' category. The widespread imprecise use of these terms has been countered in recent times by the introduction of operationally defined systems of psychiatric classification that make it possible to test the utility of these categories, but very few research workers have made use of these 'research diagnoses' in studies of social support and psychiatric disorders.

Billings & Moos (1984) compared newly referred cases of Research Diagnostic Criteria (RDC) minor and major depression (Spitzer et al 1978) with cases attending psychiatric services for a year. No differences were found between these two categories in relation to such social resources as: number of friends, number of network contacts, quality of significant relationships, etc. In a replication of the patient's primary group study (Henderson et al 1978), Brugha et al (1982) found very similar deficiencies in the social networks of patients with neurotic depression (as defined in the N class of the CATEGO4 program) (Wing et al 1974). In contrast, patients with retarded depression (class R) showed no differences from matched normal general population controls on measures of social interaction, although, as in the case of neurotic depressives, they did nominate significantly smaller primary groups. Although this finding has not been replicated in more recent work (Brugha 1986, Brugha et al 1987b), it does appear from the results of the longitudinal study, referred to in the previous section and reported in the same paper (Brugha et al 1987b), that there may be a stronger relationship between social support and recovery in 'neurotic' than in 'endogenous' cases of depression, using the PSE-CATEGO measurement and classification system.

There have been no studies in which acute and chronic cases are compared, and further work is clearly required in this area. The few results that are available, however, suggest that it is important to use reliable measures, of the kind referred to above, that permit operationally defined classification systems to be taken into consideration, when testing hypotheses about the relationship between psychiatric disorder and social support. This is because intervention strategies may differ in their effectiveness, depending upon the type of psychiatric disorder studied.

Studies conducted on major functional psychotic disorders

Reviewing the literature on social networks and social support in the schizophrenias, Henderson (1980) has pointed out that 'it has proved very difficult to know the direction of causality: whether the social variable... was altered by the psychosis or its prodromata, including premorbid personality; or whether the social variable contributed appreciably to the onset, if not the course of the disease and other people's response to it'. Additional to these fundamental difficulties is the realisation that much of the literature on social functioning in these disorders (e.g. Isele et al 1985) appears to stem from the idea that this group of patients have major deficits in social role performance which seem to be an integral part of their clinical condition. However, some authors (e.g. Wallace 1984) have tried to argue that these findings should be looked upon as indicators of vulnerability to these disorders, rather than solely as their consequences.

The possibility that people with major psychotic disorders may be unreliable sources of information about their own social worlds has been partly circumscribed by the work, discussed elsewhere in this book (Ch.6), on Expressed Emotion in schizophrenia. By conducting detailed assessments of the social behaviour of close relatives living with the patient, highly significant associations with symptomatic relapse have been demonstrated repeatedly, both in observational and experimental research. This direction of enquiry is likely to continue to yield considerable theoretical, and in all likelihood, practical benefits.

However, there remain many chronic psychotic patients who are no longer supported by their families. A number of studies have suggested that their level of social isolation is a crucial factor in determining their successful survival in the community (Grusky et al 1985, Sultan & Johnson 1985, Harris et al 1986). More rigorous research on the role of social support in the course of these often severely disabling conditions is clearly warranted. In the meantime, it is far from clear what interpretation can be placed on the association between deficits in social networks and support on the one hand, and the major, and in particular, the long-term functional psychoses on the other.

DISCUSSION

Issues arising from the theoretical and empirical literature

In this chapter, which so far has been largely concerned with reviewing the literature on personal relationships and psychiatric disorders (the empirical literature being almost exclusively concerned with non-psychotic disorders), a number of difficulties have been encountered, both in theory and in methodology. Attention now needs to be given to the implications of what has been established and to what can be said, in a very tentative way, about management principles in clinical practice as well as the wider, future implications of this work for the health and social services.

Some of the problems that have arisen in the results of empirical research can be traced back to a number of conceptual and theoretical difficulties. There are several misgivings about the theoretical basis for separating social support (and other models of social functioning) from other concepts such as adversity, personality, and non-psychotic psychiatric disorder. Some evidence has been presented for overlaps between measures, which leads to significant problems of inference. Whilst such difficulties may appear inevitable in social and psychological research of this kind, it is important that the results of empirical research should be judged carefully, in the light of these kinds of criticisms. The work of Brown et al (1975, Brown & Harris 1978), in which considerable effort was devoted to refining a measure of adversity in order to establish a clear separation from a measure of psychopathology, is a notable example of what can be achieved.

In spite of the considerable volume of recent work, it remains unclear whether the reported deficiencies in the personal relationships of psychologically disturbed and distressed individuals are causes or epiphenomena of these disorders. In particular, findings from the few experimental, as well as from some of the prospective investigations, do not provide clear evidence for a causal model in which deficiences in personal relationships (or their provisions) give rise to psychiatric disorders. However, the quality of prospective observational research is improving and more persuasive findings can be expected.

Other factors, in particular adversity and personality factors, may also play a crucial role in the association, but progress will, of course, depend on the development of better measures of personality factors. Aetiological models are likely to become increasingly complex: for example, it has already been pointed out that there may be evidence for the hypothesis that personality characteristics increase the likelihood that an individual will experience adversity (Robins 1985, Brown et al 1986, Rutter & Quinton 1984). Others have noted similar associations; Henderson et al (1981) found that the EPQ-N predicted a higher score on a life events scale, although it was not altogether clear whether this analysis was prospective. This is an interesting and important line of enquiry, since it has been pointed out above that personality factors may also influence how the individual seeks crisis support, when faced with difficulties. Unfortunately, psychologists have been almost alone in studying the dynamics of help-seeking, and their work has been almost invariably on normal subjects (Williams & Williams 1983). Not only might effective social support from others depend on the individual making known her needs, but it could also be argued that individuals who frequently convey to others their perceived needs for support, whilst rarely having the opportunity to 'give something back in return', may lose friends more quickly than they gain them. 'Being let down' can also be looked upon as 'expecting too much'. But on the other hand, inequity is almost inevitable in the personal relationships of people with major physical (and mental) handicaps. Before further large-scale intervention studies can be embarked upon, it is important to explore these issues further.

Much of the literature is also marred by the use of poorly devised measures of personal relationships and social support (Brugha 1986); good research, yielding interpretable results, is costly and time-consuming. A wide variety of measures of personal relationships have been employed, but few have the conceptual or psychometric sophistication to make them worth using in replication studies. Those embarking on new research in this area would do well to consider using existing standardised interview measures such as the ISSI, SESS, and the IMSR, rather than attempting to add further to the long list of new measures that make comparative research and replication studies a rare and distant dream. The choice of which measure to use will depend on resources, on the aim of the study, and in particular, on whether replication is being attempted. As in social psychiatry research, in general, replication studies are the exception rather than the rule; this deficiency is of especial relevance in an area where precision is difficult to achieve, and wisdom suggests that one should only rely on findings that have been repeated independently and often.

Two reasonably firm findings can be adduced from the literature. First, that perceived numerical and qualitative deficiences in close personal relationships are now well established associations of non-psychotic disorders, both in the general population and in hospital-treated cases. With certain qualifications, the same conclusion can be drawn in relation to functional psychotic disorders. Secondly, in a number of studies, these findings have been shown to exist independently of the experience of adversity. The question, therefore, is no longer 'should we count personal relationships in psychiatric disorders?', but rather, 'why do personal relationships count in psychiatric disorders?'.

Several lines of enquiry are needed. First, since these findings all derive from informants who are themselves the object of study, are they a reflection of actual social behaviour, or alternatively a reflection of negative cognitive perceptions? This question suggests a number of hypotheses and lines of research; the most challenging task, technically, is the collection of data that can be shown to represent actual social behaviour (Brugha 1986). Some measures of personal relationships, including the ISSI and the IMSR, are remarkably stable over time (Brugha et al 1987a), and attention needs to be directed towards developmental aspects of social interaction — the formation and duration of peer relationships from pre-school age onwards. Although parenting style seems to be the most popular potential influence to look at in this area (Parker 1984), developmental psychology has also emphasised the importance of the influence that the child's behaviour has on adults (Rutter & Hersov 1985). Both temperamental characteristics and early social experiences could be considered in this respect.

In spite of the tentative nature of what can already be said to be known about the relationship between social support and psychiatric morbidity, this account would be incomplete without making some attempt to consider what practical benefits can be gleaned from the theoretical and empirical literature.

Management principles

It should be clear that what follows cannot be said to be based on experimental evidence; apart from the single, and very particular, example of intervention with personal relationships in cases of schizophrenia where the patient is in high contact with a 'high EE' relative, there is in effect no such evidence to fall back on. In addition, most of what follows will primarily be relevant to people with non-psychotic disorders (i.e. psychiatric disorders in which hallucinations, delusions, or subjectively described experiences of thought disorder do not dominate the clinical presentation).

An approach that has been found to be of some use in ordinary clinical work, and which should be thought of as complementing all the usual general enquiries and investigations recommended in current clinical practice, begins with an enquiry about the patient's social network and the support it provides. Sokolove & Trimble (1986) have suggested a set of 14 questions that can be used during an interview with a patient who has been in long-term contact with psychiatric services. It can also be important to consider the nature of the psychopathology, and how this may affect and be affected by such social factors. A 'social' formulation based upon this information, a set of 'therapeutic' aims, and a consideration of the methods to be employed in attempting to achieve these aims should also precede any attempts to intervene.

Describing the social network and social supports

Customarily, description begins by adding to the information already gathered about the family — focusing on the location of members, their frequency of contact, and the kinds of transactions that occur, then moving on to a consideration of the strength of relationships in terms of 'felt attachment', the ability and tendency to confide, and the degree to which these qualities appear to be reciprocated. Where the patient is married or has a close sexual relationship, particular attention is given to this relationship under these headings. The enquiry then moves out towards the wider social network of close friends, neighbours, and work associates (particularly if they are also regarded as 'friends', 'acquaintances', 'mates', etc,. Again, it seems useful to enquire about recent social interaction, its nature and context, and in particular, whether there have been planned social events involving these others which are not ordinarily a necessary part of work or routine events in the community (e.g. church attendance). Where, as is often the case, a major significant life event has occurred recently, the transmission of information between other members of the network concerning such events can also be enquired about.

There are two elements to the enquiry about social support: the first concerns itself with action taken by the patient (help- and support-eliciting, where this seems to be appropriate), and the second concerns the behaviour and action of others. With reference to material aid (tangible support), it can be particularly revealing to enquire about the degree to which transactions of this kind occur in both directions (sometimes termed 'equity' in a dyadic relationship). In trying to make a judgement about the quality of emotional support, it is important to ask questions that reveal something of the capacity of those involved to identify sources of distress, to tolerate unpleasant news and the feelings that go with it, and to empathise with the person who is distressed. A simple set of questions can focus, on the one hand, on how easy or difficult it is for the patient to listen to someone else who has something distressing to discuss, and on the other hand to ask whether one felt that the other person was really listening and was interested in something important that one wished to discuss. When these questions focus on what actually happened during a recent crisis, they may reveal a great deal about other potentially important elements such as coping style, personality, and the degree to which elements of an individual's psychopathology directly impinge on social interaction.

Psychopathological issues

The possibility has also to be considered that symptoms such as pathological guilt, subjective retardation, irritability, and simple ideas of reference, which may be elements of the clinical picture, may significantly inhibit the quality and quantity of social interaction between a patient and his/her social network. Equally, this principle may also extend to other members of the network who are distressed or have problems in psychological functioning.

A second important issue that must be considered in relation to possible intervention strategies is the extent to which a patient's vulnerability to stress or the nature of his psychopathology may contraindicate any significant attempts to increase social stimulation (with its inevitable demands) from others. Some examples of this might include patients suffering from acute exacerbations of symptoms with a persecutory content, or those with fundamental social handicaps that greatly limit their capacity to interact with others, as for example occurs in cases of Asperger's syndrome (or schizoid personality disorder).

Formulating a management plan

Based on this kind of information about the patient's own social network and supports, it may be possible to produce a 'social formulation' that summarises the difficulties and possible routes for action.

A set of aims, both for the patient's social functioning and for those in the wider social network, should then be recorded. Common to all such situations is the aim of bringing about an improvement in the patient's own perception of the quality of transactions with others, particularly with those with whom it is appropriate to share information about feelings, worries and hopes. In addition, not only does the quality of confiding relationships appear to matter, but an extension of the range of different kinds of relationships and their functions (sometimes referred to as multiplex relationships) should be aimed for, as these also appear to be indicative of a better level of functioning. Specific methods can then be set out that are designed to try to achieve these aims (bearing in mind the need to consider both the short-term and long-term effects on the course of the psychiatric disturbance). The methods used will be familiar to those working in the field of rehabilitation — training and skill enhancement, monitoring of goals, and making use of feedback from others. For those who do not or cannot respond to these learning strategies, sheltered social amenities and the use of visual and verbal reminders and cues by staff or relatives should be provided, possibly on a long-term basis.

Clearly, the clinician (or social worker, psychologist, occupational therapist, nurse) must be open to the potential value of changing the patient's social perceptions and behaviour, and also to the value of modifying the behaviour and perceptions of others in the network. Examples of the kind of action to be taken can range from a relatively brief set of guidelines to the patient on how to make better use of potential social resources in their network, to a more detailed series of counselling sessions, incorporating both insight building and specific directions on social behaviour and social interaction with others. A series of counselling sessions also offer the important opportunity both of monitoring the results of directive advice and the possibility of modifying it in order to increase the patient's effectiveness in transactions with others. There may, of course, be some parallels between this approach and that of social skills and problem-solving training, although the important distinction between them lies in the way the approach is specifically tailored to the particular social relationships that the patient is developing with others in his network.

It may also be useful to intervene directly through others by working with a couple, a family, key members of a community, or at the place of work. An example of the latter is the way in which social isolation due to the stigma of being labelled a psychiatric patient can be overcome by making direct links with employers, key figures in personnel departments, or employee organisations. Where these strategies are effective, they may lead others in the social network to change their ideas (or perhaps more specifically their own expectations) about the patient's personality. The adoption of a more realistic and also a less negative set of attitudes may well be highly therapeutic; there are some ways in which the experimental modification of relatives' perceptions, as in the work — referred to above — of Leff and others on Expressed Emotion, may also be producing a beneficial effect in a like manner. As Mischel (1973) pointed out, one of the most curious things about the concept of personality is the tendency for people to hold strong convictions about its usefulness as a predictor of behaviour in others, in spite of their reluctance to accept such views about themselves and in the absence of any real evidence for the value of this supposition.

By extending management principles that are already used by many workers in the mental health field, it may be possible, through use of the social support/network model, to identify more effective ways of maintaining or enhancing the social integration of psychologically disturbed or impaired persons. It is to be hoped that experience gained through such efforts may provide further guidance on more specific intervention strategies that might subsequently survive the rigorous test of experiment.

Implications for the health and social services

A great deal has been written in recent years about the psychosocial management of patients and particularly, of chronic patients who may have difficulty in living outside institutions. Indeed, one of the puzzling things about the literature on social support is that the work on non-psychotic and minor disorders is almost exclusively exploratory, with a growing and impressive body of empirical knowledge, whereas that on the long-term disorders includes a great deal of discussion about policy, management, and services, but a stark paucity of empirical data.

Whittaker & Garbarino (1984) have used the social support model to urge the expansion of informal and voluntary agencies, while Gottlieb's book (1983) uses the same model to discuss rehabilitation services. Many others use the term 'social network' in discussions of policy and management (e.g. Cohen & Adler 1986, Gottlieb 1985, Taylor et al 1984, Harris et al 1986–7, Morin & Seidman 1986). Of these, perhaps the most acceptable general statement on management and policy at the present time is that of Gottlieb (1985), when he urges us to be cautious of programmes that involve the mobilisation of formal helpers (i.e. trained 'supporters') in the community, preferring instead approaches based on encouraging those who appear to need additional support to participate in self-help groups, sharing their difficulties and problem-solving strategies with 'fellow-sufferers'. Of course, there exists also a smaller group of long-term patients who will need 'support in the community' from more formal agencies with trained staff, such as social workers and community psychiatric nurses, who provide or facilitate access to a range of different forms of social and clinical care (Brugha et al 1988).

This overview of the social support literature in psychiatric disorders seems to point fairly clearly in several directions. Deficiencies in social networks and social support are a risk factor for virtually all forms of psychiatric disorder, and ultimately an explanation for this phenomenon is very likely to have a bearing on both intervention and prevention. Research based on the social network approach may identify patterns of social behaviour and organisation, whether in families, neighbourhoods, work places, or institutions that predict psychiatric morbidity and that can be modified. Research on the nature of social support, particularly in close, confiding relationships, may tell us a great deal about the form of social transactions that increase the risk of psychiatric morbidity; the work on Expressed Emotion is relevant and promising in this regard. Research into the personality characteristics that correlate with perceived deficits in social support may lead to intervention strategies that require alterations in behaviour and cognitions by means of learning techniques; they may also lead to methods of early detection of individuals who are at high risk (particularly at times of considerable life change and stress) and who may, therefore, benefit from such training at an early stage in life — e.g. during primary and secondary education, when first taking up employment, or during pregnancy. Such training might include promoting awareness and knowledge of the importance of relationships, emphasising the need to be cooperative (giving as well as accepting) and to be consciously aware of competitive behaviour in oneself and in others, as well as examining, in discussion with an appropriate peer group, the individual's own personal experiences in these areas. Accordingly, both the social environment and the individual at risk of illness might become the object of intervention on rational lines, consistent with existing, and more particularly, future observational and experimental research findings.

When knowledge of effective intervention techniques becomes

available, questions will arise about the cost of their implementation. Health, social, and quite possibly educational services may well be required to contribute. As the present cost to society, direct and indirect, of psychiatric morbidity is very considerable (Brugha 1986), we are unlikely to have to wait very long for support from studies of costs and benefits, once effective techniques have been found. In the meantime, it cannot be presumed that the methods will be simple and straight-forward — indeed, if they were, they might well have been identified long ago. It is for this reason that it would be far wiser to wait until we are sure that we have the correct prescription.

Acknowledgement

I would like to thank Paul Bebbington of the MRC Social Psychiatry Unit for his invaluable advice and criticism of earlier versions of this chapter.

Note. Since completing this chapter, the author has published three update reviews in the journal *Current Opinion in Psychiatry* which cover recent significant developments in the field since 1988 (Brugha 1988, 1989, 1990).

REFERENCES

Alderson M 1983 An introduction to epidemiology. MacMillan, London

Alloway R, Bebbington P 1987 The buffer theory of social support — a review of the literature. Psychological Medicine 17: 91-108

Andreason N C 1982 Concepts, diagnosis and classification. In: Paykel E S (ed) Handbook of affective disorders. Churchill Livingstone; Edinburgh

Andrews G, Schonell M, Tennant C 1977 The relation between physical, psychological, and social morbidity in a suburban community. American Journal of Epidemiology 105: 324-329

Andrews G, Tennant C, Hewson D, Schonell M 1978 The relation of social factors to physical and psychiatric illness. American Journal of Epidemiology 108: 27-35

Aneshensel C S, Frederichs R R 1982 Stress, support and depression: a longitudinal causal model. Journal of Community Psychology 10: 363-376

Barnes J A 1954 Class and committee in a Norwegian island parish. Human Relations 7: 39-58

Bebbington P E 1985 Aetiology of schizophrenia and affective disorders — psychosocial. In: Michels R (ed) Psychiatry. Lippincott, Philadelphia

Bebbington P E, Tennant C, Hurry J 1981 Adversity and the nature of psychiatric disorder in the community. Journal of Affective Disorders 3: 345-366

Bebbington P E, Tennant C, Sturt E, Hurry J 1984 Misfortune and resilience: a community study of women. Psychological Medicine 14: 347-364

Beck A T, Ward C H, Mendelson M, Mock J, Erbaugh J 1961 An inventory for measuring depression. Archives of General Psychiatry 4: 561-571

Berkman L F, Syme S L 1979 Social networks, host resistance and mortality. A nine year follow-up study of Alameda county residents. American Journal of Epidemiology 109: 186-204

Billings A G, Moos R H 1982 Social support and functioning among community and clinical groups: a panel model. Journal of Behavioural Medicine 5: 295-312

Billings A G, Moos R H 1984 Chronic and non-chronic unipolar depression. The differential role of environmental stressors and resources. Journal of Nervous and Mental Disease 172: 65-75

Blazer D G 1983 Impact of late-life depression on the social network. American Journal of Psychiatry 140: 162-166

Bowlby J 1969 Attachment and loss volume 1: attachment. Penguin, Harmondsworth

Bowlby J 1977 The making and breaking of affectional bonds I. Aetiology and psychopathology in the light of attachment theory. British Journal of Psychiatry 130: 201-210

Brewin C R 1985 Depression and causal attributions. What is their relation? Psychological Bulletin 98: 297-309

Broadhead W E, Kaplan B H, James S A et al 1983 The epidemiologic evidence for a relationship between social support and health. American Journal of Epidemiology 117: 621-637

Brown G W, Harris T O 1978 Social origins of depression. Tavistock, London

Brown G W, Prudo R 1981 Psychiatric disorder in a rural and an urban population: 1. Aetiology of depression. Psychological Medicine 11: 581-599

Brown G W, Ni Bhrolchain M, Harris T 1975 Social class and psychiatric disturbance among women in an urban population. Sociology 9: 225-254

Brown G W, Andrews B, Harris T, Adler Z, Bridge L 1986 Social support self-esteem and depression. Psychological Medicine 16: 813-831

Brugha T 1981 Social support, social network research and the psychiatric patient. (Mimeo, available from author)

Brugha T 1984a Needs for care: developing and evaluating services for the chronically mentally ill. Irish Journal of Psychiatry 5: 10-13

Brugha T 1984b Personal losses and deficiencies in social networks. Social Psychiatry 19: 69-74

Brugha T S 1986 Depressive disorders and personal relationships. MD Thesis. National University of Ireland, Dublin

Brugha T S 1988a Social support. Current opinion in Psychiatry 1: 206–211

Brugha T S 1988b Social psychiatry. In: Thompson C (ed) Instruments of psychiatric research. Wiley, Chichester

Brugha T S, Conroy R 1985 Categories of depression: reported life events in a controlled design. British Journal of Psychiatry 147: 641-646

Brugha T S, Conroy R, Walsh N et al 1982 Social networks, attachments and support in minor affective disorders: a replication. British Journal of Psychiatry 141: 249-255

Brugha T S, Sturt E, MacCarthy B, Potter J, Wykes T, Bebbington P E 1987a The interview measure of social relationships: the description and evaluation of a survey instrument for assessing personal social resources. Social Psychiatry 22: 123-128

Brugha T S, Bebbington P E, MacCarthy B, Potter J, Sturt E, Wykes T 1987b Social networks, social support and the type of depressive illness. Acta Psychiatrica Scandinavica 76: 664-673

Brugha T S, Wing J K, Brewin C R, MacCarthy S, Lesage A, Mumford J 1988 The problems of people in long-term psychiatric day care: an introduction to the Camberwell High Contact Survey. Psychological Medicine 18: 443-456

Brugha T S, Bebbington P E, MacCarthy B, Sturt E, Wykes T, Potter J 1990 Gender, social support and recovery from depressive disorders: a prospective clinical study. Psychological Medicine 20: 147-156

Bruhn J G, Philips B U 1984 Measuring social support: a synthesis of current approaches. Journal of Behavioral Medicine 7: 151-169

Campbell E A, Cope S J, Teasdale J D 1983 Social factors and affective disorder: an investigation of Brown & Harris's Model. British Journal of Psychiatry 143: 548-554

Caplan G 1974 Support systems. In: Caplan G (ed) Support systems and community mental health. Basic Books, New York

Cassel J 1976 The contribution of the social environment to host resistance. American Journal of Epidemiology 104: 107-123

Catalano R, Dooley C D 1977 The economic predictors of depressed mood and stressful life events in a metropolitan community. Journal of Health and Social Behaviour 18: 292-307

Cobb S 1976 Social support as a moderator of life stress. Psychosomatic Medicine 38: 300-314

Cohen C I, Adler A 1986 Assessing the role of social network interventions within an inner city population. American Journal of Orthopsychiatry 56: 278-288

Cohen C I, Sokolovsky J 1978 Schizophrenia and social networks: ex-patients in the inner city. Schizophrenia Bulletin 4: 546-560

Cohen S, Haberman H M 1983 Positive events and social supports as buffers of life change stress. Journal of Applied Social Psychology 13: 99-125

Cohen S, Wills T A 1985 Stress, social support and the buffering hypothesis. Psychological Bulletin 98: 310-357

Cooke D J 1987 The significance of life events as a cause of psychological and physical disorders. In: Cooper B (ed) Psychiatric epidemiology, progress and prospects. Croom Helm, London

Cooley C H 1909 Social organisation: a study of the larger mind. Scribner, New York

Coyne J C 1976a Depression and the response of others. Journal of Abnormal Psychology 85: 186-193

Coyne J C 1976b Toward an interactional description of depression. Psychiatry 39: 28-40

Dalgard O S 1980 Mental health, neighbourhood and related social variables in Oslo. Acta Scandinavica Psychiatrica 62, Supplement No 285: 298-304

Dalgard O S 1986 Epidemiology as a basis for preventive intervention. Acta Psychiatrica Belgica 86: 470-475

Dalgard O S, Anstorp T, Benum K, Sorensen T, Moum T 1986 Social psychiatric field studies in Oslo. Some preliminary results. Paper read at: Second International Kurt Lewin Conference, Philadelphia

D'Arcy C, Siddique C M 1984 Social support and mental health among mothers of preschool and school age children. Social Psychiatry 19: 155-162

Di Matteo M R, Hays R 1981 Social support and serious illness. In: Gottlieb B H (ed) Social networks and social support. Sage, London

Dohrenwend B S, Dohrenwend B P 1974 Overview and prospects for research on stressful life events. In: Dohrenwend B S, Dohrenwend B P (eds) Stressful life events: their nature and effects. Wiley, New York

Duncan-Jones P 1981 The structure of social relationships: analysis of a survey instrument. Part 1. Social Psychiatry 16: 55-61

Duncan-Jones P 1983 On the aetiology of neurotic illness in the general population. Paper read to MRC Social Psychiatry Unit, Institute of Psychiatry, London.

Durkheim E 1951 Suicide: a study in sociology. Trans. Spaulding J, Simpson G. Free Press, New York

Erickson G 1984 A framework and themes for social network intervention. Family Process 23: 187-198

Everitt B S, Dunn G 1983 Advanced methods of data exploration and modelling. Heinemann, London

Eysenck H J, Eysenck S B G 1964 Manual of the Eysenck Personality Inventory. London University Press, London

Faris R E L, Dunham M W 1939 Mental disorders in urban areas. University of Chicago Press, Chicago

Ferraro K, Mutray E, Barresi C M 1984 Widowhood, health, and friendship support in later life. Journal of Health and Social Behavior 25: 245-259

Firth J, Brewin C 1982 Attributions and recovery from depression: a preliminary study using cross-lagged correlation analysis. British Journal of Clinical Psychology 21: 229-230

Fischer C S 1982 To dwell among friends, personal networks in town and city. University of Chicago Press, Chicago

Frydman M I 1981 Social support, life events and psychiatric symptoms: a study of direct, conditional and interaction effects. Social Psychiatry 16: 69-78

Goldberg D P 1972 The detection of psychiatric illness by questionnaire. Oxford University Press, London

Gore S 1978 The effect of social support in moderating the health consequences of unemployment. Journal of Health & Social Behavior 19: 157-165

Gottlieb B H 1983 Social support strategies: guidelines for mental health. Sage, London

Gottlieb B H 1985 Social networks and social support: an overview of research, practice and policy implications. Health Education Quarterly 12: 5-22

Grusky O, Tierney K, Manderscheid R W, Grusky D 1985 Social bonding and community adjustment of chronically mentally ill adults. Journal of Health & Social Behavior 26: 49-63

Harris M, Bergman H C, Bachrach C C 1986 Psychiatric and non-psychiatric indicators for rehospitalisation in a chronic patient population. Hospital & Community Psychiatry 37: 630-631

Harris M, Bergman H C, Bachrach C C 1986-7 Individualised network planning for chronic psychiatric patients. Psychiatric Quarterly 58: 51-56

Hammer M 1980 Social access and the clustering of personal connections. Social Networks 2: 305-325

Hammer M 1981 Social supports, social networks, and schizophrenia. Schizophrenia Bulletin 7: 45-57

Hammer M, Makiesky-Barrow S, Guthwirth L 1978 Social networks and schizophrenia. Schizophrenia Bulletin 4: 522-545

Heard D M, Lake B 1986 The attachment dynamic in adult life. British Journal of Psychiatry 149: 430-438

Helzer J E, Robins L N, Darlene H D 1976 Depressive disorders in Vietnam returnees. The Journal of Nervous and Mental Disease 163: 177-185

Henderson S 1977 The social network, support and neurosis. British Journal of Psychiatry 131: 185-191

Henderson S 1980 A development in social psychiatry: the systematic study of social bonds. Journal of Nervous & Mental Diseases 168: 63-69

Henderson S, Duncan-Jones P, McAuley H, Ritchie K 1978 The patient's primary group. British Journal of Psychiatry 132: 74-86

Henderson S, Byrne D G, Duncan-Jones P, Scott R, Adcock S 1980 Social relationships, adversity and neurosis: a study of associations in a general population sample. British Journal of Psychiatry 136: 574-583

Henderson S, Byrne D G, Duncan-Jones P 1981 Neurosis and the Social Environment. Academic Press, Sydney

Hinde R A 1978 Interpersonal relationships in search of a science. Psychological Medicine 8: 373-386

Hinde R A 1979 Towards understanding relationships. Academic Press, London

Hirshfeld R M A, Klerman G, Andreason N C et al 1985 Situational major depressive disorder. Archives of General Psychiatry 42: 1109-1114

Holahan C J, Moos R H 1981 Social support and psychological distress: a longitudinal analysis. Journal of Abnormal Psychology 90: 365-370

Holmes T H, Rahe R H 1967 The social readjustment rating scale. Journal of Psychosomatic Research 11: 213-218

Hurry J, Sturt E 1981 Social performance in a population sample — relation to psychiatric symptoms. In: Wing J K, Bebbington P E, Robins L (eds) What is a case: the problem of definition in psychiatric community surveys. Grant McIntyre, London

Husaini B A, Neff A J 1980 Characteristics of life events and psychiatric impairment in rural communities. Journal of Nervous & Mental Diseases 168: 159-166

Husaini B A, Von Frank A 1983 Life events, coping resources and depression: a longitudinal study of direct, buffering and reciprocal effects.

Husaini B A, Neff A J, Newbrough J R, Moore M C 1982 The stress buffering role of social support and personal competence among the rural married. Journal of Community Psychology 10: 409-426

Isele R, Merz J, Malzachen M, Augst J 1985 Social disability in schizophrenia: the controlled prospective Burgholzli study I.I. Premorbid living situation and social adjustment — comparison with a normal control sample. European Archives of Psychiatry & Neurological Science 234: 348-356

Jenkins R, Mann A H, Belsey E 1981 The background, design and use of a short interview to assess social stress and support in research and clinical settings. Social Science & Medicine 15: 195-203

Joreskog K G, Sorbom D 1978 Lisrel IV: analysis of linear structural relationships by the method of maximum likelihood. International Educational Services, Chicago

Kandel D B, Davies M 1982 Epidemiology of depressive mood in adolescents. Archives of General Psychiatry 39: 1205-1212

Katz R, McGuffin P 1987 Neuroticism in familial depression. Psychological Medicine 17: 155-161

Keller M B, Shapiro R W, Lavori P W, Wolf N 1982a Recovery in major depressive disorder. Archives of General Psychiatry 39: 905-910

Keller M B, Shapiro R W, Lavori P W, Wolf N 1982b Relapse in major depressive disorder. Archives of General Psychiatry 39: 911-915

Kreitman N, Collins J, Nelson B, Troop J 1970 Neurosis and marital interaction: I Personality and symptoms. British Journal of Psychiatry 117: 33-46

La Rocco J, House J S, French J R 1980 Social support, occupational stress and health. Journal of Health & Social Behavior 21: 202-218

Leaf P J, Weissman M M, Myers J K, Tischler G L, Holzer C E 1984 Social factors related to psychiatric disorder: the Yale Epidemiologic Catchment Area Study. Social Psychiatry 19: 53-61

Liem R, Liem J 1978 Social class and mental illness reconsidered: the role of economic stress and social support. Journal of Health & Social Behavior 19: 139-156

Lin N, Dean A 1984 Social support and depression. A panel study. Social Psychiatry 19: 83-91

Lin N, Ensel W M 1984 Depression-mobility and its social etiology: the role of life events and social support. Journal of Health & Social Behavior 25 : 176-188

Lipkin M, Kupka K 1982 Psychological factors affecting health. Praeger, New York

McCullagh P, Nelder J A 1983 Generalised linear models. Chapman & Hall, London

McFarlane A H, Norman G R, Streiner D L, Roy R G 1983 The process of social stress: stable, reciprocal and mediating relationships. Journal of Health & Social Behavior 24: 160-173

Mann A H, Jenkins R, Belsey E 1981 The twelve-month outcome of patients with neurotic illness in general practice. Psychological Medicine 11: 535-550

Mehrabian A 1970 The development and validation of measures of affiliative tendency and sensitivity to rejection. Education & Psychological Measurement 30: 417-428

Miller P McC, Ingham J G 1976 Friends, confidants and symptoms. Social Psychiatry 11: 51-58

Mischel W 1973 Toward a cognitive social learning reconceptualisation of personality. Psychological Review 80: 252-283

Mitchell J C 1969 Social networks in urban situations. Manchester University Press, Manchester

Monroe S M, Imhoff D F, Wise B D, Harris J E 1983 Prediction of psychological symptoms under high-risk psychosocial circumstances: life events, social support and symptom specificity. Journal of Abnormal Psychology 92: 338-350

Morin R C, Seidman E 1986 A social network approach and the revolving door patient. Schizophrenia Bulletin 12: 262-273

Mueller D P 1980 Social networks: a promising direction for research on the relationship of the social environment to psychiatric disorder. Social Science & Medicine 14: 147-161

Murphy E 1982 Social origins of depression in old age. British Journal of Psychiatry 141: 135-142

Myers J K, Lindenthal J J, Pepper M P 1975 Life events, social integration and psychiatric symptomatology. Journal of Health & Social Behavior 16: 421-427

Nuckolls C B, Cassel J, Kaplan B H 1972 Psychosocial assets, life crises and the prognosis of pregnancy. American Journal of Epidemiology 95: 431-441

O'Connor P, Brown G W 1984 Supportive relationships: fact or fancy? Journal of Personal & Social Relationships 1: 159-175

Parker G 1984 The measurement of pathogenic parental style and its relevance to psychiatric disorder. Social Psychiatry 19: 75-81

Parker G, Barnett B 1987 A test of the social support hypothesis. British Journal of Psychiatry 150: 72-77

Parry G, Shapiro D A 1986 Social support and life events in working class women: stress buffering or independent effects? Archives of General Psychiatry 43: 315-323

Pattison E M, De Francisco D, Wood P, Frazer H, Crowden J 1975 A psychosocial kinship model for family therapy. American Journal of Psychiatry 132: 1246-1251

Paykel E S, McGuiness B, Gomez J 1976 An Anglo-American comparison of the scaling of life events. British Journal of Medical Psychology 49: 237-247

Paykel E S, Emms E M, Fletcher J, Rassaby E S 1980 Life events and social support in puerperal depression. British Journal of Psychiatry 136: 339-346

Pearlin L I, Schooler C 1978 The structure of coping. Journal of Health & Social Behavior 19: 2-21

President's Commission on Mental Health 1978 Task Panel on Community Support

Systems. In: Task Panel Reports submitted to the President's Commission on Mental Health. US Government Printing Office, Washington D C

Puig-Antich J, Lukens E, Davis M, Goetz D, Brennan-Quatrock J, Todak G 1985 Psychosocial functioning in prepubertal major depressive disorders. Interpersonal relationships during the depressive episode. Archives of General Psychiatry 42: 500-510

Radloff E S 1977 The CES-D scale: a self-report depression scale for research in the general population. Applied Psychological Measurement 1: 385-401

Robins L N 1985 The consequences of conduct disorder in girls. In: Olwens D, Block J, Radke-Yarros M (eds) Development of antisocial and prosocial behaviour: research theories and issues. Academic Press, New York

Robins L N, Helzer J E, Croughan J, Ratcliff K S 1981 National Institute of Mental Health Diagnostic Interview Schedule: its history characteristics and validity. Archives of General Psychiatry 38: 381-389

Rutter M, Hersov L 1985 Child and adolescent psychiatry — modern approaches. Blackwell, Oxford

Rutter M, Quinton D 1984 Parental psychiatric disorder: effects on children. Psychological Medicine 14: 853-880

Schaefer C, Coyne J C, Lazarus R S 1982 The health related functions of social support. Journal of Behavioral Medicine 4: 381-406

Seligman M E P, Abramson L Y, Semmel A, Von Baeyer C 1979 Depressive attributional style. Journal of Abnormal Psychology 88: 242-247

Siberfeld M 1978 Psychological symptoms and social supports. Social Psychiatry 13: 11-17

Sokolove R L, Trimble D 1986 Assessing support and stress in the social networks of chronic patients. Hospital & Community Psychiatry 37: 370-372

Solomon Z, Bromet E 1982 The role of social factors in affective disorders. Psychological Medicine 12: 123-130

Spitzer R L, Endicott J, Robins E 1978 Research diagnostic criteria: Rationale and reliability. Archives of General Psychiatry 35: 773-782

Sturt E 1981 Hierarchical patterns in the distribution of psychiatric symptoms. Psychological Medicine 11: 783-794

Sultan F E, Johnson P J 1985 Characteristics of drop-outs, remainers and refusers at a psychosocial rehabilitation programme for the chronically mentally disabled. Journal of Psychology 119: 175-183

Surtees P G 1980 Social support, residual adversity and depressive outcome. Social Psychiatry 15: 71-80

Surtees P 1984 Kith, kin and psychiatric health: a Scottish survey. Social Psychiatry 19: 63-67

Taylor R D W, Huxley P J, Johnson D A W 1984 The role of social networks in the maintenance of schizophrenic patients. British Journal of Social Work 14: 129-140

Tennant C, Andrews G 1976 A scale to measure the stress of life events. Australian & New Zealand Journal of Psychiatry 10: 27-32

Tennant C, Bebbington P, Hurry J 1981 The role of life events in depressive illness: is there a substantial causal relation? Psychological Medicine 11: 379-389

Thoits P A 1982 Conceptual, methodological and theoretical problems in studying social support as a buffer against life stress. Journal of Health & Social Behavior 23: 145-159

Tolsdorf C C 1976 Social networks, support and coping: an exploratory study. Family Process 15: 407-417

Turner R J 1981 Social support as a contingency in psychological well being. Journal of Health & Social Behavior 22: 357-367

Turner J, Noh S 1983 Class and psychological vulnerability among women: the significance of social support and personal control. Journal of Health & Social Behavior 24: 2-15

Veiel H O F 1985 Dimensions of social support: a conceptual framework for research. Social Psychiatry 20: 156-162

Wallace C J 1984 Community and interpersonal functioning in the course of schizophrenic disorders. Schizophrenia Bulletin 10: 233-257

Warheit G, Vega W, Shimizu D, Meinhardt K 1982 Interpersonal coping networks and mental health problems among four race-ethnic groups. Journal of Community Psychology 10: 312-324

Waryszak Z 1982 Symptomatology and social adjustment of psychiatric patients before and after hospitalisation. Social Psychiatry 17: 149-154

Weiss R S 1969 The fund of sociability. Trans-Action 6: 36-43

Weiss R S 1974 The provisions of social relationships. In: Rubin Z (ed) Doing Unto Others. Prentice Hall, Englewood Cliffs, N J

Weissman M M, Paykel E S 1974 The depressed woman: a study of social relationships. University of Chicago Press, Chicago

Welin L, Tibblin G, Svardsudd K et al 1985 Prospective study of social influences on mortality. Lancet i: 915-918

Wellman B 1981 Applying network analysis to the problem of support. In: Gottlieb B H (ed) Social networks and social support. Sage, London

West M, Lively W J, Reiffer L, Sheldon A 1986 The place of attachment in the life events model of stress and illness. Canadian Journal of Psychiatry 31: 202-207

Whittaker J K, Garbarino J 1984 Social support networks: informal helping in the human services. Aldine

Wilcox B L 1981 Social support, life stress, and psychological adjustment: a test of the buffering hypothesis. American Journal of Community Psychology 9: 371-386

Williams A W, Ware J E, Donald C A 1981 A model of mental health, life events and social supports applicable to general populations. Journal of Health & Social Behavior 22: 324-336

Williams K B, Williams K D 1983 Social inhibition and asking for help: the effect of number strength and immediacy of potential help givers. Journal of Personality & Social Psychology 44: 67-77

Wing J K (ed) 1982 Long-term care: Experience in a London Borough. Psychological Medicine Monograph Supplement 2

Wing J K, Bebbington P 1982 Epidemiology of depressive disorders in the community. Journal of Affective Disorders 4: 331-345

Wing J K, Sturt P 1978 The PSE-ID-CATEGO System: Supplementary Manual. (Mimeo). Institute of Psychiatry, London

Wing J K, Cooper J, Sartorius N 1974 Measurement and classification of psychiatric symptoms. Cambridge University Press, London

5. The contribution of epidemiological research to community psychiatry

T.K.J. Craig   A.P. Boardman

In their various capacities throughout the health service, research workers trained in epidemiological methods have made a substantial contribution to the current shift in the emphasis of health care, away from the institutional setting towards community-orientated services. During the twentieth century, both psychiatric care and epidemiology have moved away from the confines of the asylum out into the community at large. This parallel shift of emphasis has resulted in new theoretical insights and new forms of care, with epidemiology and community psychiatry developing a reciprocal relationship, each discipline informing the other.

Epidemiological research has helped to provide fundamental insights into at least three broad areas of relevance to developments in community psychiatry: the clarification of nosological aspects of disease, the determination of the geographical and demographic distribution of disease, (including aetiological factors), and finally, in the evaluation of the utilisation, relevance, and impact of health care services.

THE CLARIFICATION OF DIAGNOSTIC ISSUES

Classification is a primary cognitive ability of man, present from the earliest differentiation of external objects in infancy, and elaborated throughout life to the complex socialisation patterns of adulthood (Rosch 1976). All classifications serve to simplify relationships between objects and phenomena, so that these can be more easily comprehended and communicated to others. Medical classification is no more nor less than this, with the additional proviso that a successful classification should be useful in therapeutic and preventive clinical activity (Jablensky 1988).

As a branch of medicine, psychiatry shares that discipline's use of disease theory as an approach to the study of nosology, i.e. the grouping of observed symptoms into patterns or syndromes, not simply for classification, but to link them with particular aetiological factors and treatments. Such syndromal groupings are, in theory at least, not fixed, but open to rearrangement in the light of either new information or the failure to identify meaningful causal and prognostic factors. Yet despite general agreement that much of the current classification of psychiatric disorder is no more than provisional, there is considerable resistance to abandoning familiar categories, even in the face of lack of support from aetiological studies.

One current dispute which illustrates this reluctance to abandon old systems of thought and which is of immediate relevance, both to research workers and to clinicians involved in the development of community-based services, concerns the ability to distinguish the sadness felt as a response to one of life's unhappier circumstances from the depression thought to characterise a depressive illness requiring treatment.

Clinicians of the nineteenth and early twentieth century, basing their judgements on observations of hospital inpatients, concluded that such distinctions could be made with relative ease, and that environmental precipitants of depressive disorder were infrequent (e.g. Griesinger 1861). However, as psychiatrists moved out of institutions and began dealing with people who were not ill enough to require admission, they found that such absolute distinctions did not hold for the majority of their new clients. Aubrey Lewis (1938) commented that contrary to the medical textbooks of the time, his patients with depression did not conform to the descriptions of 'endogenous' and 'reactive' depression — many reactive depressions were severe and exhibited vegetative symptoms, while some endogenous illnesses were preceded by plausible environmental stressors. He went on to suggest that in the existing state of knowledge, it would be prudent to avoid including poorly substantiated speculations about causal mechanisms in taxonomic judgements. But this caution has been little heeded, and the muddle-headed thinking criticised by Lewis continues to dog our taxonomic efforts.

As recently as 1978, international classifications of depression continued to attempt to catalogue sub-types of disorder on the basis of the presence of prior stressors, despite the burgeoning evidence that such stressors could be identified as antecedents to the entire range of depressive states. This led to the anomalous situation whereby the Ninth edition of the International Classification of Diseases (WHO 1978) includes six categories of depression dealing with the response to life stress, two of which are characterised by the severe symptoms which formerly had been taken to distinguish the *'disease'* from the *'distress'* state. This is not to say that endogenous depression is a meaningless concept (as some depressive disorders do indeed seem to arise without external environmental precipitants), but rather that this lack of reactivity is neither typical of depression as a whole, nor is it an explanation of observed symptom patterns. We will never begin to understand such exceptions to the general rule so long as we prematurely build inferential aetiological agents into the diagnostic classification itself (Katschnig et al 1986, Derogatis et al 1972, Cooke 1982, see also Brown in this volume, Ch. 3). The most recent revisions of the more important national and international classifications have gone some way towards confronting this issue. The classification of depressive illnesses in the American DSM III-R (American Psychiatric Association 1987) and that contained in the impending ICD-10 (WHO 1987) are more firmly rooted in atheoretical symptomatic criteria. ICD-10 goes even further towards abandoning irrelevant theory, in that the most recent draft has dropped the category 'depressive reaction' (broadly equivalent to DSM III-R 'Adjustment disorder with depressed mood'), on the grounds that the boundaries between it and traditionally recognised depressive illness 'are too fuzzy to be useful in practice' (WHO 1987).

This shift towards a classification which is less dependent on uncertain aetiological theory owes much to the demands of epidemiological investigations. Hospital studies have the very dubious advantage of lacking any real pressure to *define* psychiatric disorder; 'cases' are simply those who enter the treatment population. But classifications of disorder based entirely on hospital patients are necessarily biased and under-representative. Goldberg & Huxley (1980) provide a particularly illuminating discussion of the pathways to psychiatric care, which illustrates the extent to which depression seen in hospital settings may be unrepresentative of the cases in the general population. On average, no more than half of those with psychiatric disorder attending general practice surgeries are recognised by their doctor as ill, and only about 5% of cases are referred to psychiatric services (see also Shepherd et al 1966). In addition, while there is a gradient of severity between community and hospital 'cases', it is also a fact than some individuals with severe disorders never pass through the referral filter. Referral has more to do with individual characteristics such as past history of treatment, perceived suicidal risk and antisocial behaviour, that with the severity of the condition per se (Brown et al 1985, Craig et al 1987).

Studies seeking to explore the aetiology of psychiatric illness must therefore move beyond consulting patients to an examination of all in-stances of disorder. Bebbington et al (1980) listed five requirements for 'caseness' definition in epidemiological research:

1. The constituent symptoms of the 'case' should be clearly and explicitly defined.
2. The definition of these symptoms should be consistent with general clinical usage.
3. A technique for eliciting and recording symptoms should be developed so that they can be reliably obtained in any population, and by implication, taught to other investigators, even if they have not been trained in a particular school of psychiatry.
4. Symptoms should be used to build specific diagnostic classes.
5. The classification rules on which diagnosis is based should be precise and explicit.

Few early epidemiological studies managed to encompass all these requirements. Some built on the assumption that the most appropriate basis for assessing psychiatric disorder is the judgement of an experienced clinician, and a number of well known epidemiological surveys used this approach with some success, e.g. the surveys near Lund, Sweden which provided point-prevalence rates for all 2550 inhabitants using psychiatrists trained in the same tradition (Essen-Moller & Hagnell 1961, Hagnell 1966). There are, however, difficulties in interpreting the results of such investigations which use idiosyncratic diagnostic classifications. Taken together with the well documented difficulties in attaining agreement on the construction of clinically meaningful diagnostic groupings, it now seems that such everyday clinical judgement is too fragile a base on which to proceed.

About the time of the first Lund survey, other workers turned in quite a different direction, seeking a solution to the poor reliability of clinical diagnosis through a conception of psychiatric disorders as a quantitative continuum, differing in degree rather than in kind. Of the two best known early surveys of this kind, one in Midtown Manhattan suggested that 815 per thousand of the general population experienced some psychiatric symptoms (Srole et al 1962), while the other, in 'Stirling county', Nova Scotia, estimated that 690 per thousand were 'genuine psychiatric cases' (Leighton et al 1963). Although these North American studies may have successfully dealt with the problems of reliability, they were unsatisfactory from the clinical viewpoint, as they did not provide prevalence estimates for phenomena which psychiatrists found clinically meaningful. Not surprisingly, therefore, the quoted rates were greeted with considerable scepticism by clinicians, who regarded these as indicative of the ubiquity of trivial complaints rather than of 'genuine' psychiatric cases.

Perhaps the most important advance came with the development of semi-structured interviews, which enabled the reliable identification of *symptoms* in non-consulting populations. Three such instruments are in common use today: the Present State Examination (PSE—Wing et al 1974), the Schizophrenia and Affective Disorder Schedule (SADS—Spitzer & Endicott 1978), and the Clinical Interview Schedule (Goldberg et al 1970). All three are interviewer-based measures of disorder, in the sense that it is the interviewer who must judge whether reported symptoms are present and how far to go with additional probes in order to elicit enough information for rating purposes. This necessitates rigorous training, which must provide sufficient knowledge to allow the interviewer to interpret the data in a clinically meaningful way. Indeed, good reliability can only be achieved if this secondary task is also accomplished (Rabkin & Klein 1987). This may seem a tall order, yet there are numerous studies attesting to the fact that it can be achieved, given suitable training and supervision (e.g. Brown et al 1985, Cooper et al 1977, Wing et al 1977).

However, the ascertainment of symptoms is only part of the task of measurement: a means has to be found to group these symptoms into clinically meaningful syndromes and diagnoses. This is achieved in two ways: first, by setting the thresholds for scoring symptoms at the level seen in consulting populations: although the PSE and SADS have been criticised on the grounds that their inclusion criteria are too severe (Dean et al 1983, Shepherd & Williams 1988), such bias acts against the inclusion of 'trivial' emotional reactions; and secondly, by developing procedures for determining thresholds for the number and patterning of symptoms, above which clinical disorder can be said to be present. Wing's group approached this issue by laying down rules, based on clinical experience, to define a number of levels of certainty that sufficient PSE symptoms are present to allow recognition of any disorder; these rules were incorporated in the CATEGO suite of computer programs (Wing et al 1974, Wing & Sturt 1978). Other groups approached the issue of establishing thresholds by utilising consensus meetings for rating, and providing detailed case vignettes of case examples (Brown & Harris 1978, Finlay-Jones et al 1980). Both techniques work well enough, but the latter retains greater flexibility for research, at the expense of considerably more time in training and supervision.

In its simplest form, the PSE is essentially a cross-sectional measure which does not take into account the course of the episode of illness. As such, it reproduces only part of the clinical diagnostic practice, where the pattern of the evolution of symptoms within episodes makes a major contribution to the final diagnostic judgement. In recent years, however, efforts have been made to deal with this more complex tack of measurement. The major methodological hurdle to overcome has been one of obtaining reliable information about symptoms which may have occurred months or even years before interview; recent studies using a modified PSE suggest that this can be achieved. For example, when a general population sample was interviewed by different interviewers, one year apart, the kappa of agreement for anxiety and depression was 0.75; if anything, respondents tended to under-estimate past pathology (Brown et al 1985). But such encouraging results are confined to approaches which rely on lengthy and detailed interviews, with careful cross-referencing between key symptoms, as well as important datable events and temporal markers (e.g. public holidays or important environmental changes such as moving house or changing jobs). Without the use of lengthy interviews and such cross-referencing, reliability is poor (Zimmerman et al 1986).

Accuracy also depends on the approach used to anchor the onset and to map the course of individual episodes. In the Bedford College PSE-based interview, a series of general probes are used to establish the likely presence of episodes before there is any detailed examination of individual symptoms. If these general probes fail to identify potential episodes, questioning proceeds with individual symptoms, covering the month prior to interview. The interviewer is instructed to feed back summary statements at regular intervals, to check whether the respondent has experienced these symptoms at earlier time periods; if so, he/she must map their onset, sequencing, and any recovery in relation to other symptoms, as well as any temporal markers. This is very different to the approach used by most other episode-based measurement systems. For example, the 'lifetime' version of the SADS, and the accompanying Research Diagnostic Criteria (RDC — Spitzer et al 1978), determine whether symptoms have occurred at any time, and then ask whether these symptoms have occurred simultaneously. This has the potential drawback that only symptoms which have already been mentioned can be included in questions about a specific episode, and it ignores temporal patterns between individual symptoms. These approaches also differ in the importance given to certain key items and on the rating thresholds for these. It comes as no surprise, therefore, to learn that these two techniques differ widely in the classifications they produce, when compared in a common population. In one such recent comparative investigation, Dean et al (1983) used a composite measure of disorder, designed to produce one-month prevalence estimates of psychiatric disorder on a number of popular diagnostic schemes. The overall 'case' rate according to the PSE-CATEGO scheme was 8.7%, compared with 13.7% by RDC criteria, and there was poor agreement about labelling: only 56% of cases of depression and 17% of cases of anxiety were identified in common by both systems, despite the minimisation of likely disagreement by utilising PSE equivalents for some RDC symptoms. Discrepancies were even greater for the other diagnostic approaches, with the Bedford College criteria providing the most conservative estimate of definite cases.

The PSE and SADS remain essentially clinical schedules, designed to be administered by trained research workers with close supervision. For large-scale population surveys, some investigators have held to the notion of developing research interviews which are sufficiently structured to permit their valid use by lay interviewers, who have relatively little training and no clinical experience. The Diagnostic Interview Schedule (DIS) was developed to provide a low-cost alternative to detailed clinical interviews in large population surveys, such as the recent Epidemiological Catchment Area (ECA) project in the United States (Robins et al 1981, 1982, 1984, Regier et al 1984, Eaton et al 1984). Although the ECA studies will undoubtedly play an influential role in the future development of American community care, such moves away from clinical semi-structured interviews are not without problems. Where both lay interviewers and clinicians have used the DIS in hospital populations, reliability has been satisfactory, but even in the relatively straightforward case of hospital inpatients, lay interviewers tend to over-diagnose obsessive-compulsive illness and under-diagnose major depressions (Helzer et al 1985). Further doubts are raised by a recent investigation which contrasted DSM-III diagnoses derived from the DIS interview with those obtained by a clinical interview based on the PSE. In this study, concordance between lay interviewers and clinicians was low for all categories other than schizophrenia and mania. Point estimates suggest that within each diagnostic category, less than half of the clinically diagnosed cases would have been given a concordant diagnosis by the DIS (Anthony et al 1985). Possible explanations for this include three issues which are fundamental to the use of highly structured interviews: their ability to implement diagnostic criteria fully; the over-inclusiveness of certain items when administered without recourse to detailed interview probes; and the reliance on subjective reports rather than the judgement of experienced clinicians as to the relevance of reported symptoms (Anthony et al 1985).

To complicate matters still further, the DIS continues a long-standing tradition of attempting to estimate lifetime prevalence. The steps that are necessary to achieve satisfactory reliability and accuracy over a period as short as a year were indicated above. Yet the DIS, with its structured approach, does not permit such complex interviewing; as with the SADS, episodes can only be established after symptoms are determined. Now, however, the drawback is even more severe, since the usual clinical freedom to probe the constituent of each episode is not permitted. As a result, vital changes in the course of an illness are liable to be missed, and symptoms which lie just outside apparent episodes can never be retrieved, nor can people be detected who formerly met full criteria but who currently display only some symptoms. Such factors probably explain the poor reliability of recording past episodes (Anthony et al 1985, Bromet et al 1986).

There must be doubts, therefore, about the clinical relevance of highly structured lay-administered diagnostic interviews. In contrast, it is possible to attain reliable and valid observations in non-consulting populations, using the sort of interview with which most practising psychiatrists are familiar. This is itself no small achievement. It has led to objective and easily transmitted diagnostic criteria, improved conceptualisations of what constitutes a 'case' of disorder, as well as having opened the way for aetiological studies.

STUDIES OF THE DISTRIBUTION OF DISEASE: THE SEARCH FOR AETIOLOGICAL FACTORS

Information about the distribution of disease in the general population is an essential first step towards identifying aetiological processes. In this chapter, the ways in which knowledge about the distribution of disease has contributed to the understanding of causal processes will be discussed in relation to suicide and schizophrenia (but see also the chapter by Brown, Ch. 3, for a discussion of affective disorder).

Suicide

Since the classic work of Emil Durkheim (1952), it has been apparent that suicide rates respond to factors within the economy and the structure of society. It has seemed to many, therefore, that a study of suicide patterns across several decades ought to throw light on possible social and clinical interventions which could literally be life-saving. But the data are complex and such epidemiological studies are fraught with pitfalls. Epidemiologists recognise three forces at play: a period effect (e.g. suicide rates in Britain fell during the second world war, an age effect (rates tend to rise with advancing age), and a cohort effect (people born in a particular generation tend to share unique rates, relative to other generations). The evidence for cohort effects are the least conclusive. Solomon & Hellon (1980) in Canada, studied the relationship between age and suicide during the period of 1951 to 1977. They noted that rates in young men (under 50 years) increased during that time and that this increase persisted within cohorts, despite the fact that overall, increasing age was not correlated with increased risk. Thus, cohorts with high initial rates preserved this into adulthood, while low-rate cohorts maintained a low rate. In contrast, Lester (1984), studying patterns in the USA between 1935 and 1975, found a significant negative correlation between rates for women at intervals of 15, 20, and 25 years, while for men, there was a positive but progressively weakening correlation at 5-, 10-, and 15-year intervals. He suggested that the results for women indicate that in any generation, there would be a finite population of people who were at a high risk of killing themselves. Cohorts with high rates in youth should show relatively lower rates as they age, as the pool of people at risk becomes depleted by death. These two studies, indicating rather different types of cohort effects, have not been widely replicated, however. In the UK, Murphy et al (1986) examined 60 years of suicide data, but found no evidence for any cohort effect in either sex. Instead, there was a climb in rates with advancing age, as well as a pronounced period effect of a decline in rates amongst men during the second world war. More recent work in the USA (Wetzel et al 1987), examining longer time periods than previous North American studies, also tends to confirm that rates can adequately explained by age and period effects alone.

In the USA, however, the relationship between age and suicide has changed in the last two decades; the fall in suicide rates amongst the elderly is counter-balanced by a rise in youthful suicide. If cohort effects can be discounted, the obvious candidate for these temporal changes in the age-distribution is some kind of period effect. In the UK, the lower risk for middle-aged and older men has been attributed to the decline in the availability of toxic domestic gas, coupled with a disinclination to adopt alternative strategies in middle and later age (Kreitman 1976, Murphy et al 1986). But there may also be wider influences at work. In the USA, there is no change in availability or use of method to explain the changes, and   it has been suggested that improvements in the medical, social, financial, and support systems of middle-aged and elderly people are the more important protective factors (Wetzel et al 1987).

The increased risk for young people in America is less easy to explain. Klerman et al (1985) report that the incidence of major depression varies by year of birth, with the onset of first depression occurring earlier in successive generations. The years of birth associated with greater risk of depression correspond reasonably closely with those of increased risk of suicide, and of course, there is a long established link between severe depression and suicide. In the USA, increased abuse of illicit drugs and alcohol in these younger age-groups probably also plays a role; indeed, some studies have been able to show marked increases in the rates of substance abuse in the suicides of young people (e.g. Fowler et al 1986). Such research is important, because the recognition of risk in people who are depressed depends largely on the ability to make specific predictions from what is known of the broader pattern of that risk. Until we know more about the epidemiological distribution of depression and suicide, it is impossible to tell whether observed changes in rates are a response to a growing number of young people with depression in our society, or whether some other factor in our environments has made depression in this group more dangerous.

Schizophrenia

In the study of schizophrenia, incidence is typically assessed in terms of the 'social onset' of the disorder, defined by an event, such as the first contact with the wider health care services (Odegaard 1946, Wing & Fryers 1976). This approach relies on the assumption that most cases of the disorder in the general population of industrialised countries are eventually seen by mental health services (e.g. Cooper 1978). On this basis, the annual inception rates for the UK lie between 11 and 14 per 100000 (Cooper et al 1987, Wing & Fryers 1976). In the USA, case register surveys have produced somewhat higher rates (e.g. Kramer 1980), although interpretation is complicated by the fact that rather more 'lenient' diagnostic criteria may have been used and some patients may have had earlier spells of unrecorded outpatient treatment (Cooper 1978). Babigian (1980), for example, suggests that application of DSM-III criteria would reduce the rates reported in some of these studies by as much as 30%.

A number of important international research programmes have utilised these methods, with additional screening procedures aimed at non-hospital services, such as those provided by religious groups or the practitioners of traditional medicine. The particular symptoms which characterise the disorder are to be found in all cultures so far examined.

No studies have yet produced convincing evidence for new varieties of disorder, nor is there evidence that the schizophrenias found in developed countries are absent in other parts of the world. Furthermore, the constellation of signs and symptoms of the disorder tends to be viewed as morbid, both by traditional practitioners of medicine (be they Western medical services or tribal healers) and by the general public, thus putting paid to the notion that such diagnosis is exclusively a consequence of labelling or the result of prolonged confinement to institutional care.

One of the more puzzling outcomes of this international research is the remarkable uniformity of incidence rates worldwide, and the suggestion that there has been little change in these rates since the mid-nineteenth century (Goldhamer & Marshall 1953, Odegaard 1971). This relative uniformity, both across time and in populations which are culturally and genetically very different, is difficult to explain. It would suggest that unless estimates are fundamentally flawed, biological and environmental risk factors are uniformly distributed all over the world, or more plausibly, that environmental differences account for minor variation around some genetically determined mean rate.

Inception rates may be more variable within particular societies (Sartorius et al 1986), but whenever such variations have been reported, they have invariably been controversial and have led, at best, to heated accusations of inappropriate labelling, or at worst, to those of racial bias. One such observation concerns increased rates among, the Afro-Caribbean population of the UK (Cochrane 1977, Dean et al 1981, Giggs 1986a). Early studies have been challenged on the grounds that they incorrectly included 'atypical' syndromes such as schizophrenia, that the sampling procedures may have been flawed (Littlewood & Lipsedge 1981), or that the observed rates are susceptible to racial bias in a society which is less tolerant of behavioural abnormalities in this sub-population (McGovern & Cope 1987, Harrison et al 1984, Ineichen et al 1984). But some recent British research (Harrison et al 1988), conducted with meticulous attention to case finding methodology, has once again recorded a higher incidence in this sub-population. This study utilised the PSE interview in possible cases that were identified by the screening methods used in a WHO multinational investigation of severe mental illness (Sartorius et al 1986). In Nottingham, rates of schizophrenia were substantially increased in the Afro-Caribbean population, particularly for second-generation (i.e. UK-born) residents. This increase is not account-ed for by any excess of 'atypical' disorder, while the nature of sectori-sation of services in the study area, together with the use of an over-inclusive screening procedure, make it unlikely that significant numbers of new cases in either the target or comparison populations were missed. The main criticism that can be levelled at this study concerns the method of determining the size of the population at risk. Up to the present time, there are no comprehensive population figures for British-born residents of Afro-Caribbean parentage in the UK; the 1981 population census (OPCS 1982) does not specifically identify the racial origin of British-born residents, so that the appropriate denominator has to be estimated indirectly. The Nottingham study obtained these estimates from the census variable 'country of origin of the head of the household', making the assumption that the majority of the at-risk population would have still been living with their parents at the time of the 1981 census. This procedure is bound to lead to an under-estimate of the denominator population which, of course, will inflate the apparent rate of disorder. However, as the authors point out, the rates are so elevated that even if the denominator is doubled, the recalculated estimates are higher than the highest previously quoted inception figures for schizophrenia.

The identification of high-risk sub-populations is a crucially important first step in the process of determining aetiology. Although it is too early to be certain about specific aetiological factors for schizophrenia in Afro-Caribbean immigrants (or indeed in any other group), the results bear upon other studies in which the interaction of inheritance and environment seem to be important. Investigations grounded in epidemiological methodology have contributed substantially to the evidence for a major genetic contribution to the aetiology of schizophrenia. The reported morbid risk for the siblings of affected probands is as much as four times that of the risk in the general population (e.g. Winokur et al 1974). Also, twin studies, in which zygosity and disorder have been independently assessed, suggest that the monozygous concordance rates (i.e. the extent to which both members of identical twin pairs develop schizophrenia) are up to three times higher than in dizygous pairs (Gottesman & Shields 1972). Furthermore, these observations cannot be explained by environmental factors alone. Children of schizophrenic patients, adopted while still very young, have an increased risk for schizophrenia (e.g. Heston 1966), and while the biological relatives of affected probands have a raised rate of disorder, the adoptive relatives show no such increased risk (Kety et al 1975). It is still not clear, however, just how the risk is transmitted. Of the current theories, monogenic explanations have greater difficulty than heterogeneity and polygenic theories in explaining the relatively stable incidence of schizophrenia, in view of the impaired fecundity of schizophrenic patients. Proponents of single-gene theories have to resort to complex hypotheses, suggesting that non-affected heterozygotes are at a biologically selected advantage by reason of factors such as increased resistance to infection (e.g. Huxley et al 1964, Kidd 1975).

On the other hand, one of the more attractive facets of the polygenic theories is their ability to take account of environmental precipitants which are unlikely to be evenly distributed within society or between cultures. Identification of such precipitants would be enhanced if it could be shown that the incidence of schizophrenia differed in different environments. Surprisingly, however, epidemiological studies have shown only small differences in the expectancy of disease between different populations or over time (Stromgren 1987). Some studies of isolated communities have noted higher expectancy rates, e.g. in the north of Sweden (Book et al 1978) and in the west of Ireland (Torrey 1980, Walsh et al 1980). Such outliers are of particular interest, as they may represent either the consequences of the out-migration of healthier members of the society or a high frequency of cousin marriages (see, e.g. Book et al 1978, Torrey 1980, Walsh et al 1980). Apart from these differences between cultures, which may be explained on methodological grounds (see Ni Nullain et al 1984), there is a consistent observation of greater expectancy among the less skilled and lower social status groups of society (e.g. Odegaard 1956, Goldberg & Morrison 1963), and in inner-city areas typified by social disorganisation and environmental decay (Faris & Dunham 1939, Freeman & Alpert 1986, Hare 1956a, Hafner & Reimann 1970). It is now reasonably clear that this excess is largely the consequence of the course of the disorder, the association being explained by the accumulation of people with chronic handicaps in the lower social strata (Dunham 1965), brought about by a downward social 'drift' after the onset of illness (Dunham 1965, Gerard & Houston 1953) or as a consequence of a pre-syndromal manifestation of the disorder (Goldberg & Morrison 1963). At the time of first admission, a significant proportion of patients live alone and have relatively few contacts with relatives and friends (Hare 1956a, Dunham 1965). This may, in part, be due to premorbid personality traits such as timidity and shyness, and is reflected in a gradual process of alienation in adolescence, with a poor early work record (e.g. O'Neal & Robins 1958, Watt et al 1984). Finally, there may be a higher rate of general mobility amongst pre-syndromal cases, which may explain the excess of illness in some immigrant populations (Malzberg & Lee 1956, Lazarus et al 1963).

More intensive studies of limited population groups suggest that parents with schizophrenic offspring show more protectiveness and concern than the mothers of normal children, echoing earlier theories that serious disturbances in family relationships or patterns of communication between parent and child might play an important aetiological role in the genesis of the disorder (e.g. Bateson et al 1956, Lidz et al 1965, Singer & Wynne 1965). But none of these early theories, which implicated aetiological processes in the families of schizophrenic patients, have received direct empirical verification. On the whole, they fail to explain why one family member should fall ill while his sibling, exposed to similarly adverse conditions remains well. The observed abnormalities may be the result of responses to altered behaviour in their child, or even an expression of the genetic constitution that is shared by both patient and immediate kin.

This is not to say that family environment is unimportant. An early study dealing with the outcome of patients discharged from hospital, showed an increased rate of relapse in those who had returned to their parents or wives, in contrast to those who had gone to live in lodgings or with more distant family (Brown et al 1958). Subsequent longitudinal studies involving direct measures of family interaction confirmed this finding. A measure based on the number of critical comments and emotional over-concern shown by family members when talking about the patient were highly predictive of relapse (Brown et al 1962, Brown et al 1972). Such high degrees of 'Expressed Emotion' (EE) could be found in any family and carries none of the implications of a deeply disturbed relationship specific to schizophrenia. Several intervention studies have now been carried out in the UK and the USA, based on the implications of this research; they suggest that either reduced contact with high-EE relatives or the modification of high EE in these relatives reduces the relapse rate substantially (e.g. Leff et al 1982, Leff & Vaughn 1985, Falloon et al 1982 and see also Ch. 6 by Leff in this volume).

Both this research and that conducted in hospital settings suggests that schizophrenic patients are particularly sensitive to emotional arousal, engendered by extensive changes in levels of stimulation (e.g. Wing 1966, Watts & Bennett 1983). Similar observations emerge from investigation of life event stress. In a classic investigation, the occurrence of life events in a group of patients suffering a relapse or first onset of schizophrenia, was compared with the occurrence of similar events in a control sample of normal people. While the proportion experiencing events remained relatively constant over a three-month period for the normal subjects, the proportion of schizophrenics experiencing at least one such event rose sharply in the three weeks prior to onset, with some 60% of patients experiencing an event thought likely to lead to significant emotional arousal in that period (Brown & Birley 1968).

To return to the Nottingham Afro-Caribbean study, it seems that a combination of genetic and social factors might account for the elevated rates of disorder. It is possible, for example, that the open immigration policies in the late 1940s and 1950s encouraged a 'drift' of people with vulnerable personalities and that they, and more importantly, their children, were subsequently exposed to a hostile and discriminatory society which conspires to obstruct efforts at integration and goal fulfilment. Experiences of discrimination and alienation are highly threatening stressors, and thus might play a part in precipitating illness in vulnerable individuals (Burke 1984, Murphy 1972). Harrison et al (1988) are rightly circumspect in their attempts to interpret their findings, but if upheld by replication, such studies can lead, not only to a better understanding of aetiological processes but also to new, better targeted service initiatives, which are in fact the *raison d'être* of clinical research activity.

PLANNING AND EVALUATING COMMUNITY CARE

Whilst epidemiological data on the incidence of disorder may be helpful in discerning aetiology, the rational planning of health care depends on the juxtaposition of information about the numbers of ill people in the general population and in contact with services. From these data, planners can begin the task of determining the extent to which existing services reach those who are ill. Epidemiological data on the prevalence and geographical distribution of disease are essential to this process, both as an indication of need and also at later stages, when they can be used to determine whether or not changes that were introduced had the desired effects of decreasing disability or of increasing access to treatment.

Identifying unmet needs

One now classic UK investigation concerned the prevalence of neuro-psychiatric disorders among school-age children living on the Isle of Wight. This survey demonstrated that although nearly 9% of the selected population were eligible for specialist referral for diagnosis, treatment or advice, rather less than 1 in 9 of these were, in fact, receiving such care (Rutter et al 1970). Similar conclusions concerning the shortfall of traditional mental health services can be drawn from interpretation of population-based studies of affective disorder (Ginsburg & Brown 1982, Goldberg & Huxley 1980, and Ch. 3 by Brown in this volume) and even of psychotic disorders. For example, in a review of the epidemiological estimates for the United States, Dohrenwend et al (1980) concluded that as many as two out of every five persons suffering from 'psychosis' had never received treatment. In short, these and other surveys indicate a massive unmet need for mental health services.

The failure to appreciate the service implications of this research evidence has often caught the planners and clinicians off their guard. New community-based services soon became saturated, often with clients whom the service did not set out to treat, and this is nicely illustrated by the current controversy surrounding the introduction of community mental health centres (CMHCs), which offer ease of access, rapid assessment, and short-term treatment as their primary goals. The first CMHC in Britain opened in 1977. By 1987, 81 were fully operational, and 136 were planned to be in service by 1989. But concerns are mounting about what treatments they actually provide and about the effects they may have on the balance of district services. Three-quarters of British centres report primary aims of rapid intervention and employ techniques of counselling or psychotherapy, while less than a third have programmes specifically devoted to the rehabilitation of people with chronic, severe mental illness. Fewer than 1 in 10 offer practical assistance in obtaining housing, employment, and income support. A quarter are without the services of psychiatrists, and a further quarter have no occupational or industrial therapists (Sayce et al 1990). With such emphasis on treatments for 'neurotic' disorders, it is hardly surprising that these centres are recruiting a new population of consulters from the large pool of people with affective disorders in the general population, and that the majority of these new cases have not previously been dealt with by psychiatric services. For example, in one district, the introduction of a CMHC to a consultant psychiatrist's catchment area resulted in a doubling of the total number of new patients after only two years' operation — a rise which had shown no signs of abating six years on (Boardman et al 1987, Boardman & Bouras 1988). The new population of patients comprised people mainly suffering from emotional disorders, variously labelled as 'transient stress disorder', and 'adjustment disorder', who hitherto had been contained within the primary care setting. In contrast, the numbers of patients with psychoses seen by the centres actually decreased in the comparable time period, despite the fact that the centres saw this population as particularly in need of their efforts. In the sense of caseness thresholds employed in most of the epidemiological studies (see Ch. 3 by Brown in this volume), there is no doubt that the majority of consulters were 'cases'. However, the issue is not whether they are deserving of treatment, but rather who should be responsible for providing this care and what safeguards need to be introduced to limit the tendency for resources to shift from more handicapped, often psychotic clients, to this new treatment population (Boardman & Bouras 1988, Sayce et al 1990).

This expansion in the treated population following the introduction of a new community service is not confined to CMHC programmes. In the decade following 1964, the Camberwell community service treated an increasing number of patients, nearly half of whom suffered from neurotic disorders (Bennett et al 1972, Wing & Fryers 1976). Similarly, the Salford case register (Wooff et al 1983) found that introducing new community psychiatric nursing teams increased register-based point-prevalence rates, indicating a latent need for care which was supplementary to that which existed prior to the introduction of the new service. Very similar experiences have been reported in other countries (e.g. Munk-Jorgensen 1985, Neilsen et al 1980).

In the face of such data, there is an understandable tendency for psychiatrists to demand precise definitions of the boundaries of their commitments, specifying which kind of patient should be seen by whom and to what end. Many would seek to involve themselves only in the care of 'major' psychiatric disorders, and exclude 'the predicaments and problems of living which do not reasonably require psychiatric intervention' (Richman & Barry 1985). But who is to define 'major' disorders, or for that matter, to decide which 'problems of living' do not reasonably require psychiatric intervention? Psychiatrists have themselves largely determined the thresholds which are serving to highlight the size of unmet needs. While it is true that knowledge of diagnosis does not denote the need for treatment, or provide any help as to what clinical action should be taken, there are few better qualified to judge this need than the experienced clinician, who, with his training in both the social and biological basis of human behaviour, 'concerns himself not only with disorders characterised by gross lesions in the brain, or with the so-called functional psychoses, but also with the wider issues surrounding neurotic and personality disorders, the origins of which reflect complex inter-actions between constitutional and precipitating factors, be these physical, psychological or social' (Rawnsley 1984). This is not to say that psychiatrists should be unaware of the therapeutic skills of other workers in allied sciences. Indeed, Richman & Barry (1985), in their cry for clearer boundaries, offer one possible solution, in calling for the reaffirmation of the role of psychiatrists as consultants to primary care practitioners; they suggest that many people with minor psychiatric disorders might be as well served by primary care workers who were given improved training and better liaison with specialist psychiatric services.

Related to these issues, concerning the introduction of new community-based services, is the need to ensure that treatments are targeted at those most in need, and that facilities are located in close geographical proximity to the residential location of the target client group. This implies some knowledge of the distribution of disease within the target population, which in turn rests on the ability to identify population characteristics that either predict need or are correlated with service utilisation. It is important to distinguish between problems of given areas of the population on the one hand, and the services provided on the other , as well as obtaining independent measures of both, since they may bear only a weak correlation to one another. The effective identification of precise geographical areas of need has both national and local consequences. Nationally, such data can help in the allocation of resources, having the potential to replace current formulae for the allocation of resources in the National Health Service. Locally, it can aid planners in decisions concerning the siting of limited resources, for instance, so as to provide access to the widest possible consumer popu-lation or to achieve greatest impact. However, the method of identifying such areas must be valid, reliable, and clearly specifiable if the placement of services is to be undertaken with any conviction.

A major problem is how to obtain trustworthy information about the likely level of psychiatric morbidity in geographically defined populations. Estimates can be obtained through population surveys, but unfortunately, there is rarely the time or resources to conduct such complex surveys across an entire health district; the best that can be achieved is an estimate based on surveys conducted in other districts or catchment areas which are similar to the area in question, in terms of the distribution of important social correlates of illness. Computerised case registers can provide reasonable estimates of prevalence and the utilization of services for severe psychiatric disorder, but such registers require considerable time and development effort before they can be relied upon. Furthermore, case registers can only reflect disorders which come to the attention of services, whereas those referred to psychiatric services represent only a minority of all who suffer from less severe forms of psychiatric illness.

In most areas, there are no extensive case registers, and no detailed population surveys have been conducted, but recent reports suggest a third possible approach to estimates of social deprivation and relative morbidity. Geographical Information Systems (GIS) are a new technology which combines computer database methods with the ability to store and manipulate socio-demographic data in map form. Such data, collected at the time of the UK national census in 1981 (OPCS 1982), can be used to highlight geographical areas of social deprivation — a factor which is believed to be associated with higher prevalence of psychiatric disorder (see Bagley et al 1973, Freeman 1985, Hare 1956b, Levy & Rowitz 1971, McCulloch et al 1967, Phillip & McCulloch 1966). This approach to predicting the geographical distribution of disease and risk has been used to classify local authorities (Webber & Craig 1978, Imber 1976), to examine residential mobility (Short 1978), and housing resource need (Thompson 1984), as well as to investigate the ecology of mental disorders (Giggs 1986b).

A recent study by the authors of this chapter set out to examine the feasibility of using such data to provide estimates needed for planning purposes. The smallest unit of UK national census data that is publicly available is the Enumeration District (ED) which consists, on average, of 150 households. Census data at the level of EDs can be used to portray chosen geographical areas, and such profiling may be done, either by examining individual census variables or by employing aggregate measures that are obtained by subjecting individual census variables to multivariate statistical analyses (e.g. principal components and cluster analytical procedures). The use of profiling permits the classification of EDs according to the extent to which they share similar distributions of selected variables chosen, for example, to reflect high levels of social deprivation. The utility of this ED classification can be considerably enhanced if existing data of the utilisation of services can be linked directly to the demographic clusters. To do this, patients attending services can be linked to the local population by placing them according to the ED in which they reside by means of their postcode (zipcode). A typical ED contains approximately 10 postcodes, and since both EDs and postcodes have defined geographical grid references, this enables the assignment of each postcode (i.e. patient) to an appropriate ED, and hence to one of the aggregate clusters.

Although the prevalence of psychiatric disorder in a given geographical area will not be known in most instances, the aggregates do reflect certain life-style indicators, which in turn correlate with physical and psychiatric disorders. Thus, the aggregates provide a morbidity estimate, and hence estimates of both met and unmet need, if it is assumed that areas with the greatest score on aggregate measures of social deprivation will also contain the greatest psychiatric morbidity (Bagley et al 1973, Levy & Rowitz 1971, McCulloch et al 1967). In this way, the method combines a rough estimate of geographical clusters of need, with an indication of service usage for members of given clusters.

Cluster analysis of 39 census variables across the EDs constituting the catchment area of a Community Mental Health Centre in South-East London (Boardman et al 1989) resulted in six clusters, which highlighted the mixed socio-demographic nature of the area served. It was predicted that sub-areas of deprivation would show the highest rates of referral, *if the services were tapping this morbidity*, and that those of highest affluence would show the lowest rates. However, this did not, in fact, appear to be the case; the service was apparently not 'reaching' deprived sub-areas, but persons from one relatively affluent part were being differentially referred to it.

The use of small-area statistics has enormous potential use in the evaluation and planning of health facilities. When aggregated into clusters, they can provide a means of identifying possible areas of need which cut across the traditionally utilised catchment area and ward boundaries. In addition, they are of particular value for creating a formula that may be used for comparison in other health districts and other health fields. Additional mapping software allows the geographical co-ordinates of area boundaries, public transport routes, or the precise siting of service delivery points to be incorporated. From this combined database, it is possible to produce a series of maps which show the spatial relationships between the clusters and these geographical boundaries (see for example Dear 1977, 1978).

The evaluation of existing services

Since the late 1950s, there has been a conspicuous effort to reduce the length of hospital stay, and the emphasis on community psychiatry has almost certainly led to a fall in the numbers of long-stay inpatients (at least for those under 65 years of age) in most industrialised countries (Freeman et al 1985). Tooth & Brook (1961), examining the rate of attrition of long-stay inpatients in England and Wales over a 5-year period, came to the conclusion that bed requirements would stabilise at about 1.8 per 1000 of the population by 1975. Whilst these figures were eagerly taken up by planners at the time, it is now clear that such estimates erred on the optimistic side, not least because of a diminishing return on active rehabilitation policies. Many of the old long-stay inpatients had severe disabilities that were only partially amenable to rehabilitation efforts, and others continued to be disabled, either by recurring episodes of psychotic symptoms or by pervasive social disablement. One survey (Sturt 1984), based on case register records, noted that over half of those patients who received periods of care amounting to a year or more in duration from residential or day care centres, remained in such settings over the 2-year period following the original census day. Many of the remainder had further readmissions during this period, and most showed a poor record of work achievement. Furthermore, the burden of care falling on relatives who now have to assume a supervisory role is considerable (Wykes et al 1982), and almost certainly plays a part in determining how long an independent life in the general community is likely to last.

These studies highlight the fact that the data derived from current statistics of the use of services require careful interpretation; they cannot of themselves provide adequate guidance for the development of future health care requirements. Such developments should, ideally, be based on the measured needs of patients and their families, linked to an ongoing evaluation and monitoring of new services (Hirsch 1988, Wilkinson & Freeman 1986, Wing & Hailey 1972).

Such precise evaluation of newly introduced community services has proven rather difficult to implement, not least because of the problems of measuring social and clinical changes in patients across a diversity of settings. One such evaluative programme, which compared a traditional hospital service with that of a newly implemented community service in order to establish differences in referral patterns, clinical outcome, and effects on patients' families, suggested that the new community-based services might well place greater burden on the relatives of certain types of patients (Grad & Sainsbury 1966, 1968). Similar studies of the efficacy of psychiatric units attached to general hospitals have been dogged by problems of comparability of the sorts of patients dealt with by these, as compared to more traditional psychiatric hospitals, particularly with regard to the relatively fewer patients with a diagnosis of schizophrenia, as compared to non-psychotic diagnoses, amongst patients of the DGH units (Hoenig 1968). In a more recent comparison of one such unit and a traditional psychiatric hospital, there was little difference in clinical outcome for two cohorts of patients with a first admission for schizophrenia, although the DGH unit imposed less strain on relatives and was associated with considerably fewer unmet needs, together with the monetary advantage of lower overall hospital costs, despite greater staff-patient ratios (Jones et al 1980). Similar examination of the efficacy of day hospital placements reveal striking differences between centres in terms of the services they offer, the extent of their occupational provision, and the extent to which they can be said to meet the real needs of the patients who attend (e.g. McCreadie et al 1983, 1984, Milne 1984).

Whether or not community-based services promote advantages over hospital-based services, other than the prevention of 'secondary' handicaps due to 'institutionalisation', remains a moot issue, championed perhaps most eloquently by Mosher (1983), who concluded from a review of the American experience that such care is cheaper and more effective than hospital admission. He suggested that the failure of community psychiatry to command greater respect lies largely at the feet of psychiatrists, who collude with society to keep patients 'out of sight' and attain greater financial rewards through inpatient care. However, Tantam (1985) has pointed to a number of issues which cast doubt on these advantages as being as great as were suggested in the United States, let alone in Britain. First, in many of the studies quoted, the patients in the experimental groups (i.e. receiving community-based care) reported fewer symptoms than their hospitalised controls. Prominent advantages were largely confined to the amount of time living in care or in sheltered employment and the extent of subsequent readmissions or contact with casualty departments — an observation which may reflect the more assiduous follow-up of the experimental patients. On the whole, these studies suggest that hospital admission remains necessary for some patients, and it is likely that consumer satisfaction would be as great in these cases if attention to after-care and support on discharge was as intensive as was evident for the experimental groups. Finally, on the issue of costs, intensive community programmes may cost more in financial terms than hospitalisation (e.g. Weisbrod et al 1980) and may carry some increased risk to a patient's safety (see e.g. Weisbrod et al 1980, Estroff 1981), although the latter remains a moot point (Stein & Test 1980, Grad & Sainsbury 1968).

CONCLUSION

The development of effective community-based services for psychiatric disorder depends largely on the intelligent interpretation of research findings concerning the distribution and course of disorder in the general population, where such services are aimed.

Attention is required, not only to basic survey information, but also to the development of systems of monitoring current therapeutic activities, and to devising quantifiable measures of the more complex concepts of medical, social, and personal 'needs', 'demands', and ultimately 'costs'. Partly through lack of foresight, partly as a consequence of inadequate support for research monitoring of clinical activities, many of our current systems of health care remain essentially articles of faith. Unfortunately, clinical and research practices are too often viewed as inherently incompatible. The setting up of novel treatments with ill-defined goals, based on inadequate scientific information and too little information about how these goals can reasonably be achieved, is surely sufficient recipe for disaster; yet if this were not enough, such innovatory schemes are threatened from other quarters as well. The failure to integrate such new services with existing clinical practice may have contributed to the fall in popularity of community mental health centres in the USA; failures to serve the needs of the chronically ill, a selective bias towards 'less severe' disorders, and isolation from the mainstream of psychiatry have made them both unpopular with psychiatrists and ineffective in preventing admission to state hospitals or in implementing the sort of crisis intervention programmes that were the reason behind their creation (Fink & Weinstein 1979, Mollica 1980, Donovan 1980, see also Ch. 19). In the UK, we may be able to avoid such undesirable outcomes by ensuring that new services are explicitly targeted on priority care groups, and are not allowed to drift away from the remainder of the psychiatric service.

Community psychiatry will continue to face an uphill task; in this struggle, it will need to base growth on sound empirical evidence, to plan and develop services for the populations and the demographic areas which most need them, and avoid, at all costs, a voluntary amputation of this far reaching limb from the body which constitutes comprehensive psychiatric care.

REFERENCES

American Psychiatric Association 1987 Diagnostic and statistical manual of mental disorders. 3rd edn Revised DSM-III-R
Anthony J C, Folstein M, Romanoski A J et al 1985 Comparison of the lay diagnostic interview schedule and a standardized psychiatric diagnosis. Archives of General Psychiatry 42: 667-675
Babigian H M 1980 Schizophrenia: epidemiology. In: Kaplan H, Freedman A M, Sadock B J (eds) Comprehensive textbook of psychiatry, 3rd edn, vol 2. Williams and Wilkins, Baltimore
Bagley C, Jacobson S, Palmer C 1973 Social structure and the ecological distribution of mental illness, suicide and delinquency. Psychological Medicine 3: 177-187
Bateson G, Jackson D, Haley J, Weakland J 1956 Towards a theory of schizophrenia. Behavioural Science 1: 251-264
Bebbington P, Hurry J, Tennant C 1980 Recent advances in the epidemiological study of minor psychiatric disorders. Journal of the Royal Society of Medicine 73: 315-318
Bennett D H, Birley J L T, Hailey A, Wing J K 1972 Non-residential services for the mentally ill, 1964-1971. In: Wing J K, Hailey A H (eds) Evaluating a community psychiatric service. Oxford University Press, London: pp 141-158
Boardman A P, Bouras N 1988 Monitoring the usage of the Mental Health Advice Centres in Lewisham. Health Trends (in press)
Boardman A P, Bouras N, Cundy J 1987 The Mental Health Advice Centres in Lewisham. Service usage: trends from 1978 to 1984. National Unit for Psychiatric Research & Development Research report No 3. Lewisham Hospital, London
Boardman A P, Craig T K J, Openshaw S, Andrews V, Rhind D 1989 The uses of small area census data in the evaluation of the usage of a community psychiatric clinic (in press)
Book J A, Wetterberg L, Modrzewska K 1978 Schizophrenia in a North Swedish geographical isolate, 1900-1977. Epidemiology, genetics and biochemistry.Clinical Genetics 14: 373-394
Bromet E J, Dunn L O, Connell M M, Dew M A, Schulberg H C 1986 Long-term reliability of diagnosing lifetime major depression in a community sample. Archives of

General Psychiatry 43: 435-440

Brown G W, Birley J L T 1968 Crises and life changes and the onset of schizophrenia. Journal of Health & Social Behavior 9: 203-214

Brown G W, Harris T O 1978 Social origins of depression: a study of psychiatric disorder in women. Tavistock, London

Brown G W, Carstairs G M, Topping G 1958 Post-hospital adjustment of chronic mental patients. Lancet ii: 685-689

Brown G W, Monck E M, Carstairs G M, Wing J K 1962 Influence of family life on the course of schizophrenic illness. British Journal of Preventive & Social Medicine 16: 55-68

Brown G W, Birley J L T, Wing J K 1972 Influence of family life on the course of schizophrenic disorders: a replication. British Journal of Psychiatry 121: 241-258

Brown G W, Craig T K J, Harris T O 1985 Depression: distress or disease? Some epidemiological considerations. British Journal of Psychiatry 147: 612-622

Burke A W 1984 Racism and psychological disturbance among West Indians in Britain International Journal of Social Psychiatry 30: 50-68

Cochrane R 1977 Mental illness in immigrants to England and Wales. Social Psychiatry 12: 25-35

Cooke D J 1982 Life events and psychological distress: some problems in design and analysis. In: Main C J (ed) Clinical psychology and medicine: a behavioural perspective. Plenum press, New York

Cooper B 1978 Epidemiology. In: Wing J K (ed) Schizophrenia: towards a new synthesis. Academic Press, London

Cooper J E, Copeland J R N, Brown G W, Harris T O, Gourlay A J 1977 Further studies on interview training and inter-rater reliability of the Present State Examination (PSE). Psychological Medicine 7: 517-523

Cooper J E, Goodhead T, Craig T, Harris M, Howat J, Korer J 1987 The incidence of schizophrenia in Nottingham. British Journal of Psychiatry 151: 619-626

Craig T K J, Brown G W, Harris T O 1987 Depression in the general population: comparability of survey results. British Journal of Psychiatry 150: 707-708

Dean C, Walsh D, Downing H, Shelley E 1981 First admission of native-born immigrants to psychiatric hospitals in South-East England 1976. British Journal of Psychiatry 139: 506-512

Dean C, Surtees P G, Sashidharan S P 1983 Comparison of research diagnostic systems in an Edinburgh community sample. British Journal of Psychiatry 142: 243-256

Dear M 1977 Locational factors in the demand for mental health care. Economic geography 58: 223-240

Dear M 1978 Planning for mental health care: a reconsideration of public facility location theory. International Regional Science Review 3: 93-111

Derogatis L R, Klerman G R, Lipman R S 1972 Anxiety states and depressive neurosis: issues in nosological discrimination. Journal of Nervous & Mental Disease 155: 392-403

Dohrenwend B P, Dohrenwend B S, Gould M S, Link B, Neugebauer R, Wunsch-Hitzig R 1980 Mental illness in the United States: epidemiological estimates. Praeger, New York

Donovan C M 1980 Problems of psychiatric practice in community mental health centres. American Journal of Psychiatry 139: 456-460

Dunham H W 1965 Community and schizophrenia: an epidemiological analysis. Wayne State University Press, Detroit

Durkheim E 1952 Suicide. Routledge & Kegan Paul, London

Eaton W W, Holzer C E, Von Korff M et al 1984 The design of the epidemiologic catchment area surveys. Archives of General Psychiatry 41: 942-948

Essen-Moller E, Hagnell O 1961 The frequency and risk of depression within a rural population group in Scandinavia. Acta Psychiatrica Scandinavica 37, Supplementum 162: 28-32

Estroff S E 1981 Making it crazy. University of California Press, Berkeley

Falloon I R H, Boyd J L, McGill C W, Razani J, Moss H B, Gilderman A M 1982 Family management in the prevention of exacerbations of schizophrenia. New England Journal of Medicine 306: 1437-1440

Faris R E L, Dunham H W 1939 Mental disorders in urban areas. University of Chicago Press, Chicago

Fink P J, Weinstein S P 1979 Whatever happened to psychiatry? The deprofessionalisation of community health centres. American Journal of Psychiatry 136: 406-409

Finlay-Jones R, Brown G W, Duncan-Jones P, Harris T O, Murphy E, Prudo R
1980 Depression and anxiety in the community. Psychological Medicine
10: 445-454

Fowler R C, Rich C L, Young D 1986 San Diego suicide study: II. Substance abuse in
young cases. Archives of General Psychiatry 43: 962-965

Freeman H 1985 The scientific background. In: Freeman H L (ed) Mental health and the
environment. Churchill Livingstone, London

Freeman H, Alpert M 1986 Prevalence of schizophrenia in an urban population. British
Journal of Psychiatry 149: 603-611

Freeman H, Fryers T, Henderson S 1985 Mental health services in Europe. World Health
Organisation

Gerard D L, Houston L G 1953 Family setting and the social ecology of schizophrenia.
Psychiatric Quarterly 27: 90

Giggs J 1986a Ethnic status and mental illness in urban areas. In: Rathwell T, Phillips D
(eds) Health, race and ethnicity. Croom Helm, London

Giggs J A 1986b Mental disorders and ecological structure in Nottingham. Social Science &
Medicine 23: 945-961

Ginsburg S, Brown G W 1982 No time for depression: a study of help seeking among
mothers of pre-school children. In: Mechanic D (ed) Monographs in psychosocial
epidemiology 3: Symptoms, illness behaviour and help-seeking. Neale Watson Academic
Publications, New York

Goldberg D, Huxley P 1980 Mental illness in the community. The pathway to psychiatric
care. Tavistock, London

Goldberg E M, Morrison S L 1963 Schizophrenia and social class. British Journal of
Psychiatry 109: 785-802

Goldberg D P, Cooper B, Eastwood R R, Kedward H B, Shepherd M 1970 A standardised
psychiatric interview for use in community surveys. British Journal of Preventive and
Social Medicine 24: 18-23

Goldhamer H, Marshall A 1953 Psychosis and civilisation. Glencoe Free Press, Illinois

Gottesman I I, Shields J 1972 Schizophrenia and genetics: a twin study vantage point.
Academic Press, New York & London

Grad J, Sainsbury P 1966 Evaluating the community psychiatric service in Chichester:
results. Millbank Research Fund Quarterly 44: 246-277

Grad J, Sainsbury P 1968 The effects that patients have on their families in a community
care and control psychiatric service. British Journal of Psychiatry 14: 265-278

Griesinger W 1861 Die Pathologie und Therapie der psychischen Krankheiten. 2nd edn.
Braunschweig, Wreden. Translated as mental pathology and therapeutics by Robertson
C L, Rutherford J, New Syndenham Society, London 1867

Hafner H, Riemann H 1970 In: Hare E H, Wing J K (eds) Psychiatric epidemiology.
Oxford University Press, London

Hagnell O A 1966 A prospective study of the incidence of mental disorder. Scandinavian
University Books

Hare E H 1956a Family setting and the urban distribution of schizophrenia. Journal of
Mental Science 102: 753

Hare E H 1956b Mental illness and social conditions in Bristol. Journal of Mental Science
102: 349-357

Harrison G, Ineichen B, Smith J, Morgan H G 1984 Psychiatric hospital admissions in
Bristol. II. Social and clinical aspects of compulsory admission. British Journal of
Psychiatry 145 : 605-611

Harrison G, Owens D, Holton A, Neilson D, Boot D 1988 A prospective study of severe
mental disorder in Afro-Caribbean patients. Psychological Medicine 18: 643-657

Helzer J E, Robins L N, McEvoy L T et al 1985 A comparison of clinical and diagnostic
interview schedule diagnoses. Archives of General Psychiatry 42: 657-666

Heston L L 1966 Psychiatric disorders in foster home reared children of schizophrenic
mothers. British Journal of Psychiatry 112: 819-825

Hirsch S 1988 Psychiatric beds and resources: factors influencing bed use and service
planning. Gaskell Publication. Royal College of Psychiatrists, London

Hoenig J 1968 The de-segregation of the psychiatric patient. Proceedings of the Royal
Society of Medicine 61: 115-120

Huxley J, Mayr E, Osmond H, Hoffer A 1964 Schizophrenia as a genetic morphism. Nature 204: 220-250

Imber V 1976 A classification of English Personal Social Service Authorities. Statistical and Research Report Series No 16. DHSS HMSO, London

Ineichen B, Harrison G, Morgan H G 1984 Psychiatric hospital admissions in Bristol. II. Geographical and ethnic factors. British Journal of Psychiatry 145: 600-604

Jablensky A 1988 Methodological issues in psychiatric classification. British Journal of Psychiatry 152, Supplement 1: 15-20

Jones R, Goldberg D, Hughes B 1980 A comparison of two different services treating schizophrenia: a cost-benefit approach. Psychological Medicine 10: 493-505

Katschnig H, Pakesch G, Egger-Zeidner E 1986 Life stress and depressive subtypes: a review of present diagnostic criteria and recent research results. In: Katschnig H (ed) Life events and psychiatric disorders: controversial issues. Cambridge University Press, London

Kety S S, Rosenthal D, Wender P H, Schulsinger D F, Jacobsen B 1975 In: Fieve R R, Rosenthal D, Brill H (eds) Genetic research in psychiatry. Johns Hopkins University Press, Baltimore

Kidd K K 1975 In: Fieve R R, Rosenthal D, Brill H (eds) Genetic research in psychiatry. Johns Hopkins University Press, Baltimore

Klerman G L, Lavori P W, Rice J et al 1985 Birth-cohort trends in rates of major depressive disorder among relatives of patients with affective disorder. Archives of General Psychiatry 42: 689-693

Kramer M 1980 The rising pandemic of mental disorders and associated chronic diseases and disabilities. Acta Psychiatrica Scandinavica, Supplementum 285: 382-396

Kreitman N 1976 The coal gas story. British Journal of Preventive & Social Medicine 30: 86-93

Lazarus J, Locke B Z, Thomas D S 1963 Migration differentials in mental disease: state patterns in first admissions to mental hospitals for all disorders and for schizophrenia. New York, Ohio and California, as of 1950. Millbank Memorial Fund Quarterly 41: 25-42

Leff J, Vaughn C 1985 Expressed emotion in families. Guilford Press, New York

Leff J, Kuipers L, Berkowitz R, Everelin-Vries R, Sturgeon D A 1982 A controlled trial of social intervention in the families of schizophrenic patients. British Journal of Psychiatry 141: 121-134

Leighton D C, Harding J S, Macklin D B, MacMillan A M, Leighton A H 1963 The character of danger. Basic Books, New York

Lester D 1984 Suicide risk by birth cohort. Suicide & Life Threatening Behavior 14: 132-136

Levy L, Rowitz L 1971 Ecological attributes of high and low rate mental hospitalisation areas in Chicago. Social Psychiatry 6: 20-28

Lewis A J 1938 States of depression: their clinical and aetiological differentiation. British Medical Journal ii: 875-878

Lidz T, Fleck S, Cornelison A 1965 Schizophrenia and the family. International University Press, New York

Littlewood R, Lipsedge M 1981 Some social and phenomenological characteristics of psychotic immigrants. Psychological Medicine 11: 289-302

McCreadie R G, Oliver A, Wilson A, Burton L L 1983 The Scottish survey of 'new chronic' inpatients. British Journal of Psychiatry 143: 564-572

McCreadie R G, Robinson A D, Wilson O A 1984 The Scottish survey of chronic day-patients. British Journal of Psychiatry 145: 626-630

McCulloch J W, Philip A E, Carstairs G M 1967 The ecology of suicide behaviour. British Journal of Psychiatry 113: 313-319

McGovern D, Cope R V 1987 The compulsory detention of males of different ethnic groups, with special reference to offender patients. British Journal of Psychiatry 150: 502-512

Malzberg B, Lee E S 1956 Migration and mental disease. Social Science Research Council, New York

Milne D 1984 A comparative evaluation of two psychiatric day hospitals. British Journal of Psychiatry 145: 533-537

Mollica R F 1980 Community mental health centres: an American response to Kathleen Jones. Journal of the Royal Society of Medicine 73: 863-870

Mosher L R 1983 Alternatives to psychiatric hospitalization: why has research failed to be translated into practice? New England Journal of Medicine 309: 1579-1580

Munk-Jorgensen P 1985 Cumulated need for psychiatric service as shown in a community psychiatric project. Psychological Medicine 15: 629-635

Murphy H B 1972 The evocation role of complex social demands. In: Kaplan A R (ed) Genetic factors in schizophrenia. Thomas, Springfield, Illinois: pp 407-421

Murphy E, Lindesay J, Grundy E 1986 60 years of suicide in England and Wales: a cohort study. Archives of General Psychiatry 43: 969-976

Nielsen J, Biorn-Henrikson T, Nielson J 1980 Psychiatric illness and use of psychotropic drugs in the geographically delimited population of Samso, Denmark. Acta Psychiatrica Scandinavica 285, Supplementum 62: 97-102

Ni Nullain M, Buckley H, McHugh B, Ottare A, Walsh D 1984 Methodology of a study of mental illness in Ireland. Irish Journal of Psychiatry 5: 4-9

Odegaard O 1946 A statistical investigation of the incidence of mental disorder in Norway. Psychiatric Quarterly 20: 381

Odegaard O 1956 The incidence of psychoses in various occupations. International Journal of Social Psychiatry 2: 85-104

Odegaard O 1971 hospitalized psychoses in Norway: time trends 1926-1965. Social Psychiatry 6: 53-58

Office of Population Censuses & Surveys 1982 Census 1981. HMSO, London

O'Neal P, Robins L N 1958 Childhood patterns predictive of adult schizophrenia. American Journal of Psychiatry 115: 385-391

Phillip A E, McCulloch J W 1966 Uses of social indices in psychiatric epidemiology. British Journal of Preventive & Social Medicine 20: 122-126

Rabkin J G, Klein D F 1987 The clinical measurement of depressive disorders. In: Marsela A J, Hirschfeld R M J, Katz M M (eds) The measurement of depression. Guilford Press, New York

Rawnsley K 1984 Psychiatry in jeopardy. British Journal of Psychiatry 145: 573-578

Regier D A, Myers J K, Kramer M et al 1984 The NIMH epidemiologic catchment area program. Archives of General Psychiatry 41: 934-941

Richman A, Barry A 1985 More and more is less and less: the myth of massive psychiatric need. British Journal of Psychiatry 146: 164-168

Robins L N, Helzer J E, Croughan J, Ratcliff K S 1981 National Institute of Mental Health Diagnostic Interview Schedule: its history, characteristics, and validity. Archives of General Psychiatry 38: 381-389

Robins L N, Helzer J E, Ratcliff K S, Seyfried W 1982 Validity of the Diagnostic Interview Schedule, Version II: DSM-III diagnoses. Psychological Medicine 12: 855-870

Robins L N, Helzer J E, Weissman M M 1984 Lifetime prevalence of specific psychiatric disorders in three sites Archives of General Psychiatry 41: 949-958

Rosch E 1976 Classification of real world objects: origins and representation in cognition. In: Ehrlich S, Tislving E (eds) La Memoire Semantique. Bulletin de Psychologie, Paris

Rutter M, Graham P, Birch H G 1970 A neuropsychiatric study of childhood. Clinics in developmental medicine 35/36, Heinemann, London

Sartorius N, Jablensky A, Korten A 1986 Early manifestations and first contact incidence of schizophrenia in different cultures. Psychological Medicine 16: 909-928

Sayce L, Craig T K J, Boardman A P 1990 Social Psychiatry (In Press) Community Mental Health Centres in Britain.

Shepherd M, Williams P 1988 Primary care as the middle ground for psychiatric epidemiology. Psychological Medicine 18: 263-267

Shepherd M, Cooper B, Brown A C, Kalton G W 1966 Psychiatric illness in general practice. Oxford University Press, Oxford

Short J R 1978 Residential mobility in the private housing market of Bristol. Institute of British Geographers, New Series 3: 533-547

Singer M T, Wynne J 1965 Thought disorder and family relations of schizophrenics: results and implications. Archives of General Psychiatry 12: 201-212

Solomon M I, Hellon C P 1980 Suicide and age in Alberta, Canada, 1951 to 1977. A cohort analysis. Archives of General Psychiatry 37: 511-513

Spitzer R L, Endicott J 1978 Schedule for affective disorders and schizophrenia (SADS).

Biometrics Research, Evaluation Section, New York State Psychiatric Institute, New York

Spitzer R L, Endicott J, Robins E 1978 Research diagnostic criteria: rationale and reliability. Archives of General Psychiatry 35: 773-782

Srole L, Langer T S, Michael S T, Opler M K, Rennie T A C 1962 Mental health in the metropolis. McGraw Hill, New York

Stein L I, Test M A 1980 Alternative to mental hospital I: conceptual model, treatment program, and clinical evaluation. Archives of General Psychiatry 37: 392-397

Stromgren E 1987 Changes in the incidence of schizophrenia? British Journal of Psychiatry 150: 1-7

Sturt E 1984 Community care in Camberwell: a two-year follow-up of a cohort of long-term users. British Journal of Psychiatry 145: 178-186

Tantam D 1985 Alternatives to psychiatric hospitalisation. British Journal of Psychiatry 146: 1-4

Thompson R 1984 Towards a new area perspective: social area analysis of the 1981 census. Planning Division, Policy & Research Report 84/1 Southwark, a London Borough

Tooth G C, Brook E M 1961 Trends in the mental hospital population and their effects on future planning. Lancet i: 710-713

Torrey E F 1980 Schizophrenia and civilisation. Jason Arouson, New York

Walsh D, O'Hare A, Blake B, Halpenny J V, O'Brien P F 1980 The treated prevalence of mental illness in the Republic of Ireland — the three county case register study. Psychological Medicine 10: 465-470

Watt N F, Anthony E J, Wynne L C, Rolf T C 1984 Children at risk for schizophrenia — a longitudinal perspective. Cambridge University Press, New York

Watts F N, Bennett D H 1983 Introduction: the concept of rehabilitation. In: Watts F N, Bennett D H (eds) Theory and practice of psychiatric rehabilitation. Wiley, Chichester

Webber R J, Craig J 1978 Socioeconomic classification of local authority areas. Studies in medical and population subjects No 35, OPCS, HMSO, London

Weisbrod B A, Test M A, Stein L I 1980 Alternative to mental hospital II: economic cost-benefit analysis. Archives of General Psychiatry 37: 400-405

Wetzel R D, Reich T, Murphy G E, Province M, Miller J P 1987 The changing relationship between age and suicide rates: cohort effect, period effect or both? Psychiatric Developments 3: 179-218

Wilkinson G, Freeman H L 1986 Provision of mental health services in Britain: The Way Ahead. Royal College of Psychiatrists, London

Wing J K 1966 Social and Psychological changes in a rehabilitation unit. Social Psychiatry 1: 21-28

Wing J K, Fryers T 1976 Statistics from the Camberwell and Salford registers 1964-1974. MRC Social Psychiatry Unit, London and Dept of Community Medicine, University of Manchester

Wing J K, Hailey A M 1972 Evaluating a community psychiatric service: the Camberwell register 1964-1971. Oxford University Press, London

Wing J K, Sturt E 1978 The PSE-ID-CATEGO system Supplementary Manual. MRC Social Psychiatry Unit, London

Wing J K, Cooper J E, Sartorius N 1974 The measurement and classification of psychiatric symptoms: an instruction manual for the Present State Examination and CATEGO programme. Cambridge University Press, London

Wing J K, Nixon J M, Mann S A, Leff J P 1977 Reliability of the PSE (9th edn) used in a population study. Psychological Medicine 7: 505-516

Winokur G, Morrison J, Clancy C, Crowe R 1974 Iowa 500: the clinical and genetic distribution of hebephrenic and paranoid schizophrenia. Journal of Nervous & Mental Disease 159: 12-19

Wooff K, Freeman H L, Fryers T 1983 Psychiatric service use in Salford: a comparison of point-prevalence ratios 1968 and 1978. British Journal of Psychiatry 142: 588-597

World Health Organisation 1978 Mental disorders: glossary and guide to their classifications in accordance with the 9th Revision of the International Classification of Diseases. World Health Organisation, Geneva

World Health Organisation 1987 10th revision of the international classification of diseases. Chapter V: mental behavioural and developmental disorders. World Health Organisation, Geneva

Wykes T, Sturt E, Creer C 1982 Practices of day and residential units in relation to the social behaviour of attenders. In: Wing J K (ed) Long term community care: experience in a London borough. Psychological Medicine Monograph, Supplement 2
Zimmerman M, Coryell W, Pfohl B, Stangl D 1986 The validity of four definitions of endogenous depression. II. Clinical, demographic, familial and psychosocial correlates. Archives of General Psychiatry 43: 234-244

6. Schizophrenia: social influences on onset and relapse

J. Leff

If schizophrenia was purely a genetically transmitted condition, then preventive efforts such as genetic counselling and, ultimately, genetic engineering would be employed against it. Current evidence, however, indicates that while there is certainly a genetically transmitted component, this accounts only partially for the development of the disease. The highest estimates of the heritability index reach 70% to 80%. It is most likely that schizophrenia represents the final common pathway for a number of different pathogenic factors, including a genetic predisposition (Shields 1967), perinatal brain damage (Kasanin et al 1934), and other acquired structural pathology, e.g. in conjunction with temporal lobe epilepsy (Slater et al 1963). Attempts have been made to identify biological measures that mark a predisposition to schizophrenia. There is quite strong evidence from studies of children of a parent with schizophrenia for an excess of 'soft' neurological signs in individuals at risk (Marcus et al 1985). The findings on psychophysiological abnormalities are conflicting, although Dawson & Nuechterlein (1984) concluded from a review of the published work that genetically defined high-risk subjects do exhibit electrodermal hyper-responsivity. Whatever the biological basis of the illness may be, careful investigations over several decades have revealed an important role for social factors, both in the onset and in the relapse of schizophrenia. Hence, there is ample opportunity for appropriate social management to improve the outlook for patients, although preventive measures so far remain elusive.

INFLUENCES IN CHILDHOOD

Social factors operating in the patient's childhood are very difficult to identify, because it is not possible to recognise an individual who will later develop schizophrenia. Hence, the majority of enquiries of this kind involve the retrospective reconstruction of family relationships and attitudes. This is a very dubious procedure, as it relies on the memories of both relatives and patients, which are bound to be influenced by the fact that a serious illness has appeared in a family member. However, an ingenious way of avoiding this source of bias was employed by two groups of workers — O'Neal & Robins (1958) and Waring & Ricks (1965). They exploited the fact that child guidance clinics were established in the United States in the first decades of this century, and that a proportion of the children who were seen at the clinics later developed schizophrenia. These children were identified in a follow-up study, and matched with control children who also attended the same clinics but were not subsequently admitted to a psychiatric hospital. It was then possible to compare the records of the two matched groups of children, made at a time when no one knew which of them might later develop schizophrenia.

O'Neal & Robins found that the pre-schizophrenic children, compared with their matched controls, showed significantly more pathological lying, physical aggression, eating disorders, phobias, tics, and mannerisms. However, only a single difference was identified in the parent - child relationship; the pre-schizophrenic children were more often dependent on their mothers than the controls, as shown by a fear of letting the mother out of sight. From data collected in their study of child guidance clinic records, Ricks & Nameche (1966) also found that prolonged over-dependence of the child on the parent was common, exemplified by the parent bathing the child even in adolescence, isolating the child from its peers, and not allowing the child privacy. Waring & Ricks (1965) found, in addition, that children who later developed schizophrenia more often came from homes which were characterised by 'emotional divorce', i.e. the parents living under the same roof but in a state of mutual withdrawal.

These studies concur in finding excess dependence in pre-schizophrenic children and over-protectiveness in their parents. However, the direction of cause and effect is obscure, since the nature of this relationship may be determined by some quality of the child, rather than being initiated by the parents. A number of alternative models, incorporating genetic and environmental influences, were proposed by Hirsch & Leff (1975) to account for these findings. There will be occasion to refer back to these results when the nature of parental attitudes towards patients with an established schizophrenic illness is considered below.

In addition to child guidance clinic records, the accounts kept of children's behaviour at school have been exploited by American research workers. Using a similar strategy, Lewine et al (1978) identified children who later became schizophrenic, and compared their school records with matched children who grew up to be psychiatrically healthy. The pre-schizophrenic children were judged to be less secure, personable, and considerate of others, as well as more introverted and submissive than the group of matched normals. The school records did not include information on parent - child relationships. However, they do provide further evidence of minor, non-specific behavioural abnormalities in pre-schizophrenic children, which could readily affect the parents' attitudes to the child, long before the appearance of an identifiable schizophrenic illness.

SOCIAL CAUSATION OR SOCIAL DRIFT?

One of the pioneering epidemiological studies of schizophrenia was conducted by Faris & Dunham (1939) in the city of Chicago. They screened all first admissions to hospital and found that patients with schizophrenia were concentrated in the centre of the city, in the 'zone in transition' — the area immediately surrounding the commercial and entertainment centres of the city, which was threatened by the development of office blocks and stores. Hence, the houses were deteriorating, rents were low, and many dwellings were subject to multiple occupancy. Faris & Dunham proposed two contrasting explanations: either the poor living conditions in the zone in transition predisposed to schizophrenia, or else pre-schizophrenic individuals selectively migrated to this area. The latter became known as the 'social drift' hypothesis.

The argument was taken a stage further by Hare (1956), who applied similar epidemiological techniques to the city of Bristol. He replicated the finding that patients admitted for the first time with schizophrenia were concentrated in the centre. However, the association with socio-economic factors was narrowed down by studying the characteristics of individual wards of the city. Hare was able to show that the distribution of schizophrenia was not associated with poverty or with overcrowding, but was linked with the proportion of single-person households.

Before this issue of possible geographical drift was examined further, a related topic was investigated by Goldberg & Morrison (1963). They started from the observation that on first admission, schizophrenic patients cluster in the lower socio-economic classes, but once again, the dilemma is whether poverty produces schizophrenia or pre-schizophrenics drift down the social scale. Goldberg & Morrison argued that if the drift hypothesis is correct, then the social class distribution of the patients' fathers should be identical with that of the general population. They included a number of precautions against sources of bias, and discovered that whereas the patients were over-represented in the lower socio-economic classes, this was not true of their fathers. Hence, their data support the notion of a pre-schizophrenic descent into more impoverished conditions. In looking at individual case histories, they found that it was common for an unexpected deterioration in schoolwork to supervene in mid-adolescence; this is consonant with the findings by Lewine et al of various behavioural disturbances in pre-schizophrenic schoolchildren.

After some decades of controversy, a major contribution to the evidence for geographical drift was made by Dunham (1965), whose work with Faris initiated the argument. His later study was conducted in the city of Detroit, in which he selected a central city area, Cass, and compared it with a peripheral suburb, Conner-Burbank. As anticipated, he found a first-admission rate for Cass that was over double that for Conner-Burbank, but he then divided the patients on the basis of residence in their particular suburb for more or less than five years. When only those patients with at least a 5-year residence were considered, the admission rates for the two suburbs were found to be virtually identical. Thus, the excess of schizophrenic patients admitted from Cass had all arrived in the centre of the city within the preceding five years.

The body of research on social class and schizophrenia was reviewed by Kohn in 1973. He pointed out that the association between schizophrenia and low social class failed to hold up when small towns were examined, as in his own study with Clausen of Hagerstown, Maryland (Clausen & Kohn 1959). He noted that, in general, the larger the city studied, the stronger the correlation between rates of schizophrenia and indices of social class. An obvious explanation would be that pre-schizophrenic individuals leave small towns and rural areas and move to large cities, where they experience their first episode of illness while living in poor socio-economic conditions. Dunham's (1965) study supports this formulation. Kohn concluded that there is overwhelming evidence for an unusually high rate of schizophrenia in the lowest socio-economic strata of urban communities, but that the interpretation of this is equivocal.

The relationship between social class and schizophrenia appears to be different in the third world. Warner (1985) reviewed a number of studies carried out in India, all of which found a higher prevalence of schizophrenia in higher castes, compared to lower ones; regrettably, however, there have not been comparable studies of their incidence. The caste differences in prevalence could reflect social influences on the course of the disorder, rather than on its aetiology — e.g. those of higher caste might live longer, so that they do not throw light on the controversy over social drift.

To summarise, it is very likely that a major cause of the social class differences in the incidence of schizophrenia is the migration of pre-schizophrenic individuals to the isolated living conditions prevailing in the centre of cities. However, it remains a possibility that some factors implicit in low socio-economic status contribute to the aetiology of schizophrenia.

ACUTE STRESS AND ONSET

The idea that stress can produce psychiatric illness has a long lineage, but it is only recently that technical developments in the measurement of stress have enabled scientific evidence to be gathered. A major advance has been in the area of life events. No definition exists that would allow the immediate distinction between an event and a non-event, but happenings that are classed as events occur over short periods of time and are assumed to demand some unusual effort at psychological adjustment. The early investigators constructed lists of what they considered to qualify as life events, and asked respondents to check if any event on the list had happened to them within a specific time period. This is a relatively crude approach, which was subsequently refined in a number of ways. The most sophisticated instrument has been developed by Brown (Brown & Birley 1968; Brown 1974); it consists of an interview which is conducted with the patient and/or a key relative, and which is linked with a manual of definitions of life events. Events categorised as stemming from the patient's disturbed behaviour, e.g. quarrelling with a relative, are excluded. The remaining events are classified as 'independent' or 'possibly independent' when the patient's disordered behaviour might conceivably have given rise to them. The psychological impact an event is likely to have on the subject is assessed by taking into account everything that is known about the individual's circumstances. For instance, the impact of the death of a mother-in-law depends crucially on the nature of the subject's emotional relationship with her; this rating is known as 'contextual threat', and can be made with a high degree of reliability after a course of training.

The final precaution instituted by Brown's group is the accurate and conservative dating of the onset of illness; only patients with a clearly datable onset of illness are included in their studies. This avoids the danger of circularity, whereby prodromal changes in the patient's behaviour might give rise to alterations in their life, which could be identified as events.

Brown first used these techniques to study schizophrenia, although the contextual threat ratings were not developed until he embarked on his later studies of depression. Brown & Birley (1968) compared a group of 50 schizophrenic patients with 325 healthy individuals; the patients and an informant for each were asked about the occurrence of events in the 12 weeks before the onset of the episode of schizophrenia, while for the healthy controls, the period covered by the enquiry was the 12 weeks preceding the interview. They found that the proportion of controls experiencing an independent event was 14% for each of the four 3-week periods making up the 12 weeks. The patients showed a similar pattern, except for the 3-week period immediately before the onset of schizophrenia, when the proportion reporting an independent event jumped to 46%. In view of the methodological precautions taken to avoid circularity, this finding can reasonably be interpreted as implicating life events in the causation of episodes of schizophrenia. In Brown & Birley's sample of schizophrenic patients, 15 were experiencing their first-ever episode; the proportion of these reporting an event in the final three weeks was not different from that of the other patients. Hence, it appears that the role played by life events is as important for the first episode of schizophrenia as for subsequent attacks.

These findings have been confirmed by other investigators (Leff et al 1973, Leff & Vaughn 1980), but by far the most substantial replication has been conducted by the World Health Organisation (WHO). Brown & Birley's Life Events Interview and Manual were modified for use in both developing and developed countries, and were applied to samples of schizophrenic patients who were making their first contact with psychiatric services. A total of 371 patients was included from centres in eight countries, located in Aarhus, Agra, Cali, Chandigarh, Honolulu, Ibadan, Nagasaki and Prague. A significant clustering of life events was found in the three weeks before onset for patients in six of the eight centres. In the Honolulu centre, the same temporal clustering was evident, but the number of patients included (13) was too small for a statistical analysis. Only in Ibadan was the result not replicated, and there were some doubts about the comprehensiveness of the data collected in that centre (Day et al 1987).

The association between life events and the onset of episodes of illness is by no means peculiar to schizophrenia. Brown and his colleagues have found life events to precede episodes of depression in a number of studies (e.g. Brown & Harris 1978), as have other workers (Bebbington et al 1984). The same techniques have been applied to non-psychiatric conditions, and life events have been found to cluster in the few weeks before myocardial infarction (Connolly 1976) and before abdominal pain leading to appendicectomy at which a healthy appendix is found (Creed 1981). It is evident that life events can precipitate a wide variety of pathological conditions, but there is some indication of specificity in the time period over which they appear to operate; whereas clustering of these events occurs during some three months or more before episodes of depression, the crucial period in schizophrenia is three weeks. However, this same short period was identified in the studies of myocardial infarction and appendicectomy. Brown & Harris (1978) claimed that whereas events with a severe degree of threat are associated with onset of depression, events of little or no long-term threat are implicated in the onset of schizophrenia. However, the contextual threat ratings for the schizophrenic material were made retrospectively, using data not collected specifically for that purpose. Leff & Vaughn (1980) classified events as desirable, undesirable, and neutral, and found that undesirable events were no more common in depressed than in schizophrenic patients. Although specificity does not lie in the timing or the nature of events, it is possible that it is to be found in the mode of interaction of events with other forms of stress. This theme will be explored here after discussion of the influence of the family on schizophrenia.

FAMILY INFLUENCES ON THE COURSE OF SCHIZOPHRENIA

The problems of identifying family factors that are related to the first appearance of schizophrenia have been considered above. The relative success of the research covered in this section is largely attributable to the fact that it has concentrated on factors influencing the course of illnesses that are already established; this strategy avoids the biases inherent in the retrospective reconstruction of family relationships. Relatives' attitudes towards the patient are measured in the current situation by means of a semi-structured interview — the Camberwell Family Interview (CFI). This was originally developed by Brown & Rutter (1966), and then modified by Vaughn & Leff (1976b); it consists of questions about the patient's symptoms and behaviour, and covers the three months prior to the interview. The purpose of the interview is not evident to the subject, and indeed it is not possible for the interviewer to rate it as it is proceeding. Ratings are made from an audio-tape of the interview and depend crucially on vocal aspects of speech, including rate, volume and tone. There are five principal scales for rating Expressed Emotion (EE): critical comments, hostility, over-involvement, warmth and positive remarks. Inter-rater reliability reaches high levels on all scales after a 2-week training course; training is not considered complete until trainees reach a reliability of at least 0.8 on each scale.

The fact that the EE ratings are made from an interview with the relative and yet are assumed to reflect ongoing behaviour between relative and patient, might be considered a drawback of the technique. However, recent work has shown that criticism, as measured by the CFI, is closely related to critical remarks made by the relative to the patient in direct interactions (Strachan et al 1986, Szmukler et al 1987). These direct observations of behaviour do not show such a close correspondence with over-involvement as elicited by the CFI, but this is probably because the EE rating of this component takes into account behaviour that the relative reports outside the interview situation, e.g. excessive self-sacrifice shown by not encouraging the patient to draw unemployment benefit to which he is entitled. In this respect, the CFI covers a more comprehensive range of behaviour than is likely to be observed during a direct interaction with the patient.

In an early study, Brown et al (1972) found that in a 9-month period following discharge, a high level of criticism, the presence of hostility, and high over-involvement were each related to relapse of schizophrenia. On the other hand, high warmth was related to a good outcome over the same period, and this latter finding is of great importance, since it indicates that relatives can influence the course of schizophrenia in a beneficial way. It also contradicts the conclusion, incorrectly drawn by some from this body of work, that relatives of schizophrenic patients ideally should suppress all emotion. There is evidence from psychophysiological studies that some relatives actively support schizophrenic patients and enable them to tolerate stress better (Tarrier et al 1979).

In the Anglo – American studies using the CFI, hostility was virtually confined to relatives who also scored high on criticism. Thus, an index of EE can be constructed by using a cut-off point of six or more critical comments or a score of three or more on the over-involvement scale. The number of critical comments made during the interview are simply summed, while over-involvement is scored on a global scale, extending from 0 to 5. Patients returning to live with high-EE relatives were found by Brown et al (1972) to have a relapse rate of over 50% in nine months, compared with only 16% for those in low-EE homes (p < 0.001). These findings were almost exactly replicated by Vaughn & Leff (1976a), studying a similar population in South East London. More surprisingly, very similar relapse rates in high- and- low EE homes have been recorded by Vaughn et al (1984) for a sample of Californian schizophrenic patients. A WHO study of relatives' EE in North India also demonstrated a significant link with the outcome of schizophrenia, although the overall relapse rate is lower than in the Anglo-American studies, partly because all patients were making their first contact with the services. The relapse rates were 31% for those in high-EE homes and only 9% for low-EE homes (exact p = 0.04) (Leff et al 1987). Thus, the association between relatives' EE and the course of schizophrenia has been found to hold true for a variety of cultural settings.

Nine months is, of course, a very short interval in the lifetime of a schizophrenic patient. Leff & Vaughn (1981) extended the follow-up period to two years, and found that beyond the 9-month point, the high-EE patients relapsed at almost twice the rate of low-EE patients. By the end of two years, the overall relapse rates were 62% and 20% respectively (exact p = 0.015).

A study of first-admitted schizophrenic patients by MacMillan et al (1986) also found a significant association between relatives' EE and outcome of schizophrenia over two years. However, in contrast to Vaughn & Leff (1976a), these researchers found that the association was no longer significant when the effects of neuroleptic medication and duration of onset were taken into account.

Thus, the association between EE and relapse appears to persist over a considerable period of time, although the way in which it is mediated is the subject of controversy.

Within the high-EE group, the studies by Leff and Vaughn identified two protective factors: regular maintenance treatment with neuroleptic drugs, and low social contact between the relative and patient. The latter was measured by a time budget of a typical week, constructed from patients' and relatives' accounts; the amount of time the patient and relative spend in the same room together is summed to give the number of hours of face-to-face contact (as it is termed) and an arbitrary cut-off point of

35 hours a week is applied. Patients in low contact with high-EE relatives were found to have a significantly lower relapse rate than those in high contact.

In the British studies, the two protective factors had an additive effect, with the result that if patients were in low contact *and* took regular neuroleptic drugs, their relapse rate was lower than if only one protective factor was present. In the Californian study, the effect was different — i.e. interactional; neither drugs nor low contact on their own lowered the relapse rate, but both together resulted in a significant reduction in relapses. However, in both the British and American studies, patients in high-EE homes who employed the two protective factors together, had a relapse rate as low as that of patients in low-EE homes.

These associations between high EE and a high relapse rate, and between low contact, prophylactic medication, and a low relapse rate have all been derived from naturalistic observations. As such, they are open to a number of different interpretations. It could be argued, for example, that patients who exhibit disturbed behaviour both provoke criticism and over-involvement in relatives, and are thus more likely to relapse. In fact, that possibility was explored both by Leff & Vaughn and by Brown et al.

Brown and his colleagues (1972) first controlled for the degree of behavioural disturbance of the patients, and found that the association between EE and relapse was only slightly reduced. Then they controlled for EE, with the result that the association between disturbed behaviour and relapse fell to zero. Finally, they looked separately at the patients who had not shown behavioural disturbance prior to the key admission. Within this group, the relapse rate in high-EE homes was 64%, compared with 20% in low-EE homes ($p < 0.01$), showing that EE is strongly related to relapse even when there is no disturbed behaviour to mediate the relationship.

Vaughn & Leff (1976a) used a different statistical approach to the same problem, constructing a correlation matrix with the variables that were most closely related to relapse. Disturbance of behaviour on admission was actually related negatively to relapse ($r = -0.20$), so that when it was partialled out, the correlation between EE and relapse increased from 0.45 to 0.52.

These data strongly indicate that disturbed behaviour does not mediate the relationship between relatives' high-EE attitudes and patients' propensity to relapse, but numerous other factors, including some not measured in these studies, could theoretically be responsible.

The same argument can be applied to the apparently protective effect of drugs and low contact, i.e. that patients with a good premorbid personality are more likely to take drugs regularly and to have a wide circle of friends outside the home, and that their favourable outcome is a consequence of their personality strengths. Of course, the issue regarding drugs has been resolved by a number of controlled trials (e.g. Leff & Wing 1971, Hogarty & Goldberg 1973) which have demonstrated convincingly that maintenance neuroleptics exert a genuine protective effect against schizophrenic relapse. It was clear that a similar experimental approach was required to resolve the ambiguities surrounding the role of family factors in the course of schizophrenia.

EXPERIMENTAL INTERVENTION IN FAMILIES OF SCHIZOPHRENIC PATIENTS

A controlled trial was mounted by Leff et al (1982, 1985) with the primary aim of lowering relatives' EE and/or face-to-face contact, to determine whether this would have an impact on the patients' relapse rate. An additional aim of the trial was an evaluation of the effectiveness of social intervention in the families, but this was secondary to the accumulation of evidence on the direction of cause and effect. It was not considered ethical to withhold maintenance drugs, since their effectiveness had been clearly established. Therefore, a group of patients was chosen who were at a high risk of relapse even when on regular medication, in order to give some opportunity for the demonstration of an effect of social treatments. Data from the earlier naturalistic studies indicated that the highest-risk group on maintenance drugs were those in high face-to-face contact with high-EE relatives, who experienced a 50% relapse rate over nine months. If it proved possible to lower EE and/or contact in this group, a relapse rate of between 12% and 15% would be expected, assuming that these factors did indeed exert a causal influence on outcome.

Patients who were suitable for the trial by virtue of being diagnosed as schizophrenic by the CATEGO program (Wing et al 1974) and of being in high contact with high-EE relatives, were prescribed long-acting neuroleptic drugs where possible. Of the 24 patients included in the trial, 21 were maintained on these preparations. Families were randomly assigned to an experimental or a control group: the latter received no help from the research team, although they could have been offered any form of support by the clinical staff responsible for the patients. In fact, only one control relative (a wife) was given help of the frequency and intensity provided for the experimental relatives.

The experimental families received a package of social treatments comprising a brief education programme (Berkowitz et al 1984), a relatives' group (Berkowitz 1984), and family sessions, in which the patient and key relatives in the household were included. An eclectic approach to family treatment was adopted, with the use of behavioural, structural, and strategic interventions. Both the education and the family sessions were held in the patients' homes, while the group took place at a hospital. In order to reduce face-to-face contact, use was also made of day centres, day hospitals, hostels, and classes run by local authority

Table 6.1 Outcome of patients in a trial of social intervention who remained on maintenance neuroleptic drugs.

Group	Relapse rates	
	9 months	2 years
A Control	5/10 50%	7/9 78%
B Experimental	1/12 8%	2/10 20%
C Experimental in which aims were achieved	0/9 0%	1/7 14%
A vs B	exact p = 0.032	exact p = 0.017
A vs C	exact p = 0.017	exact p = 0.020

social services. The programme continued intensively for nine months, after which follow-up interviews were conducted on both experimental and control families. Some contact was maintained with the majority of the experimental families until two years after the patients' discharge, when a further follow-up was carried out.

The experimental group comprised 13 relatives, of whom 7 were found to have become low-EE at the 9-month assessment. There were also 13 high-EE, high-contact relatives in the control group, only two of whom became low-EE over the same period (exact p = 0.043). Face-to-face contact was reduced to below 35 hours per week for six experimental relatives, compared with three control relatives — a non-significant difference. A reduction of EE and/or contact from high to low was achieved in 9 of the 12 experimental families. The relapse rates in the various groups are shown in Table 6.1 for both the 9-month and 2-year follow-ups (Leff et al 1982,1985).

Patients who continued taking neuroleptic drugs and who lived in families in which one or both of the aims of intervention were achieved, suffered no relapses during the first nine months, and a 14% relapse rate over the whole two years. This compared very favourably with the rates for the control group — 50% and 78% for the two follow-ups, respectively. These data provide evidence for a genuine protective effect against relapse of low EE and low contact, and conversely, for the deleterious influence on the course of schizophrenia of high EE and high contact.

Use of relapse rates as the outcome measure underestimates the psychiatric morbidity in this trial, since several patients made suicidal attempts and two of these were successful. The two suicides were in patients in the experimental group, while three control patients made suicidal attempts serious enough to warrant admission; the suicides of the experimental patients could not be directly linked with any return of schizophrenic symptoms, but nevertheless, they undoubtedly represent failures of management. When these are included with the overt schizophrenic relapses, the treatment failure rate becomes 40% in the experimental group, which is about half the rate for the control patients (78%), but is not significantly different.

These data suggest that the effectiveness of social intervention, although clear-cut at the 9-month follow-up, may not have been sustained over the whole 2-year period; they raise doubts about the usefulness of incorporating work with relatives of schizophrenic patients into routine clinical practice. However, it is not an isolated study, and four other similar trials have been published, three conducted in the United States, and one in Britain.

The first to be completed was that by Goldstein et al (1978), followed by the trials of Anderson et al (1981), Falloon et al (1982), Hogarty et al (1986), and Tarrier et al (1988). In all four studies, schizophrenic patients were maintained on neuroleptic medication, and were randomly assigned to an experimental group, which received some form of family intervention, and a control group, in which the relatives were offered either limited assistance or none at all. In the studies of Falloon et al and of Hogarty et al, the control patients were given supportive individual management. The forms of family treatment used in the five studies reviewed here are referred to by different names, but a close look at their components reveals more similarities than differences.

Education about schizophrenia

This could be considered the most innovatory component in these programmes, since it runs directly counter to the traditional therapeutic approach to families. Conventional family therapists view the patient's symptoms as a communication about the distress experienced by the whole family, with the expectation that as the family's functioning improves, the symptoms will disappear. The common use of the term 'the designated patient' indicates that it is the entire family that is seen as 'sick', and that any member could well have presented symptoms that signalled the need for help. By contrast, in the four studies we are comparing, schizophrenia was presented in the education programmes as an illness in its own right, which can be influenced by family factors, but which has an existence independent of the family.

Goldstein and his colleagues spent the first one and a half sessions, out of their brief programme of six sessions, exploring each family member's experience of the events prior to and during the patient's psychotic episode. An emphasis was placed on the connection between stressful events and the development of symptoms; in describing sources of stress, they included pervasive conflicts between the patient and significant others. The input of information was not as comprehensive or structured as in the four later studies, which included facts about the aetiology, symptoms, course, and management of schizophrenia. However, they each imparted the education in a different setting: Falloon and his team saw the patient and relatives at home, Leff's group held sessions in the home for the relatives only, while Hogarty and his colleagues initially excluded the patients, and later on involved them in day-long multiple-family workshops. The relative efficacy of these different approaches — in particular, the advisability of including patients in education sessions, and the stage of the illness at which this is best done — need to be investigated empirically. Tarrier et al (1988) included one group in their trial who received education only; these patients did no better than the controls, indicating that education needs to be part of a package which incorporates other interventions.

Problem-solving activities

For Falloon's team, this is the central prop of their intervention. They first watch each family attempt to resolve problems, and having identified their deficiencies, attempt to remedy them; the aim is to teach the families to adopt a structured approach (Falloon et al 1984). This comprises six steps: 1. identify a specific problem; 2. list alternative solutions; 3. discuss advantages and disadvantages of each solution; 4. choose the best solutions; 5. plan how to implement the chosen solution; 6. review the outcome of their efforts at a later date. Tarrier and his colleagues were closest to Falloon's group in their emphasis on the behavioural management of the family. The other three studies each included the essence of this approach, viz — the setting of clear, specific, and attainable goals, and the seeking of agreement from the family that they would attempt to achieve them. However, while in these studies this was viewed as one component among many, to Falloon and his colleagues, it was the pre-eminent and crucial intervention. This does not simply represent a difference in emphasis, but reveals a fundamental ideological split between Falloon (Falloon & Pederson 1985), who holds that the successful adoption of efficient problem-solving techniques is necessary and sufficient to improve family functioning, and the other groups, who view an improvement in the family's disturbed emotional relationships as equally vital. This important issue could be resolved by appropriate studies, and will no doubt be examined in future work.

Improving communication

This is not mentioned by Goldstein's team in their account of their intervention, but featured as an aim in the other studies. In each, relatives were encouraged to voice appreciation of and praise for specific actions of other family members. Attempts were also made to improve the clarity of communication, where this was required, and to encourage individuals to listen carefully to what others were saying. Falloon's intervention appears to differ from the others in its focus on the communication of negative feelings, such as anger, hurt, disappointment, or sadness in an effective manner. The expression of anger was deliberately curbed by Leff's team, as a part of the next aim to be considered.

Lowering expressed emotion

This was one of the two main aims of Leff's team, and their education programme was planned as one approach to achieving it, since it had been found in previous studies that critical comments were chiefly directed at the negative symptoms of schizophrenia (Leff 1976). It was hoped that teaching relatives that the negative symptoms were an integral part of the illness, and not deliberately provocative behaviour, would ameliorate critical attitudes; in addition, both structural and behavioural methods of family therapy were utilised in an attempt to alter disturbed family relationships. The three other teams also tried to modify high-EE characteristics of relatives, although their techniques differed. Falloon's therapists modelled low-EE behaviour, Hogarty's group emphasised positive behaviour and took a structural approach in reinforcing interpersonal and intergenerational boundaries, while Goldstein's team attempted to resolve pervasive conflicts in the family and to reduce relatives' expression of criticism.

Lowering expectations

Goldstein's team approached this aim most directly, and informed relatives and patients early in their intervention that full recovery of social functioning could take from six months to one year. They discouraged premature efforts to pressurise patients into activities beyond their ability at the time. However, this requires the therapist to judge what the patient is capable of at any moment, and a course has to be steered between over-ambitious goals and expectations that are too low. Hogarty's group took a similar approach, while both the other teams employed the strategy of setting the patient very small tasks and of encouraging the relatives to praise small advances.

In the intervention by Leff's group, there was a particular focus on negative symptoms, since these had been found to attract the bulk of relatives' critical remarks. Families were told that although positive symptoms usually recede or disappear after a few weeks of treatment, negative symptoms can take between one and two years to show improvement.

Reducing contact

This was the second main aim in Leff's study, and was achieved by organising the placement of patients in sheltered daytime activities, while relatives were encouraged to take on part-time or full-time jobs. Attempts were also made to engage patients and relatives in separate leisure pursuits, but only rarely was a patient able to move out of the home into sheltered accommodation. Hogarty's and Tarrier's teams used similar strategies, but this aim is only briefly referred to in Goldstein's study, and receives no mention in the trial of Falloon et al.

Expanding social networks

The social networks of relatives of schizophrenic patients tend to decrease in size with the duration of the illness (Anderson et al 1984). This withdrawal is probably a consequence of a sense of guilt and sensitivity to the stigma attached to schizophrenia. Of the five groups, Hogarty's laid the greatest emphasis on endeavours to enhance the families' social networks. This was partly achieved through the day-long workshop, which brought a number of families together; a similar benefit was derived by relatives attending a group run by Leff and his colleagues. Falloon's team also held multiple-family groups for some of their therapeutic work, and only Goldstein et al and Tarrier et al omit this activity from their account of their programme.

In summary, the interventions of Leff's and of Hogarty's groups appear to be most similar, while Falloon's team differs in laying a heavier emphasis on problem-solving and improving communication; this is also the main focus of Tarrier. Goldstein's programme is not as comprehensive as the other four, and it is probably relevant that his was the first to be instituted. This comparison of the five modes of intervention reveals more similarities than differences, despite the varied theoretical orientations of their instigators, and it is, therefore, not surprising to find closely similar relapse rates emerging from all these studies. Short-term follow-ups were conducted over periods varying from six months to one year; the relapse rates in the control groups ranged between 41% and 53%, while in no study did the experimental patients have a relapse rate exceeding 12%. The two-year follow-ups have been completed in the studies of Leff et al (1985), Falloon et al (1985) and Hogarty et al (1987) and show a continuing advantage for the experimental patients over the control patients, although this was not significantly different in the former trial.

It cannot be inferred from the similarity of the outcome findings of these five studies that the many components shared by the various intervention programmes are all essential for their success. A question of great practical importance is whether it is necessary to work with the patients, the relatives, or both in order to achieve the maximum therapeutic effect. From this point of view, the studies of Falloon's group, of Hogarty's group and a recent trial by Leff et al (1989) are of particular relevance. Falloon et al (1985) set up a control group in which the patients received a behavioural programme, while the relatives were offered little assistance. The control patients did very poorly, even though they were maintained on medication; in fact, their outcome was no better over nine months and two years than the controls in Leff's study, who received nothing other than routine outpatient care. Hogarty et al (1986) employed a more complex design; in addition to a control group of patients who received drug alone, three other groups were treated, respectively, with drug plus social skills training, drug plus family treatment, and all these treatments combined. At the 1-year follow-up, 41% of the control patients had relapsed, compared with 19% of those receiving family treatment in addition, and 20% of those in the social skills training group. Both these rates are significantly lower than that of the control group. However, no patient who received the combination of drug and the two psychosocial treatments relapsed — an even better outcome.

These findings appear to contradict the results of Falloon's study, in which behavioural treatment appeared to add little or nothing to the effect of maintenance drugs. However, this difference was resolved when Hogarty et al repeated their analysis for only those patients who were compliant with the drug regimen. With this more restricted sample, the significant advantage for family treatment remained, whereas that for social skills training disappeared. It can be concluded that the advantage conferred on the patients who received social skills training is largely attributable to better drug compliance. This cannot be the case with family treatment, which is adding a significant benefit to the effect of maintenance drugs. In Falloon's study, behavioural treatment was aimed at the acquisition of general living skills, whereas in Hogarty's study it was targeted at behaviours that were likely to provoke high-EE attitudes in relatives.

The results of the studies by Falloon's and Hogarty's groups indicate that if drug compliance is assured, further clinical benefit can only be achieved by therapy directed at the whole family, and is maximised if additional training is given to the patient. In Hogarty's trial, it was found that regardless of the treatment received, no patient relapsed in a household which changed from high to low EE. This suggests that at least part of the therapeutic effect of family treatment given can be attributed to its success in lowering relatives' EE. In a second trial of intervention, Leff et al (1989) specifically dealt with the issue of whether patients needed to be included in the social treatment in order to benefit. They compared a relatives' group, from which patients were excluded, with family sessions during which the patient was present; both sets of relatives received an education programme initially. It was found that compliance with the relatives' group was poor, but in those families in which relatives did attend, the patients did as well as with family sessions.

Having shown that experimental amelioration of the family environment is possible, and does indeed lead to a reduction in the relapse rate of schizophrenia, we can turn to the issue of the specificity of the relationship between high-EE attitudes and the course of schizophrenia.

RELATIVES' EXPRESSED EMOTION AND NON-SCHIZOPHRENIC CONDITIONS

In their naturalistic study of EE, Vaughn & Leff (1976a) included a group of patients with depressive neurosis, to examine the specificity of the association with the outcome of schizophrenia. The sample of depressed patients differed from the schizophrenic group in that virtually all of them were living with a spouse, whereas half the schizophrenic patients were still in their parental home. Over-involvement is fairly common in parents of schizophrenics, but rare in spouses, so that it was only found in one relative of a depressed patient. However, criticism was as commonly expressed by the relatives of the depressed patients as by those of the schizophrenics. The cut-off point of six critical comments was applied to depressives' relatives, and failed to predict outcome over nine months; however, when the threshold for high criticism was lowered to two comments, a significant difference in outcome emerged between the resulting groups of patients. Thus, it appeared that patients with depressive neurosis were even more sensitive to criticism from relatives than were schizophrenic patients. This adjustment of the cut-off point for high criticism was quite arbitrary, but has found support in a recent study of EE and depression by Hooley (1985), who exactly replicated the methods and findings of Vaughn & Leff (1976a).

Other studies of non-schizophrenic conditions have been completed or are in progress. Havstad (1979) found that the criticism level of spouses predicted whether obese women would maintain a weight loss through dieting. A study comparing family therapy with individual therapy for anorexia nervosa has shown that high-EE attitudes of relatives are associated with failure to complete a course of family therapy (Szmukler et al 1985). An association has also been established between high-EE attitudes in parents and uncontrolled epilepsy in children (S Brown, personal communication). It is evident that high-EE attitudes are by no means exclusively characteristic of relatives of schizophrenic patients, and that they are linked with the course of a variety of psychiatric and non-psychiatric conditions, although the direction of cause and effect has yet to be established in each case. We have seen that neither life events nor relatives' EE are specific in their influence on schizophrenic patients. Where then does the specificity lie?

THE SEARCH FOR SPECIFICITY IN SOCIAL FACTORS

The most obvious answer is that the biological fault in schizophrenia, whether inherited or acquired, determines the characteristic psycho-pathological response to a variety of stressful situations. However, in the absence of any detailed knowledge about the nature of the presumed fault, this statement remains speculative. It is therefore worth searching further through the social data in an attempt to identify some specific features.

Although the link between life events and onset of episodes of illness is not peculiar to schizophrenia, it is possible that the period over which the psychological impact becomes manifest might be characteristic. All the studies of life events and schizophrenia have found that clustering occurs within a relatively short time before onset — between two to five weeks. By contrast, the time period over which events seem to exert their effect in bringing about depression, extends from three months to one year (Brown & Harris, 1978). However, the briefer period over which events operate as triggers of schizophrenic episodes is not characteristic only of that illness, since similar short time-spans are found to be important in myocardial infarction (Connolly 1976), and in abdominal pain leading to appendicectomy (Creed 1981).

We have already seen that the part played by EE differs between depressive neurosis and schizophrenia; over-involvement is of little or no importance in the former, while depressed patients are liable to relapse at lower levels of criticism than schizophrenic patients. Further data on EE in other psychiatric conditions are needed before these differences can be given much weight. Another difference between these two illnesses concerns the relationship between EE and face-to-face contact. Among the schizophrenic patients, low face-to-face contact with high-EE relatives was associated with a reduced relapse rate, and the intervention trial provided evidence that this was a genuine protective effect. By contrast, low face-to-face contact with a highly critical relative was linked with an *increased* relapse rate for depressed patients (Vaughn & Leff 1976a); for this group of patients, who were virtually all living with a spouse, low contact was interpreted as an indication of a poor marriage enduring for some time. In this interpretation, low contact and high criticism are seen as two facets of an unsatisfactory marital relationship.

The relationship *between* life events and relatives' EE has also been scrutinised; here again, differences were found between patients with depression and with schizophrenia. In Vaughn & Leff's (1976a) comparison of schizophrenic and depressed neurotic patients, a history of life events was taken, in addition to the EE assessments. It was found that in the schizophrenic group, patients admitted from high-EE homes had a low rate of independent events (5%) in the three weeks before onset, whereas patients from low-EE homes had a high rate (56%) (exact p = 0.0007). By contrast, depressed patients from highly critical homes had an event rate of 76% in the three months before onset, compared with only 33% of those from homes with a low level (exact p = 0.036). These data were interpreted as indicating that the onset or relapse of schizophrenia is associated with *either* the presence of high-EE relatives *or* with an independent life event. For the depressed patients, however, the pattern is quite different; in the majority, it is the *conjunction* of a critical relative and an independent life event that is associated with the onset of a depressive episode (Leff & Vaughn 1980).

In considering the social factors that have been found to be associated with the onset or relapse of schizophrenia, some indications of specificity have emerged, particularly when the interactions between life events, relatives' EE, and face-to-face contact are studied. There are clear differences between schizophrenia and depressive neurosis in respect to these relationships. However, a wider range of diagnostic conditions needs to be studied before firmer conclusions can be drawn.

THE RELATIONSHIPS BETWEEN SOCIAL FACTORS AND MAINTENANCE DRUGS

The data collected by Vaughn & Leff (1976a) on life events and EE related to schizophrenic patients, virtually all of whom were *not* taking regular maintenance neuroleptics; in fact, of the 37 patients studied, only six were receiving prophylactic drug treatment. The findings for the patients off medication are shown in Table 6.2, along with comparable data from the Chandigarh study of EE (Leff et al 1987).

The relationship between life events and EE is evidently very similar for both London and Chandigarh schizophrenic patients who are off medication, but these data leave unanswered the question of this relationship for patients on regular neuroleptic drugs. Material relevant to this issue was collected in the course of the trial of social intervention (Leff et al 1982); 14 patients living in high-EE homes remained on medication throughout the 9-month follow-up period, and of those, six relapsed and eight remained well. All but one of the relapsed patients had experienced an independent life event in the three weeks before relapse, whereas three of the eight well patients reported an event in the three weeks before the follow-up interview. This difference is not significant, but becomes so if events posing a trivial threat, or none at all are excluded; this results in the elimination of one event (brother started first

Table 6.2 The relationship between EE and independent life events in the three weeks before onset or relapse of schizophrenia. Patients off medication

	Number of patients with life event	Number of patients with no life event	Proportion with event
London			
High-EE home	1	14	6.7%
Low-EE home	9	7	56.3%
			exact p = 0.004
Chandigarh			
High-EE home	1	6	14.3%
Low-EE home	17	13	56.7%
			exact p = 0.05

job) from the group of well patients. As a consequence, the event rates became 83% for relapsed patients and 25% for those remaining well (exact p = 0.049). This finding indicates that patients living with high-EE relatives and protected by regular medication are often precipitated into relapse by the occurrence of a threatening event (Leff et al 1983). This contrasts with the patients in high-EE homes not taking medication, who do not appear to require an event to bring about a relapse.

These relationships can be summarised as follows: in patients who are unprotected by medication, either the acute stress of a life event or the chronic stress of a high-EE home can provoke an episode of schizophrenia. Patients on regular medication are protected against one or other stress, but the pharmacological protection is inadequate to buffer them against a combination of the acute and chronic stresses.

These statements have clear therapeutic implications. Maintenance neuroleptics appear to be indicated for patients in low-EE homes to protect them against the impact of life events, and drugs are highly effective in this respect, as evidenced by a group of 15 patients in low-EE homes maintained on prophylactic medication for two years with only a single relapse. However, there may also be other effective ways of protecting patients against life events. For instance, if an event can be anticipated, the psychological impact might be reduced by enabling the patient to rehearse the actions to be taken and to work through in advance the feelings likely to be aroused: this approach needs to be evaluated scientifically.

For patients living in high-EE homes, prophylactic medication alone is evidently an inadequate treatment, particularly if they are in high contact with their relatives. Additional measures of the kind used in the intervention studies described above are indicated here.

So far, we have discussed outcome solely in terms of relapse, implying a worsening of the florid or positive symptoms of schizophrenia. However, it is also necessary to pay attention to the negative symptoms.

THE NATURE OF NEGATIVE SYMPTOMS

Whereas the positive symptoms are *distortions* of normal experience or behaviour, the negative symptoms represent the *absence* of normal behaviour (Leff 1982); it is hardly surprising, therefore, that many relatives fail to recognise them as products of an illness, and consequently blame the patients for them. The negative symptoms include low motivation, lack of initiative, loss of interest in happenings in the patient's immediate environment and the wider world, withdrawal from social contacts, restriction of conversation, and blunting of affect. Such a clinical picture was common in the back wards of psychiatric hospitals during the custodial era; in fact, it was assumed by many to be a product of the atmosphere in such places, in which patients were rewarded for inactivity and silence. The pioneering study by Wing & Brown (1970) demonstrated wide variations between three psychiatric hospitals in the amount of activity provided for patients, and commensurate differences in the prevalence of negative symptoms. Since then, there has been continuing controversy over the extent to which such symptoms are induced by a deprived social environment, as opposed to being an integral part of the schizophrenic process. The advent of community care in the 1950s demonstrated that it was also possible for schizophrenic patients to develop severe negative symptoms outside psychiatric institutions, but this phenomenon appears to depend on the maintenance of an atmosphere in the home equivalent to that in custodial institutions. This is usually not because the relatives are content to allow the patient to spend much of the day lying on his bed, sleeping, or staring at the ceiling; on the contrary, they are often desperate to change the situation, but cannot find a way to do so. Such relatives can be greatly helped by the kind of interventions employed by Leff et al (1982).

A study by Johnstone et al (1985) has made an important contribution to the controversy over the nature of negative symptoms. They compared patients remaining for long periods in a psychiatric hospital who had diagnoses of either schizophrenia or manic-depressive psychosis, with schizophrenic patients living in the community. Cognitive function was assessed with a standardised test, and both inpatient groups were found to be equally impaired, in comparison with the schizophrenic patients living outside hospital. However, the manic-depressive patients showed significantly fewer negative symptoms than the schizophrenic inpatients, whose scores did not differ from those of the schizophrenic outpatients. This evidence supports the view that cognitive impairment is associated with long-term hospital care, regardless of psychiatric diagnosis. By contrast, negative symptoms do not appear to be an inevitable consequence of years spent in an institution, but are more closely linked with the long-term outcome of schizophrenia, regardless of whether patients are inside or outside hospital.

These data could be interpreted as indicating that negative symptoms are an integral component of the schizophrenic process. However, it is quite common to see one or more of the negative symptoms presenting during an acute florid episode of schizophrenia, and then to observe them recede as the episode resolves. In general, however, the time-course of negative symptoms is considerably more prolonged than that of positive symptoms; patients who are discharged from hospital free of positive symptoms, often retain negative symptoms for between one and two years after discharge. It is important to warn relatives about this; otherwise, they become impatient with the lack of progress, and develop critical attitudes towards the patient, which impede recovery.

It is possible to view negative symptoms as a strategy employed by patients, either consciously or unconsciously, to reduce environmental stimulation to a minimum. By these means, patients may protect themselves against further episodes of florid symptoms, but at the same time increase the likelihood of a chronic defect state. Although social withdrawal may remove patients from potentially dangerous situations, it can lead to a worsening of positive as well as negative symptoms. Cooklin et al (1983) found that auditory hallucinations occurred much more frequently when the schizophrenic patient was alone than in the presence of an interviewer — 55% of the time, compared with 9% (p > 0.001). Patients commonly report that their auditory hallucinations recede when they are engaged in workshop activities.

This observation is supported by an experiment conducted by Wing & Freudenberg (1961), who studied two groups of chronic schizophrenic patients, resident in hospital for more than two years. Two conditions of supervision of work were alternated: 'passive' — just seeing that the work went smoothly, and 'active' — giving praise and encouragement, and setting goals. It was found that not only did the patients respond to active supervision with a marked increase in output, but immobility, mannerisms, and restlessness decreased during periods of active supervision. Thus, encouragement and goal-setting improved symptoms of both the negative and positive variety. However, it is important to note that the improvements observed in the workshop setting did not extend to behaviour on the ward; this failure of improvements to generalise from the target setting to other situations is characteristic of schizophrenia.

IMPLICATIONS FOR MANAGEMENT

The evidence reviewed indicates that schizophrenic patients are highly responsive to features of their social environment. Both acute stress, in the form of life events, and chronic stress, generated in a high-EE home, can induce episodes of florid schizophrenic symptoms. Neuroleptic drugs confer only partial protection against the stress of close contact with a high-EE relative, so that in addition to prescribing drugs, it is necessary to make efforts to alter the family environment. Low-EE relatives actively support patients, and sustain them through stressful periods of change, though maintenance drugs are still needed as an adjunct in these situations. It is possible for therapists to act like low-EE relatives in enabling patients to weather the psychological stress of life events.

While being sensitive to high levels of stimulation, schizophrenic patients also do badly if under-stimulated; both negative and positive symptoms are exacerbated by an environment deprived of meaningful stimuli. Rehabilitation programmes are based on this premise, but care has to be taken to find the appropriate level of stimulation for each patient. It is all too easy for professional staff to develop high expectations for a patient, to exert a great deal of pressure for improvement, and thereby to produce a relapse of florid symptoms. There are high-EE individuals among staff, as well as among the relatives of patients. It is helpful, though, to provide a structured environment in which the patient learns the habits that are second nature to healthy people: getting up in the morning, washing and dressing, preparing a meal, and going out to a work-like activity during the day.

It is crucial for success to appreciate two problems that affect the learning of new behaviour by schizophrenic patients. Unlike patients with other psychiatric conditions, they fail to generalise from the learning situation, so that the skills they acquire there are not exhibited in other similar situations. To deal with this problem, it is necessary to ensure that the situation in which learning is being fostered is as similar as possible to the situation in which the skills will be demanded. Greatest success is achieved if the patients are taught the skills in the actual situation in which they will operate; for example, it is best if patients can be taught to purchase items in the shops closest to their homes.

The other problem peculiar to schizophrenic patients is that when the reward for the behaviour is withdrawn, the learned behaviour often disappears. Healthy people and other psychiatric patients appear to derive sufficient reward from their own satisfaction in achievement to maintain new skills, when praise from the teacher is no longer available. This is not the case with patients suffering from schizophrenia. Consequently, to sustain progress, it is necessary to continue to provide lavish praise and encouragement, even for the attainment of very small advances. It is this kind of social environment, provided by low-EE relatives and many professional staff, that can benefit even the most severely disabled schizophrenic patient.

REFERENCES

Anderson C M, Hogarty G, Reiss D H 1981 The psychoeducational family treatment of schizophrenia. In: Goldstein M J (ed) New developments in interventions with families of schizophrenics. Jossey-Bass, San Francisco

Anderson C M, Hogarty G, Bayer T, Needleman R 1984 Expressed emotion and social networks of parents of schizophrenic patients. British Journal of Psychiatry 144: 247-255

Bebbington P, Sturt P, Tennant C, Hurry D 1984 Misfortune and resilience: a community study of women. Psychological Medicine 14: 347-365

Berkowitz R 1984 Therapeutic intervention with schizophrenic patients and their families: a description of a clinical research project. Journal of Family Therapy 6: 211-233

Berkowitz R, Eberlein-Fries R, Kuipers L, Leff J 1984 Educating relatives about schizophrenia. Schizophrenia Bulletin 10: 418-430

Brown G W 1974 Meaning, measurement and stress of life-events. In: Dohrenwend B S, Dohrenwend B P (eds) Stressful life-events: their nature and effects. Wiley, New York

Brown G W, Birley J L T 1968 Crises and life changes and the onset of schizophrenia. Journal of Health & Social Behaviour 9: 203-214

Brown G W, Harris T 1978 Social origins of depression. Tavistock, London

Brown G W, Rutter M 1966 The measurement of family activities and relationships: a methodological study. Human Relations 19: 241-263

Brown G W, Birley J L T, Wing J K 1972 Influence of family life on the course of schizophrenic disorders: a replication. British Journal of Psychiatry 121: 241-258

Clausen J A, Kohn M L 1959 Relation of schizophrenia to the social structure of a small city. In: Pasamanick B (ed) Epidemiology of mental disorder. American Association for the Advancement of Science, Washington, DC

Connolly J 1976 Life events before myocardial infarction. Journal of Human Stress 2: 3-17

Cooklin R, Sturgeon D, Leff J 1983 The relationship between auditory hallucinations and spontaneous fluctuations of skin conductance in schizophrenia. British Journal of Psychiatry 142: 47-52

Creed F 1981 Life events and appendicectomy. Lancet i: 1381-1385

Dawson M E, Nuechterlein K H 1984 Psychophysiological dysfunction in the developmental course of schizophrenic disorders. Schizophrenia Bulletin 10: 204-232

Day R, Neilsen J A, Korten A et al 1987 Stressful life events preceding the acute onset of schizophrenia: A cross-national study from the World Health Organization. Culture, Medicine & Psychiatry 11: 123-206

Dunham H W 1965 Community and schizophrenia: an epidemiological analysis. Wayne State University Press, Detroit

Falloon I R H, Pederson J 1985 Family management in the prevention of morbidity of schizophrenia: the adjustment of the family unit. British Journal of Psychiatry 147: 156-163

Falloon I R H, Boyd J L, McGill C W, Razani J, Moss H B, Gilderman A M 1982 Family management in the prevention of exacerbations of schizophrenia: a controlled study. New England Journal of Medicine 306: 1437-1440

Falloon I R H, Boyd J L, McGill C W 1984 Family care of schizophrenia: a problem-solving approach to the treatment of mental illness. Guilford, New York

Falloon I R H, Boyd J L, McGill C W et al 1985 Family management in the prevention of morbidity of schizophrenia: 1. Clinical outcome of a two-year longitudinal study. Archives of General Psychiatry 42: 887-896

Faris R E L, Dunham H W 1939 Mental disorders in urban areas. University of Chicago Press, Chicago

Goldberg E M, Morrison S L 1963 Schizophrenia and social class. British Journal of Psychiatry 109: 785-802

Goldstein M J, Rodnick E H, Evans J R, May P R A, Steinberg M R 1978 Drug and family therapy in the aftercare treatment of acute schizophrenics. Archives of General Psychiatry 35: 1169-1177

Hare E H 1956 Mental illness and social conditions in Bristol. Journal of Mental Science 102: 349-357

Havstad L F 1979 Weight loss and weight loss maintenance as aspects of family emotional processes. Ph D Thesis. University of Southern California, Los Angeles

Hirsch S R, Leff J P 1975 Abnormalities in parents of schizophrenics. Maudsley Monograph No 22. Oxford University Press, London

Hogarty G E, Goldberg S C and the Collaborative Study Group 1973 Drug and socio-therapy in the aftercare of schizophrenic patients: one-year relapse rates. Archives of General Psychiatry 28: 54-64

Hogarty G E, Anderson C M, Reiss D J et al 1986 Family psycho-education, social skills training, and maintenance chemotherapy in the aftercare treatment of schizophrenia. I. One-year effects of a controlled study on relapse and Expressed Emotion. Archives of General Psychiatry 43: 633-642

Hogarty G E, Anderson C M, Reiss D J 1987 Family psychoeducation, social skills training and medication in schizophrenics: the long and the short of it. Psychopharmacology Bulletin 23: 12-13

Hooley J 1985 Criticism and depression. D Phil Thesis, Oxford

Johnstone E C, Owens D G C, Frith C D, Calvert L M 1985 Institutionalism and the outcome of functional psychoses. British Journal of Psychiatry 146: 36-44

Kasanin J, Knight E, Sage P 1934 The parent – child relationship in schizophrenia. Journal of Nervous & Mental Diseases 79: 249-263

Kohn M L 1973 Social class and schizophrenia: a critical review and a reformulation. Schizophrenia Bulletin 1: 60-79

Leff J P 1976 Schizophrenia and sensitivity to the family environment. Schizophrenia Bulletin 2: 566-574

Leff J P 1982 Chronic syndromes of schizophrenia. In: Wing J K, Wing L (eds) Psychoses of uncertain aetiology. Handbook of Psychiatry 3. Cambridge University Press, Cambridge

Leff J P, Vaughn C 1980 The interaction of life events and relatives' expressed emotion in schizophrenia and depressive neurosis. British Journal of Psychiatry 136: 146-153

Leff J P, Vaughn C 1981 The role of maintenance therapy and relatives' expressed emotion in relapse of schizophrenia: a two year follow-up. British Journal of Psychiatry 139: 102-104

Leff J P, Wing J K 1971 Trial of maintenance therapy in schizophrenia. British Medical Journal 3: 599-604

Leff J P, Berkowitz R, Shavit N, Strachan A, Glass I, Vaughn C 1989 A trial of family therapy v. a relatives' group for schizophrenia. British Journal of Psychiatry 154: 58 - 66

Leff J P, Hirsch S R, Gaind R, Rohde P D, Stevens B C 1973 Life events and maintenance therapy in schizophrenic relapse. British Journal of Psychiatry 123: 659-660

Leff J P, Kuipers L, Berkowitz R, Eberlein-Fries R, Sturgeon D 1982 A controlled trial of social intervention in the families of schizophrenic patients. British Journal of Psychiatry 141: 121-134

Leff J P, Kuipers L, Berkowitz R, Vaughn C, Sturgeon D 1983 Life events, relatives' expressed emotion and maintenance neuroleptics in schizophrenic relapse. Psychological Medicine 13: 799-807

Leff J P, Kuipers L, Berkowitz R, Sturgeon D 1985 A controlled trial of social intervention in the families of schizophrenic patients: two year follow-up. British Journal of Psychiatry 146: 594-600

Leff J P, Wig N, Ghosh A et al 1987 Influence of relatives' expressed emotion on the course of schizophrenia in Chandigarh. British Journal of Psychiatry 151: 166-173

Lewine R, Watt N, Prentky R, Fryer J 1978 Childhood behaviour in schizophrenia, depression, personality disorder and neurosis. British Journal of Psychiatry 133: 347-357

MacMillan J F, Gold A, Crow T J, Johnson A L, Johnstone E C 1986 The Northwick Park study of first episodes of schizophrenia. IV Expressed Emotion and relapse. British Journal of Psychiatry 148:133-143

Marcus J, Hans S L, Lewow E, Wilkinson L, Burack C M 1985 Neurological findings in high-risk children: childhood assessment and 5-year follow-up. Schizophrenia Bulletin 11: 85-100

O'Neal P, Robins L N 1958 Childhood patterns predictive of adult schizophrenia: a 30 year follow-up study. American Journal of Psychiatry 115: 385-391

Ricks D F, Nameche C 1966 Symbiosis, sacrifice and schizophrenia. Mental Hygiene (New York) 50: 541-551

Shields J 1967 The genetics of schizophrenia in historical context. In: Coppen A, Walk A (eds) Recent developments in schizophrenia. Headley Bros, London

Slater E, Beard A W, Glithero E 1963 The schizophrenia-like psychoses of epilepsy. British Journal of Psychiatry 109: 95-150

Strachan A M, Leff J P, Goldstein M J, Doane J A, Burtt C 1986 Emotional attitudes and direct communication in the families of schizophrenics: a cross–national replication. British Journal of Psychiatry 149: 279-287

Szmukler G I, Eisler I, Russell G F M, Dare C 1985 Anorexia nervosa: Parental expressed emotion and dropping out of treatment. British Journal of Psychiatry 147: 265-271

Szmukler G, Berkowitz R, Eisler I, Leff J, Dare C 1987 Expressed emotion in independent and family settings: a comparative study. British Journal of Psychiatry 151: 174-178

Tarrier N, Vaughn C, Lader M H, Leff J P 1979 Bodily reactions to people and events in schizophrenia. Archives of General Psychiatry 36: 311-315

Tarrier N, Barrowclough C, Vaughn C et al 1988 The community management of schizophrenia: a controlled trial of a behavioural intervention with families to reduce relapse. British Journal of Psychiatry 153: 532-542

Vaughn C E, Leff J P 1976a The influence of family and social factors on the course of psychiatric illness: a comparison of schizophrenic and depressed neurotic patients. British Journal of Psychiatry 129: 125-137

Vaughn C E, Leff J P 1976b The measurement of expressed emotion in the families of psychiatric patients. British Journal of Social & Clinical Psychology 15: 157-165

Vaughn C E, Snyder K S, Freeman W, Jones S, Falloon I R H, Liberman R P 1984 Family factors in schizophrenic relapse. Archives of General Psychiatry 41: 1169-1177

Waring M, Ricks D 1965 Family patterns of children who become adult schizophrenics. Journal of Nervous & Mental Diseases 140: 351-364

Warner R 1985 Recovery from schizophrenia: psychiatry and political economy. Routledge

& Kegan Paul, London

Wing J K, Brown G W 1970 Institutionalism and schizophrenia. Cambridge University Press, London

Wing J K, Freudenberg R K 1961 The response of severely ill chronic schizophrenic patients to social stimulation. American Journal of Psychiatry 118: 311-322

Wing J K, Cooper J E, Sartorius N 1974 The description and classification of psychiatric symptoms: an instruction manual for the PSE and Catego system. Cambridge University Press, London

7. Schizophrenia: the problems of handicap

J.L.T. Birley

Schizophrenia is one of the most disabling of all forms of psychiatric illness. Its low incidence and high prevalence mark it as a condition affecting people typically in early adulthood and, in some cases, lasting for the rest of their lives. The long-stay populations of psychiatric hospitals have consisted largely of people suffering from schizophrenia, who have thus made a major contribution to the character of these places. 'Institutionalism', however, is a product of the interaction between the patient and the staff: studies of this process (Wing & Brown 1970) have shown that both staff attitudes and the facilities and programmes provided, can all have a considerable effect on the patients' disabilities. Current trends for providing care for patients in less 'closed' systems, outside large institutions, have been influenced to some extent by these studies, but to a greater extent by fluctuations in society — of attitudes, social welfare, and employment — which up to now have advanced the process of 'community care', (although in the future they might reverse it). This chapter will be concerned first with the nature of the handicaps found in persons suffering from schizophrenia, and secondly with a consideration of how their prevention and treatment can be provided in a system which is less dependent on long-term inpatient care.

CLASSIFICATION OF HANDICAP

'Handicap', as used in this chapter, is an umbrella term covering both physical, psychological, and social difficulties, although in other systems it has been used in a more specific way to describe the social and environmental consequences of disablement (Wood & Badley 1978). It is not a satisfactory term, as it can be taken to mean a static, constant condition — which might apply to mental handicap or to some physical disabilities such as loss of a limb — but in the case of schizophrenia (and in many other conditions), is usually variable and requiring a flexible approach to prevention and treatment. The classification of handicaps can be based on their 'origin' or on the 'mechanism', but for our present purposes, both need to be considered.

THE ORIGINS OF HANDICAP

Wing's classification (1975) is based on the origins of handicap; it is a useful one, since it indicates both possible and impossible lines of treatment. Although it is a classification which can apply to any condition (e.g. epilepsy, diabetes), rather surprisingly, it does not appear to have been used for other purposes. It proposes three categories:

1. Premorbid handicap

These are disabilities which have pre-existed the illness itself. They may be related to the illness (e.g. having a parent who also suffers from schizophrenia, or having long-term difficulty in making friends) or may be unrelated but contributing to the overall handicap, e.g. being of low intelligence, physically disabled, or having a violent father.

2. Primary handicap

These are the disabilities that are thought to arise directly from the psychiatric illness itself. They include the so-called 'positive' symptoms of schizophrenia, such as experiencing hallucinations, believing in and acting on delusions, or having a distorted view of internal and external reality, as well as the 'negative' ones of retardation, withdrawal, inactivity, and poverty of thought and speech. In addition and often equally disabling, are symptoms of depression, irritability, restlessness, anxiety, and poor concentration which may affect both psychological and social function.

3. Secondary handicap

These are the disabilities arising from having been mentally ill, currently or in the past. They include those which may follow treatment, such as dependency and loss of skills as a result of 'institutional' care, either in hospital or in a restricted environment at home, or lethargy and other effects of drugs. Secondly, a person's psychiatric illness may have profound effects on other people, in particular relatives, other carers, and employers. Secondary handicaps thus comprise a wide range of physical, psychological, and social disadvantages.

It is important to recognise the extent of interaction between these types of handicap. For instance, many studies have indicated the association between certain types of premorbid personality and types of symptomatology: e.g. 'poor premorbid adjustment' is typically associated with 'nuclear, first rank symptoms'. A shy young bachelor, living with very concerned and critical relatives, with persistent symptoms, loss of life skills, and a need for heavy medication, typifies this sort of interaction. The value of Wing's approach is that it gives some indications for appropriate intervention; some of the secondary handicaps can be tackled by changing the attitudes and behaviour of other people, as well as, or instead of, the patient's.

Another approach to the classification of handicap, complementary to Wing's, is to look in more detail at the 'mechanisms' which may have brought them about. This remains an important area for research (Cutting 1985).

COGNITIVE DISTURBANCE

Many studies have described the poor attention and concentration found in persons suffering from schizophrenia (Frith 1979, Oltmanns & Neale 1982, Hemsley 1978, 1985). It has been suggested that this may be due to a failure to 'filter out' both internal and external information which is normally 'edited' at an unconscious level. Withdrawal by the patient is seen as a means of 'coping', to reduce input from the environment, while treatment by drugs may remedy this 'defect in editing' — there is good evidence that they improve cognitive function and reduce withdrawal (Oltmanns et al 1978). Another approach is to 'tranquillise' the patient with a structured, supportive, and not too demanding regime which strikes the right balance between over- and under-stimulation.

COGNITIVE DISTORTION

A deluded patient's view of the world may dominate his actions completely, but this is comparatively rare; delusions and hallucinations are usually 'partial' and are often related to specific situations or topics. Most patients retain some ability to cope with reality and enjoy doing so; indeed, to encourage this is the cornerstone of treatment. However, in pursuit of this aim, the degree of the patient's distortion and misinterpretation of the environment, including the behaviour and language of others, experienced by the patient, may be seriously underestimated.

FAILURE TO RECOGNISE SOCIAL OR AFFECTIVE CUES

People who later develop schizophrenia are often described as having been previously shy, with difficulties in making friends, lack of interest in having them, and being 'awkward' in company. There is also some evidence that patients may have difficulty in recognising 'social signals' from others who may be communicating their feelings by posture, facial expression, or words (Walker 1984, Cutting 1981). Thus, they fail to recognise information from other people or misinterpret it, and are in the position of a person in a foreign country, not understanding the language and habits of the natives, or of a colour-blind person trying to read traffic signals. Whether this difficulty is specific to facial and affective signals, or merely a more general problem of focusing attention, remains to be clarified.

SENSITIVITY TO FAMILY ATMOSPHERE

The shyness and unsociability of many patients have made it difficult, if not impossible, for them to leave the family circle. When this is compounded with the other disabilities of the illness, the patient becomes locked into the family, in a way which is distressing and often intolerable for all concerned. For everyone, family ties have a special power, but sufferers from schizophrenia and their families are particularly at the mercy of these bonds. Similar highly-charged situations may occur in other 'family groups', e.g. wards, sheltered workshops, or hostels, but they are generally less frequent, less intense, and more easily remedied.

RETARDATION AND REDUCTION IN DRIVE

This is a common disability, although the mechanism responsible for it is not known; attempts have been made recently, however, to account for this and other 'negative symptoms' in terms of a subtle form of brain damage (Crow 1980, 1983). Whilst thought, speech, and movement are all affected, it is not clear whether the reduction is in 'drive' or in 'ability to be motivated'. Nevertheless, patients may still be activated by certain situations, such as a structured regime and rewards, and it is remarkable how, on particular occasions (e.g. in response to dancing, singing, or games), apparently severely retarded patients 'come to life'. Many psychiatric hospital cricket teams, in the past, are said to have included a 'catatonic' patient who, once on the field, was transformed into a fast bowler!

SELF-NEGLECT

Some patients seem to take remarkably little notice of the state of their bodies, clothes, and surroundings, or if they do, seem unable to maintain their minimal care; this creates obvious difficulties in leading an independent existence outside hospital. The patient's person or surroundings, or both, become dirty, dishevelled, and smelly. This, at best, is off-putting to others — in Goffman's terms, it prevents the patient from passing as normal — while at worst, it is a threat to health and hygiene. However, self-neglect is not necessarily correlated with depression and demoralisation; a cheerful and proud worker may live in a chaotically dirty flat. Another may emerge from a room where rotting food lies all over the floor, but be smartly dressed and a popular piano player at a nearby social club.

MOOD DISTURBANCE

Just as some patients may have difficulty in interpreting other people's emotions, so they have difficulty in expressing their own. There is often a restriction in the range of moods, and at times the mood is not appropriate to the situation or to the context of their speech. This is a further handicap, which is often embarrassing for relatives and increases the problems of communication with others; mutual misunderstandings can lead to frustration and anger, or to withdrawal.

VULNERABILITY

Vulnerability refers to the way in which a person copes with stress, or anticipated stress, including life changes; persons suffering from schizophrenia are particularly sensitive to these. The assessment of vulnerability depends first on what is known about the patient's past reactions to stress or change, and secondly on his current social and psychiatric state; this information needs to be known for planning future treatment. Sometimes life changes, if successfully managed, can reduce a patient's vulnerability, e.g. acquiring a friend or looking after an ailing parent who had previously been providing most of the care.

THE EXPERIENCE OF PATIENTHOOD

Wing's 'secondary' handicaps include the experience of patienthood — the realisation of and adaptation to the fact that a person or a member of his family is mentally ill. This process is a long and painful one, and requires continued information and support, which cannot possibly be taken in at a single point in a person's career as a patient. A common reaction is one of guilt, alienation, and shame. The word 'schizophrenia' has a particularly ominous meaning, with its suggestions of a 'split mind', violence, and unpredictability — a view which may be reinforced by popular articles and programmes. Continued disability leads to a sense of loss, e.g. of old ambitions and skills. Drug treatment may lead to further disability, a staring gaze, and reduced movement of the face and arms, or abnormal movements, which are often noticed more by others than by the patient. Studies on 'stigma', as felt by psychiatric patients, suggest that it is highly related to continued disability and its accompanying demoralisation (Gove 1975).

THE PREVALENCE OF DISABILITY IN POPULATIONS SUFFERING FROM SCHIZOPHRENIA

The prevalence of disability clearly depends on the sample which is studied. Samples of patients in various forms of current psychiatric care illustrate this.

Cheadle et al (1978) reported on an outpatient sample, drawn from the Salford Case Register of patients who were in contact with the psychiatric service during 1974. Long-stay (those in hospital more than 12 months) patients were excluded, as were those aged over 65; 190 patients (71%) were seen from an original sample of 269. The Present State Examination (PSE), (Wing et al 1974) was used and a striking finding was the comparatively high prevalence of 'neurotic' symptoms: worrying, depressions, and tensions, were found in 30–50% of the sample. Specifically 'schizophrenic' symptoms were less common, and although three-quarters of the patients were unemployed, those who were employed reported fewer symptoms; 82% of the sample were receiving medication — mostly phenothiazines.

McCreadie (1982) reported a prevalence study of schizophrenia in a largely rural part of South-West Scotland. The overall prevalence was 2.38 per 1000 [1.73 per 1000 if the stricter 'Feighner criteria' (Feighner et al 1972) were used]. Of the 133 patients, 28% were inpatients, 17% day patients, 32% outpatients, and 23% were attending only their general practitioners. Three-quarters of the patients were receiving medication. The patients' symptoms were rated on the Manchester Scale (Krawiecka et al 1977) and their behaviour on the Wing Scale (Wing 1961). The most common symptoms were flatness of affect (45%), retardation (33%), poverty of speech (29%), anxiety (28%), delusions (23%), and depression (23%). The most frequent behaviour problems were social withdrawal (61%), restricted leisure interests (50%), limited conversation (48%), slowness of movement (33%), underactivity (30%), and poor care of personal appearance (24%). Thirty per cent of the patients had some symptoms or signs of parkinsonism and another 30% showed some signs of tardive dyskinesia; in 10%, these conditions coexisted. As might be expected, the inpatients were the most disabled and those attending their general practitioners the least disabled. Of the total sample, 75% (68% of the men) were unemployed, compared to 12% (13% of the men) in the general population; 18% were attending the hospital's industrial or occupational therapy department.

Watt et al (1983) reported a 5-year follow-up study of 121 inpatients from a semi-rural catchment area; the particular strength of this study was the completeness of its follow-up (99%) in a sample drawn from a known population. One-third of the sample were first admissions, and for these, as expected, the outcome was better than for the total sample. Of the first admissions, 58% had a good outcome in terms of no or minimal impairment, even though over half of this 'unimpaired' group had experienced recurrent episodes. For another third, impairment had increased. A better outcome was reported for women than for men, both in the first-admitted and readmitted patients. On the basis of comparison with previous cohort studies from the same area, it was suggested that improved outcome between 1931 and 1975 for patients suffering from schizophrenia had been confined to women only.

Johnstone et al (1984) reported a follow-up study of 120 patients with a 'Feighner' diagnosis of schizophrenia who had been discharged from a hospital in North London during the years 1970–1974. Of the 105 patients traced, 77 were interviewed — 11 in hospital and 66 at home — with their families (49), alone (7), or in sheltered accommodation (10). Information from informants, mostly relatives, was obtained in 42 cases. Of these 66 patients, 36 (55%) had a clearly abnormal mental state and only 26% were regarded as normal; 25 (38%) were impaired in their personal care and 27 (41%) were in open employment or day centres.

Only 11 were attending a psychiatric clinic and some dissatisfaction was expressed about their difficulties by the relatives, who nevertheless reported considerable concern, the most common being over the future for the patient when they died. They were dissatisfied with the health services, feeling that these were interested in patients when they first become ill, but lost interest as time passed. The informants felt that those concerned did not realise how great a burden was being placed upon relatives when patients were discharged from hospital. They regretted the frequent changes in staff associated with the patient, and 'would have valued the possibility of contact, albeit occasionally over the years, with a constant figure who was familiar with the facts of the patient's case'. Yet the patients did not want to go back to hospital and only in rare cases did the relatives wish them to return there.

In summary, therefore, recent British studies indicate a favourable outcome in up to one-half of schizophrenic patients, in terms of absence of persistent disability — but with recurrent episodes — and a poor outcome for a third of the patients. Women may have a better outcome than men. However, studies of cohorts of admissions (mostly read-missions) paint a gloomier picture of persisting disability, affecting employment and daily living; this is reflected in population prevalence studies. The symptomatic experiences of patients are mainly of reduction in activity and withdrawal — the 'clinical poverty syndrome' — together with a considerable amount of psychological distress arising from 'non-specific neurotic symptoms'. Drug side effects, generally mild, are found in about 50% of patients. Many relatives report continuing difficulties and distress, but their proposals for help are formulated not in terms of readmission, except in times of crisis, but in terms of long-term, consistent, and responsible support — the same comments as those reported in Creer & Wing's (1974) classic study 'Schizophrenia at home'.

VERY LONG-TERM PROGNOSIS

Mention should also be made of follow-up studies over a very long period

— a lifetime prognosis of schizophrenia. There are clearly problems of sampling and completeness of data, with a possible tendency of the survival of the 'fittest' to give an optimistic bias to the results. Nevertheless, recent studies, covering periods of more than 20 years (Bleuler 1978, Ciompi 1980, Harding et al 1987) indicate a gradual improvement in the survivors, with up to 'full recovery being reported in 50–60% of patients'. These findings suggest that the care of the patient during the early years of the illness needs to combine reducing damage with ensuring survival.

HOW SPECIFIC ARE THESE HANDICAPS TO SCHIZOPHRENIA?

It is of both theoretical and practical importance to consider how specific are certain psychological handicaps to schizophrenia. On the whole, the evidence suggests that they are not, except for those which are 'specific' in a tautological sense — i.e. that they are required to make the diagnosis of schizophrenia in the first place. Invalidism, loss of skills, and dependence can be found in all forms of long-term disability. The psychiatric symptoms of loss of drive, self-neglect, and apathy are found in persons suffering from brain damage, alcoholism, drug addiction, head injury, and chronic depressive states, to name but a few. It has already been remarked that many of the most troublesome complaints for patients are the 'non-specific' ones of tension, worrying, poor concentration, and depression; psychological tests of various types of cognitive deficit have not identified any which are 'specific' to schizophrenia (Oltmanns & Neale 1982). In a survey of chronic patients attending a large urban after-care clinic in Chicago, Summers & Hersh (1983) found no differences in symptomatology and social functioning between patients suffering from schizophrenia and those with other diagnoses. Their results 'suggest the startling conclusion that once it is known that a patient is chronic, knowledge of living situation or social performance indicates more about the patient's functioning than does the knowledge of diagnosis'. Most workers in the field of psychiatric rehabilitation would agree with this. Schizophrenia may lead to more of its sufferers developing a chronic handicap than those with other psychiatric conditions, but the reasons for this may have as much to do with the previous personality and adjustment of the patient as with the particular nature of the neuropsychological disturbance. Certainly, affective psychoses make a considerable contribution to chronic psychiatric disability (Bebbington 1982). In their survey of 'new long-stay patients', Mann & Cree (1976) found that affective psychosis was the second most common diagnosis in this group, accounting for 16%, compared with 44% suffering from schizophrenia.

THE CONTRIBUTION OF 'INSTITUTIONALISM' TO THE HANDICAPS OF SCHIZOPHRENIA

In the past, the great majority of patients suffering from schizophrenia in industrialised countries were admitted to hospital, and a proportion were detained for long periods of time, some of them indefinitely. The studies of Wing & Brown (1970) showed that the symptoms of such patients were related to their ward environment; in particular, severe withdrawal and 'clinical poverty' could be correlated with an impoverished environment and a monotonous and inactive regime. This classic monograph recorded that patients improved as the hospital regime improved and deteriorated as the hospital's activity declined, yet a question remains about the degree of improvement. For instance, in the 'worst' hospital, Severalls, which made the greatest strides over four years, of 82 women patients assessed in 1960, only 24 (29%) were in the moderate handicap categories(1,2). In 1964 this proportion was doubled to 58%, but that left another 42% still seriously handicapped. Wing & Brown concluded that a 'substantial proportion, although by no means all of the morbidity shown by long-stay schizophrenic patients in mental hospitals, is a product of their environment'. Their findings suggested that some of these patients' handicaps can be reduced, but not eliminated, by a suitable regime. In particular, the aim should be to 'prevent the developments of secondary handicaps and provide a series of sheltered environments in which patient's assets will be maximised and disabilities least evident'.

In a study comparing long-term inpatients with discharged patients who had avoided further long-term hospitalisation over a period of at least five years, Johnstone et al (1981) found that both groups were equally handicapped in terms of symptomatology and behaviour. The only differences — when allowance had been made for age and total duration of illness — were to be found in cognitive tests, the inpatients being more impaired. These results were said to show that even 'uninstitutionalised' patients have severe handicaps, which cannot be ascribed to institutional care. Another way of interpreting their results, however, is that the care provided outside hospital was no better or worse than that provided in the institution. Nevertheless, the challenges remain. Can a form of care be provided which combines the best of both worlds — the support and shelter of the institution with the variety, opportunity, and autonomy of the 'outside world'?

SOME ASPECTS OF TREATMENT AND MANAGEMENT

General

The aim of any treatment or rehabilitation regime is to bring about an as near as possible return to normal function, and to help the patient both to adjust to his disability and to make efforts to overcome it. Often, much less than this is achieved, but patients with untreatable disability may learn to adapt and live outside hospital and to manage in spite of severe handicap. From the beginning, treatment, and later rehabilitation, should be a co-operative effort between the professional team, the patient himself, and other people concerned, particularly the family. But rehabilitation is what has to be done when treatment fails; it is an attempt to improve the patient's functioning through a condensation of skills training, counselling, and environmental manipulation, together with efforts to develop and maintain a long-term support system. There is a central problem in maintaining high-quality care over a long period of time, which depends on staff morale and enthusiasm when little progress seems to be made. Shepherd (1988a) has drawn attention to certain factors which seem to play a part in this: good team work (Watts & Bennett 1983), involvement in decision-making (Raynes et al 1979), effective support for staff (Mendel 1979), the provision of clear feedback of results (Woods & Cullen 1983), the need for 'holiday'(Elliot 1977), and true understanding of the nature of the problem (Allen & Mendel 1982). All these help, but there is no easy answer.

Bleuler (1978) has emphasised: first, the importance of relating to the 'person behind the psychosis' and to that person's healthy aspects; secondly, the value of calming actions and influences, both personal, social, and pharmacological; and thirdly, the value of sudden changes — in general, social, or somatic conditions — in leading to the 'mobilisation of hidden resources'. The 'dose' of such changes, both in terms of 'extent' and 'suddenness', may need to be controlled, but the value of opportunities 'to display and mobilise hidden resources' cannot be over-estimated. For instance, a very disorganised and uncontrollable man who has been a psychiatric inpatient for over 10 years, nevertheless enjoys the weekly trip to the local swimming baths and the snack afterwards at a cafe, where his behaviour is quite appropriate. More profound and lasting changes may occur where patients take on, perhaps unexpectedly, caring responsibilities for a pet, a child, or an ailing parent.

Meeting the demands of existence and surviving in a particular society are powerful measures of social control. However differently from each other most men and women may feel, think, or act in some ways, there are many other ways in which, in a given situation, their behaviour is remarkably similar. A person suffering from schizophrenia may be preoccupied with many bizarre ideas and experiences, but yet behave as an ordinary citizen when given the opportunity to walk the treadmill of existence, with its trivial rounds and common tasks. Therefore, one aim of treatment for the reduction of handicap is that a patient should be exposed to the rewards, disappointments, and demands of 'normal life'. At the same time, a patient may be handicapped in ways which make some of the demands of ordinary life very difficult, if not impossible to meet. There is an 'optimum dose' of social demands which varies both between patients and, over time, for any particular patient; the ingredients of this 'dose' need to be considered and adjusted. Failure to maintain this dose may lead to lethargy and apathy, while demanding too much may precipitate a psychotic relapse, even after some years of quiescence (Stone & Eldred 1959, Wing et al 1964).

Community life for the person handicapped by schizophrenia requires a range of opportunities: educational, occupational, and residential. While these have developed slowly, both in Britain and other societies, they are nowhere complete. There are excellent services, but their distribution is patchy, both nationally and throughout the world. It has been found that hospital readmission rates are more dependent on the nature of social support and interpersonal conflict than on the physical nature of the living situation (Goldstein & Caton 1983). It seems important to show that Expressed Emotion and interpersonal relations remain at a low level in all living situations, and not just in the family (Berkowitz & Heinl 1984), while services must be provided in a way that avoids staff 'burnout' (Shepherd 1988b). Since the disabled individual's need for treatment and support varies in kind and extent over time, there should be no services for patients or families defined in terms of their high-, medium-, or low-dependency needs. Instead, staff should not be tied to facilities or buildings, but should work directly with patients and families, who would get the help they need when and where they need it and for as long as necessary. There is much talk of 'normalisation', which suggests that psychiatrically disabled people should be treated in ways that are socially valued (Wolfensberger 1972). At the same time, we must recognise the reality that handicap requires an adapted environment to provide for an accommodation between the needs and outlook of the handicapped and those of the non-handicapped (Criswell 1968).

Support

Everybody needs support and those disabled by schizophrenia perhaps need it even more — from family, friends, and professional staff. There are three types of 'support': first, 'affective', involving a relationship which includes concern, understanding and encouragement as well as, at times, control; secondly, 'educational', teaching patients to cope with practical and emotional problems — from their rent to their hallucinations; and thirdly, 'replacement', when certain tasks, practical or emotional, are actually taken over or provided by somebody else — self-care, medication, or caring for a child.

At different times, a person suffering from schizophrenia may need different types of support from 'institutional sources'. In terms of 'affective support', many patients have remarkably small social networks

(Pattison et al 1975), and probably have difficulty in maintaining and coping with large ones. Nevertheless, they seem to appreciate a 'familiar group', even though perhaps preferring to remain fringe members (Beels 1981, Cohen & Sokolovsky 1978). In a study of patients attending an in-patient unit as 'day patients' (Mitchell & Birley 1983), it was found that many patients suffering from schizophrenia had attended regularly for years but had not made much, if indeed any, intimate contact with the staff or other patients. A friendly but undemanding group seemed to suit them, as judged by their frequent attendance. Staff may need to be made aware that such 'fringe group' patients are deriving benefit from attending, even though they do not appear to participate very much, if at all, in the 'therapeutic programme'.

Such individuals may have difficulty in using the available services, so that 'case management' is much favoured in some countries (Intagliata 1982), although the term has been criticised for calling individuals cases and suggesting that a professional is in fact a manager, while Test (1979) has suggested that for the disabled patient, a core services team is more necessary than individual case management. This offers more continuous cover and co-ordination than an individual worker can provide — team planning brings more points of view to bear on the solution of the problem and it helps prevent staff 'burn-out', since members help and support each other. Nevertheless, case management can be an important component of care, as a continuing support to patients in assessing and co-ordinating services, although it is useless if there is a basic lack of facilities (Shepherd 1988b).

A 'fringe' group, however, comprises only a small proportion of patients, many of whom require a more intimate relationship; the development of trust is often a slow process and there are particular problems in the formation of a relationship with one individual: first, this may be too intense and may switch at times to one of delusional force; and secondly, on practical grounds, the not infrequent changes of staff may lead to a 'make and break' pattern which everybody finds un-comfortable and unhelpful. There is therefore something to be said for a relationship to be built up with a group of staff, although at any one time one member may be particularly involved. For many patients, however, relationships with other patients are as valuable and often more long-lasting than relationships with staff. Shanks & Atkins (1985) reported a series of 22 marriages, each between two patients, and showed that they were generally supportive to both partners. For others, 'be-friending schemes' have been very helpful; these have recruited and selected volunteers drawn from the local community, who are usually given an introductory course on ways of helping people with chronic handicaps. They need to be administered and the volunteers continually supported by a responsible person — usually a social worker, nurse, or voluntary help organiser.

'Educational support'

Although there has been much interest in remedying deficits in social skills, the gains in this field have been rather limited for patients suffering from schizophrenia — perhaps because of the nature of their handicaps and the lack of generalisation from specific training situations (Shepherd 1980, 1986, Liberman et al 1987). The emphasis has therefore moved to dealing with particular problems, such as budgeting, domestic skills, or symptom control. Effective training of this kind requires an accurate assessment of the problem, some motivation, both from the teacher and the taught, and a carefully thought out and executed programme. It has to be related to the patients' own perceived needs; for instance, it is a waste of time to teach cooking to a bachelor who intends to continue getting his meals at a local cafe.

In the United States, social skills training has formed the basis of rehabilitation (Anthony et al 1984, Anthony & Liberman 1986), but a review of 50 studies concluded that while it may be effective, it is little better than other possible treatments (Shepherd 1986). Even Liberman, a strong advocate of such treatment, concludes that 'the data are far less convincing that such interpersonal strenghtening actually reduces the probability of relapse or symptom exacerbation and increases community tenure and quality' (Liberman et al 1987). He concludes that patients with limited potential for acquiring and generalising functional skills may benefit more from social support and prosthetic environments. It is obviously easier to train people in instrumental rather than in social skills, for success in the latter depends on knowing how to use such skills, which is a difficult task for someone suffering from schizophrenia. Skills training needs to become something that is done *with* the patient and not *to* him, so that professionals who prescribe solutions to their view of the patient's difficulties are unlikely to be effective.

Education can comprise a wider field than merely survival or social or domestic skills; some understanding of the nature of their illness and of the treatments available is of help to many patients. In addition, education can be used in its more traditional sense of 'widening a person's horizons', since boredom and monotony often seem to be adopted by patients as a way of life. This may be seen as partly protective, but such a life-style may go on for much longer than is really necessary. Many treatment facilities now have links with local schools and colleges, who run courses in, e.g. 'expanding horizons', specific training, welfare rights, and 'enhanced leisure'.

'Replacement' support is the provision of functions which the patient cannot perform for himself; this may vary from self-control to budgeting. One of the problems in management is how to provide such replacement in an accurate and specific way, rather than in a 'package' which may be unnecessarily large. A patient who cannot manage money may still be able to survive independently if his daily or weekly budget is controlled by, for instance, a social worker or other staff member at a day centre. Another, whose room rapidly deteriorates to dangerously unhygienic levels, may still be capable of going to work and could be maintained by regular visits by a cleaner who does not object to dealing with greasy carpets and mouldy refrigerators. Adjusting the amount of replacement support, often a matter of negotiation, can only be done when there is, first, a working relationship with the patient, and secondly, a fairly wide range of services, often provided not by different statutory organisations but by a group of people who are prepared to do a variety of different tasks. A 'sheltered house' may be better accepted, locally, by cleaning out its untended garden and talking to the neighbours over the fence, than by calling on them in a more formal manner and preaching the virtues of community psychiatry. However, the administrative arrangements under which staff are employed may not allow such flexibility, and in such cases, the help of volunteers can be particularly valuable.

Occupation

Inpatient studies (Wing & Brown 1970) demonstrated convincingly that the provision of structured occupation was of great benefit to people suffering from psychiatric illness, but for those living outside hospital, the situation is rather different. Coping with the demands of ordinary existence provides its own occupation and structure, but in addition, other work opportunities need to be available. These should not only provide occupation, but also allow opportunities for patients to leave their homes during the day, thus avoiding 'institutionalisation at home' as well as the burdens which some families and patients impose on each other. The practicability of providing such activities, at least from statutory sources, must depend on geography. They are appropriate and possible for urban areas with good public transport, but in rural areas, accessibility may be more important than the requirements of individual patients. Such activities are usually provided in day centres in Britain, in psychosocial rehabilitation centres in the United States, and in Living Skills centres in Australia.

As living independently is not the sole aim of rehabilitation, so paid employment is not the only goal of vocational rehabilitation; only a small number of people will be fit for open employment in today's economic situation. However, work can be valuable in situations which do not lead to economic employment and there is a tendency to provide it in service-orientated occupations or small 'firms', which may be more fully integrated into the community than are some traditional sheltered workshops. Many such hospital-based workshops, faced with an ageing and more chronic population, and relying on a too narrow use of paid work, have become pale shadows of their former selves (Dick 1984). There has been a tendency to look to leisure activities as the solution, but

Kelvin (1980) recognised that this is not sufficient, since it does not in any way replace the important psychological functions of work (Jahoda 1982). For some patients, occupation rather than employment will be a realistic aim, but that occupation should match the needs and interests of the patient as far as possible. Unskilled work often seems boring and monotonous to occupational therapists and middle-class doctors, but these are subjective estimates, and the work may not have the same meaning to the patient who is being paid to do something that is required by his society.

The prospects of employment for people handicapped by schizophrenia, in a country with a large number of healthy people all out of work, are poor. Therefore, for many, occupation rather than employment will be the realistic aim, but the nature of the occupation will need to match the needs and interests of the patient so far as possible. The opportunity to earn some extra money will often be an over-riding consideration, even though the work may be rather monotonous. However, every advantage should be taken of schemes which allow a person to earn a full wage, with the help of some form of government subsidy, e.g. in a sheltered factory for the disabled or in a scheme which allows a person to be subsidised while working in open employment, at least for a probationary period.

It is most important that occupation of some sort is made available for the most handicapped patients and that these are not forgotten in enthusiasm for 'rehabilitation', which is in fact confined to a flourishing factory occupied by less disabled patients. One of the challenges for those working in day centres is to provide programmes which the patients find rewarding. Hospital studies of token economy programmes (Hall et al 1977, 1983) have indicated that their effectiveness depended as much on the general atmosphere generated by the programme as on the actual token economy rewards. The same is probably true of day centres; the best seem to provide not only work but a social support group, encouragement of individual and group talent (e.g. a magazine), self-help (e.g. jumble sales), support (e.g. darts matches), and excursions (e.g. an annual holiday). Even so, much will depend on the way in which these day centres are run. A study of four day centres found varying degrees of institutional practice in these community settings (Shepherd & Richardson 1979).

Housing

The provision of accommodation is a practical exercise in adapting to, and compensating for, the handicaps associated with schizophrenia. In Britain, at least 20 options are offered by hospitals, local authority social services, and housing departments, together with voluntary organisations and private provision (Garety 1988); the need for autonomy and privacy have to be balanced against the need for supervision, company, and practical support. In assessing these, it is important not to assume that everything has to be provided 'under one roof'; as a general rule, in fact, such an arrangement should be avoided if at all possible. Some supervision, practical support, and company can be provided by various forms of day care, rather than in the home. Supervision within the domestic setting may be required to help with withdrawal and inertia, poor self-care, and difficulties between various residents, but these problems may not require the presence of 24-hour residential staff; they can generally be managed by visiting staff, especially in the morning and evenings. 'Home helps' can act as extra cleaners and some local authorities designate some of them specially to assist the mentally ill. Many day centres have their own washing, bathing, and laundry facilities for their clients.

With moderately handicapped patients, the provision of privacy — 'a room of one's own' — is a valuable support for many patients suffering from schizophrenia, particularly if they are assured that they can stay as long as they like, provided they keep to the 'house rules' (Birley 1974). Shared accommodation leads to difficulties in matching flat-mates and, particularly, in introducing new members into an established group when a vacancy occurs. A further advantage in several countries of not having residential staff is that it allows ordinary housing to be used without any official 'change of use', thus avoiding a local planning enquiry and allowing for the creation of an 'invisible hostel'.

However, such accommodation does not provide adequate supervision for all patients, even when day care is included: some will require residential supervision, and a small proportion with severe and chronic disability will require 24-hour nursing care. Although this is care of a hospital type, it need not be provided in a ward, but can be in a domestic setting; two such experimental hostels in England have been described recently (Wykes 1982, Goldberg et al 1985).

Particular emphasis needs to be given to the management and staffing of sheltered housing. At present, this is provided in Britain by a variety of different organisations including private enterprise, housing associations, voluntary organisations, local authorities, and health authorities. Piecemeal development has its advantages, particularly in providing variety and innovation, but some coherent overall planning is also needed so that an appropriate range of facilities is available in any district. In addition, these facilities must be efficiently managed with respect to selection of residents and staff, collecting rents, and ensuring adequate routine supervision as well as appropriate action in emergencies. Some statutory authority should have the responsibility of inspecting and re-licencing(or de-licencing) sheltered housing facilities at regular intervals. There is a risk that a 'scandal' or a tragedy occurring in sheltered housing could provide the wherewithal for a backlash against 'community care'.

Special approaches to the family

The age of onset of schizophrenia covers the period of adolescence, courtship, sexual maturity, and bonding, the creation of a new family, and the development of independence; all these processes may be seriously damaged by the illness. In addition, some previous degree of social shyness or awkwardness has commonly been present in the case of both sexes, as has bachelorhood for men. Patients are thus very likely to remain dependent upon their families, particularly on parents, but also at times on spouses (if the marriage does not break up), or on children. At the same time, schizophrenia seems to be associated with a high degree of sensitivity to the social environment, both in the home and in the institution (Wing & Brown 1970, Brown et al 1972). With the move to 'partial care', more patients are living with their relatives, and the family situation thus requires particular attention.

The considerable demands made on families have been frequently described (Stevens 1972, Creer & Wing 1974, Arey & Warheit 1980, Creer et al 1982), but although the overall impression is one of 'burden', the picture is by no means totally bleak and some studies report a good deal of satisfaction and appreciation by relatives (Stevens 1972, Collis & Ekdawi 1984), in terms of help and company. Creer et. al. (1982) found that 60% of the relatives they interviewed were content with their responsibilities, but the interviewing team themselves felt that over one-third of the relatives required more practical help, and over one-quarter needed to be involved with the plans that were being made for the patient, as well as needing more advice on the management of the patient's difficult behaviour.

In Sydney, Australia, Hoult has used crisis teams made up from 7 nurses, a psychologist, and a psychiatrist or a social worker for a population of around 100 000: 3 workers are available on the day shift and 2 on the evening shift, 7 days a week. From 23h to 08h, one of the evening staff remains on call. Mobile community treatment teams are also being implemented for the support of the more refractory chronic patients. These teams are reported to be popular with families because the staff spend considerable time talking to the patients and the relatives, giving explanations and practical advice, and because the relatives know that they can get help at any time (Hoult & Reynolds 1984).

The special approaches which have been devised to improve 'the family atmosphere' and their successful use have been described by Falloon et al (1985) and by Leff et al (1985). However, these have a rather different approach from some other forms of 'family therapy', being problem-orientated, tackling a wide range of specific difficulties arising in a particular family, and avoiding any imputation of blame on the relatives, who are often already preoccupied with guilt about their family's predicament. These treatments need to be provided in a setting of continued support by an accessible service; a common complaint of relatives is of being abandoned, particularly at times of crisis and of not knowing whom to approach. Tunnell et al (1988) reviewed four models of the education of families, together with the provision of skill training or professional support (Anderson et al 1986, Goldstein & Kopeikin 1981, Falloon et al 1984); multiple family groups have been described by Berkowitz et al (1981). There are differrences, though, as to whether or not the patient is included in the group: neither Tunnell et al nor Berkowitz et al included the patient.

Medication

A considerable body of evidence is now available to indicate that treatment with phenothiazine and similar drugs is of value to people suffering from schizophrenia, both in terms of reduction of symptoms and distress, and long-term stability. Patients who stop their drugs, either as part of a trial or through 'non-compliance', are more liable to relapse (Johnson et al 1983). At the same time, approximately one-third of patients respond rather poorly to drug therapy and another proportion — more in a first-admission sample than in readmissions — do not require long-term maintenance treatment. To some extent, the need for drugs may depend upon the social circumstances of the patient, both in terms of the long-term 'emotional atmosphere' of his surroundings and of the more short-term impacts of life events. There is also the risk of side effects of drugs, some of which can be serious. A recent study (Curson et al 1985) found, as have many others, that maintenance medication may not prevent relapse, but that the relapses may be delayed and their frequency reduced; this in turn allows for the return of some social stability and progress in social adjustment.

From these considerations, it follows that maintenance treatment must be provided in the setting of individual concern for each patient and regularly reviewed, both in terms of developing side effects and in terms of social progress and of changes in the patient's social situation. It is in this setting that problems of compliance can be reduced (Falloon 1984), but nevertheless, all surveys report some problems of compliance, due to a mixture of absolute refusal, some unwillingness, and failures in the system of follow-up (Johnson & Freeman 1973, Curson et al 1985).

Control

Of particular concern in the community management of schizophrenia is the issue of control. A small proportion of patients are habitually unco-operative and actively avoid treatment, while a larger proportion may have occasional periods (often associated with relapse) in which more control is required. Violence to others or to themselves is rare but well recognized, and so is the gradual drift to destitution, petty crime, and prison or unsavoury lodging houses (Taylor 1982, Taylor & Gunn 1984, Lamb & Grant 1982, Leach & Wing 1980). Unless the psychiatric services make efforts to exert control, they will be criticised for looking after the 'easiest' patients, while leaving the 'most difficult' to cause trouble and distress both to themselves and to others. At the same time, these services are meant to be replacing a system which has often been regarded as 'too controlling', both by the public and by the staff themselves. There may thus be a reluctance by staff to intervene and to make sure that an 'uncontrollable' patient can be properly cared for.

In general, the most important sources of control are: first, the patient's efforts to cope with the ordinary demands of everyday life and his own social circle; secondly, the relationship he has with the service which is looking after him; and thirdly, the actual control, organisation, and efficiency of the service itself. These are all, to some extent, inter-related. If a service is well managed and efficient, it can, to some extent, control the 'dose' of 'ordinary demands' made on the patient, so that it is beneficial rather than overwhelming. At the same time, the service will provide people whom the patient and his circle can regard as reliable and understanding, who are technically competent for the tasks assigned to them, and who themselves know to whom they should consult and report. The organisation of the more diffuse service required to look after patients in a variety of settings, communications within this service, and the technical competence of its staff are all crucial ingredients in the management of patients handicapped by schizophrenia. Managerial language usually speaks of the need for clear management structure, defined goals, and regular reviews. But equally important is a sense of trust and respect between all those in the system — patients, families, staff, and the public — which is by no means the same as universal agreement.

Psychiatrists are also empowered to take compulsory action for the care of patients, with the agreement of others who need to be consulted (usually family or social workers), and can admit and detain patients for treatment. These powers are certainly needed occasionally in the treatment of schizophrenia, but to be most effective, they have to be used within the setting of the other controls already mentioned. In England and Wales, the Mental Health Act (1983) makes it clear that compulsory action can be taken on behalf of the health of the patient or his safety and/or the safety of others. Although it does not specify physical danger, it allows compulsory intervention when this is indicated on clinical rather than on criminal grounds. The timing of compulsory intervention is important; if possible, it should only be used when the patient has reached a stage which he will recognise, either at the time or later on, as justifying such a drastic step.

With increased emphasis on care in the 'least restrictive setting', should control, in a legal sense, be confined to hospital care, or should it follow the patient to his home or hostel? It might be justifiable to insist on treating a patient's acute relapse at home, but without admission. There is a small group of patients who habitually relapse after stopping their medication, causing both themselves and their families (or fellow residents in sheltered accommodation) a great deal of trouble and distress. Should it be possible to continue to treat them compulsorily, after they have left hospital? The legal, ethical, and practical issues in this question need to be fully debated, since the future of 'community care' for some patients suffering from schizophrenia will certainly depend on separating 'compulsory treatment' from 'hospital treatment'.

Patients' techniques of coping

It always seems to be assumed that the patient is helpless in the face of schizophrenia, but Breier & Strauss (1983) believe that to some extent, patients may influence the course of their disorder. One of their female patients asked why professionals never enquired about what she did to influence her illness, and subsequent interviews revealed that many individuals with schizophrenia had developed strategies which they felt helped them to control their psychotic symptoms (Strauss et al 1987). Further work on these lines is proceeding (Boeker 1987, Brenner et al 1987, Suellwold 1982), but so far, there has been little discussion which combines the families' problems of coping with their patient member with his/her problems of coping with the family situation.

CONCLUSIONS

Handicapped patients living in the community require access to a wide range of services, and their rehabilitation is determined by the way these services are provided and co-ordinated. While there are good local services, there are many gaps in the provision. In the United States, where de-institutionalisation has gone further than in the United Kingdom, services are very fragmented and this, together with the effects of handicap, has led to the problems seen in new young chronic patients (Pepper & Ryglewicz 1984). Even in the UK, there is emphasis in recent studies on the needs, met and unmet, of high-contact patients, 50–70% of whom have a diagnosis of schizophrenia and are being cared for in day treatment (Brugha et al 1988). It was shown that while psychotropic medication and shelter were provided, advice on coping and on some other forms of social treatment were rarely available. Such long-term attenders had no major clinical problem, but had difficulty surviving in the community because of skills deficiency, for which provision was not being made. Psychiatry cannot, and should not, take responsibility for solving all these problems, but there is a need for knowledgeable leadership which depends on understanding how psychiatric handicap affects the individuals, and to what extent care is needed (Lamb 1986). It is the psychiatrist's responsibility to explain this to patients, to families, to legislators, and to the public at large.

REFERENCES

Allen C, Mendel W M 1982 Chronic illness and staff burnout: revised expectation for change in the supportive-care model. International Journal of Partial Hospitalisation 1: 191–199

Anderson C M, Reiss D J, Hogarty G E 1986 Schizophrenia and the family. Guilford Press, New York

Anthony W A, Liberman R P 1986 The practice of psychiatric rehabilitation: historical, conceptual and research base. Schizophrenia Bulletin 12: 542-559

Anthony W A, Cohen B F 1984 Psychiatric rehabilitation. In: Talbot J A (ed) The chronic mental patient: five years later. Grune & Stratton, Orlando

Arey S, Warheit G J 1980 Psychosocial costs of living with psychologically disturbed family members. In: Robins L N, Wing J K (eds) The social consequences of psychiatric illness. Brunner/Mazel, New York

Bebbington P 1982 The course and prognosis of affective psychoses. In: Wing J K, Wing L (eds) Handbook of psychiatry Vol. 3. Psychoses of uncertain aetiology. Cambridge University Press, Cambridge

Beels C C 1981 Social support and schizophrenia. Schizophrenia Bulletin 7: 58-72

Berkowitz R, Heinl P 1984 The management of the schizophrenic patient: the nurses view. Journal of Advanced Nursing 9: 23-33

Berkowitz R, Kuipers L, Eberlein-Vries R, Leff J 1981 Lowering expressed emotion in relatives of schizophrenics. In: Goldstein M J (ed.) New developments in intervention with families of schizophrenics. Jossey-Bass, San Francisco

Birley J L T 1974 A housing association for psychiatric patients. Psychiatric Quarterly 58: 568-571

Bleuler M 1978 The schizophrenic disorders, long term patient and family studies. Translated by Clemens S M. Yale University Press, New Haven

Boeker W 1987 Self-help among schizophrenics: problem analysis and empirical studies. In: Strauss J S, Boeker W, Brenner H D (eds) Psychosocial treatment of schizophrenia. Huber, Toronto

Breier A, Strauss J S 1983 Self-control in psychotic disorders. Archives of General Psychiatry 40: 1141-1145

Brenner H D, Boeker W, Mueller J, Spichtig L, Wuergler S 1987 Auto-protective efforts among schizophrenics, neurotics and controls. Acta Psychiatrica Scandinavica 75: 405-414

Brown G W, Birley J L T, Wing J K 1972 Influence of family life on the course of schizophrenic disorders: a replication. British Journal of Psychiatry 121: 241-258

Brugha T S, Wing J K, Brewin C R et al 1988 The problems of people in long-term psychiatric day care. Psychological Medicine 18: 443-456

Cheadle A J, Freeman H L, Korer J R 1978 Chronic schizophrenic patients in the community. British Journal of Psychiatry 132: 221-227

Ciompi L 1980 The natural history of schizophrenia in the long term. British Journal of Psychiatry 136: 413-420

Cohen C I, Sokolovsky J 1978 Schizophrenia and social networks: ex-patients in the inner city. Schizophrenia Bulletin 4: 546-560

Collis M, Ekdawi M 1984 The relatives' story. Netherne Hospital, Coulsdon, Surrey

Creer C, Wing J K 1974 Schizophrenia at home. National Schizophrenia Fellowship, 79 Victoria Road, Surbiton, Surrey

Creer C, Sturt E, Wykes T 1982 The role of relatives. In: Wing J K (ed) Long term community care: experience in a London Borough. Psychological Medicine Monograph No. 2

Criswell J K 1968 Considerations on the permanence of psychiatric rehabilitation. Rehabilitation Literature 29: 162-165

Crow T J 1980 Molecular pathology of schizophrenia: more than one disease process.

British Medical Journal 1: 66-68

Crow T J 1983 Is schizophrenia an infectious disease? Lancet i: 173-175

Curson D A, Barnes T R E, Bamber R W, Platt S D, Hirsch R, Duffy J C 1985 Long term depot maintenance of chronic schizophrenic out-patients. The seven year follow up of the Medical Research Council fluphenazine/placebo trial. British Journal of Psychiatry 146: 646-680

Cutting J C 1981 Judgement of emotional expression in schizophrenics. British Journal of Psychiatry 139: 1-6

Cutting J C 1985 The psychology of schizophrenia. Churchill Livingstone, London

Dick D 1984 Occupation or work: the real issue. In: Herbst K (ed) Rehabilitation: the way ahead or the end of the road? Mental Health Foundation, London

Elliot P A 1977 The effect of holidays on a token economy regime. British Journal of Psychiatry 130: 481-483

Falloon I R H 1984 Developing and maintaining adherence to long term drug taking regimes. Schizophrenia Bulletin 10: 412-417

Falloon I R H, Boyd J L, McGill C W 1984 Family care of schizophrenia. Guilford Press, New York

Falloon I R H, Williamson M, Razani J, Moss H B, Gilderman A M, Simpson G M 1985 Family versus individual management in the prevention of morbidity in schizophrenia. Clinical outcome of a two-year study. Archives of General Psychiatry 42: 887-896

Feighner J P, Rodins E, Goze S B, Woodruff A, Winokur G, Munoz R 1972 Diagnositc criteria for use in psychiatric research. Archives of General Psychiatry 26: 57-63

Frith C D 1979 Consciousness, information processing and schizophrenia. British Journal of Psychiatry 134: 225-235

Garety P 1988 Housing. In: Lavender A, Holloway F (eds) Community care in practice. Wiley, Chichester

Goldberg D P, Bridges K, Cooper W, Hyde C, Sterling C, Wyatt R 1985 Douglas House: a new type of hostel ward for chronic psychotic patients. British Journal of Psychiatry 147: 383-388

Goldstein J M, Caton C L M 1983 The effects of the community environment on chronic psychiatric patients. Psychological Medicine 13: 193-199

Goldstein M J, Kopeikin H S 1981 Short- and long-term effects of combining drug and family therapy. In: Goldstein M J (ed) New developments in interventions with families of schizophrenics. Jossey-Bass, San Francisco

Gove W L 1975 Labelling and mental illness: a critique. In: Gove W R (ed) The labelling of deviance. Wiley, New York

Hall J N 1983 Ward-based rehabilitation programmes. In: Watts F N, Bennett D H(eds) Theory and practice of psychiatric rehabilitation. Wiley, London

Hall J N, Baker R D, Hutchinson K 1977 A controlled evaluation of token economy procedures with chronic schizophrenic patients. Behaviour Research & Therapy 15: 261-283

Harding C M, Brooks G W, Ashikaga T, Strauss J S, Breier A 1987 The Vermont longitudinal study of persons with severe mental illness. II: Long-term outcome of subjects who retrospectively met DSM-III criteria for schizophrenia. American Journal of Psychiatry 144: 727-735

Hemsley D R 1978 Limitations of operant procedures in the modification of schizophrenic functioning: the possible relevance of studies of cognitive disturbance. Behaviour Analysis Modification 2: 165-173

Hemsley D R 1985 Schizophrenia. In: Bradley B P, Thompson C (eds) Psychological application in psychiatry. Wiley, London

Hoult J E, Reynolds I 1984 Schizophrenia: a comparative trial of community-oriented and hospital-oriented psychiatric care. Acta Psychiatrica Scandinavica 69: 359-372

Intagliata J 1982 Improving the quality of community care for the chronically mentally disabled: the role of case management. Schizophrenia Bulletin 8: 655-674

Jahoda M 1982 Employment and unemployment: a social psychological analysis. Cambridge University Press, Cambridge

Johnson D A W, Freeman H L 1973 Drug defaulting by patients on long-acting phenothiazines. Psychological Medicine 3: 115-119

Johnson D A W, Pasterski G, Ludlow J M, Street K, Taylor R D W, 1983 The discontinuance of maintenance neuroleptic therapy in chronic schizophrenic patients:

drug and social consequences. Acta Psychiatrica Scandinavica 67: 339-352

Johnstone E C, Owens D G C, Gold A, Crow T J, Macmillan J F 1981 Institutionalisation and the defects of schizophrenia. British Journal of Psychiatry 139: 195-203

Johnstone E C, Owens D G C, Gold A, Crow T J, Macmillan J F 1984 Schizophrenic patients discharged from hospital — a follow up study. British Journal of Psychiatry 145: 586-590

Kelvin P 1980 Doing without work. In: What directions for psychiatric day services? MIND, London

Krawiecka M, Goldberg D, Vaughn M 1977 A standardised psychiatric assessment scale for rating chronic psychotic patients. Acta Psychiatrica Scandinavica 55: 299-308

Lamb H R 1986 Some reflections of treating schizoprenics. Archives of General Psychiatry 43: 1007-1011

Lamb H R, Grant R W 1982 The mentally ill in an urban county jail. Archives of General Psychiatry 39: 17-22

Leach J, Wing J K 1980 Helping destitute men. Tavistock, London

Leff J, Kuipers L, Berkowitz R, Sturgeon D 1985 A controlled trial of social intervention in the families of schizophrenic patients: two year follow up. British Journal of Psychiatry 146: 594-600

Liberman R P, Jacobs H E, Boone S E et al 1987 Skills training for the community adaptation of schizophrenics. In: Strauss J S, Boeker W, Brenner H D (eds) Psychosocial treatment of schizophrenia. Huber, Toronto

McCreadie R G 1982 The Nithsdale Schizophrenia Survey. I. Psychiatric and social handicaps. British Journal of Psychiatry 140: 582-585

Mann S, Cree W 1976 'New' long stay patients: a national sample of fifteen mental hospitals in England and Wales 1972/1973. Psychological Medicine 6: 603-616

MenFdel W M 1979 Staff burn-out: diagnosis, treatment and prevention. New Directions in Mental Health Services 2: 75-79

Mitchell S F, Birley J L T 1983 The use of ward support by psychiatric patients in the community. British Journal of Psychiatry 142: 9-15

Oltmanns T F, Neale J M 1982 Psychological deficits in schizophrenia: information processing and communication problems. In: Wing J, Wing L (eds) Handbook of psychiatry 3. Psychoses of uncertain aetiology. Cambridge University Press, Cambridge: p 55

Oltmanns T F, Ohayon J, Neale J M 1978 The effect of anti-psychotic medication and diagnostic criteria on distractability of schizophrenia. Journal of Psychiatric Research 14: 81-89

Pattison E M, Defrancisco D, Wood P, Frazier H, Crowder J 1975 A psychosocial kinship model for family therapy. American Journal of Psychiatry 132: 1246-1251

Pepper B, Ryglewicz H (eds) 1984 Advances in treating the young adult chronic patient. New directions in mental health services No. 21 Jossey-Bass, San Francisco

Raynes N, Pratt M, Roses S 1979 Organisational structure and care of the mentally handicapped. Croom Helm, London

Shanks J, Atkins P 1985 Psychiatric patients who marry each other. Psychological Medicine 15: 377-382

Shepherd G 1980 The treatment of social difficulties in special environments. In: Feldman M P, Orford J (eds) Psychological problems: the social context. Wiley, Chichester

Shepherd G 1986 Social skills training and schizophrenia. In: Hollin C, Trower P (eds) Handbook of social skills training Vol. 2. Pergamon Press, Oxford

Shepherd G 1988a Practical aspects of the management of negative symptoms in preventing disability and relapse in schizophrenia. International Journal of Mental Health 16: 75-97

Shepherd G 1988b The contribution of psychological interactions to the treatment and management of schizophrenia. In: Bebbington P, McGuffin P (eds) New initiatives in schizophrenia research. Heinemann Medical, London

Shepherd G, Richardson A 1979 Organisation and interaction in psychiatric day centres. Psychological Medicine 9: 573-579

Stevens B 1972 Dependence of schizophrenic patients on elderly relatives. Psychological Medicine 2: 17-32

Stone A A, Eldred S H 1959 Delusion formation during the activation of chronic schizophrenic patients. Archives of General Psychiatry 1: 177-179

Strauss J S, Harding C M, Hafez H, Lieberman P 1987 The role of the patient in recovery from psychosis. In: Strauss J S, Boeker W, Brenner H D (eds) Psychosocial treatment of schizophrenia. Huber, Toronto

Suellwold L 1982 Zum einfluss von sekundaerreaktionen auf die langzeitentwicklung schizophrener psychosen. In: Beckmann H (ed) Biologische Psychiatrie. Thieme, New York

Summers F, Hersh S 1983 Psychiatric chronicity and diagnosis. Schizophrenia Bulletin 9: 122-132

Taylor P J 1982 Schizophrenia and violence. In: Gunn J, Farrington D P (eds) Abnormal offenders, delinquency and the criminal justice system. Wiley, London

Taylor P J, Gunn J 1984 Violence and psychosis. In: Risk of violence among psychotic men. British Medical Journal 288: 1945-1949

Test M 1979 Continuity of care in community treatment. In: Stein L (ed) Community support systems for the long-term patient. Jossey-Bass, San Francisco

Tunnell G, Alpert M, Jacobs J, Osiason J 1988 Designing a family psycho-education program to meet community needs: the NYU-Bellevue project. International Journal of Mental Health 17: 75-98

Walker E 1984 Recognition and identification of facial stimuli by schizophrenics and patients with affective disorders. British Journal of Clinical Psychology 23: 37-44

Watt D C, Katz K, Shepherd M 1983 The natural history of schizophrenia: a five-year prospective follow up of a representative sample of schizophrenics by means of a standardised clinical and social assessment. Psychological Medicine 13: 663-670

Watts F N, Bennett D H 1983 Management of the staff team. In: Watts F N, Bennett D H (eds) Theory and practice of psychiatric rehabilitation. Wiley, Chichester

Wing J K 1961 A simple and reliable sub-classification of schizophrenia. Journal of Mental Science 107: 862-875

Wing J K 1975 Impairment in schizophrenia: a rational basis for social treatment. In: Wirt R D, Winokur G, Ruff M (eds) Life history research in psychopathology Vol 4. University of Minnesota Press, Minneapolis

Wing J K, Brown G W 1970 Institutionalism and schizophrenia. Cambridge University Press, Cambridge

Wing J K, Bennett D H, Denham J 1964 Industrial rehabilitation of long-stay schizophrenic patients. Medical Research Memorandum No. 42. HMSO, London

Wing J K, Cooper J E, Sartorius N 1974 The measurement and classification of psychiatric symptoms. Cambridge University Press, Cambridge

Wolfensberger W 1972 The principle of normalisation in human services. National Institute of Mental Retardation, Toronto

Wood P H N, Badley E M 1978 An epidemiological appraisal of disablement. In: Bennett H E (ed) Recent advances in community medicine. Churchill Livingstone, Edinburgh

Woods P A, Cullen C 1983 Determinants of staff behaviour in long-term care settings. Behavioural Psychotherapy 11: 4-13

Wykes T 1982 A hostel ward for 'new' long-stay patients: an evaluative study of 'a ward in a house'. In: Wing J K (ed) Long-term community care: experience in a London borough. Psychological Medicine Monograph Supplement 2

8. Depression: social approaches to treatment

E.S. Paykel   D.L. Marshall

INTRODUCTION

There is a striking contrast between depression and schizophrenia in the literature on the social approaches to the treatment of these two disorders. Social aspects of causation have received considerable attention — for depression, in respect of life events, social support, and social background; for schizophrenia, there have been studies on life events, institutional environment, family setting, and expressed emotion. These studies of schizophrenia have had direct implications for management, with a well-formulated clinical literature supported by high-quality research studies of the optimal hospital environment, effects of rehabilitation, patterns of community care, use of hostels, and interventions in families.

For depression, the literature on social aspects of treatment is sparse. There are few direct clinical discussions and even fewer treatment trials; we are aware of only one previous systematic review (Bennett 1982). However, the use of support and social networks, early intervention in crises, work with families, attention to employment and rehabilitation, and admission to community day care or residential resources are part of everyday treatment. Supportive contact and ventilation of problems for mild depression, and short hospital admission for more severe depression are probably among the most powerful therapeutic influences available. Most of the assumptions and clinical guidelines for such social interventions remain implicit rather than explicit.

Depression is largely a community problem. Hospital admission rates for severe affective disorder approximate to 1 in a 1000 of the general population, annually (Bebbington 1978). Case register studies in the 1960s of all psychiatric contacts for depression produced annual referral rates of 3 per 1000 (Juel-Nielsen et al 1961, Grad de Alarcon et al 1975), suggesting that two-thirds of psychiatrically treated depressives are treated as outpatients. There is an additional case load of patients who are initially treated in hospital but whose care continues in the community.

This conclusion becomes even more striking when the boundaries are taken further. In the UK, the 1971 National Morbidity survey of general practice (OPCS 1974) reported a one-year consultation rate for depression of 35.5 per 1000, while recent general population studies have obtained prevalences of 6–9% in women (Bebbington et al 1981, Dean et al 1983). Goldberg & Huxley (1980) estimated that most subjects with psychiatric disorder in the community see their general practitioner in the same year, although in about half of these, the disorder is unrecognised.

The historical trend from the late 1950s onwards, away from hospital admission to community care, has reinforced this pattern, as has another documented change — towards more ready acceptance of psychiatric treatment by patients, their families, and their doctors. This has led to milder disorders receiving treatment. Rosenthal (1966) studied patients admitted to the Massachusetts Mental Health Center between 1945 and 1965, and showed that an increased proportion had affective diagnoses, with a progressive shift from severe psychotic depressions to depressive reactions. Over this period, there was a great expansion of outpatient psychiatric services.

In this chapter, we will discuss social influences on depressive disorders and their course, as well as social and community approaches to the management of both acute and chronic disorders.

SOCIAL INFLUENCES ON DEPRESSION

Life events and social support

Studies of life events in the onset of depressive disorders are discussed earlier in this volume, and in reviews elsewhere (Paykel 1982, Paykel & Hollyman 1984). Eleven studies, making comparisons of treated depressives with general population controls, have shown that depressives experience more events prior to onset. A wide variety of threatening events is involved, although there is weak specificity for losses and separations. Depressions with an endogenous symptom pattern appear to be almost as closely related to life stress as do those without it. The overall effect is moderate in magnitude — greater than for schizophrenia, but less than for parasuicide.

Among factors modifying the effects of life events, other social influences are also important. In the well known Camberwell study of Brown & Harris (1978), three out of the four vulnerability factors — presence in the home of young children, absence of a confidant, and lack of work outside the home — were potentially modifiable current social influences. In their subsequent study in the Outer Hebrides (Brown & Prudo 1981), an additional social influence — absence of church-going — which reflected non-integration in the community, was important. There is considerable further evidence from epidemiological studies that absence of social support renders subjects more liable to symptoms (Sarason & Sarason 1985), although two subsequent studies did not confirm Brown's other modifying factors (Costello 1982, Solomon & Bromet 1982).

Direct studies of Brown's factors in samples of patients rather than in general population cases have been relatively few, but have tended to be confirmatory. Roy (1981a, b, c & d), in a series of studies, replicated Brown's vulnerability factors in both British depressed women and Canadian subjects, but did not examine interaction with life events. Billings et al (1983) found that depressives had quantitatively and qualitatively deficient social support networks, compared with community controls. Slater & Depue (1981) found that subjects who had attempted suicide were more often living without a confidant than were primary depressive controls, but in the majority of cases this was because of an earlier 'exit' event; events and social circumstances may be confounded. In cases of sub-clinical depression, six weeks post-partum, Paykel et al (1980) found that the effects of a stressful life event were moderated by social support variables, particularly a poor marital relationship with impaired communication and little help from the husband.

In recent years, economic recession has produced a considerable increase in unemployment in many developed countries, and has focused attention on its harmful social and medical consequences. Gainful employment remains one of the most important determinants of role and status in Western society, but in studies of unemployment and psychiatric morbidity, it may be difficult to disentangle cause and effect without a prospective design. Indirect evidence comes from associations between periods of economic recession and high levels both of suicide and of admissions to psychiatric hospitals (Brenner 1979, Barling & Handel 1980, Dooley & Catalano 1980). Some prospective follow-up studies of subjects exposed to the threat or occurrence of job loss have demonstrated increases in minor psychiatric symptoms such as depression and anxiety (Banks & Jackson 1982, Jenkins et al 1982). These findings suggest that in general symptoms are caused by unemployment, rather than preceding it. Employment-related events also emerge as an important group in more general studies of life events.

Women are often considered less at risk from unemployment than the conventional male breadwinners, but some of the evidence does not support this. Lack of employment outside the home was identified by Brown & Harris (1978) as a vulnerability factor in the development of depression, and since that time, social and economic pressures on women to go to work have increased further. Amongst the young unemployed studied by Banks & Jackson (1982), females scored consistently higher than males on the GHQ. Parry (1986) found a complex interaction in effects on symptoms between work outside the home and social class.

Voluntary retirement is a socially sanctioned loss of employment which is sometimes seen as opening the door to a new era of leisure. Nevertheless there are studies which support the view that it is a life crisis, with increased mortality, and physical and psychiatric morbidity, including depression (Martin & Doran 1966, Haynes et al 1977, Hinds 1963, Silverman 1968).

Crisis theory and coping styles

Caplan's crisis theory (1964) provides a useful integration of the impact of events with vulnerability and coping mechanisms. A crisis is said to occur whenever an individual's available repertoire of coping skills is insufficient to meet the threat to psychological stability imposed by a particular set of circumstances. The result is an increase in anxiety and a search for a new means of coping with the threat. If this is successful, the crisis resolves, with the individual having extended his repertoire of coping mechanisms. If it is unsuccessful, the state of disequilibrium persists, with the development of symptoms of anxiety, depression, or even psychosis.

Caplan believes that crises are typically self-limiting, with a duration of 4–6 weeks that does not depend on therapeutic intervention. A crisis period, he emphasises, contains both elements of psychological distur- bance and opportunities for personal growth. During a crisis, the individual engages in problem-solving behaviour, in successive phases, each depending on the outcome of the previous one. First, the difficulty is sensed; then attention is directed to it, and the problem further defined; next, possible solutions are generated and considered, together with their likely consequences; then a solution is chosen and applied. In a sort of recapitulation, the problem-solver frequently returns to earlier stages in the process to verify the effectiveness of the selected solution (Merryfield et al 1962, Guilford 1967).

Up to a point, anxiety and arousal are regarded as assisting in the process of focused problem-solving. However, for those with a poor repertoire of coping skills on which to base the search for new solutions, or in circumstances of great threat, anxiety may become crippling, and the individual unable to concentrate on anything beyond the symptoms he is experiencing. The generation of solutions may then depend on the timely intervention of others.

Coping behaviour itself has received less attention, and studies of it have usually relied upon subjects recalling how they reacted to past stressful situations or imagining how they would respond to hypothetical events. Classification of types of response has been attempted by several authors (Folkman & Lazarus 1980, Pearlin & Schooler 1978). There is some agreement that coping may either be directed externally towards the problem itself, or internally towards regulating the emotional responses to the problem. Within this basic classification, many specific examples of coping responses have been listed. Amongst those which aim to modify the threatening situation, Pearlin & Schooler included negotiation between marital partners, the use of punitive discipline in parenting, and optimistic action in the work setting. Internally-directed coping behaviour includes defensive manoeuvres such as avoidance, intellectualisation and denial, and cognitive adjustments which allow a more optimistic framing of the situation, such as positive comparisons with the problems of other people or other occasions, and selective ignoring of the negative aspects of the threatening situation.

Pearlin & Schooler (1978) considered that the coping repertoire of an individual results from the combination of his social resources (support network), general psychological resources (cognitive style), and specific coping responses (behaviours evoked specifically by threatening life situations). They found that people tended to make use of different specific responses in different areas of their lives, suggesting that what served to resolve a difficulty in one role area might be ineffective in another. General psychological resources appeared to be more effective in economic and occupational problems, and specific responses in family and marital problems. Women employed fewer specific coping responses than men overall, but more of those involving selective ignoring — a response type which tended to exacerbate stress in the role areas of marriage and parenting. Social class and economic status also affected the range and efficacy of coping resources and responses: the better-off and better educated are at an advantage, particularly in occupational and economic problems.

Social influences on course of depression

Studies of social factors on the course and outcome of depression have been fewer than those of onset, but they are accumulating. Indirect evidence from controlled trials of social work, family crisis therapy, or psychotherapy can be interpreted as showing that social support improves outcome. As with onset, direct evidence of effects of social support in patients is scanty. Surtees (1980), in a follow-up study of depressed patients, found that poor social support — on a composite measure of contacts, living group, and confiding relationships — was associated with poorer outcome. However, in a follow-up of elderly depressives (Murphy 1983), absence of social support, as measured by marital status, living alone, or intimacy of relationships, did not predict poor outcome.

A larger body of data exists regarding effects of life events on the outcome of depression. Two separate effects on outcome have in fact been studied: those of life events at the onset of depression and those of concurrent events occurring during treatment and follow-up. The first is an aspect of endogenous depression, but it is important to consider it separately, since absence of precipitant stress is only weakly related to the endogenous pattern of symptoms (Paykel 1982). Overall, studies have not found a very consistent effect of the onset of life events on outcome:

Lloyd et al (1981), in a drug trial, found that these did not influence outcome. In unpublished analyses from a controlled trial of phenelzine, amitriptyline; and placebo (Rowan et al 1982), we found a weak trend for outcome to be worse, particularly on amitriptyline, where major life events had occurred. In elderly depressives, Murphy (1983) found that life events at onset did not predict outcome at one year. However, Tennant et al (1981), in cases identified in a community survey, found that remission over the next month was more likely where there was a threatening life event in the three months before onset. Such milder cases may involve something more like a normal transient reaction to stress.

Events concurrent with treatment are more relevant to this chapter, and appear to have greater effects. Three studies have involved short-term follow-up studies of 4–6 weeks. Lloyd et al (1981) found that patients with poor outcome were more likely to have experienced undesirable events, physical illnesses, illnesses of family members, and events outside their own control. In our controlled trial (Rowan et al 1982), events had no significant effect on outcome, but were infrequent. In community cases, Tennant et al (1981) found that remission was more likely to take place over a month where there had been a neutralising event, counteracting the effect of an earlier threatening event. In two further studies involving intermediate follow-up periods of 6–8 months, Surtees (1980) found that greater event stress was associated with worse outcome, while Paykel & Tanner (1976) found undesirable life events associated with relapse over eight months. In longer-term follow-up studies, Murphy (1983) found that outcome over one year in elderly depressives was worse if there had been a severely threatening event, particularly a physical illness; it was also worse with chronic health difficulties. Giel et al (1978), in a 5-year follow-up of neurotic subjects in the community, found worse outcome where there were independent threatening events or difficulties in the last year of the follow-up. Overall, these studies consistently indicate that concurrent events are important for outcome; negative events produce worse outcome; neutralising events, one class of positive events, produce better outcome.

Pathways to care

The distressed individual often follows a tortuous path to help. The first need is for the person or someone close to recognise the distress, impairment of function, or other abnormalities, such as a physical symptom. Help may then be sought from either informal or formal agencies. Appropriate action relies upon an accurate assessment of the true nature of the disorder by the caring agents — whether in general practice, social services, or in religious or other counselling bodies. Specialist psychiatric help by secondary referral is relatively rare. Goldberg & Huxley (1980) estimated from the literature that from a median 1 year prevalence of psychiatric morbidity in the community of 250 per 1000 (higher than some estimates), 230 would attend their GPs, of whom 140 would be recognised as having a psychiatric disorder. From these, 17 would be referred to psychiatrists, and six of these would be admitted to hospital. The figures for depression cited earlier in this chapter suggest very similar ratios for referral from general practice to psychiatrists and for admission; although in the USA, Weissman et al (1981) found that only about a third of depressives identified in the community received any treatment.

Factors influencing self-recognition of depression have not been well studied. Women appear more likely than men to acknowledge personal problems (Kessler et al 1981), including depressive symptoms (Yokopenic et al 1983). The latter authors studied other variables; most important was the severity of the depression, but nevertheless, nearly one-third of those with high symptom levels reported having no problems. A higher level of education was also associated with better recognition of depressive problems, and with their differentiation from other problems.

Family and friendship networks are important in the further progress towards outside help. Yokopenic et al found that most respondents spoke to friends and relatives about personal problems; where the discussion included the subject of counselling, there was greater subsequent use of mental health services. This was also the case if there was previous experience, personal or second-hand, of such services. The other major influence on help-seeking was, again, severity of symptoms. Amongst those who did not seek psychiatric help, the great majority gave as the reason for this that they could handle their problems by themselves or with a friend's help. A small proportion mentioned practical obstacles such as lack of time, money, or transport, or a negative attitude towards specialist help and a fear of stigmatisation.

Horwitz (1978) interviewed 120 patients with various psychiatric disorders about their efforts to obtain assistance from members of their close social network. Spouse relationships only provided positive support in 20% of cases, and were held at least partly responsible for the psychiatric symptoms by more than 50% of subjects. Individuals with marital conflict showed a greater tendency to seek help from friends or other family members. Parents and siblings were approached less frequently than friends; family members were more likely to provide practical assistance, while friends were more likely to suggest professional consultation. Women approached more than twice as many network members as did men, especially outside the nuclear family. There is little evidence beyond the anecdotal about variation across cultures in help-seeking behaviour.

General practitioners vary widely in their tendency to make a psychiatric diagnosis. Goldberg & colleagues have divided this variation into two elements: 'bias', or the tendency of individual doctors towards consistently diagnosing psychiatric disorder; and 'accuracy', or the degree to which the doctor's judgement of the patient as psychiatrically ill corresponds to independent assessment (Goldberg & Huxley 1980). In studies undertaken both in Manchester (Marks et al 1979) and in the USA, the two elements were found to be largely independent. Bias related particularly to the doctor's empathy, emphasis on psychiatry, sensitivity to verbal cues relating to psychological distress, and, negatively, to being a high-status practitioner. Accuracy of diagnosis was determined more by interview skills and academic ability.

Goldberg has studied mixed psychiatric disorders, and focussed particularly on factors in the doctor, while Freeling et al (1985) specifically studied depression, and factors in the patient. They compared symptom ratings and history in patients with major depression according to Research Diagnostic Criteria who were not recognised by general practitioners, on the one hand, with those who were recognised, on the other. Differences were relatively few, but unrecognised depressives tended to have less overt symptomatology, with less evidence of depressed mood, appearance of depression, or insight; they also had longer illnesses, and these were more related to physical disorder, which might focus attention away from the depression.

Factors affecting referral of depressives to psychiatrists by general practitioners can be inferred from comparisons of depressed patients treated either in general practice or by psychiatrists. Severity appears to be an important determinant. General practice depressives have been found to be less severely ill (Fahy 1974, Davies & Blashki 1973) and less endogenous in symptoms (Pilowsky & Spence 1978) than psychiatric inpatient depressives. A more relevant comparison of general practice with outpatient depressives (Sireling et al 1985) gave similar findings. General practice assessment and treatment is often a staged process, with several successive consultations leading to progressively greater interventions, as failure to improve occurs; psychiatric referral may follow failure to respond to antidepressants.

Weissman et al (1981) studied the treatment received overall by depressives identified in the community, in New Haven, Connecticut. They were twice as likely to have been treated with a minor tranquilliser in the previous year (34.5%) than with an antidepressant (17.2%). Women were more likely to have received treatment than men, and the upper social classes more than the lower. Help was provided by non-mental health professions (e.g. clergy, non-psychiatric social workers, nurses) almost as often as by mental health professionals.

Depressed individuals receiving inadequate or inappropriate treatment for their depression make considerable demands on health and social services (Hoeper et al 1979, Houper et al 1979). Weissman et al (1981) found that depressives who had received no treatment for emotional problems in the previous year made many more visits to non-psychiatric doctors than those with other or no psychiatric disorder.

TREATMENT OF THE ACUTE EPISODE

Social assessment

Social treatment of depression is rarely a sole treatment; it is a facet of good management which applies to every case, although it may be of particular value in some.

The first step should be social assessment — a clinical procedure which has received relatively little explicit literature discussion. Attention should be paid to the social setting in which the depressive lives; preceding life events and chronic stresses; absence of social supports; marital and family relationships; the work setting; social disabilities and relationship problems consequent on depression; and coping resources and repertoires. More than the stresses at the onset of the episode, it is the current social scene which is important for management.

Factors leading to presentation should also be considered. Often a key event, or a change in the perception of the patient, family, and referring general practitioner have led to psychiatric referral, which only becomes fully explicable when this trigger can be identified. Some family aspects may only become apparent after a home visit.

Bennett (et al 1976, 1982) has discussed the value of the family conference, with as many family members as possible present together with the patient. This not only gives an opportunity for direct observation and assessment of the family setting, with its stresses and strains, but also provides a forum in which members can express their perception of the illness, expectation of treatment, and hopes for the future, as well as an exploration of difficult or taboo subjects such as fears of suicide. This does not necessarily lead to family therapy; a single interview may be sufficient to elicit and impart a great deal of information. Problems in coping with the depressed member can be communicated, the background of the illness explored, and the team's assessment of the problem, treatment plan, and prognosis explained. Reassurance can be given and hope instilled.

Choice of treatment setting

Choice of treatment setting is a choice of social environment. It should take into account the depressed individual's immediate need for support and dependency, as well as the capacities of family and friends, while avoiding reinforcement of the sick role and inhibition of innate strengths and coping skills. The range of settings available to the psychiatrist spans a spectrum from independent living to partial and full hospital care. Paykel et al (1970) studied depressed patients in four kinds of treatment settings in New Haven, Connecticut: outpatient clinics, day hospitals, brief crisis admission units, and inpatient wards. Across these settings, differences in symptoms were dominant: a progressive increase in the level of hospitalisation was paralleled by a progressive severity of illness, including suicidal tendencies. Inpatients were also more likely to show endogenous symptoms, while day hospital patients were more often of intermediate severity, with chronicity and anxiety. However, among different inpatient units — university general hospital, community mental health centre, state mental hospital — the distinguishing features were primarily social, particularly social class.

Social criteria should also rank highly in the decision as to whether to admit to hospital; a caring, supportive, and perceptive family setting can enable severely depressed patients to be cared for in the community or at a day hospital. The usual organisation of psychiatric services in Britain, with teams providing comprehensive care to a catchment area across a range of facilities, provides particular advantages for choosing appropriate settings for individual patients.

Admission to hospital provides a potent social treatment for severe depression with respite from outside stress, support from many helpers, time to reassess problems and solutions, and relief to a disordered family; dramatic remission may occur without drug treatment. While the patient is in hospital, support may be needed for those left at home, ranging from supportive psychotherapy to practical interventions such as arranging for a home help to visit, or for children's attendance at play group. As treatment progresses, contact with the family will enable sharing of information, planning of trial periods at home, and then discharge, with guidance as to how to relate to the returned member, as well as the roles of continued medication and follow-up.

Brief admission

Hospital admission is also recognised to have disadvantages. It puts the patient in a strange, disorientating, and depersonalising environment, with its own alien set of rules. It tends to lower self-esteem, and may lead to stigmatisation. It breaks ties with the family, the social setting, and work, rendering return to them more difficult. It fosters dependency, the sick role, and institutionalisation. Awareness of these problems has led to exploration of alternatives. Depression is better suited to these alternatives than is schizophrenia, because of the possibility of rapid remission, with less residual social disability.

One modification is to minimise the length of hospital admission. Several controlled trials have examined the efficacy and practicability of brief hospital stays, in comparison with the longer standard admission, but most of these have been limited to schizophrenics, or have not separated depressives in their analyses of the data. In London, Hirsch et al (1979) randomly allocated 127 patients, of whom 60% had a diagnosis of neurosis or affective psychosis, to either standard or brief care. It proved impossible to apply the policy indiscriminately, but early discharge was achieved in a considerable proportion of the experimental group. The brief care patients did as well as the control group on measures of clinical outcome, social performance, behaviour as reported by relatives, and family burden. Improvement was most marked during the first two weeks after admission, irrespective of the type of treatment, and was maintained at 14 weeks' follow-up. Readmission rates in the following year were no higher for the brief care patients, and the only service of which they made more use following discharge was the day hospital; greater attendance almost made up for the days saved on in-patient care.

Similar findings have emerged from other studies of brief hospital care in the United States. Herz et al (1975, 1977) assigned 175 newly admitted inpatients to either standard or brief care, with or without transitional day hospitalisation; fewer than 40% were non-schizophrenics. Patients without a responsible adult at home were excluded. Brief-care was associated with no increase in symptoms of family burden, and some benefit, largely accruing from the patient's quicker return to a normal role. The brief-care programmes were less expensive, both to the hospital services and the family. Brief-care patients required no more admissions during the next two years than did the standard care group. Glick et al (1976) randomly assigned patients to short- or long-term hospital care: non-schizophrenic patients (25% of them depressive) in the short-term group improved more rapidly than those in the long-admission group, and were functioning as well at the time of their discharge after 3–4 weeks, as were patients in the long-term group, after 3–4 months. Patients with a diagnosis of affective disorder were rated as more impaired at admission, and more improved at discharge than other diagnostic groups, regardless of the length of stay.

Overall, these three studies are consistent in suggesting that outcome is as good for brief as for longer admission. The definition of brief hospital care is variable, though, and it may be that the critical factor is not length of stay but the intensity of inpatient treatment. Staff and relatives may respond to a policy of brief care by mobilising and applying their resources more rapidly and effectively, and the patient too may attempt to prepare for an earlier return home. Brief treatment, when well deployed, is often intensive treatment.

Day hospitals

Day hospitals provide another alternative form of care which has undergone great expansion in the last 30 years, and depressives comprise a substantial proportion of all patients treated in day hospitals (Paykel et al 1970). Craft (1958) carried out a retrospective case record analysis, including 43 matched pairs of female depressives. Using the indices of length of admission, and condition at discharge and 5-month follow-up, day care was found to be as effective as inpatient treatment and slightly shorter. In another early study, Smith & Cross (1957) matched 38 neurotic day patients with a similar number of inpatients, and found no significant differences on a variety of outcome measures. Zwerling & Wilder (1964) randomly allocated newly admitted inpatients to inpatient or day care, and were able to treat 40% of the latter group without subsequent recourse to full admission. In another randomised controlled trial, Herz et al (1971) found day hospitals superior to inpatient care, but the study included relatively few depressives.

A recent British study (Dick et al 1985a) specifically included patients with neurotic disorders, adjustment reactions, or personality disorders; more than half received the diagnosis of depressive neurosis. Patients admitted as emergencies were randomly allocated to continuing in patient or day hospital care. Day hospital treatment was associated with greater patient satisfaction and equally good clinical outcome, and was less costly than inpatient care, despite contact being, on average, twice as long. Information about the 167 subjects who were interviewed but excluded from the study is instructive as to the limitations of both forms of treatment (Dick et al 1985b): 39 were considered too well to warrant inclusion, 25 were considered suitable but were unwilling to accept early transfer to the day hospital, and 101 were felt to be too ill, including some with a high risk of suicide.

These studies all compared day hospital and inpatient treatment. An alternative comparison by Tyrer & Remington (1979) examined the clinical and social outcome of 106 neurotic patients, none seriously ill enough to warrant inpatient care, after allocation to either one of two types of day care or to outpatient treatment. No differences were found, except that there were more drop-outs from day hospital treatment, and outpatient care was generally preferred by the patients. The general trend in all these studies of treatment settings is that the least degree of hospital care compatible with the patient's clinical and social state emerges as the preferable one.

Domiciliary care

A logical extension is found in the many projects which have attempted to substitute some form of domiciliary care for admission to hospital. Since a variety of models has been used, though, the evaluative studies are often not directly comparable. Some common themes emerge in the characteristics of the experimental services: they usually consist of fairly intensive, home-based treatment programmes, carried out by multidisciplinary teams providing 24-hour cover; emphasis is placed on meeting short-term needs whilst reinforcing good coping behaviour, and on the involvement of the family in these processes; community support and rehabilitation resources are developed and utilised according to individual needs; and hospital facilities are available for back-up.

Some of these studies fall on the borderline with preventive crisis intervention, and are described in a later section. Amongst the methodological problems (Tantam 1985) in studies of depressives are a tendency for suicidal patients to be excluded from the experimental group, and the frequency with which patients in the domiciliary group require admission to hospital during the studies (typically 20–30%). It is also important to take into account the high levels of enthusiasm amongst workers in innovative treatment programmes as well as the value and practicability of 24-hour cover. Also, the comparison groups may not sometimes be of high quality, or may have been admitted over-readily, so that admission can easily be reduced.

Test & Stein (1980) used an experimental programme which included training and support in daily living activities, and also intensive assistance in finding and coping with employment; team members had daily contact with patients and their employers or supervisors. Comparisons with standard admission showed a reduction in the length of time in hospital (including for relapse), more time in sheltered care rather than unemployment, but no clear benefit in costs. Gains were quickly lost after the end of the referral programme. Hoult et al (1983) used a 24-hour community service, and achieved great reduction in admission, compared with a standard service, with better clinical outcome, less cost, no more family burden, and greater consumer satisfaction.

In the UK, several papers have suggested that domiciliary services can reduce bed usage, without detriment to clinical outcome or significantly increased burden on families (Scott 1980, Jones 1982). Most of these services have treated a spectrum of psychiatric disorders.

DEPRESSION AS A LONG-TERM PROBLEM

Follow-up studies

It has been increasingly realised that depression is not simply an acute disorder, but is responsible for a considerable amount of continuing morbidity in the community, with persistent minor symptoms, a risk of major relapses, and considerable social disability and handicap.

An American follow-up study has provided a recent picture of short-term prognosis; about 60% of patients had recovered within four months of treatment, but rates then declined sharply, and after one year, 26% had still failed to recover (Keller et al 1982a). There was also a considerable risk of relapse; 38% of recovered patients relapsed within 40 weeks of recovery (Keller et al 1982b). Prognosis was worse in the case of more severe depression, with longer duration of illness and where the acute depression was superimposed on an earlier chronic or recurrent condition. Clinically, the problem is often not that of the patient with severe affective disorder, but of persisting milder depressions in the community, showing only partial recovery (Paykel et al 1974).

The problem of the chronic milder depressive is also recognised in an important recent American diagnostic concept — dysthymic disorder. DSM III criteria specify a persisting pattern of at least two years' symptoms, without remission for more than a few weeks and without sufficient severity to reach a major depressive episode. Major episodes may be superimposed on this pattern.

Longer-term course has been reviewed by Coryell & Winokur (1982). Most long-term follow-up studies still date from an era before modern treatment, and it is difficult to be sure that they are now valid; they show that more than 50% of subjects have a further episode, with recurrences more common in those with bipolar disorders, among whom at least 25% show chronic disability.

Social disability

These studies have predominantly used symptom measures, but major social disability may also occur with depression. Weissman & Paykel (1974) studied 40 depressed women, mainly outpatients, and made comparisons with normal controls. At the height of the depression, there was pervasive disability of social function, characterised by impairment of role function at work, in housework, and as a parent; increased interpersonal friction with family members (particularly husband); inhibited communication; increased dependency on and withdrawal into the family; as well as dissatisfaction, and distress. In this sample, symptomatic improvement was fairly rapid, but social improvement much slower, particularly in respect of marital friction and impaired communication. Some disability persisted, mainly reflecting previous personality and stressful situations preceding the depression. Other investigations have given similar findings. In an early descriptive study, Cassidy et al (1957) found job loss, marital discord, business failures, and automobile accidents, all of which were regarded as consequences of the depression, although the distinction from precipitant life events was not clear. Deykin et al (1966) and Jacobson & Klerman (1966) reported conflict between depressed women and their adult children. Eisemann (1984) found impairment in the leisure activities of depressives, compared with controls; there were significant correlations with personality measures. The impact on children has also received detailed study (Ghodsian et al 1984). Impairment in work and social activity are widely recognised as characteristic of depression and are incorporated into symptom rating scales such as those of Hamilton (1967) and Beck (1961). In a follow-up study of male patients from Veterans Administration Hospitals, Honigfeld and Lasky (1962) reported, that within 20 weeks, there was a return to baseline levels in family and interpersonal adjustment, but a striking tendency to vocational impairment, in a time of economic recession.

Marital relationships of depressives have also received special study; reported findings illustrate the complex interplay of social function and symptoms, since poor marital relationships may be both consequences and also pre-existing causes of depression. Hinchcliffe et al (1978) studied intensively the impaired communication between depressed in-patients and their spouses. Merikangas et al (1979) found changes in the balance of power, as recovery took place, with patients achieving increased influence in joint discussion. Spouses appeared to affect the outcome of treatment with amitriptyline; non-responders' spouses were initially more depressed and anxious than those of responders. Rounsaville et al (1980) followed up depressed women over four years, and found a tendency for marital disputes to persist and also to give a worse prognosis to the depression while Merikangas (1984) reported a tendency for depressed patients to have depressed spouses, and a high rate of divorce on follow up.

Bipolar disorder particularly causes social damage because of its recurrent nature, the additional damage to occupational, marital, and family relationships resulting from the disinhibition and reckless behaviour of mania, and the inconsistencies consequent on fluctuating mood. Mayo et al (1979) have described the impact on children, while Targum et al (1981) found that 53% of the spouses of bipolar patients indicated that they would not have married, and 47% that they would not have had children if they had known more about the disorder.

The continuing morbidity in the community throws an appreciable load on services. Gillis & Egert (1973) found that depression was over represented in a sample of long-term outpatient attenders, compared with new patients. They drew attention to a group of long-standing depressed women, comprising about a fifth of their small sample, whose depression was resistant to treatment, most commonly in a setting of adverse and unchangeable family circumstances.

Prevention of relapse

Social aspects of treatment are potentially relevant to the prevention of relapse. If possible, the adverse circumstances which contributed towards the development of the depression should not be allowed to persist or recur; the patient who has made a good recovery in hospital should not return to a home in which the hostile or stressful situation which was left behind remains unchanged. Even where admission has been avoided, adjustments made by the family during the crisis period to improve support and resolve conflicts may be forgotten, once clinical improvement has occurred. Social or financial pressures may lead to a precipitate return to work, and in the early part of recovery, friends and acquaintances may, with the best of motives, encourage a degree of social contact and activity for which the individual is not yet ready. The recovering depressive may allow himself to be drawn into these problems as a result of a natural desire to return to a normal level of functioning as soon as possible. The psychiatrist should recognise forces that militate towards early relapse, and should intervene appropriately. In the longer term, where there are major defects in the patient's social support network, remedial action may be taken: contact can be established with self-help groups or community resources; children can be placed in play groups or creches, and voluntary work can be organised for the patient if employment on the open market is sparse. Intensive social work involvement may be necessary in cases of marital conflict, of severe deprivation, of homelessness, or when children have been received into care.

These activities will at the very least facilitate a smooth transition to a full level of functioning in the community, but whether they can directly prevent early relapse is not clearly proven. In one of the few studies to examine the question (Weissman et al 1974, Paykel et al 1976), recovering depressed women in New Haven were randomly assigned to continue amitriptyline or to withdraw from it after two months, with or without psychotherapy from social workers. There was a considerable incidence of relapse after drug withdrawal, which was halved by continuing the drug; psychotherapy improved social adjustment, but did not affect relapse. In these circumstances of early drug withdrawal, the effect of drug treatment on relapse may be so large as to swamp other effects. However, most such studies show an appreciable incidence of relapse, even with drug continuation. In the New Haven study, relapses were related to life events (Paykel & Tanner 1976), in an effect which appeared to be independent of drug treatment.

Rehabilitation and management of chronic disorder

Incomplete resolution, chronic symptoms, and poor social functioning may be residual features of a persisting illness, or may reflect pre-morbid handicaps such as inadequate or unstable personality, poor social adjustment, or a limited coping repertoire. Some lasting handicaps may be secondary to having been ill, rather than consequences of persistent symptoms. These handicaps include the effects of institutionalisation, loss of employment, and the damage done to social and personal relationships during the period of impaired health.

Despite these problems, there is little literature on the rehabilitation of chronic depressives, which contrasts with the considerable published body of work and wide range of resources directed towards chronic schizophrenia. We must therefore borrow concepts from this work, and consider their applicability to the problems of chronic depression.

Wing & Morris (1981) regard the disablement seen in chronic psychosis as containing both medical and social components. A proportion is said to be due to residual psychiatric symptoms, a proportion to social disadvantage, and a proportion to the individual's reaction to these symptoms and disadvantages. The process of rehabilitation involves 'identifying and preventing or minimising these causes while, at the same time, helping the individual to develop and use his or her talents, and thus to acquire confidence and self-esteem through success in social roles'. Wing & Morris emphasise the individual nature of handicap and, therefore, the importance of a thorough assessment of each case with the setting of appropriate goals; what is a realistic target for one patient may be totally unattainable by another. A limited achievement in absolute terms may represent relative success for the individual concerned. Progress should be by a series of small steps, each lying within and reinforcing the individual's competence.

In depressive illness, severe handicap develops much less frequently than in schizophrenia. Some patients with affective disorder become part of the long-stay population of psychiatric hospitals — possibly representing a higher proportion of such patients as the prevention of handicap in chronic psychosis improves (Mann & Cree 1976, Abrahamson & Brenner 1979). Thus, the full range of facilities employed in the rehabilitation of chronic functional psychosis is likely to be needed for at least some chronic depressives. Within the hospital setting, the patients may need to learn or re-learn basic skills in the areas of work, social functioning, leisure, and daily living.

The chronic depressive living in the community may also need a range of services. A day hospital may provide both invaluable support to the patient and relief to care-givers, whether they be family or the staff of sheltered accommodation, while continuing specific rehabilitation measures. Non-medical resources such as social services day centres, workshops, family centres, and self-help organisations are well suited to meet the needs of chronic depressives with social handicap, avoiding inappropriate medicalisation of problems. This also applies to residential facilities.

In the development of psychiatric rehabilitation services, much emphasis has been placed on occupational activities. Work has obvious value as a normative social activity, providing the individual with income, role, and status, and rehabilitation for work has been shown to be effective in reducing handicap in many cases of chronic schizophrenia (Wing & Brown 1970). Equally in chronic depression, it seems probable that a gradual progression towards employment, with supervision, support, and the experience of social interactions, will lessen the depressive withdrawal, loss of role, and low self-esteem.

There has been little evaluation of rehabilitation programmes for depression. Chwast & Lurie (1966) demonstrated a reduction of social estrangement in a resocialisation programme for former depressed in-patients, but there was no control group, leaving the contribution of the therapeutic programme in doubt.

Social skills training

A behavioural treatment with strong social and rehabilitative components which has been applied in depression is social skills training. A number of behavioural theories relate depression to reduced reinforcement. Lewinsohn (1975) has pointed out that reinforcement comes from social relationships, and has suggested that many depressives lack the social skills necessary to gain adequate social reinforcement.

Shipley & Fazio (1973) found that social skills training produced more improvement in depression than occurred in a waiting list control group, in students with depressive symptoms. Bellack et al (1983) compared social skills training, psychotherapy, amitriptyline, and amitriptyline plus social skills training in depressed female outpatients. There was a tendency for greater improvement with social skills training, particularly on measures of social skills. However, Zeiss et al (1979), comparing three treatments — social skills training, cognitive therapy, and treatment designed to increase frequency and enjoyment of pleasure activities — found equal improvement without specific effects on different dependent variables. Social skills elements are incorporated into many varieties of behavioural and cognitive-behavioural therapies.

ROLES OF OTHER PROFESSIONAL AND VOLUNTARY WORKERS IN DEPRESSION

Social work

Treatment of depression in the community is not the exclusive province of doctors. Multi-disciplinary teams allow co-ordinated division of workload, with preservation of specialist skills, but the contribution of non-medical workers extends to agencies well outside this team structure.

Social work has an important role. Deykin et al (1971), in a descriptive account of the treatment of depressed women, emphasised the value of case work in: maintaining the integrity of the family unit by preventing alienation of the sick member; allowing the patient to retain some responsibilities whilst permitting temporary dependence; and educating and supporting other members of the caring network in their unaccustomed roles, but guarding against their becoming entrenched.

The social worker may also explain and monitor the effects of pharmaco-therapy. Psychotherapeutic techniques may be incorporated into case work, and Deykin et al suggest that a patient's motivation for insight-directed therapy after the symptoms have resolved is greater where there are more ongoing social and marital stresses.

Corney (1981) carried out a controlled trial of social work in the management of female depressives in general practice. In acute depression, the outcome was generally good, but where this was superimposed on chronic depression, involvement of a social worker produced greater improvement than in a control group, on measures of social functioning and overall clinical outcome. The social workers provided their normal range of services, including support, counselling, and help for practical problems. The results were consistent with those of Cooper et al (1975), who found that chronic neurotic patients mainly suffering from affective disorders who received social work help improved significantly more than did a control group. The New Haven study of psychotherapy from social workers has already been referred to (Weissman et al 1974, Paykel et al 1976).

Community psychiatric nursing

A major development in Britain in the last 15 years has been the employment of psychiatric nurses within the community. Community psychiatric nurses (CPNs) may fulfil a variety of roles in assessment and acute care, and especially in aftercare. Parnell (1978) surveyed 147 community psychiatric nursing services in 1975; 72% of case loads were of former inpatients. Ranking second among diagnoses was depression, comprising 18% of caseloads, although well behind the 45% figure for schizophrenia. CPNs can be valuable in the treatment of depression, with a variety of roles. In acute treatment, they can assess home circumstances and the quality of family relationships, establish good communication with the family, and provide active support to patients. In longer-term care, a supportive relationship can be forged with both patient and family.

Paykel & Griffiths (1983) described an evaluative controlled trial in non-psychotic patients, about half of them depressives, including many long-term outpatient attenders. Patients were randomly assigned for continuing treatment to domiciliary care by CPNs as their key workers, or to outpatient visits to psychiatrists. Nursing care was predominantly in the patients' homes, and contacts with family members — in addition to the patient — were common. Activities were mainly supportive, with reassurance, ventilation, clarification, and advice, but over time, became increasingly psychotherapeutic. The two modes of care showed equal efficacy on symptoms, social functioning, and family burden. CPNs achieved both more discharges and produced high levels of satisfaction; a cost-benefit analysis showed them to be the cheaper alternative in direct costs of care, although the differences were not great.

One of the particularly beneficial aspects for the more chronic patients in this study appeared to be in the stability of contact provided by the community psychiatric nurse. In outpatient follow-up clinics, patients are most often seen by junior psychiatrists, who rotate frequently between posts for training needs. A group of long-term patients develops, who are seen infrequently and briefly, but who resist discharge, and may develop symptoms if it is threatened. Often, it seems that the contacts are partly symbolic, in that the patient still feels under care, and partly social, in that they provide a transaction in an otherwise socially impoverished and isolated life. Frequently changing staff never have the opportunity to get the measure of the patient, formulate a treatment plan, and carry it through against resistance; it is much easier, in the hurried circumstances of a large case load, to prescribe medication and set the next appointment as far off as possible, in the knowledge that after a few such appointments, it will be the next doctor's turn. Only stable contact over time permits proper assessment, construction of a therapeutic plan, and development of a trusting relationship which may allow the patient to gradually relinquish dependency and move forward.

Other professional and voluntary workers

Other professional and voluntary groups also contribute to the acute and long-term management of depression. District midwives and health visitors are in a good position to recognise depression in women with new-born babies or young children, and to assist in their resolution, often by crisis work. Similar skills may be required in dealing with the elderly depressed — another large group whose symptoms easily escape the doctor, but who are often well-known to district nurses.

Among voluntary services, the best known in Britain is the telephone counselling and befriending service provided by the Samaritans. The development of this organisation in the UK coincided with a fall in the national suicide rate. Bagley (1968) found that 15 county boroughs served by branches of the Samaritans had significantly lower suicide rates than matched control towns; however, the way in which these control towns were selected has been criticised, and a study employing a variety of alternative methods failed to show any effect due to the Samaritans (Jennings et al 1978). Experience with suicide prevention services else-where in the world shows that they provide crisis intervention to a wide variety of clients, of whom those with high suicidal risk may be only a small proportion, and the value of these services needs to be judged on wider criteria.

The church and religious organisations of all denominations also have a role in providing care for the distressed individual in the community.

Activities in pastoral counselling are now extensive. Finally, self-help groups may be valuable in providing mutual support for long-term sufferers. Among recent developments of this kind in Britain has been The Manic Depression Fellowship.

INTERACTIONS OF PHYSICAL AND SOCIAL TREATMENTS

In practice, social treatments are usually not administered alone, but in combination with drug treatment. The empirical evidence for the effects of combining different forms of treatment comes mainly from a related area — controlled studies of psychotherapy. The effects of psychotherapy can be regarded as in part mediated by social support. The theoretical issues have been reviewed by Uhlenhuth et al (1969) and by Klerman & Schechter (1982). More than with social treatments, it has often been suggested that combining psychotherapy and drugs might be detrimental — drug therapy might impair progress in psychotherapy by focusing on somatic issues, while psychotherapy might impair a drug-induced symptom remission by stirring up conflicts. The correct experimental model to test combined effects is the factorial design with four groups: no treatment (or placebo), drug therapy, psychosocial therapy, and combined treatment with both modalities.

A series of studies of depression has put this issue to rest, at the same time showing that impaired social function in depression can be improved therapeutically. In the New Haven study (of depressed women) already cited (Weissman et al 1974, Paykel et al 1976), continuation of drug therapy prevented relapse, and psychotherapy improved both social functioning and interpersonal relationships. The two effects were largely independent, but the greatest benefit was from receiving both treatments. In a second study (Friedman 1975), depressives received acute treatment with amitriptyline, conjoint marital therapy, a combination of the two, or placebo. Amitriptyline produced the greatest improvement in symptoms, and marital therapy in marital relationships, while the combination produced an additive effect, with some evidence of a potentiating interaction. The third study (Covi et al 1974) employed a similar design, but with group therapy instead of marital therapy, and imipramine instead of amitriptyline. Imipramine produced a strong therapeutic benefit on symptoms, and group therapy, a weak effect on social function. The effects of the combination were mainly additive.

These three studies also found that the main effect of psychotherapy was on social effectiveness, rather than on symptoms. A fourth study (DiMascio et al 1979) employed acute treatment with amitriptyline, individual psychotherapy from psychiatrists, a combination of the two, and no treatment. Both treatments produced strong effects on symptom remission, but the combination again produced the best effect.

None of these four studies showed any evidence that either treatment modality impaired the effects of the other. All suggested the value of the combination, either directly on symptoms, or more commonly, with different targets — medication for symptoms, and psychosocial therapies for social benefit. Social intervention, in the form of social work and involvement with families to discuss treatment plans, may also aid compliance in the taking of medication.

PREVENTION

Depression has social causes, and might be amenable to social prevention. However there has not yet been a direct demonstration of the primary prevention of any functional psychiatric disorder, i.e. prevention of the development of the disease. Because most psychiatric disorders have multifactorial aetiologies in which any specific factor is responsible for only a small amount of variance, it is possible that prevention will be more profitably aimed at preventing single factors operating across a range of disorders, rather than in preventing single disorders. Possible approaches involve the removal of risk factors and events which are known to be associated with subsequent depression. Many of these lie within the political and socioeconomic arenas, if they can be prevented at all.

Long-term separation from and deaths of parents are risk factors for the development of depression, or for its severity, with at least weak effects (Bowlby 1961, Brown & Harris 1978, Birtchnell 1978). Some separations are avoidable, and the effects of others may be lessened by providing an effective mother-substitute (Rutter 1972). Advances in health care have reduced the incidence of untimely deaths of young parents, but the effects of these on subsequent depression are unknown.

Risk factors associated with social and material deprivation are difficult to prevent. The case for social action to amelioriate overcrowding, urban decay, male unemployment, or Brown's vulnerability factors is better made on general grounds than on those of preventing clinical depression. However, some measures to reduce the isolation of young mothers are feasible: community facilities such as mother-and-baby groups in settings like GPs' surgeries; enlistment of health visitors to encourage the use of them (Tomson 1983); provision of advice about contraception; and information about part-time jobs, as well as other alternatives to the housewife role. The efficacy of such measures might be more in preventing mild than severe disorders, but would nevertheless be very worthwhile.

Many of the recent life events associated with depressive onset, such as departures of children from the home and bereavement, seem inevitable consequences of the life cycle, and are not in themselves preventable. Nevertheless, the occurrence of a life event can be regarded as a signal of a period of increased risk, when intervention may be profitable. Studies which have attempted to anticipate the psychological effects of threatening life events and to dissipate them by means of counselling or other interventions have suggested good results, although they have not directly tested the prevention of clinical depressive sequelae. These include counselling in bereavement (Parkes 1980, Raphael 1977), in pregnancy, and before major surgical operations (Carpenter et al 1968). Much of this work could best be done by non-psychiatrists, including nurses, social workers, GPs, or voluntary workers (Parkes 1979).

Rather than primary prevention, however, this is secondary prevention — modification of the course of illness by intervention before the full clinical picture has evolved. It is partly from this basis and partly from crisis theory that the movement towards crisis intervention has arisen. The principal goal of intervention is to resolve the immediate crisis and to restore equilibrium and function, at least to pre-crisis levels (Aguilera & Messick 1982). Crisis intervention depends on early recognition and prompt response. Jacobson et al (1968) have described two distinct approaches: the individual and the generic. The former emphasises detailed assessment of the specific needs and psychological mechanisms of the individual in crisis, with individualised problem-solving efforts which also involve other members of the family or social network. The more common generic approach assumes that individuals' responses to crisis situations follow certain common patterns, which can provide a framework for therapeutic interventions (Tyhurst 1957). Thus, studies have elucidated the typical phases of the bereavement reaction (Parkes 1972, Kubler-Ross 1969), the response of a mother to the birth of a premature baby (Kaplan & Mason 1965), as well as reactions to life-threatening illness (Janis 1958), marital breakdown, migration, and retirement. A generic approach does not entail as much detailed assessment, and may be suitable for less skilled workers.

The few controlled evaluations of crisis intervention that have been undertaken relate to activities that are in fact intermediate between secondary prevention and treatment of the developed disorder. In the Colorado study (Langsley et al 1969), patients were randomly assigned, either to a psychiatric hospital for treatment, or to management of the crisis at home by a mobile family crisis team. This and other similar studies (Scott 1973, Fenton et al 1979) have generally shown that the crisis intervention subjects spend considerably less time away from their accustomed roles and less time in hospital, and have an equally good clinical outcome. Other members of the supportive network might be expected to experience increased stress as a result, but these findings suggest that crisis intervention, with the emphasis on home care, results in no greater family burden than does hospital admission (Langsley et al 1969, Fenton et al 1979).

A limited number of services of this sort have been set up in Britain, usually by the district psychiatric facilities, and sometimes in association with walk-in clinics. The need to be accessible and to respond rapidly requires a location in the community served. Services have also been initiated by social workers and by psychologists with training in counselling techniques (Holland 1979). Telephone crisis hotline services, manned by volunteers including the Samaritans, and some community self-help groups may serve similar functions.

CONCLUSIONS

In contrast to the literature on schizophrenia, and on depressive causation, there has been relatively little explicit attention to the social aspects of the management of depression. Nevertheless, it is an important part of care, and there is much literature which implicitly bears on it.

Depression is largely a community problem, with high rates identified in surveys and the vast majority of cases outside hospital. Social factors, particularly life events and social support, have been clearly shown to have considerable effects on causation and on course, and they provide some theoretical basis for treatment formulations. Pathways to care are complex and influenced by many factors.

Treatment of the acute episode requires social assessment: major environmental relief may be provided by hospital admission or by day hospital care. However, within the limits of what is compatible with the patient's clinical state and social setting, controlled trials of brief admission, day hospital care, outpatient attendance, and domiciliary care in the community suggest that the least level of removal from the community is the one which is preferable.

Depression is not only an acute problem but a longer-term one, associated with a moderate amount of chronicity in the community, relapse, recurrence, and social morbidity. Since impaired marital relationships may be both the cause and the consequence of the disorder, work with families may assist both in the return of patients to normal life in the community and in the amelioration of problems. Rehabilitation approaches may be important, although they have been much less clearly formulated than for schizophrenia. A wide variety of professional and non-professional workers may contribute to all these efforts.

Interactions regarding psychosocial and pharmacological therapies have been studied in controlled trials. They consistently demonstrate that the two kinds of treatment reinforce each other, with some tendency for them to have different targets: drug treatments for symptoms, and psychosocial treatments for social and interpersonal functioning.

Social aetiology raises the possibility of social prevention, although primary prevention has not yet been demonstrated for any functional psychiatric disorder. Counselling, crisis intervention, and other forms of social support may offer approaches to modifying the transition from normal reaction to frank disorder, as well as the further course and consequences of the disorder. However, there have been too few evaluative studies for firm conclusions to be drawn as yet as to how much can be achieved in this way.

REFERENCES

Abrahamson D, Brenner D 1979 A study of the 'old long-stay' patients in Goodmayes Hospital. Report to the DHSS, London

Aguilera D C, Messick J M 1982 Crisis intervention. Theory and methodology. Mosby, St. Louis

Bagley C 1968 The evaluation of a suicide prevention scheme by an ecological method. Social Science & Medicine 2: 1–14

Banks M H, Jackson P R 1982 Unemployment and risk of minor psychiatric disorder in young people; cross-sectional and longitudinal evidence. Psychological Medicine 12: 789–798

Barling P W, Handel P J 1980 Incidence of utilisation of public mental health facilities as a function of short-term economic decline. American Journal of Community Psychiatry 8: 31–39

Bebbington P E 1978 The epidemiology of depressive disorder. In: Kleinman A M (ed) Culture, medicine and psychiatry. Reidel, Dordrecht, pp 297-341

Bebbington P E, Tennant C, Hurry J 1981 Adversity and the nature of psychiatric disorders in the community. Journal of Affective Disorders 3: 345–366

Beck A T, Ward C H, Mendelson M, Mock J, Erbaugh J 1961 An inventory for measuring depression. Archives of General Psychiatry 4: 561–571

Bellack A S, Hersen M, Himmelhoch J M 1983 A comparison of social skills training, pharmacotherapy and psychotherapy for depression. Behavioural Research & Therapy 21: 101–107

Bennett D 1982 Social and community approaches. In: Paykel E S (ed) Handbook of affective disorders. Churchill Livingstone, Edinburgh, pp 346–357

Bennett D, Fox C, Jowell T, Skynner A C R 1976 Towards a family approach in a psychiatric day hospital. British Journal of Psychiatry 129: 73–81

Billings A G, Cronkite R C, Moos R H 1983 Social-environmental factors in unipolar depression: comparisons of depressed patients and nondepressed controls. Journal of Abnormal Psychology 92: 119–133

Birtchnell J 1978 Early parent death and the clinical scales of the MMPI. British Journal of Psychiatry 132: 574-579

Bowlby J 1961 Child care and the growth of love. Pelican, London

Brenner M H 1979 Mortality and the national economy. Lancet i: 568–573

Brown G W, Harris T 1978 The social origins of depression: a study of psychiatric disorder in women. Tavistock, London

Brown G W, Prudo R 1981 Psychiatric disorder in a rural and an urban population: 1. Aetiology of depression. Psychological Medicine 11: 581–599

Caplan G 1964 Principles of preventive psychiatry. Basic Books Inc, New York

Carpenter J, Aldrich C K, Boverman H 1968 The effectiveness of patient interviews: a controlled study of emotional support during pregnancy. Archives of General Psychiatry 19: 110–112

Cassidy W L, Flanagan N B, Spellman M, Cohen M E 1957 Clinical observations in manic depressive disease: a quantitative study of 100 manic depressive patients and 50 medically sick controls. JAMA 104: 1535–1546

Chwast J, Lurie A 1966 The resocialization of the discharged depressed patient. Canadian Psychiatric Association Journal 11: 5131–5140

Cooper B, Harwin B G, Depla C, Shepherd M 1975 Mental health care in the community: an evaluative study. Psychological Medicine 5: 372–380

Coryell W, Winokur G 1982 Course and outcome. In: Paykel E S (ed) Handbook of affective disorders. Churchill Livingstone, Edinburgh, pp 93–106

Costello C G 1982 Social factors associated with depression: a retrospective community study. Psychological Medicine 12: 329–339

Covi L, Lipman R, Derogatis L et al 1974 Drugs and group psychotherapy in neurotic depression. American Journal of Psychiatry 131: 191–198

Craft M 1958 An evaluation of treatment of depressive illness in a day hospital. Lancet ii: 149–151

Davies B, Blashki T 1973 Course of depression: a comparison of depression in general practice and hospital. In: Classification and prediction of outcome of depression. F K Schattaner, Stuttgart

Dean C, Surtees P G, Sashidharan S P 1983 Comparison of research diagnostic systems in an Edinburgh community sample. British Journal of Psychiatry 142: 247–256

Deykin E Y, Jacobson S, Klerman G L, Solomon M 1966 The empty nest: psychosocial aspects of conflict between depressed women and their grown children. American Journal of Psychiatry 122: 1422–1426

Deykin E Y, Weissman M M, Klerman G 1971 Treatment of depressed women: therapeutic issues with hospitalised patients and out-patients. British Journal of Social Work 1: 277–291

Dick P, Cameron L, Cohen D, Barlow M, Ince A 1985a Day and full time psychiatric treatment: a controlled comparison. British Journal of Psychiatry 147: 246–250

Dick P, Ince A, Barlow M 1985b Day treatment: suitability and referral procedure. British Journal of Psychiatry 147: 250–253

DiMascio A, Weissman M M, Prusoff B A, Neu C, Zwilling M, Klerman G L 1979 Differential symptom reduction by drugs and psychotherapy in acute depression. Archives of General Psychiatry 36: 1450–1456

Dooley D, Catalano R 1980 Economic change as a cause of behavioural disorder. Psychological Bulletin 87: 450–468

Eisemann M 1984 Leisure activities of depressive patients. Acta Psychiatrica Scandinavica 69: 45–51

Fahy T J 1974 Depression in hospital and in general practice: a direct clinical comparison. British Journal of Psychiatry 124: 240–242

Fenton F R, Tessier L, Struening E L 1979 A comparative trial of home and hospital psychiatric care. Archives of General Psychiatry 36: 1073–1079

Folkman S, Lazarus R 1980 An analysis of coping in a middle aged community sample. Journal of Health & Social Behaviour 21: 219–239

Freeling P, Rao B M, Paykel E S, Sireling L I, Burton R H 1985 Unrecognised depression in general practice. British Medical Journal 290: 1880–1883

Friedman A S 1975 Interaction of drug therapy with marital therapy in depressed patients. Archives of General Psychiatry 32: 619–637

Ghodsian M, Zajicek E, Wolkind S 1984 A longitudinal study of maternal depression and child behaviour problems. Journal of Child Psychological Psychiatry 25: 91–109

Giel R, Ten Horn G H M M, Ormel J, Schudel W J, Wiersuma O 1978 Mental illness, neuroticism and life events in a Dutch Village sample: a follow-up. Psychological Medicine 8: 235–243

Gillis L, Egert S 1973 The psychiatric outpatient, clinical and organizational aspects. Faber and Faber, London

Glick I D, Hargreaves W A, Drues J, Showstack J A 1976 Short vs long hospitalisation. A controlled study: III. Inpatient results for non-schizophrenics. Archives of General Psychiatry 33: 78–83

Goldberg D, Huxley P J 1980 Mental illness in the community. Tavistock, London

Grad de Alarcon J, Sainsbury P, Costain W R 1975 Incidence of referred mental illness in Chichester and Salisbury. Psychological Medicine 5: 32–54

Guilford J P 1967 The nature of human intelligence. McGraw-Hill, New York

Hamilton M 1967 Development of a rating scale for primary depressive illness. British Journal of Social & Clinical Psychology 6: 278–296

Haynes S G, McMichael A J, Tyroler H A 1977 The relationship of normal involuntary retirement to early mortality amongst US rubber workers. Social Science & Medicine 11: 105–114

Herz M I, Endicott J, Spitzer R L, Mesnikoff A 1971 Day versus inpatient hospitalisation: a controlled study. American Journal of Psychiatry 127: 1371-1382

Herz M I, Endicott J, Spitzer R L 1975 Brief hospitalisation of patients with families: initial results. American Journal of Psychiatry 132: 413–418

Herz M I, Endicott J, Spitzer R L 1977 Brief hospitalisation: a 2 year follow-up. American Journal of Psychiatry 134: 502–507

Hinchliffe M K, Hooper D, Roberts F J 1978 The melancholy marriage, depression in marriage and psychosocial approaches to therapy. Wiley, New York

Hinds S W 1963 The personal and sociomedical aspects of retirement. Royal Society of Health Journal 83: 281

Hirsch S R, Platt S, Knights A, Weyman A 1979 Shortening hospital stay for psychiatric care: effect on patients and their families. British Medical Journal 1: 442–446

Hoeper E W, Nycz G R, Regier D A 1979 The importance of mental health services to general health care. Ballinger, Massachusetts

Holland S 1979 The development of an action and counselling service in a deprived urban area. In: Meacher M (ed) New methods of mental health care. Pergamon, Oxford

Honigfeld G, Lasky J J 1962 One-year follow-up of depressed patients treated in a multi-hospital drug study. Diseases of the Nervous System 23: 555–562

Horwitz A 1978 Family, kin and friend networks in psychiatric help-seeking. Social Science & Medicine 12: 297–304

Hoult J, Reynolds I, Charbonneau-Powis M, Weekes P, Briggs J 1983 Psychiatric hospital versus community treatment: the results of a randomised trial. Australian & New Zealand Journal of Psychiatry 17: 160–167

Jacobson G, Strickler M, Morley W E 1968 Generic and individual approaches to crisis intervention. American Journal of Public Health 58: 339

Jacobson S, Klerman G L 1966 Interpersonal dynamics of hospitalized depressed patients' home visits. Journal of Marriage & The Family 28: 94–102

Janis I L 1958 Psychological stress; psychoanalytical and behavioural studies of surgical patients. Wiley, New York

Jenkins R, Macdonald A, Murray J, Strathdee G 1982 Minor psychiatric morbidity and the threat of redundancy in a professional group. Psychological Medicine 12: 799–807

Jennings C, Barraclough B M, Moss J R 1978 Have the Samaritans lowered the suicide rate? Psychological Medicine 8: 413–422

Jones D 1982 The Borders Mental Health Service. British Journal of Clinical & Social Psychiatry 2: 8–12

Juel-Nielsen N, Bille M, Flygenring J, Helgason T 1961 Frequency of depressive states within geographically delimited population groups: incidence (the Aarhus County investigation). Acta Psychiatrica Scandinavica 53: 35–50

Kaplan D M, Mason E A 1965 Maternal reactions to premature birth viewed as an acute emotional disorder. In: Parad H J (ed) Crisis intervention. Family Service Association of America, New York

Keller M B, Shapiro R W, Lavori P W, Wolfe N 1982a Recovery in major depressive disorder, analysis with the life table and regression models. Archives of General Psychiatry 39: 905–910

Keller M B, Shapiro R W, Lavori P W, Wolfe N 1982b Relapse in major depressive disorder, analysis with the life table. Archives of General Psychiatry 39: 911-915

Kessler R C, Brown R L, Broman C L 1981 Sex differences in psychiatric help-seeking: evidence from 4 large-scale surveys. Journal of Health & Social Behaviour 22: 49–64

Klerman G L, Schechter G 1982 Drugs and psychotherapy. In: Paykel E S (ed) Handbook of affective disorders. Churchill Livingstone, Edinburgh, pp 329–337

Kubler-Ross E 1969 On death and dying. Macmillan, New York

Langsley D G, Flomenhaft K, Machotka P 1969 Follow-up evaluations of family crisis therapy. American Journal of Orthopsychiatry 39: 753

Lewinsohn P M 1975 The use of activity schedules in the treatment of depressed individuals. In: Thoreson C E, Krumboltz J D (eds) Counselling methods. New American Library, New York

Lloyd C, Zisook S, Click M, Jaffe K E 1981 Life events and response to antidepressants. Journal of Human Stress 7: 2–15

Mann S A, Cree W 1976 'New' long-stay psychiatric patients: a national sample survey of 15 mental hospitals in England and Wales 1972. Psychological Medicine 6: 603–616

Marks J, Goldberg D P, Hillier V F 1979 Determinants of the ability of general practitioners to detect psychiatric illness. Psychological Medicine 9: 337–353

Martin J, Doran A 1966 Evidence concerning the relationship between health and retirement. Sociological Review 14: 329

Mayo J A, O'Connell R A, O'Brien J D 1979 Families of manic-depressive patients: effect of treatment. American Journal of Psychiatry 136: 1535–1539

Merikangas K R 1984 Divorce and assortative mating among depressed patients. American

Journal of Psychiatry 141: 74–76

Merikangas K R Ranelli C J, Kupfer D J 1979 Marital interaction in hospitalized depressed patients. Journal of Nervous & Mental Disease 167: 11, 689–695

Merrifield P R 1962 The role of intellectual factors in problem solving. Psychological Monographs 76 (10)

Murphy E 1983 The prognosis of depression in old age. British Journal of Psychiatry 142: 111–119

Office of Population Censuses and Surveys (OPCS) 1974 Morbidity statistics from general practice. Second National Study 1970–75. Studies on medical and population subjects No. 26. HMSO, London

Parkes C M 1972 Bereavement; studies in grief in adult life. Tavistock, London, New York

Parkes C M 1979 The use of community care in prevention. In: Meacher M (ed) New methods of mental health care. Pergamon Press, Oxford

Parkes C M 1980 Bereavement counselling: does it work? British Medical Journal 281: 3–6

Parry G 1987 Paid Employment, life events, social support and mental health in working-class mothers. Journal of Health & Social Behaviour 27: 193–208

Paykel E S 1982 Life events and early environment. In: Paykel E S (ed) Handbook of affective disorders. Churchill Livingstone, Edinburgh, pp 146–161

Paykel E S, Griffith J H 1983 Community psychiatric nursing for neurotic patients: the Springfield controlled trials. Research monographs in nursing series. Royal College of Nursing, London

Paykel E S, Hollyman J A 1984 Life events and depression — a psychiatric view. Trends in Neurosciences 7: 478-481

Paykel E S, Tanner J 1976 Life events, depressive relapse and maintenance treatment. Psychological Medicine 6: 481–485

Paykel E S, Klerman G L, Prusoff B A 1970 Treatment setting and clinical depression. Archives of General Psychiatry 22: 11–21

Paykel E S, Klerman G L, Prusoff B A 1974 Depressive prognosis and the endogenous-neurotic distinction. Psychological Medicine 4: 57–64

Paykel E S, DiMascio G L, Klerman G L, Prusoff B A, Weissman M M 1976 Maintenance therapy of depression. Pharmakopsychiatrie Neuro-Psychopharmacologie 9: 127–136

Paykel E S, Emms E M, Fletcher J, Rassaby E S 1980 Life events and social support in puerperal depression. British Journal of Psychiatry 136: 339–346

Pearlin L, Schooler C 1978 The structure of coping. Journal of Health & Social Behaviour 19: 2–21

Pilowsky I, Spence N D 1978 Depression inside and outside the hospital setting. British Journal of Psychiatry 132: 265–268

Raphael B 1977 Preventive intervention with the recently bereaved. Archives of General Psychiatry 34: 1450–1454

Rosenthal S H 1966 Changes in a population of hospitalised patients with affective disorders. American Journal of Psychiatry 6: 671–681

Rounsaville B J, Prusoff B A, Weissman M M 1980 The course of marital disputes in depressed women: a 48-month follow-up study. Comprehensive Psychiatry 21: 111–117

Rowan P R, Paykel E S, Parker R R 1982 Phenelzine and amitriptyline: effects on symptoms of neurotic depression. British Journal of Psychiatry 140: 475–483

Roy A 1981a Vulnerability factors in depression in men. British Journal of Psychiatry 138: 75–77

Roy A 1981b Specificity of risk factors for depression. American Journal of Psychiatry 138: 959–961

Roy A 1981c The role of past loss in depression. Archives of General Psychiatry 38: 301–302

Roy A 1981d Risk factors and depression in Canadian women. Journal of Affective Disorders 3: 65–70

Rutter M 1972 Maternal deprivation reassessed. Penguin, Harmondsworth

Sarason I G, Sarason B R (ed) 1985 Social support: theory, research and applications. Martinus Nijhoff, Dordrecht

Scott R D 1973 The treatment barrier. British Journal of Medical Psychology 48: 45

Scott R D 1980 A family orientated and psychiatric service to the London Borough of Barnet. Health Trends 12: 65–68

Shipley C R, Fazio A F 1973 Pilot study of a treatment of psychological depression. Journal of Abnormal Psychology 82: 372–376

Silverman C 1968 The epidemiology of depression. Johns Hopkins University Press, Baltimore

Sireling L I, Freeling P, Paykel E S, Rao B M 1985 Depression in general practice: clinical features and comparison with out-patients. British Journal of Psychiatry 147: 119–126

Slater J, Depue R A 1981 The contribution of environmental events and social support to serious suicide attempts in primary depressive disorder. Journal of Abnormal Psychology 90: 275–285

Smith S, Cross E G W 1957 Review of 1000 patients treated at a psychiatric day hospital. International Journal of Social Psychiatry 2: 292–298

Solomon Z, Bromet E 1982 The role of social factors in affective disorder: an assessment of the vulnerability model of Brown and his colleagues. Psychological Medicine 12: 123–130

Surtees P G 1980 Social support, residual adversity and depressive outcome. Social Psychiatry 15: 71–80

Tantam D 1985 Alternatives to psychiatric hospitalisation. British Journal of Psychiatry 146: 1–4

Targum S D, Dibble E D, Davenport Y B, Gershon E S 1981 The family attitudes questionnaire, patients' and spouses' views of bipolar illness. Archives of General Psychiatry 38: 562–568

Tennant C, Bebbington P, Hurry J 1981 The short-term outcome of neurotic disorders in the community: the relation of remission to clinical factors and to 'neutralizing' life events. British Journal of Psychiatry 139: 213–220

Test M A, Stein L I 1980 Alternative to mental hospital treatment. Archives of General Psychiatry 37: 409–412

Tomson P R V 1983 Depression, a preventable illness? Practitioner 227: 153–158

Tyhurst J A 1957 Role of transitional states — including disasters — in mental illness. Symposium on Preventive and Social Psychiatry. Walter Reed Medical Centre

Tyrer P J, Remington M 1979 Controlled comparison of day hospital and outpatient treatment for neurotic disorders. Lancet i: 1014–1016

Uhlenhuth E H, Lipman R S, Covi L 1969 Combined pharmacotherapy and psychotherapy. Controlled studies. Journal of Nervous & Mental Diseases 148: 52–64

Yokopenic P A, Clark V, Aneshensel C S 1983 Depression, problem recognition, and professional consultation. Journal of Nervous & Mental Disorders 171: 15–23

Weissman M M , Paykel E S 1974 The depressed woman: a study of social relations. University of Chicago Press, Chicago, London

Weissman M M, Klerman G L, Paykel E S, Prusoff B A, Hanson B 1974 Treatment effects on the social adjustment of depressed outpatients. Archives of General Psychiatry 30: 771–778

Weissman M M, Myers J K, Thompson D 1981 Depression and its treatment in a US urban community 1975–1976. Archives of General Psychiatry 38: 417–421

Wing J K, Brown G W 1970 Institutionalism and schizophrenia. Cambridge University Press, London

Wing J K, Morris B 1981 Clinical basis of rehabilitation. In: Wing J K, Morris B (eds) Handbook of psychiatric rehabilitation practice. Oxford University Press, Oxford, pp 3-16

Zeiss M, Lewinsohn P M, Munoz R F 1979 Nonspecific improvement effects in depression using interpersonal skills training, pleasant activity schedules, or cognitive training. Journal of Consulting & Clinical Psychology 47: 427–439

Zwerling I, Wilder J F 1964 An evaluation of the applicability of the day hospital in treatment of acutely disturbed patients. Israel Annals of Psychiatry 2: 162–185

NOTE: This chapter was prepared in 1985 and therefore does not include any references to later published work.

9. Psychiatric disorders in old age

S. Jolley   D. Jolley

INTRODUCTION

The psychiatric disorders of old age and the service to be delivered to those who suffer from them deserve particular consideration because of:

1. The nature of the disorders and their relationship to normal ageing and to physical ill-health.
2. The prevalence of the disorders and the increasing numbers of old people.
3. The social characteristics of the aged population.
4. The existence of other health and welfare services that focus on the elderly.

THE PSYCHIATRIC DISORDERS OF OLD AGE

'Normal' ageing — survival into the sixth, seventh, and eighth decades of life and beyond — carries with it an expectation that drive and energy will be reduced from their peaks in the prime of life, (Jolley and Jolley 1990). The number of contacts with other people that are sought and achieved is reduced, whilst the quality of established relationships may become more intense and more important. Emotions are usually less turbulent, and impulses slower, to give rise to action which may be, therefore, less often ill-considered. Intellectual processes are slower; old people take on new information or ways of looking at things with less enthusiasm and flexibility than is characteristic of youth, yet performance in the face of problems may remain excellent, supported by a wealth of accumulated experience and often the old fashioned virtue of wisdom (Bromley 1966).

Folklore recognises that changes occur in the senium, but does not declare with any certainty where divergence from previous personal style becomes pathological. This acceptance and tolerance of 'differences' in the elderly is both a weakness and a strength for those old people who develop psychiatric disorders: a weakness in that their problems may not be recognised, but a strength in that they are less likely to be rejected by their local community.

Of the psychiatric disorders that arise in the senium, the dementias are the most characteristic, being extremely rare among younger people. Progressive loss of intellect and emotional control, and deterioration of other aspects of personality, leaving the sufferer eventually unable to cope with the basic requirements of dressing, feeding, and appropriate disposal of excretory products make these amongst the most dreadful of conditions. The major dementing illnesses — Senile Dementia of the Alzheimer Type (SDAT), 'multi-infarct' or arteriosclerotic dementia, Pick's Disease, and Huntington's Chorea — are looked on as degenerative disorders, yet it is very common for their presentation and course to be influenced by other intercurrent illnesses, which in themselves are treatable. More rarely, a dementing syndrome may be entirely symptomatic, and the identification of underlying, usually physical factors and their treatment lead to complete resolution of the symptoms (Lishman 1978, Jolley 1981, Dodwell 1986).

Delirium or confusional states have long been recognised to be caused by physical pathology in predisposed individuals, while advanced age, with or without the addition of a dementing process, is a major predisposing factor. Their rapid onset, fluctuating florid symptomatology, and rapid resolution when underlying problems can be identified and corrected, make them a model of the kind of illness where physician and psychiatrist may collaborate to everyone's benefit (Jefferys & Denham 1985).

Physical factors frequently contribute to the aetiology of mood disorders in old age. For most people in industrialised countries of recent generations, most of their years have been spent free of the uncertainty that severe, chronic, or life-threatening physical illness can bring, and Bergman (1971, 1978) found that of the various stresses common among old people, it was physical illness or disability, often borne for the first time, that best predicted the emergence of 'neurotic' symptomatology. Continued physical ill-health is an important factor in maintaining depressive symptoms (Post 1962, Baldwin & Jolley 1986), but perhaps the greatest difficulty presented by this relationship between physical illness and symptoms of anxiety and depression lies in recognising the presence of a psychiatric disorder that has potential for treatment and resolution in its own right. It is all too easy to dismiss the mood disorders as understandable, even inevitable, and thereby commit the patient to further unnecessary suffering.

The inter-relationship between physical factors and the psychiatric disorders of old age is further illustrated by the persistent persecutory states (Post 1966) or schizophrenias of late life. Failure of the special senses of hearing and vision is widely recognised to predispose to paranoid states, while failing health in general, and consequent reduced mobility and restricted contact with the outside world also seem to possess this potential.

Relatively few people turn to alcohol or drugs of addiction for the first time in old age. When they do, and when they use these to an excess sufficient to produce problems, it is often possible to identify the presence of an underlying mood disorder, which may have its origins in worries about physical illness or the other hardships that ageing has brought (Jolley & Hodgson 1985a).

In addition to those who suffer from disorders that arise in late life, there are patients who survive into the senium with long-standing or relapsing psychiatric illnesses; normal ageing and age-related physical disorders then have pathoplastic effects on the symptomatology and overall clinical needs. Chronic schizophrenia often loses its most florid and troublesome symptomatology, but behavioural disorder and evidence of organic impairment may supervene (Crowe et al 1980). Recurrent mood disorders sometimes become more disabling, as periods between illnesses shorten and the durations of illnesses lengthen (Beck 1967). People with truculent, intolerant personalities that had found some sort of peace in middle-age may re-emerge with illnesses, while age-related hardships throw them — once again or for the first time — into the hands of others to provide necessary care and attention. Difficulties with inter-personal relationships throughout life have often left these people bereft of close family, yet these same difficulties persist to fuel new battles and heartaches for the senium.

PREVALENCE OF PSYCHIATRIC DISORDER IN OLD AGE

The size of the old-age population

Epidemiological studies in various parts of the world identify between 5% and 10% of those aged 65 years and older as suffering from dementia (Kay et al 1964, Eastwood & Corbin 1985). Within the old-age population itself, the condition is age-related, ranging from 4% at 65–69 years to 60% in the over 85-years-old (Nielsen 1962). There is reason to believe that the prevalence of dementia at all these ages is increasing, for survival amongst sufferers is now longer than in the 1950s, whilst the incidence is probably being sustained (Gruenberg 1978).

Neurotic disorders are more common than the dementias (mild to moderate symptoms being found in 25% of community samples), although major mood disorders are present in only 2–3% of the elderly, and the status and significance of the dysphoria associated with physical ill-health requires further study (Post & Shulman 1985). Present thinking, supported both by these surveys and by referral and admission rates, suggests that neurotic problems and major mood disorders become less common in very old age, but it is uncertain whether this pheno-menon is real or partly a function of bias in the observers.

Persistent persecutory states and other paranoid disorders are rare (reported prevalence 0–2%). However, the general vigour of paranoid subjects and their attitude towards the world means they may be missed by systematic surveys (Sheldon 1948). When attempts are being made to provide relevant services to a community, though, the significance of these disorders may appear disproportionate to this supposed rarity because of the social difficulties that such people often cause. Similarly, alcohol-related problems and drug abuse are barely perceptible in epidemiological surveys, but become more apparent the closer and longer a specialist service becomes available to an elderly population.

At present, roughly 15% of the 56.5 million population of the United Kingdom is elderly (aged 65 years or older); this represents a dramatic change from the situation at the beginning of this century, when only 4.6% of the 38.2 million population was of a similar age. In absolute numbers, 1.8 million elderly, of whom 0.5 million were over 75 years, has become 8.8 million with 3.7 million aged over 75 — an increase by a factor of five for the elderly as a whole and of seven for the over-75 age group. Projections for the future suggest that the numbers of very elderly, particularly those over 85 years, will continue to increase during this century, and many other European countries have achieved an age-structure similar to that of the United Kingdom. In the newer developed nations such as Australia, Canada, and the USA, the proportion of elderly is about two-thirds that of the UK, and the USSR is similar to these 'partially developed' nations. In the poorer countries of Africa, Asia, and South America, the situation is not very different from that which prevailed in Europe 90 years ago, only 5% of their populations being old. However, the rate of change in these countries is very rapid indeed, and the transformation that occurred over three or four generations in the UK may be achieved there within one or two. The predicted increase in the numbers of old people in the third world over a matter of 20 years is 40% (CSO 1986, Arie & Jolley 1982).

The social circumstances of old people (UK)

Ninety four per cent of old people in the UK live in private households; 40% are alone, and the same proportion are with one other person, who is often an equally elderly spouse (CSO 1979). On average, their housing is less well equipped, less well maintained, and less fully utilised than the stock of younger people. Some live in ghetto-like circumstances in less favoured parts of the cities, which have been deserted by the younger, more vigorous, and more successful members of their kin. Others risk the hazards of relocation in retirement to seek new lives in sheltered housing complexes or in the bungalow estates of seaside resorts or rural spas. There too, they find their company heavily laced with others who are elderly and prone to become dependent and die. Retirement sets the elderly apart from the mainstream of life in two ways, limiting their disposable income, and often enmeshing them in a tangle of grants, means-tested benefits, or 'charitable' handouts, yet leaving them free to explore time and territory that are used by others only when work is done (Stevenson 1981). Despite all this, many old people remain well integrated within their families. The opportunities of their new life are often found to be very stimulating, and those who stay on in the decaying areas that they had known in better times play a large part in maintaining local lore (Townsend 1957).

HEALTH AND WELFARE SERVICES FOR THE ELDERLY

The elderly are by far the greatest consumers of local authority welfare services in Britain. Home helps, originally conceived as support for nursing mothers, have found their main enduring role with the elderly frail. 'Meals on wheels' had their origins in the communal feeding centres of wartime, but have found a life long beyond that and now reach out to hundreds of thousands of old people who can neither cope for themselves nor get to neighbourhood luncheon clubs. Social work may have been seen in the recent past as simply providing care and attention for elderly clients, and some of this has been delegated to assistants or wardens, but skilled social work intervention is now recognised to be appropriate to the complex problems that people commonly encounter in old age. Aids and adaptations to property, as well as equipment to improve mobility and communication, may all be provided by UK local authorities — a far cry from the times when all that could be offered was the 'indoor relief' of the workhouse (Townsend 1962). Whilst residential care remains an important and expensive component of local authority provision, large public assistance institutions are now almost unknown, having been replaced by purpose-built or adapted smaller homes with 20 to 40 places, often located in pleasant and easily accessible situations.

Primary health care in Britain has been transformed from its rather seedy image of isolated, unsupported, and out-of-date practitioners in the 1950s to a much more dynamic appearance in the 1980s. General practices are now usually organised in groups, often working from health centres and having the benefits of multidisciplinary teams that include district nurses, health visitors, and sometimes a social worker or other specialist personnel. Their work with old people is more often based on contact at home than is usual for younger patients, and many practitioners develop a particular interest in their elderly population, some organising screening clinics, and others an 'at risk' register of people to be visited regularly (Williamson 1985). Contact with the elderly constitutes roughly 30% of the workload of an average practice; over 90% of the over-75s are seen within the routine workings of a practice over a 12-month period and those few not seen are, on average, remarkably fit and self-sufficient (Williams 1984).

All hospital specialties, other than paediatrics and maternity, see and treat large numbers of old people; well over a million discharges and deaths per year from non-psychiatric wards in England are of patients aged 65 years or more. On the other hand, in absolute numbers, specialist geriatric medical services may seem relatively unimportant (200,000 deaths and discharges per year) (DHSS 1980), but there is no doubt that their significance is immense for the very frail and the very old with multiple pathologies (Isaacs 1981). Developing from an unpromising base in chronic sick wards, geriatric medical services have spread across the UK to become the most spectacular medical growth area of the post-war period (Anderson 1985). They are in constant interaction with primary health care, other medical and surgical specialties, and local authorities. Their hallmarks are assessment, treatment, and rehabilitation based on work in the community, outpatient clinics, and day hospitals, as well as using beds which increasingly are in District General Hospitals (DGHs).

In addition to these statutory services, a range of resources sponsored by voluntary organisations or the private care sector has been available in parts of Britain for some time; contributions from these agencies are now becoming more widespread and of increasing significance (Hall 1985). In some other industrialised countries, private or voluntary facilities, e.g. those provided by religious orders, play a much greater role.

PSYCHIATRIC DISORDER AND THE NEED FOR AND USE OF SERVICES

The epidemiological studies undertaken in Newcastle-upon-Tyne during the 1960s and early 1970s have been used to provide understanding of another dimension — the need for and use of services by the domiciliary-based population. Bergmann and his colleagues (Foster et al 1976) assessed as a most vulnerable group those living alone, aged over 75 years, and suffering from a psychiatric disorder. The needs of people with dementia were reasonably well identified, but only about half of these requirements were being met; comparison with those who were registered blind is illuminating, for over 80% of their needs were met. The elderly with neurotic symptoms would also have benefited from help, but this was recognised, and met in only 25% of instances. An earlier study has reported on the use of hospital and local authority beds over a follow-up period of up to four years (Kay et al 1970). Again, the presence of psychiatric disorder predicted increased use of these facilities, although it is interesting that most of the extra usage by demented patients was in geriatric medical wards and local authority homes, rather than in psychiatric hospitals. The less spectacular increased bed usage by probands with 'functional' psychiatric disorders was also greater in geriatric facilities than in psychiatric hospitals.

These observations confirm the view that the most important role for specialist psychiatric services with the elderly is in collaboration with other agencies. The principles of bringing psychiatric expertise into a community, and the special potential of such services for work with the elderly had been expounded by Carse et al (1958). In the face of the potentially overwhelming mass of elderly patients in need of care, because of dementia and other psychiatric disorders, they considered this style of work to be the only one that would allow psychiatric services to survive as active treatment facilities. The significance for as yet, unchanged mental health services of the numbers of old people predicted for the second half of this century had already been identified by Lewis (1946). Yet it took courage to galvanise the understanding derived from these observations into the actual delivery of services to the old people who needed them. The series of papers which analysed the differences between a community-orientated service for Chichester and an institution-based service for nearby Salisbury supported the potential of the community approach to reach out to the elderly and yet avoid being overwhelmed (Grad & Sainsbury 1965, Sainsbury et al 1965, Sainsbury & Grad 1970, Grad et al 1975). One weakness of these studies, though, was the lack of information concerning the work of social services and geriatric medicine in the two districts — an omission which has recently been made good in a study of the elderly referred to all specialist agencies (Wilkin et al 1985).

However, it required more than a scholarly appreciation of predictable needs from population trends to provide appropriate services on a national scale in Britain. Scandals in the care of old people accommodated in institutions, large and small, (Committees of Inquiry 1969, 1975) also played their part in this. The exposition, probably overstated, of the hazards to life when elderly patients were misplaced in inappropriate sectors of the health care system increased this impetus (Kidd 1962); it encouraged the formulation of national targets for ratios of beds and day places for old people with organic psychosyndromes (DHSS 1970, 1972). Perhaps most important of all, though, charismatic doctors were attracted into providing integrated services for the elderly, and psychogeriatric medicine emerged from the status of an oddity, practised by a handful of enthusiasts, to national recognition with a register of over 200 specialists (Norman 1982, Wattis & Arie 1984, Jolley 1986).

The principles of a psychogeriatric service are:

1. To be available to those in most need
2. To be flexible in designing solutions to individual problems
3. To make decisions only after careful assessment in the situation where problems present
4. To communicate and collaborate with other significant workers
5. To accept responsibility for solutions and be prepared to think again.

These were laid down by Arie, and were tested in his Goodmayes Service (Arie 1970); 20 years on, few would wish to vary from these principles, though styles of practice are not uniform. The kind of territory to be covered is clearly influential, for a tightly grouped city population presents different needs from a rural one with multiple smaller townships, while islands and peninsulas present their own peculiar problems of geography. Certainly in the early stages and often for the forseeable future, the inheritance from previous services is very important, both in the siting of the institutional elements of service and in the patterns of expectations, prejudices, and potential for collaboration which exist in the area. In addition, the availability of key personnel and the personal views and styles of the individuals that come together to constitute the local team determine the face it will present to the community it will serve (Jolley & Arie 1978, HAS 1982).

A SERVICE IN ACTION

Most old people in the UK live in towns or cities, and although practice in retirement areas may be different in emphasis, an account of our work in South Manchester provides a fairly representative example of how facilities and staff are brought together. The development of this service illustrates the interpretation and modification of principles on the anvil of practicability.

Territory and population

South Manchester is the largest of three health districts in the city. Straddling the River Mersey, which divides it into two roughly equal sectors, the area of eight by six miles accommodates 190 000 people, of whom 28 000 were aged 65 years or older in 1975, rising towards 31 000 by the late 1980s. The northern sector has been made up from a number of townships and villages that have been merged together during this century by building between established centres, but these older areas retain individual character and remain important to residents for shopping, education, entertainment, church-going, etc. Over 40% of the housing is owner-occupied, while social service and health provision are of at least average levels for the city as a whole (Manchester JCC 1985). The southern sector, however, is less affluent: there is only one long-established village of any size, and that is sited just south of the river. Up to the 1930s, the remainder of the area provided market garden produce to the city, with a few small hamlets housing the sparse population. Since then, a sustained building programme has created a large but well designed and reasonably resourced public housing estate. Thus, the population south of the river is equivalent in size and similar in age-structure to that in the northern sector, but less than 10% are owner-occupiers of their homes; social and health indices demonstrate some patches within the estate to be among the least privileged in the city (Manchester JCC 1985). Despite the differing histories of the elderly in these two populations, it is interesting that family support networks are not dissimilar, for many families on the southern estate have moved there together from inner city clearance areas. They have often negotiated exchanges of housing, to be more easily available to each other, and having settled, these families appear to remain in the area. Families in the north have longer established associations with the area, but some of their more able young people tend to move to other towns or cities.

There is an established expectation in this Manchester community that members of families will help each other at times of difficulty, and this is certainly understood when elderly people are in need. Neighbours are usually prepared to be 'fetchers and carriers', although they will only rarely become involved with caring of a more personal nature. However, organised voluntary activity has been rare, other than in patches in the northern sector. Social Services are provided by a city council that in the past could be proud of its history of taking the welfare of the elderly to heart: home helps (10.5 per 1000 aged 65 plus), meals on wheels (20 000 per annum per 1000 aged 65 plus), and other supports to old people at home were amongst the most generous in the country until budget cuts in 1988. Day centres, luncheon clubs, and education classes are available to offer sustenance, diversion, and company. Residential homes offer 25 places for every 1000 population aged 65 and older, in purpose-built or converted property that is well sited, and well equipped and staffed (Wilkin et al 1982). Primary health care is provided from 51 general practice centres by doctors with list sizes averaging 2200, and is supported by district nurses (0.32 per 1000 population), health visitors (0.17 per 1000 population), and other staff. There is a large district general hospital (DGH) sited in each of the sectors, and both have substantial and active geriatric units; 300 beds in the north together with 40 day hospital places, and 130 beds in the south. Since 1971, district psychiatric services had been devolved from large mental hospitals north of the city to a unit with 160 beds and 80 day hospital places, at the larger DGH in the nothern sector. From here, an active community-orientated service has been developed (Jolley 1976).

First steps

In the earlier years of the National Health Service, there were difficulties in reaching agreement between different services about who should do what for the elderly frail with mental disorders, particularly the dementias. General psychiatry had adopted a reluctant, rather defensive posture to this client-group, and the pattern of expectations that resulted meant that most care remained with families, local authority social workers, general practitioners, and geriatric physicians; there was only occasional help from local psychiatrists, with recourse sometimes to the old mental hospitals for placement of particularly difficult patients. The first step towards improving matters were taken in late 1975, with the appointment of a consultant psychogeriatrician, and the establishment of a core-team (secretary, community psychiatric nurse (CPN), and social worker). It was decided to follow Arie's principles (see above) to provide a specialist service to the elderly mentally ill of the district (Jolley et al 1982).

Priorities were:

1. To define a client group: these would be people aged 65 or older presenting with psychiatric disorders, and referred from primary health care or other specialists for help or advice; their home addresses would be within South Manchester or one of the residential homes that accepted people from the district. Patients graduating into old age under the care of another psychiatrist would usually remain with that consultant. Patients referred with home addresses outside the district might be seen for assessment and advice, but could not be offered a comprehensive service. On the other hand, patients from within the district of younger ages who were considered 'psychogeriatric' by other agencies, usually because of a diagnosis of presenile dementia, would be accepted if other services felt this was appropriate.

2. To accept referrals from the very start and 'get something going', despite lack of resources.

3. To get to know the other agencies working with the elderly in the district by going out to meet them, working with them, learning from them, and offering help and advice from a specialist viewpoint.

4. To improve the facilities available to the specialist service, in terms of the number, arrangement, and siting of beds, day hospital places and outpatient clinics, and the number and range of staff able to go out into the community.

5. To monitor the service's experience and the ideas coming from other centres, and to modify its practice as seemed appropriate in the light of these.

During the first month of operation, the service received only cross-referrals for ward consultations from other hospital specialists. Thereafter, general practitioners (GPs) began to refer directly, and within a couple of months, a pattern was established which has continued ever since — two-thirds of referrals coming from primary care and one-third from other specialists, mainly geriatric physicians. There are now roughly 550 new referrals each year, 450 patients are carried over from previous years in active management, and a further 60 are re-referred after a period out of contact. Between 50–60% are suffering from organic psychosyndromes, 25% are depressed, 10% have paranoid illnesses, and the balance of cases is made up of anxiety states, alcohol or drug dependence, personality disorders, and the occasional person referred who seems quite normal.

Three-quarters of referrals are women, three-quarters are over 75 years, 55% are living alone at the time of referral, 30% live in a private household with someone else, and 15% are already in some form of long-term care.

Of the 51 general practices in the district, 38 provided referrals either directly or via other specialists during 1976, and these have continued to be the practices to which the service relates more frequently. Two of the other 13 practices have ceased to exist, while the rest are sited on the periphery, so that many of their patients live in other districts. No systematic study of GPs' responses to their elderly patients has been undertaken, but it is known that 40% of those referred to the specialist service were receiving regular visits from the practice prior to referral (Wilkin et al 1984). Local GPs are not ignorant of the depressive states and dementias that disable their elderly patients (Williamson et al 1964); on the contrary, most have a well developed instinct for detecting adverse change, and remain interested in collaborative management with the specialist service. Three of these practitioners now work as clinical assistants, and are thus an integral part of the specialist psychogeriatric service.

Responses

First contact is with the secretariat. Housed in the psychogeriatric unit, and working closely with its doctors, social workers, and CPNs, the secretaries are the ears, eyes, and voice of the unit; through a simple but careful recording system, they carry an up-to-date knowledge of who is doing what for whom, and where and when. Once a request for help is received and adequate details of the problem and current attempts to solve it or support the old person have been recorded, a senior doctor goes out, either within a matter of minutes, hours, or a day or two (depending upon the urgency), to assess the situation and begin a programme of management. The service's axiom is that patients are most likely to receive strength and reassurance from their current situation — own home, residential home, or general medical or geriatric ward. It aims to provide understanding of their difficulties, followed by help to lessen the current problems, without losing established confidences, knowledge, and support. A great deal can be achieved by a competent psychiatrist establishing the history, examining the mental state, and acquiring an understanding of the patient's physical health, nursing needs, and available social supports at home. The power for reassurance that comes from this exhibition of interest and professional analysis is considerable. In some instances, it is necessary to gain further information or advice, or to arrange for extra help to be given by the local or team social worker — but the potential of the home situation to guide the outcome towards a best-possible solution is always given the highest respect. Residential homes that cater for groups of 20–40 elderly frail people are looked upon as especially important. Although the service's response to individuals referred from these homes is similar to that given to people in private households, it is frequently found that several residents of one become its patients, so that regular visiting, research, and programmes of in-house seminars have proved worthwhile (Jolley et al 1980a).

If patients need to be removed from their present home territory, this is explained carefully, their agreement is obtained if at all possible, and the disturbance of their usual routine kept to a minimum. A complete understanding of their physical health may only be possible after thorough examination and investigation, and with the advice of a geriatric physician. This can be achieved in an outpatient clinic at the local hospital, and takes less than a morning of the patient's time (Jolley et al 1980b); the foundation of knowledge obtained then allows further intervention to be pursued with greater confidence by follow-up at home. The twin tactics are of treating and managing the patient's abnormal mental state, while at the same time listening to, learning from, educating, and supporting the carers. Yet sometimes, the stresses are too severe, or some tasks too complicated or difficult to carry on at home, without help at the hospital.

Attendance at a day hospital maintains the patient's base in her own bed at night, but allows some respite for carers (most important for those caring for the demented). It can also provide the warmth of company, as well as professional treatment for patients who are bereft of meaningful contacts; this is most important for solitary individuals with persistent mood disorders (Hodgson 1984).

The day hospitals are very active facilities, staffed by committed nurses, doctors, occupational therapists, physiotherapists, a chiropodist, and a hairdresser. In addition, they hold a dynamic balance between care in the community and care as inpatients for those with persistent or progressive disorders. The day hospital facility for the physically able, non-demented elderly is part of the General Psychiatry Day Hospital at the DGH, situated in the northern sector, which is an integral part of the main psychiatric unit for the district. These patients are capable of self-care, and most have suffered major mood disorders which are prone to recur and/or have left persistent affective problems; 19 of the 24 patients currently attending are women, and 15 of them live alone.

Separate day hospital provision is available for patients suffering from dementia; there is one such day hospital for the northern sector and another for the southern. The former is situated on the main DGH campus and is an integral, perhaps dominant feature of the psychogeriatric unit there. The day hospital in the southern sector has

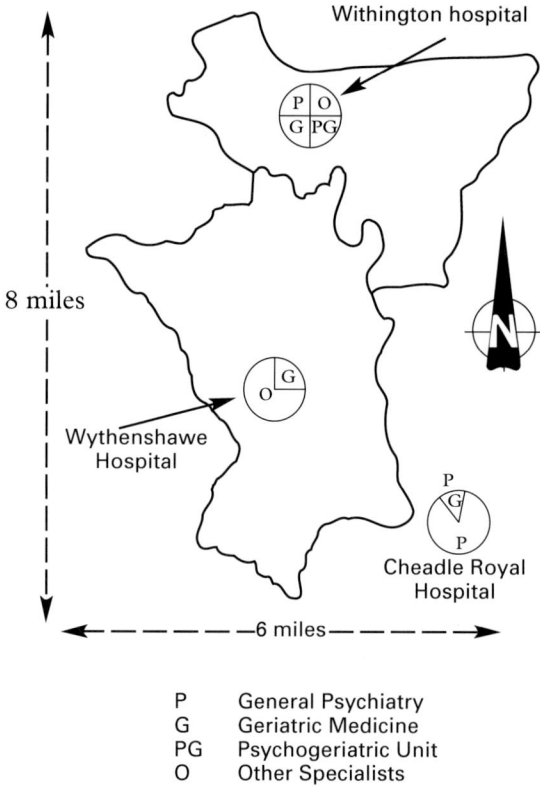

Fig. 9.1   Location of hospital facilities. P = general psychiatry; G = geriatric medicine; PG = psychogeriatric unit; O = other specialties.

been created from a converted ward in a small private mental hospital, sited half a mile to the east of the area served. This is a temporary arrangement between the National Health Service and the private hospital, since the ideal placement will be on the local DGH site (Fig.9.1). In any working week, roughly 45 patients attend each of these day hospitals, although most only do so for two or three days between Monday and Friday. Of those currently attending from the northern sector, 25 are living with relatives, 10 live alone, and 10 attend from Old People's Homes.

Regular multidisciplinary rounds are held every week in these day hospitals, not only to review the current state of patients attending and the programmes of activity being made available, but also to check through the caseloads (of about 40 patients each) of the social workers and CPNs. Further or earlier review by a doctor will be offered if this seems necessary, or attendance arranged at a day hospital, or admission programmed to hospital or a residential home. These liaison rounds ensure that the balancing function of the day hospitals between community and hospitals is efficiently maintained.

Inpatient assessment is available in a 16-bed ward of the DGH in the northern sector, sited in the same pavilion building as the day hospital and the continuing care ward for demented patients. A further 10 beds are available for physically able elderly patients with affective and other 'functional' disorders, in a 32-bed ward in the general psychiatric unit on this DGH campus. Admission is determined by the severity or complexity of symptoms, set against the competence and resilience of the support available at home; most admissions are of one to three months' duration. Very active collaboration is offered by the geriatric physicians, and this includes a regular ward round on the psychogeriatric assessment ward; 90% of patients passing through the general psychiatry ward and 80% of those from the assessment ward return to their own homes. Of the remainder, most move on to residential care, with only about 5% becoming long-stay patients, and 2–3% dying during the assessment period.

Continuing care is virtually confined to patients suffering from profound dementing disorders, usually complicated by severe behavioural problems based in the previous personality or by disinhibition from progression of the brain disease. Sensory deficits and other physical disabilities, almost always including incontinence of urine and sometimes faeces, are common. These individuals have progressed beyond the capabilities of care at home, either with (53%) or without day hospital support, and/or have proved too difficult for residential or nursing home care (15%). There is a 28-bed ward attached to the day hospital for demented patients in the nothern sector and a 23-bed ward attached to that in the southern sector. This association of continuing care wards and day hospitals is immensely important; there is a considerable overlap in the range of disabilities among both inpatients and day patients, but the latter include some who are relatively able (Fig.9.2, Robinson 1965, Wilkin & Jolley 1978). Thus, the intermingling of the two populations greatly enriches the milieu of the inpatient units, the more so because Monday – Friday is different from Saturday–Sunday. Day patients bring with them, both through their own presence and that of the ambulance drivers and escorts, gossip from home, and comments about the weather, and the state of traffic and shops. This potential for mutual support between day hospital and continuing-care beds is not possible if the two are sited separately, nor can it be achieved by a travelling day hospital. Although these other approaches may have some advantages as temporary measures in the early development of services, balanced units including beds and day places, sited in centres of population, provide the best long-term solution. Sometimes a day patient will be admitted to a bed for a 'relief' or 'holiday' period, and eventually some will become

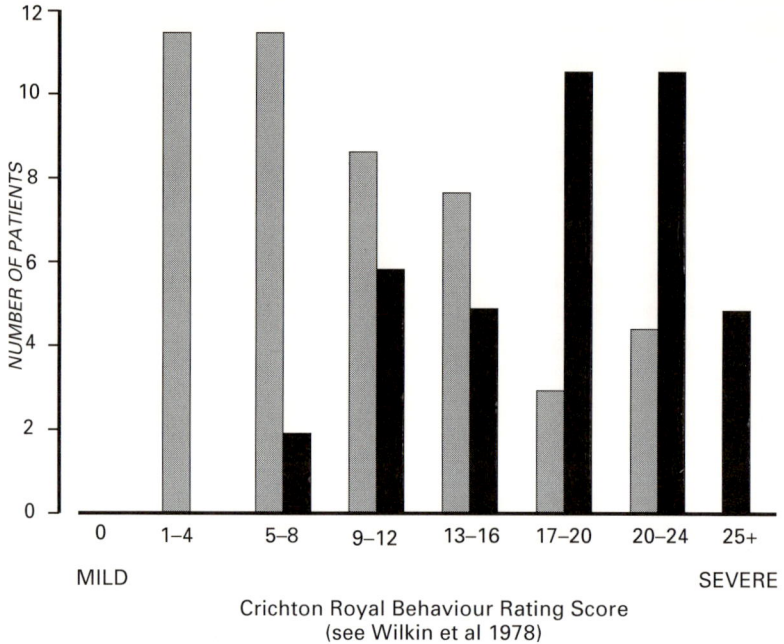

Fig. 9.2   Behavioural characteristics of patients attending the day hospital for dementia ▨ and inpatients on the continuing care wards ▨. Data combined from the Cheadle Royal and Withington Units. One week in 1983.

permanent residents. Yet they have come to feel at home with the place, while their relatives have grown to trust it and have gained the respect of staff as more than equal partners in the struggle to preserve the dignity and well-being of a dementing individual.

Continuing care beds are an essential component of the total service to the local community — not a place to put people away, out of sight and out of mind. They offer to other parts of the service an assurance that, when difficulties become too great to be handled with composure and compassion and are not remediable with the known range of treatments, there is a safe place, where the patients can be accepted and cared for. These are patients who require skilled and sustained care from a team of professionals, which is equipped to respond to their profound physical, social, and psychiatric disabilities. Models which assume them to have characteristics that require only minimal staff and equipment are misinformed and doomed to failure (Stillwell et al 1984). The psychogeriatric service offers thorough clinical understanding, which includes reassessment by doctors, nurses, occupational therapists, and physiotherapists; there is also the contribution of social workers, based on both their own observations and those of visitors, relatives, and friends of the patient, who are encouraged to feel that the wards are open to them at any time. As far as possible, activities which will maintain and re-develop the skills and emotions that remain, are organised each day, often in the company of similarly disabled day patients. Much use is made of reminiscence techniques, and among the best received activities are the frequent short trips around the locality in the unit minibus, which was purchased with funds raised by staff, friends and relatives, supplemented generously by the 'Help the Aged' charity.

Yet appropriate care and management of this group of individuals, who progress through a variable yet harrowing, deteriorating course to an early death, is not an easy task. Incontinence, falls, bruises, fractures, convulsions, pica, sexual and emotional disinhibition including physical attacks (rarely) and distracted wandering, represent regular features of their lives and cannot, with the best techniques in the world, be entirely avoided. However, these must not become the sole preoccupations of the ward, for they are balanced by islands of preserved talent, character, and affection that makes the life worth living, if they can only be explored.

Treatment and support

Treatments practised by the specialist service range across the boundaries of home, residential care, outpatient clinic, day hospitals, and wards. They are designed to help patients either directly or through their supporters, or through a modification in their immediate environment.

Patient-centred treatments begin with a thorough appraisal of their current status, previous lives, coping-styles, and weaknesses. Physical health must be maintained or improved to the best possible level and this may require medication, which must be in appropriate doses, presented in suitable containers, and taking account of possible interaction with other prescriptions (O'Malley et al 1985). Spectacles, hearing aids, and walking sticks all have their places. Occasionally major operations are required, but the dentist and chiropodist are more regularly needed, and physiotherapy has much to contribute. Psychotherapy in its simplest form is offered in the establishment of trust and understanding between patient and doctor (or other members of the team). Deeper involvement is necessary for relatively few patients, but group therapy and support are very effective with those suffering from persistent affective symptoms, who may attend either the day hospital at the main psychiatric unit or a regular group organised by the team social workers at a church hall in the southern sector.

The psychotropic medication used by the service is simple; benzodiazepines are generally avoided, since they tend to disinhibit and confuse more readily than achieve tranquillity. Anxiety, agitation, restlessness, and difficulty in getting off to sleep may all respond to major tranquillisers used in low/moderate doses: perphenazine 2 mg, haloperidol 1–2 mg, promazine syrup 50–100 mg nocte, and chlorpromazine syrup 50–100 mg nocte. Their effects must be monitored and the situation reassessed, if matters are not improving or are getting worse. Parkinsonian side effects are relatively infrequent and should be treated only if and when they arise. Higher doses of major tranquillisers and/or the use of the more potent compounds (chlorpromazine, thioridazine, trifluperazine, haloperidol, pimozide, fluperazine, flupenthixol), occasionally in depot form, are required when persecutory ideas, delusions, and hallucinations are prominent. Care must be taken by clinicians to avoid becoming so determined to eradicate these phenomena that the patient's drive, sparkle, and ability to cope and survive are steam-rollered out of existence. There are quite a number of paranoid old people who are better when left medication-free, for they do not suffer much and cause little bother, as long as they are known and understood.

Antidepressants are used with an appreciation of their potential for side effects, but an even greater respect for the suffering, morbidity, and mortality that is associated with severe depressive states in old age. Thus, dothiepin in doses ranging from 25–150 mg and imipramine or amitriptyline in doses from 10–125 mg daily account for 90% of the psychogeriatric service's prescriptions (Baldwin & Jolley 1986). If these are failing or the constellation of symptoms is life-threatening, then electroconvulsive therapy is used to good effect in most cases (Benbow 1985). This treatment is given to inpatients only — a precaution which seems appropriate in most old people.

Supporters also need to be understood. An appreciation that goes further than their current situation and personal contribution to the patient's welfare will examine their previous life experiences, coping-style, and weaknesses. Feelings toward the patient and other actual or potential helpers are also important, as well as concern for their own physical or mental health. On more than one occasion, the referral to our service has been occasioned when a carer, having struggled on by denying her own serious symptoms, has become very ill, or another family member has become aware of the difficulties. Sometimes, treatment of such illnesses gives the carer a new lease of life.

There is a place for explaining to carers the nature and prognosis of disorders, but this may be overrated, having more face validity than real potential to sustain a situation. Practical help with difficult tasks is much more worthwhile and may be undertaken at home or by taking the patient out for periods of time, to a day hospital or for short admissions. Where maintenance of precarious survival at home (e.g. a demented patient living alone and being supported by others) is all-important, then help at home and minimal recourse to treatment away from it is the best formula. However, when home includes a resident carer who will benefit from time to herself (himself), then 'time away' is more useful. In addition, there is no doubting the power of shared feelings and experiences in sustaining efforts and enthusiasm that may be faltering. Thus, CPNs, social workers, and doctors spend time in listening to carers on an individual basis, and in addition, groups of carers meet on a regular basis with each other and with staff of the combined continuing-care wards and day hospitals.

Changes in the patient's living situation may sometimes be worth achieving: difficulties and worries about an overgrown garden or a family home that has fallen into disrepair are usually best managed by finding resources that will allow the garden to be tidied, or the house made safe and comfortable, or perhaps by steps to encourage the use of part of it rather than the whole. Moving to a new home is a major undertaking. There are some old people who have moved every few years throughout their lives, doomed to be discontented wherever they are placed, and going on to ever less satisfactory accommodation that has been found wanting by others. For a few, a move to be nearer to a son or daughter may have advantages, and the attractions of 'sheltered' accommodation are increasing as violence to old people becomes more widespread and is given sensational publicity. Nevertheless, moving away from a home or neighbourhood that an individual has known and often loved, if unknowingly, for four or five decades is a very stressful event; it is therefore not pursued as a possible solution to the difficulties of many of the patients presenting to us with established psychiatric disorders.

Much more significant is the use of residential care for those patients whose home resources are insufficient to provide for the everyday needs of someone suffering from a dementia or (more rarely) a persistent or recurrent mood disorder. Unlike warden-supervised accommodation, which can offer little more than bricks and mortar with a hard-pressed warden, residential care offers regular attention, food, warmth, clothing, bedding, direction, and reassurance from staff who are available around the clock, and mainly do the work because they enjoy it (Evans et al 1981). It may not be what an individual had planned for her last days, but when the time comes, some modification of self-image may be a small price to pay for reassuming a cloak of dignity, safety, and comfort, albeit one woven largely by others.

Four case vignettes are presented below to illustrate how the principles have worked out in practice:

Widower: ex-army

Mr A had very blue hands. His arteriopathy was causing dementia, within which he would be variably confused, but retaining a mischievous sense of humour and a liking for ladies. His appearance — trouserless at his uncurtained bay window, or in front of the house on warm days, — generated local complaints and fear. Increasing physical frailty and a very overgrown privet hedge eventually overcame these exhibitions, but he could still contrive, with his false leg and poor balance, to fall under or on top of his female domiciliary helpers. Several of these were alarmed into attending in pairs or leaving the situation altogether. His salvation was the devoted advocacy and monitoring of the psychogeriatric service principal social worker, combined with his eventual home help — a robust lady who, together with her sister who would attend if the former was on holiday, sustained him until he was found dead. He had been known to us for five and a half years, of which no time at all was spent as an inpatient: contact with him and his family at home by social workers, CPNs, and doctors, interacting with district nurses and home help, was the main form of care. Occasional visits to the day hospital for a clean up, chiropody, and the company of attractive nurses added some spice and leaven to his last years.

Mrs B and the kidnap

'Endings' in psychogeriatric practice can be somewhat surprising or mystifying, as they can be in psychotherapy. Mrs B first had to be 'ambushed' into hospital by one of the CPNs because she was standing as if petrified — full of indecision, and believing her face had turned to gangrene. She was a thin, remarkably determined lady, who had married a man 'with one foot in the grave', much to her mother's displeasure. Widowed early and childless, she never regretted her happy union, although it had left her isolated in late life. The psychotic depression responded to treatment and she returned to defy hypothermia in her gently decaying house for many years. She said she owed her life to the hospital, and brought herself gratefully along to the day hospital several times a week ever after, until the last winter, when she was clearly becoming unwell. She had become mildly confused and very cold. Her obsessional traits and fears, which were always pronounced at home but never at hospital, were binding her to the house, and it was only after days of intense supervision and persuasion that she was prised away by the team social worker, whom she knew very well.

The next day brought a serious myocardial infarction; it took weeks of gentle rehabilitation on the assessment ward for her to recover, and to adjust herself to the notion that she could not endure home again. With her active participation, a home was found in social services accommodation, and she went there, to make the best of a future she would rather not have faced, partly because it involved the loss of some of her capital, which she had left to a family friend who called her 'auntie'. It was by this heir that she was kidnapped ('taken out to tea') from the local authority home into a private home in an adjacent health district, which was declared to be a little less costly to her estate. The considerable contact which the heir had with nurses on the ward, social workers, and consultant during Mrs B's rehabilitation was not the means to that particular end. She had been known to the service for six years, of which only 22 weeks in two admissions had been spent as an inpatient. Support at home by social workers and CPNs and visits from a unit doctor were supplemented by attendance at the day hospital over 5 years and 30 weeks. She never allowed home helps, district nurses, or meals on wheels to cross her front door.

A lady who knows she is right, and everyone else (almost) is not

Mrs C is a very intelligent, meticulously dressed woman, partially sighted since childhood and schooled at home. She was an admirable worker for a time, and later was content with her respectful and wealthy husband. She presented to us in widowhood with a florid persecutory state, living in her flat, experiencing auditory hallucinations and occasionally visual ones. She believes herself to be the focus of envy and resentment, which results in retributive actions from other residents. She 'responds' in like manner — by creating noise, but maintains a haughty silence when going in and out of the building. She was once, some years ago, admitted compulsorily, after presenting a physical danger to a man who went to remonstrate and whom she believed to be a persecutor of a different order. Subsequent treatment with a depot phenothiazine vastly improved her mental state, but she never had insight into the need for treatment, and when it induced a mobility problem, she never forgave the service. She permits monthly contact with a CPN who delivers pimozide, which are taken, and she permits review by a consultant every two to three months. Exasperated reports are periodically received from the housing association about irritation expressed by other residents and the warden, but an uneasy truce has so far been maintained. Of the eight years in which she has been known, only six weeks has been spent in hospital.

A Welsh schoolmistress

Miss D is a retired teacher, delightfully modest and rather puritanical in philosophy. In retirement, she suffered recurrent severe depressive illness with marked episodes of agitation, diurnal variation in mood, and ideas of worthlessness, requiring repeated inpatient treatment. These illnesses responded well to ECT, but not to drug treatment, to which she became progressively more sensitive. Between admissions, she attended the psychiatric day hospital twice a week. Mildly elated episodes developed between depressions, but did not require treatment. Physical disability in the form of severe bouts of arthritis, and gastrointestinal upsets from hiatus hernia and oesophageal stricture caused her great despondency and shame at depending on others and 'being a nuisance'. She lived in a flat and had a fond niece nearby, who nursed her through progressive disability with the support of the senior CPN and the day hospital, until a further episode of depression, with totally disorganising spells of agitation and panic, provoked her readmission. A recent element of forgetfulness had been developing and was overtaken by recurrent small strokes, causing confusion, poor balance, and brief pareses. Miss D's insight and natural shyness resulted in great distress about her decline, and she was further upset when a more serious CVA resulted in an admission that will be 'till death do us part', for her variable mood, poor cognitive status, and physical disabilities could not be managed elsewhere with any confidence. To the surprise of her niece and Miss D herself, she quickly became contented and even happy in the gentle and committed atmosphere of her long-stay ward where, despite her profound modesty, she enjoys a little bit of superiority. Of the 5 years 4 months we had known her prior to this terminal admission, a total of 36 weeks in 5 admissions had been spent as an inpatient. Day hospital support had sustained her for most of the interim, complemented by the availability throughout of social worker, CPN, and psychogeriatric doctor.

Modifications now and in the future

This psychogeriatric service pledged itself to monitor its own experiences and make changes if they seemed indicated, but so far, major fault has not been found with the original strategy. Time has allowed the negotiation of many improvements in the facilities of the specialist unit, while unforeseen and uncontrollable pressures have enforced certain other changes. The major steps in the evolution of these are summarised in Table 9.1.

The appointment of a second consultant, together with more realistic numbers of CPNs and social workers, allowed the development of separate northern and southern sector teams from 1982. These teams began to work more effectively with the area-based general social workers and in local authority homes for the elderly, and a beginning was made in the southern sector toward regular reviews of patients managed in common with GPs (Jolley & Hodgson 1985b). This is achieved by keeping a register of patients referred from each practice and reviewing their current management at meetings at the health centre or surgery, at which the consultant, social worker, and CPN can be available at regular 3-monthly intervals. At the same time, the appointment of GPs as clinical assistants in the combined day hospital and continuing-care unit of the southern sector increased the understanding and mutual trust between the specialist and primary helath care services. Follow-up outpatient clinics, held originally at the main psychiatric unit, have undergone a transformation since it was realised that transport problems meant that only 10 patients or less could be seen in each clinic, whilst the need had increased to 20, and that patients might spend up to eight hours waiting for transport and attending the clinic, where their contact with the doctor would usually be no more than 15 minutes. A mobile clinic, involving junior as well as senior psychiatrists, means that more patients can be seen more cheaply, more effectively, and with less onus on the patients. A

Table 9.1 Summary of changes in the facilities available to the service 1976-1987. Population 'at risk': 28 000 rising to 31 000 aged 65 years +.

Year	1976	1978	1979	1982	1985	1987
Patients seen per year	550	600	740	890	1000	1100
New referrals	530	360	360	490	550	504
Carried from previous years	20	240	380	400	450	596
Staff in the community						
Consultants	1	1	1	2	2	1
Community psychiatric nurses (CPNs)	1	2	2	5	5	5
Social workers	1	1	2	5	5	3
Withington Hospital (N Sector DGH)						
General Psych (old age)						
Inpatient beds	10	10	10	10	10	10
Day patient places	10	10	10	10	10	6
Outpatient clinics	new/fu	new/fu	new/fu	new/fu	new at hosp, fu in community	
Psychogeriatric Unit						
Inpatient beds	–	20	36	36	44	44
Day patient places	–	15	15	15	30	30
Wythenshawe Hospital						
(S Sector DGH)	–	–	–	–	–	–
Cheadle Royal Hospital						
Inpatient beds	42	42	42	23	23	23
Day patient places	–	–	–	12	12	12

clinic list of 20–24 patients is drawn up for the northern sector for one week and for the southern sector the next. Patients are informed by letter that a doctor from the service will be visiting them at home during the morning of the clinic within the hours 09h 30–12h 30 and are asked to let us know if it is not a convenient time. A consultant and three doctors in training, undertake these home visits by car, returning to the unit to review their findings and plans for further management over a sandwich lunch. In most instances, there is 100% attendance at this 'clinic', and the training experience is widely appreciated by the younger doctors.

For the future, the local aspirations of the service are to improve and extend its activity in the southern sector, and to make a more significant contribution to the activities of the University Department of Psychiatry and to developments within the rest of the North Western Health Region. All three teaching districts now have effective services, as have at least three other districts in the region, but it is recognised that there are hazards in the nature of the work and in the rate at which change is occurring. Frail elderly patients suffering from psychiatric disorders that impair their interpretation of the world and reduce their ability to speak for themselves, are particularly at risk of mismanagement. Scandals in large institutions were among the factors stimulating the creation of specialist services for the elderly. Yet the creation of a larger private residential care sector in Great Britain has already spawned its own breed of scandals in small institutions (Hoyland 1986), and community care for the elderly has been described as potentially care 'on the cheap' by neglect (Opit 1977). It is not only elderly patients who are at risk, though, for the efforts of those who struggle, with the best of intentions and skills, to balance their clients' wishes for independence against the risks their infirmities produce, are all too easy to misunderstand and misrepresent. Sensational journalism sells newspapers but the memory of the media is very short-lived, and their efforts seem very rarely to be constructive.

Thus, there should be a major national commitment of resources to train people, monitor their achievements, and identify the difficulties they encounter in this humane work. Research that will identify fruitful approaches and techniques to deal most effectively with problematic situations is also needed. For the most part, though, such developments have not yet taken place, crushed mainly by fiscal restraint.

THE INTERNATIONAL PERSPECTIVE

The balance between care of the elderly in the community and in institutions — hospitals, nursing homes, and rest homes — currently shows more community bias in the UK than in most other industrialised countries, where a greater proportion of retired people move into institutional care of one sort or another. There is widespread interest in the British geriatric and psychogeriatric movements; visitors come to see these services from all over the world, and courses organised under the auspices of the British Council attract participants from both developing and the older industrialised countries. There is evidence that treatable psychiatric disorders may be diagnosed as 'dementia' when active psychiatric expertise is not easily available (Copeland & Gurland 1985); in these circumstances, patients may therefore go untreated, suffer unnecessarily protracted morbidity, and spend unnecessary time in expensive yet restrictive care.

Psychogeriatric services in several other countries are described below, to provide a context for this account of a British service.

Australia

In Australia, it has been said that 'geriatric' psychiatry is in its adolescence (Williams 1987); so far, very few psychiatrists are engaged in full-time work with the elderly. The demography of Australia is different from that of the UK, but now seems to be following the same pattern, though some 30 years later. In 1981, there were 1.46 million persons aged 65 or over, a number which on present trends is projected to grow to 2.26 million (12% of the population) by 2001, and to 3.48 million (nearly 16%) in 2021. Those aged 80 or more were 0.26 million in 1981, projected to grow to 0.56 and then 0.79 million; females preponderate strongly in this very old group (Snowdon 1987). Also, the proportion of people from non-English-speaking backgrounds is expected to double to 22% by the year 2000, but there is a lack of bilingual health professionals, and management by English-speaking staff may be very difficult, particularly with the onset of dementia. Preston (1986) has calculated that the prevalence rate in Australia of moderate and severe dementia is about 6%, but rising to 7.5% by the year 2000; this means that the number of persons with dementia would double between 1981 and 2001, continuing to rise in the following two decades. Unlike the UK, perhaps half of those with moderate or severe dementia in Australia are in institutions. In Hobart, Kay et al (1985) found major depression present in 10.28% of the elderly (but 15% of those aged over 80), which are much higher rates than those reported from the USA.

Distance is an impediment to the delivery of specialist services, not only to smaller communities but even within the sprawling suburbs of larger cities, which may be 50 km from few psychogeriatric centres (Williams 1987). About 30% of the total of public and private psychiatric beds is occupied by people aged 65 or over, but only 10% of discharges are of people in this age range. Most Australian psychiatrists are in private practice and probably see relatively few elderly people; the fee-for-service system makes organised teamwork with other professionals or regular home assessment almost impossible. As in the USA, many elderly people were transferred or redirected from mental hospitals to private nursing homes through deinstitutionalisation policies; about two-thirds of such patients are demented and at least one-third depressed(Snowdon & Donnelly 1986). However, few nursing homes are visited by psychiatrists or other mental health professionals; they mostly have 20–100 beds and may be run privately or on a non-profit basis, with government subsidies. General hospital psychiatric units and community mental health centres mostly provide little service to the elderly, and although geriatric assessment teams are being established, these do not usually include psychiatric personnel. The need for specialist training seems to be overwhelming.

Switzerland

The situation of psychogeriatrics in Switzerland has been reported by Wertheimer (1986); as a confederate state with 23 cantons, this country shows a great variety of health care arrangements. In the national population, 15% are aged 65 or over, and of these, 17% are over 80, but there are large variations in age-structure between cantons, Basel-Stadt having more than 20% elderly. Of the five medical schools, only Geneva and Lausanne have so far established specific psychogeriatric services. Lausanne opened a 150-bed psychogeriatric hospital in 1961, but this quickly became overburdened, and an outpatient centre was then established, from which a multidisciplinary team has operated to intervene in patients' homes or institutions; subsequently, two day hospitals were added to the service, which has a catchment population of 250 000. It is supplemented by various paramedical and social services which visit patients' homes; geriatric physicians participate in this psychogeriatric service, whilst in Geneva, psychogeriatricians operate in the geriatric hospital and university hospital centre, but there are no joint assessment centres. In the rest of the country, specialisation by psychiatrists in the care of the elderly is developing steadily, and most psychiatric services have special units; both psychogeriatric and geriatric day hospitals exist in the four largest cities. Long-stay institutions (semi-private or private) often accept psychogeriatric patients for day care, on a flexible basis. Overall, Wertheimer (1986) reports that both the specialty and services for the psychiatric needs of old people are developing steadily.

Belgium

Those aged 65 and older in Belgium comprise 14.3% of the national population, and this proportion is expected to increase slightly: however, between 1981 and 2000, the age-group 85 and over, is projected to grow by 50%, two-thirds of these being females. In 1981, 26% of those aged over 65 were living alone and almost 25% were living with children. National planning of health services was negatively affected by economic difficulties in the 1970s, but legislation in 1977 specified 0.3 beds per 1000-population in psychiatric hospitals for severe psychogeriatric cases. So far, few specific services exist for psychogeriatric patients and few psychiatrists specialise in this work. Subsequently, norms were fixed of 2 beds per 1000 in nursing homes and 3.5 beds for 'geriatric care', but no proportion of these was specified for psychogeriatrics. Almost 5% of the elderly population are resident in old people's homes, but interest is growing in the development of sheltered housing. Belgium contains one institution of outstanding quality — Ten Kerselaere — which includes beds for 30 psychogeriatric patients. This is designed on the principle of an integrated 'village', covering every level of dependency from total hospital care to sheltered housing. The remarkable buildings include enclosed gardens, aviary, cafe, beauty parlour, chapel, shops, and exhibits, all encouraging sociability and the preservation of living skills (Baro & Dom 1986).

FUTURE DEVELOPMENTS

It seems likely that psychogeriatric teams or their equivalent, will eventually be organised in most developed parts of the world. However, there is still much more that needs to be done in the UK, not only in spreading present good practice, but also in improving and increasing the depth and quality of services provided. Yet enthusiasm for work in the community should not detract from the need of the very elderly and very vulnerable for comprehensive supervision, which can often be best provided in a suitably equipped and supported residential home. The Dutch experience has been that providing more nursing homes with strictly defined criteria for entry does not in itself satisfy the needs; waiting lists remain stubbornly large and long. An active community service does much to rationalise the use of scarce resources, but the enthusiasm with which places have recently been taken in the expanding private homes sector in the UK confirms that residential/institutional provision had been limited mainly because people were unable to afford to pay for the care that they and their families felt would be most appropriate (Central Statistical Office 1986).

Under the Government's recently announced proposals for community care (Department of Health 1989) the lead agency will be the Local Authority, as suggested by Griffiths. Local Authorities will assume responsibility for the care element of public support for people in private and voluntary residential and nursing homes. Local Authorities will become the conduit for funds that previously flowed directly to individuals through board and lodging allowances in the social security system. A single budget will cover the costs of care, thus removing the perverse incentives which led public agencies to maximise the use of social security to finance residential care. Local Authorities will assess individual needs in collaboration with medical and nursing agencies. In order to prevent the Local Authorities expanding their provider role, however, they will continue to bear the full cost of accommodating people in Local Authority homes.

The emphases of personal and family life are changing: time devoted to labour and breadwinning can be less, while time at home, always a privilege, is being given greater status. The post-war decades that overvalued the qualities of youth are giving way to a period when the virtues of wisdom and experience are being reconsidered. The elderly retired, having lived quietly and gratefully in their twilight years, now show evidence of new-found confidence to speak out for their own best interests. It may well be that these themes will come together, so that older people are even more strongly supported within the structure of normal family life, and that changes in mood, intellect, and vitality will be less passively accepted as inevitable because of age. The roles of welfare services and of primary health care must continue to develop, probably gaining in vitality and range by infusions from voluntary and privately financed ventures. Positive, creative, new developments should foster prevention, education, and improved health and welfare of the whole community, rather than just better responses to established problems. In this, specialist services for the elderly and for the mentally ill need to be transformed from institution-based last resorts to readily available teams with human faces, who are able to provide both knowledge of new developments and competence with well tried strategies. As such, they will be most acceptable and most potent.

REFERENCES

Anderson F 1985 An historical overview of geriatric medicine: definition and aims. In: Pathy J (ed) Principles & practice of Geriatric Medicine. Wiley, Chichester
Arie T 1970 The first year of the Goodmayes psychiatric service for old people. Lancet ii: 1179-1182
Arie T, Jolley D J 1982 Making services work; organisation and style of psychogeriatric services. In: Levy and Post (eds) The psychiatry of late life. Blackwell, Oxford
Baldwin R C, Jolley D J 1986 The prognosis of depression in old age. British Journal of Psychiatry 149: 574-583
Baro F, Dom R 1986 Psychogeriatrics in Belgium: an overview. In: Maletta G J, Pirozzolo F J (eds) Assessment of treatment of the elderly neuropsychiatric patient. Praeger, New York
Beck A T 1967 Depression: clinical, experimental and theoretical aspects. Staples Press, London
Benbow S M 1985 Electroconvulsive therapy in psychogeriatric practice. Geriatric Medicine 1: 19-22
Bergmann K 1971 The neuroses of old age. In: Kay D W K, Walk A (eds) Recent developments in psychogeriatrics. Headley Brothers, Ashford
Bergmann K 1978 Neurosis and personality disorder in old age. In: Isaacs A, Post F (eds) Studies in geriatric psychiatry. Wiley, New York
Bromley D 1966 The psychology of human ageing. Penguin, Harmondsworth
Carse J, Panton N, Watt A 1958 A district mental health service: the Worthing experiment. Lancet i: 39-42
Central Statistical Office 1979 Social Trends 9. HMSO, London
Central Statistical Office 1986 Social Trends 16. HMSO, London
Committee of Inquiry into Allegations of Ill-Treatment of Patients and other Irregular Activities of the Ely Hospital Cardiff 1969 Cmnd 3975. HMSO, London
Committee of Inquiry on the Transfer of Patients from Fairfield Hospital to Rossendale Hospital 1975. Report to the North West Regional Health Authority
Copeland J R M, Gurland B J 1985 International comparative studies. In: Arie (ed) Recent advances in psychogeriatrics. Churchill Livingstone, London
Crowe T J, Frith C D, Johnstone F C, Owen D G 1980 Schizophrenia and cerebral atrophy. Lancet i: 1129-1130
DHSS 1970 Psychogeriatric assessment units. Circular HM (70) 11
DHSS 1972 Service for mental illness related to old age. Circular HM (72) 71
DHSS 1980 Health and personal social service statistics for England 1978. HMSO, London
DHSS 1989 Statement by Kenneth Clarke, Secretary of State for Health, London
Dodwell D 1986 Alzheimer's disease; the clinical picture. In: Pitt (ed) Dementia. Churchill Livingstone, London
Eastwood R, Corbin S 1985 Epidemiology of mental disorders in old age. In: Arie (ed) Recent advances in psychogeriatrics. Churchill Livingstone, London
Evans G, Hughes B, Wilkin D, Jolley D J 1981 The management of mental and physical impairment in non-specialist residential homes for the elderly. Research Report No 4. Psychogeriatric Research Unit, Withington Hospital, Manchester
Foster E M, Kay D W K, Bergmann K 1976 The characteristics of old people receiving and needing domiciliary services. Age & Ageing 5: 345-355
Grad J, Sainsbury P 1965 An evaluation of the effects of caring for the aged at home. In: Psychiatric disorders in the aged, World Psychiatric Association. Manchester, Geigy
Grad J, Sainsbury P, Costain W R 1975 The incidence of referred mental illness in Chichester and Salisbury. Psychological Medicine 5: 35-54
Gruenberg E M 1978 The epidemiology of senile dementia. In: Schoenberg (ed) Advances in neurology 19. Raven Press, New York
Hall M R P 1985 Delivery of health care in the United Kingdom. In: Pathy (ed) Principles

and practice of geriatric medicine. Wiley, Chichester

Health Advisory Service 1982 The rising tide: developing services for mental illness in old age. HAS, Sutton

Hodgson S P 1984 Day hospital for dementia: safety net for a high wire act? In: Reed, Lomas (ed) Psychiatric services in the community: developments and innovations. Croom Helm, London

Hoyland P 1986 Wide abuse in private homes for elderly. The Guardian 29 April

Isaacs B 1981 Is geriatrics a specialty? In: Arie (ed) Health care of the elderly. Croom Helm, London

Jefferys P, Denham M 1985 Acute confusional states. In: Hildick-Smith (ed) Neurological problems in the elderly. Balliere Tindall, London

Jolley D J 1976 Evaluation of a psychiatric service based on a district general hospital. International Journal of Mental Health 5: 22-26

Jolley D J 1981 Dementia: Misfits in need of care. In: Arie T (ed) Health care of the elderly. Croom Helm, London

Jolley D J 1986 Register of Psychogeriatrics. Newsletter of the section of psychiatry of old age. The Royal College of Psychiatrists, London

Jolley D, Arie T 1978 Organisation of Psychogeriatric services. British Journal of Psychiatry 132: 1-11

Jolley D J, Hodgson S P 1985a Alcoholism in the elderly: a tale of women and our times. In: Isaacs (ed) Recent advances in geriatric medicine. Vol 3. Churchill Livingstone, London

Jolley D J, Hodgson S P 1985b Moving closer to primary care in psychogeriatric practice. Paper presented to The Royal College of Psychiatrists Spring Quarterly Meeting

Jolley D J, Jolley S P 1990 Psychiatry of the elderly. In Pathy (ed) Principles and practice of geriatric medicine, second edn. Wiley, Chichester

Jolley D J, Kondratowicz T, Wilkin D 1980a Helping the disabled in old people's homes. Geriatric Medicine November, pp. 74-76

Jolley D J, Kondratowicz T, Brocklehurst J C 1980b Psychogeriatric out-patient clinic. Paper presented to the British Geriatric Society, Douglas, Isle of Man

Jolley D J, Smith P, Billington L, Ainsworth D, Ring D 1982 Developing a psychogeriatric service. In: Davis Coakley (ed) Establishing a geriatric service. Croom Helm, London

Kay D W K, Beamish P, Roth M 1964 Old age mental disorders in Newcastle-upon-Tyne: I Prevalence. British Journal of Psychiatry 110: 146-158

Kay D W K, Bergmann K, Foster E M, McKechnie A A, Roth M 1970 Mental illness and hospital usage in the elderly. Comprehensive Psychiatry 1: 26-35

Kay D W K, Henderson A S, Scott R et al 1985 The prevalence of dementia and depression among the elderly living in the Hobart community. Psychological Medicine 15: 771-778

Kidd C B 1962 Misplacement of the elderly in hospital. British Medical Journal ii: 1491-1495

Lewis A 1946 Ageing and senility: a major problem of psychiatry. Journal of Mental Science 92: 150-170

Lishman W A 1978 Organic psychiatry. Blackwell, Oxford

Manchester Joint Consultative Committee (Health) 1985 Health Inequalities and Manchester

Nielson J 1962 Geronto-psychiatric period prevalence investigation in a geographically delimited population. Acta Psychiatrica Scandinavica 38: 307-330

Norman A 1982 Mental illness in old age: meeting the challenge. Policy studies in ageing No. 1. Centre for Policy on Ageing, London

O'Malley K, Meagher F, O'Callaghan W 1985 The pharmacology of ageing. In: The principles and practice of geriatric medicine. Wiley, Chichester

Opit L J 1977 Domiciliary care for the elderly sick — economy or neglect? British Medical Journal i: 30-33

Post F 1962 The Significance of affective symptoms in old age. Maudsley Monograph No 10. Oxford University Press, London

Post F 1966 Persistent persecutory states of the elderly. Pergamon Press, Oxford

Post F, Shulman K 1985 New views on old age affective disorders. In: Arie (ed) Recent advances in psychogeriatrics. Churchill Livingstone, London

Preston G A N 1986 Dementia in elderly adults: prevalence and institutionalisation. Journal of Gerontology 41: 261-267

Robinson R A 1965 The organisation of a diagnostic and treatment unit for the aged in a mental hospital. In: Psychiatric disorders in the aged.World Psychiatric Association. Geigy, Manchester

Sainsbury P, Grad J 1970 The psychiatrist and the geriatric patient. Journal of Geriatric Psychiatry 4: 23-41

Sainsbury P, Costain W R, Grad J 1965 The effects of community service on the referral and admission rates of elderly psychiatric patients. In: Psychiatric disorders in the aged. World Psychiatric Association, Geigy, Manchester

Sheldon J H 1948 The social medicine of old age. Oxford University Press, London

Snowdon J 1987 Psychiatric services for the elderly. Australian & New Zealand Journal of Psychiatry 21: 131-136

Snowdon J, Donnelly N 1986 A study of depression in nursing homes. Journal of Psychiatric Research 20: 327-333

Stevenson O 1981 The frail elderly — a social worker's perspective. In: Arie (ed) Health care of the elderly. Croom Helm, London

Stillwell J A, Hassall C, Rose S 1984 Changing demands made by senile dementia on the National Health Service. Journal of Epidemiology & Community Health 38: 131-133

Townsend P 1957 The family life of old people. Penguin, Harmondsworth

Townsend P 1962 The last refuge. Routledge & Kegan Paul, London

Wattis J, Arie T 1984 Further developments in psychogeriatrics in Britain. British Medical Journal ii: 778

Wertheimer J 1986 Psychogeriatrics in Switzerland. Gerontopsychiatry (original in Japanese)

Wilkin D, Jolley D J 1978 Mental and physical impairment in the elderly in hospital and residential care. Nursing Times 74: 29

Wilkin D, Evans G, Hughes B, Jolley D J 1982 The implications of managing confused and disabled people in non-specialist residential homes for the elderly. Health Trends 14: 98-100

Wilkin D, Durie A, Wade G, Jolley D, Stout I 1984 Specialist services for the elderly: a study of referrals to geriatric, psychiatric and social services. Research Report No. 5, Psychogeriatric Unit Research Section, Withington Hospital, Manchester

Wilkin D, Hughes B, Jolley D J 1985 Quality of care in institutions. In: Arie (ed) Recent advances in psychogeriatrics. Churchill Livingstone, London

Williams E I 1984 Characteristics of patients aged over 75 not seen during one year in general practice. British Medical Journal 228: 119-121

Williams S 1987 Geriatric psychiatry in Australia. International Journal of Geriatric psychiatry 2: 67-69

Williamson J 1985 Preventive aspects of geriatric medicine. In: Pathy (ed) Principles and practice of geriatric medicine. Wiley, Chichester

Williamson J, Stokoe I H et al 1964 Old people at home: their unreported needs. Lancet i: 1117-1120

10. Alcohol problems in the community

J. Orford

INTRODUCTION

In the last two decades there has been not only an increasing recognition of the existence of alcohol problems on a large scale, but also a radical change in our understanding of these problems and in the pattern of responses to them. From an early understanding that alcohol consumption could become, for some individuals, so excessive and addictive that it appeared disease-like (captured in the slogan 'alcoholism is a disease'), awareness has expanded in a number of directions.

First, former stereotypes of 'alcoholism' have been challenged by an awareness that excessive and difficult-to-control alcohol use is by no means confined to men around middle-age; it occurs amongst all age groups including teenagers and the elderly, and amongst women as well as men. This broadening of the picture has made it difficult to adhere to fixed conceptions about 'alcoholism', because different sex and age groups differ in many respects, including their motives for drinking, the settings in which they drink, the attitudes of family and friends towards their drinking, the rapidity with which restrained drinking can develop into excessive drinking, and the solutions to these problems which individuals prefer. For example, women with drinking problems are less likely than men to have a long history of heavy drinking (e.g. Orford & Keddie 1985).

Secondly, with this awareness has also come the realisation that individuals with drinking problems are not a discrete group, who are easily distinguished from their fellow citizens. Ledermann's (1956) demonstration that alcohol consumption was continuously distributed within a population (the distribution typically following a skewed, or roughly log normal curve), as well as population surveys of drinking problems such as Cahalan & Room's (1974) in the USA and Edwards et al's (1972) in the UK, did much to dispel the myth that people could be divided into those who were heavy or problematic drinkers and those who were not. Figure 10.1, taken from a report of the Office of Health Economics, illustrates some of the complexities. Not all those who are dependent on alcohol are experiencing problems related to their use of it, and not all those who are experiencing problems are amongst the heaviest

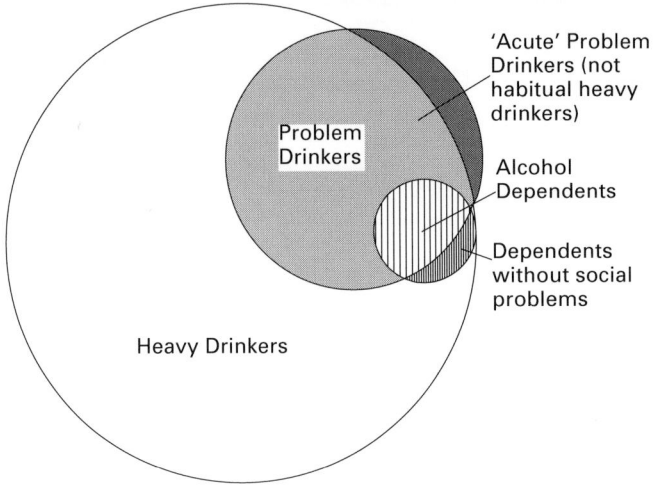

Fig. 10.1 The terminology of drinking

drinkers. Indeed, the figure probably understates the complications, since not all those who are dependent on alcohol are necessarily very heavy drinkers. Nor should it be assumed that alcohol dependence is easily defined.

The concept of the 'alcohol dependence syndrome' (ADS), proposed by Edwards & Gross (1976), has now been adopted as standard nomenclature in the International Classification of Diseases, and replaces the term 'alcoholism'. The ADS has three components, each of which exists on a continuum: altered behaviour (e.g. heavier, more regular and less socially restrained drinking), altered psychobiological response (e.g. increased tolerance and withdrawal symptoms), and altered subjective experience (e.g. increased desire and preoccupation).

An important additional component of the new awareness has been growing recognition of the existence of forms of individual or social damage or harm related to alcohol, but not necessarily linked with a high level of alcohol dependence in those who cause or experience this harm. These alcohol-related disabilities (ARDs), as they have come to be known (Edwards et al 1977), range from accidents and absenteeism to gastritis and liver cirrhosis. The large majority of people with ARDs are unknown to specialist agencies dealing with alcohol problems, but are very likely to come the way of non-specialist social and medical services. An awareness of this fact, probably more than any other, has eroded our former exclusive preoccupation with the severest forms of alcohol dependence, usually treated within the specialised psychiatric unit. Such clinical preoccupation has been further undermined by the compelling evidence that alcohol-related harm, in particular the rate of deaths from

Table 10.1   Alcohol trends in Britain 1956–1986

	1956	1966	1976	1986
Admissions to mental illness hospitals and units in England and Wales with a main diagnosis of alcohol misuse[a] (per 100 000 population)	Not available	15.24	29.4	37.5
Offences of drunkenness in England and Wales[b] (per 100 000 population[c])	158[d]	233[d]	282	186
Deaths from liver disease and cirrhosis in the UK[e] (per 100 000 population)	3.59[f]	3.93	5.28	6.72[g]
UK alcoholic drink released for home consumption (litres absolute alcohol per capita, 15 years and over)	4.9	6.0	9.1	9.2

[a] — includes alcoholism (1966, 1976), alcohol dependence syndrome (1986), non-dependent abuse of alcohol (1986), and alcoholic psychosis
[b] — includes findings of guilt and cautions, and includes simple drunkenness and drunkenness with aggravation
[c] — aged 15 and over (1952, 1962), 14 and over (1976, 1986)
[d] — figures are for 1952 and 1962 respectively
[e] — includes cirrhosis of the liver, alcoholic or other (all years), and alcoholic fatty liver, acute alcoholic hepatitis, chronic hepatitis, alcoholic liver damage, biliary cirrhosis, and other chronic non-alcoholic or unspecified liver disease (1985 only)
[f] — figure is for 1958
[g] — figure is for 1985

liver cirrhosis, is correlated with national alcohol consumption (e.g. Kendell 1979).

These various trends combined make a convincing argument that alcohol problems cannot be dealt with satisfactorily in clinical isolation, but should be viewed as community problems, understandable in the context of how a range of problems are generated by the consumption of alcohol within a community, and of how the community responds to them.

Finally, these changes in understanding have taken place against a background of apparently rising trends in alcohol consumption and alcohol-related harm. Table 10.1 illustrates the rise in alcohol-related mental hospital admissions and drunkenness offences, deaths from liver cirrhosis, and alcohol consumption, in the UK (some of the figures relate to England and Wales only) from the mid-1950s to the mid-1980s. In general, the sharp rise over this period was followed by a flattening out or decrease in the trends for these indices in the 1980s. Table 10.2 shows that the general trend towards increased alcohol consumption from the 1950s to the 1970s was an international phenomenon, by no means confined to Britain.

The remainder of this chapter will consider two questions: where and in what form are alcohol problems likely to be found in the community?; and what might be the nature of a community response to these problems? Unlike problems which can be defined largely in medical or clinical terms, community problems can only be considered within the context of a certain community. In writing this chapter, I have particularly had in mind a notional community in England or Wales, of approximately a quarter of a million people, served by a District Health Authority. When discussing a possible district service, I have drawn particularly upon my own experience of one such locality (Exeter) in the south west of England, but the general principle of understanding the range of alcohol problems within a community, and of devising a comprehensive response to them, may apply to any area of an industrialised country.

ALCOHOL PROBLEMS WITHIN A COMMUNITY

It is clear from the above that no single estimate of the number of people in any community who have drinking problems will suffice. However, on the basis of information presently available, the picture shown in Figure 10.2 is the best approximation. There are some regional differences even within England and Wales, with some evidence of more heavy drinking in

Table 10.2   Changes in consumption of alcoholic beverages in Europe 1950–1976

	1950	1976	% change 1950–1976
France	17.2	16.5	−4
Portugal	—	14.1	
Spain	—	14.0	
Luxembourg	6.8	13.4	+ 97
Italy	9.2	12.7	+ 38
West Germany	2.9	12.5	+ 331
Austria	5.0	11.2	+ 124
Hungary	4.8	10.7	+ 123
Switzerland	7.9	10.3	+ 30
Belgium	6.3	10.2	+ 62
Czechoslovakia	4.0	9.2	+ 130
Denmark	3.6	9.2	+ 156
Ireland	3.3	8.7	+ 164
United Kingdom	4.9	8.4	+ 71
Netherlands	2.1	8.3	+ 295
East Germany	1.2	8.3	+ 592
Poland	3.0	8.2	+ 173
Finland	1.7	6.4	+ 276
Sweden	3.6	5.9	+ 64
Norway	2.2	4.3	+ 95

Source: Moser 1980. Consumption expressed as average annual consumption of 100% ethanol equivalent per annum.

the north and west than in the east and south (Wilson 1980). However, a reasonable average expectation for the country as a whole is that: approximately 90 adults per 1000 will, if directly asked relevant questions, admit to regular heavy drinking; 30 will admit to more than the occasional problem related to their use of alcohol; the number known to medical and social agencies to have problems related to alcohol will be very much less; and the number admitted to psychiatric hospitals or units for the treatment of alcohol problems much smaller still.

Table 10.3 lists the various institutions, agencies, and organisations, both statutory and voluntary, formal and informal, whose personnel, either knowingly or unknowingly, are likely to meet individuals with drinking problems or members of their families. Almost all these agents are to be found in every locality, or at least in neighbouring large towns which serve the locality. The list is a large one, although probably not comprehensive; it reflects the fact that forms of alcohol-related harm include the medical, social and legal, and affect all ages including the very young and the elderly. The list covers a formidable array of personnel who should have some familiarity with, and some understanding of the nature of drinking problems in order to respond appropriately to those amongst their clients, patients, customers or members whose problems are at least partly related to their consumption of alcohol.

The list is by no means confined to those who work within medical, social or penal establishments. It includes, for example, magistrates, who deal with a large amount of drunkenness offending, often with a sense of frustration and an awareness of the ineffectiveness of the system. Like the police, most magistrates welcome innovations such as detoxification centres, to which the police can take people who are drunk in public whom they might otherwise have taken to the police station and thence

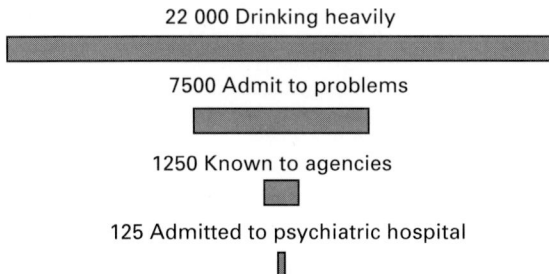

22 000 Drinking heavily

7500 Admit to problems

1250 Known to agencies

125 Admitted to psychiatric hospital

* Not to scale

Fig. 10.2   Likely annual prevalence of heavy and problem drinking in an average health district in England and Wales (Source: Oxford, 1987)

Table 10.3 Community agents in a position to detect and respond to drinking problems

General practice	A range of physical disorders, including gastritis, peptic ulcer and obesity in men; and family and social problems including effects on spouses and children, work attendance, accidents etc
Health visitors, district nurses	The same range of disorders and problems, but these agents may be particularly likely to see problems in family members
General hospital staff	A range of alcohol-related disorders and injuries, in various departments including gastroenterology and accident and emergency
Psychiatric hospital staff and community mental health staff (CMH teams, community psychiatric nurses etc)	Excessive drinking with a wide range of mental health problems including anxiety, depression, and other drug misuse
Social services	Excessive drinking with a wide range of family and social problems, especially family violence, problems experienced by the elderly, and some housing problems
Services for children or adolescents and their families (incl medical, psychiatric, social, voluntary)	Excessive drinking in a parent is a common cause of abuse and neglect of children and adolescents, and a common accompaniment of childhood disorders of various kinds
Services for the elderly	Now recognised that the elderly are a high-risk group for excessive drinking associated with bereavement, loneliness, and psychological disorder such as anxiety and depression
Clergy and voluntary organisations (incl citizens' advice, Samaritans, Relate, Women's Aid)	Particularly likely to be approached by family members affected by excessive drinking, and by problem drinkers in despair
Local authority housing departments	Drinking problems sometimes come to notice by way of rent arrears or disputes with neighbours. Housing departments also have a role in helping tenants who are undergoing treatment or who need accommodation during a period of rehabilitation
Probation services	A high proportion of clients with drinking problems, especially those with many petty offences. Also, many younger offenders whose offences are complicated by very heavy drinking
Magistrates courts	Ditto. Plus a large volume of drunkenness offending dealt with largely by fining. Plus drunken driving offences

Table 10.3 (*cont'd*)

Prison	Large proportions of remand prisoners and those serving short sentences, some for non-payment of small fines, plus a proportion of long-term prisoners
Police	Public drunkenness, incl drunken driving, other offences committed by problem drinkers, control of licenced premises incl under-age drinking, domestic disputes
Lawyers	Problem drinking is a common reason for legal separation and divorce especially, and one of the factors in many cases of violence towards wives and children
Single, homeless people, and casual users of night shelter, reception centre, and cheap commercial hostel accommodation	High rates of problem drinking in these groups
The workplace (incl employers, personnel officers, industrial medical officers, company nurses and colleagues)	Drinking problems very often come to notice first in the workplace as a result of absenteeism, accidents, and poor work performance. Some forms of employment are particularly associated with excessive drinking, including the licenced trade, shipping, hotel and catering, and the construction industry
Teachers	Drinking problems in young people may affect attendance and school performance. A sizeable minority of school pupils will also be affected by the excessive drinking of a parent
Licenced premises, especially public houses	Landlords and barstaff observe much heavy drinking at first hand, are often required to discipline excessive drinkers, and can take a responsible and helpful attitude towards individuals
Family and friends	Many quite serious problems are fully known only by family and sometimes by friends. The ways they react may be influential in helping to resolve the problem

to court. Along with their colleagues in the probation service, magistrates are equally likely to welcome schemes, such as those which are now possible in Britain under Schedule 11 of the Criminal Justice Act 1982, for placing offenders whose offences are drink-related on a probation order, with a requirement that the offender attend a short course of alcohol education as an alternative to any other sentence (e.g. Coventry Probation Service 1982).

The list also includes those who, because of their position in the work place, are able to influence people whose drinking problems manifest themselves in that setting. Responding to drinking problems there, couples humanitarian concern for the individual with a utilitarian concern for efficiency and productivity. The costs to industry of excessive drinking are estimated to be very considerable indeed (Table 10.4), while the workplace has a number of possible advantages as a location in which drinking problems can be confronted constructively. Work performance is often a relatively early indicator that drinking has become harmful; supervisors are in a position to detect, and to carry some influence with individuals who have drinking problems, and keeping a job can be made contingent upon receiving appropriate treatment. However, in practice, the experience of specialist practitioners has been that work supervisors and colleagues often shield those with drinking problems, and fail to confront the issues until it is too late and the employee loses his/her job. As a result, the appropriate aim is to encourage companies or employers to draw up, as a result of discussion between management, unions and medical and personnel officers, company-based policies for dealing with drinking problems (Hore & Plant 1981). In the UK, firms with such policies include British Telecom, British Rail and GEC.

Health Authorities in the UK are obvious candidates for the adoption of alcohol policies for their employees, and indeed many such authorities now have such policies in force or in preparation. The best of these cover individual employee assistance, alcohol education for all new and existing employees, and guidelines for the serving of alcoholic drinks on authority premises. College and university campuses are other settings where alcohol policies might usefully be adopted; much more thought has been given to this question in the USA than in the UK (e.g. Sherwood 1987).

Alcohol problems in the family setting

There are three other settings which will be dealt with in more detail here: drinking problems present themselves very frequently in all of them, and each offers opportunities for positive intervention, although these are very often missed. The first is the family setting.

Wives

Studies in the UK, USA, and a number of other countries have shown that women married to men with drinking problems sometimes describe a great deal of severe, and often long-standing hardship, which includes concern over the husband's job and financial security, social embarrassment, reduction of social contacts, failure of the husband to keep up personal appearances, rows and quarrels, a poor sex life and infidelity, possessiveness and jealousy directed towards the wife, damage to

Table 10.4   Total resource costs of alcohol misuse in England and Wales (1983 prices)

	£m
The social cost to industry	
a. Sickness absence	641.51
b. Housework services	42.23
c. Unemployment	144.74
d. Premature death	567.70
The social cost to the National Health Service	
a. Psychiatric hospitals, inpatient costs (alcoholic psychosis, alcohol dependence syndrome, non-dependent abuse of alcohol)	17.90
b. Non-psychiatric hospitals, inpatient costs (alcoholic psychosis, alcohol dependence syndrome, alcoholic cirrhosis and liver disease)	7.87
c. Other alcohol-related diseases, inpatient costs	68.58
d. GP visits	1.51
Society's response to alcohol-related problems	
a. Expenditure by National Alcohol Bodies	0.55
b. Research	0.49
The social cost of material damage	
a. Road traffic accidents (damage)	89.20
The social cost of criminal activities	
a. Police involvement in traffic offences (excluding road traffic accidents)	4.54
b. Police involvement in road traffic accidents (includes judiciary and insurance administration)	11.89
c. Drink-related court cases	15.79
Total (including unemployment and premature death)	1614.50
Total (excluding unemployment and premature death)	902.06

Source: McDonnell & Maynard 1985.

household objects or furniture, physical violence in the family, and involvement with the Police (Orford 1985a). There is good evidence also that wives living with men who are drinking excessively report raised levels of psychological and psychosomatic symptoms (Bailey 1967). Much of the uncertainty and marital distress associated with drinking problems is no different in kind from that associated with other causes, and it is easy both for family members themselves and for others who come in contact with them to miss the contribution that excessive drinking may be making.

The connection between excessive drinking and marital violence has been explored in a number of studies. In one (Orford et al 1976), 72% of wives reported sometimes being threatened by their husbands, 45% having been beaten by them, and 27% ever having experienced their husband attempting to injure them seriously. Other studies have asked women seeking refuge because of violence about their husbands' drinking. In one such British study (Gayford 1975), 100 battered wives reported a high rate (57% regularly drunk) of problem drinking amongst their husbands. A similar study in the USA (Eberle 1982) focussed on battering incidents themselves: 16% of battered women reported excessive drinking by their husbands during each of four recent incidents which they were asked to describe, and only 19% of these men were thought not to have been drinking during any of the four incidents described.

Husbands

Although most treatment agencies now report that around one in three of those seeking help for drinking problems are women, and in recent years new women members of Alcoholics Anonymous have been almost as numerous as new male members (Robinson 1979), there has been relatively little study of husbands married to women with drinking problems. However, one Swedish study (Dahlgren 1979) found a higher rate of serious conflict in the family when the wife was the identified problem drinker: husbands of women with drinking problems were less likely to be described as 'understanding', and more likely to be described as 'strongly disapproving' by their partners, than were wives of men with drinking problems. Also, in common with a number of other studies, a high proportion (50% in this study) of husbands of women with drinking problems were thought to have drinking problems themselves.

Children

Until quite recently, the possible stresses experienced by children living in families with alcohol problems were relatively neglected. The stresses, which again are mainly not specific to such families and therefore quite likely not to be attributed to parental drinking, include chronic exposure to a poor family atmosphere, with much parental marital tension and discord, disruption of joint family activities, and a restriction on meeting friends or reciprocating invitations because of embarrassment (Wilson 1982).

Preliminary data from the University of Exeter study of young adults (between the ages of 16 and 35) who had a parent with a drinking problem are shown in Tables 10.5 and 10.6. Table 10.5 shows a much higher rate of recalled family violence for those who came from families with parental drinking problems than for the comparison group. This was the case for violence directed at the child, but the difference was particularly marked for parent-to-parent violence. Table 10.6 shows some of the experiences recalled by subjects in this study: involvement in parental fights and quarrels, the pressure to side with one parent against the other, and the disruption of family arrangements are particularly to be noted.

Mayer & Black (1977) considered the possibility of a specific relationship between parental alcohol problems and child abuse. They were able to cite three previous studies, all American, two of which found high rates of excessive drinking amongst parents of abused children (30% or more), whilst the other found no significant incidence of alcohol problems amongst a group of families in which child abuse had occurred. In Mayer & Black's own study of parents with either alcohol or opiate addiction problems, physical abuse of at least one child in the family had occurred in 13% of the families, but the potential for abuse, as indicated by reported loss of control, had occurred in 31%. To date, there have been very few studies of the prevalence of alcohol problems amongst the clients of social work agencies, and those studies that have been carried out have been on a small scale. One such study in Edinburgh found that 17 out of 40 current social work clients had alcohol-related problems. These were more likely to be in families where children were thought to be 'at risk' and were more likely to be those cases that were long-term (open for at least a year, and thought likely to remain open for some time) (Lothian Regional Social Work Dept 1981). A second study, recently carried out in Exeter, asked 34 social workers covering 6 districts

Table 10.5 Percentage of 16-35 year old children of problem drinking parents, and comparisons, who recall family violence during their upbringing

	Children of problem drinkers N=168 %	Comparisons N=81 %
Parent to parent violence		
Serious and regular violence over a prolonged period	12	1
Any serious and regular violence	12.5	1
Any serious and prolonged violence	21	1
Any regular and prolonged violence	26	4
Any serious violence	29	7
Any regular violence	27	5
Any prolonged violence	48	6
Any violence	66	21
Parent to self violence		
Serious and regular violence over a prolonged period	9	4
Any serious and regular violence	11	5
Any serious and prolonged violence	14	6
Any regular and prolonged violence	18	5
Any serious violence	20	10
Any regular violence	21	6
Any prolonged violence	30	15
Any violence (excluding controlled corporal punishment)	41	19
Any violence (including controlled corporal punishment)	59	77

Source: Data from the study described by Velleman & Orford 1984.

Table 10.6   Negative childhood experiences (NCEs)

	Offspring N=165 %	Comparisons N=79 %
Arrangements going wrong	50.3	25.0
Lack of social life for family	67.9	38.8
Moving house a lot	27.3	18.8
Being on own a lot	47.3	25.0
Forced to participate in parents' rows	44.8	8.8
Being pulled between parents	51.5	20.0
Worry re parent losing job	22.4	3.8
Fear of having to do without	22.4	6.3
Keeping secrets from one parent to protect the other	33.9	10.0
Putting parent to bed	28.5	1.3
Having to take care of parent	27.3	7.5
Having to act older	61.8	21.3

Source: Data from the study described by Velleman & Orford 1990.

about those families amongst their clients where there had been child abuse or risk of abuse. Of 123 such families, 32 (26%) were stated to have drinking problems. Half of these families were without a non-drinking or normal-drinking adult, either because the family had a single parent or because both parents were thought to have drinking problems (Mather 1988).

Although there are some exceptions, most studies have reported a whole range of ill-effects occurring more frequently amongst children of excessively drinking parents than amongst children in general; this is particularly so for younger children. For example, compared to control groups, they have been reported to show a high incidence of school problems, difficulty in concentrating, conduct problems and truancy from school, poor school performance, high rates of emotional problems such as anxiety and depression, developmental disorders, and fewer means of coping with emotional upset. Other reports have suggested that they become intoxicated more often than controls, and that they may be somewhat more prone to drinking and drug problems, both as young people and as adults (Wilson 1982, el-Guebaly & Offord 1977, Orford & Velleman 1990). This inter-generational transmission of drinking problems may have both genetic (Goodwin 1976) and environmental causes.

Thus, the family setting is one in which drinking problems are particularly likely to present themselves, often in the form of non-specific stress reactions shown by other members of the family. Under these circumstances, it is particularly likely that the contribution of excessive drinking will be missed when an agency is making an assessment of a family, or of individual members of it. One recent local agency survey found that only one person with problems attributed to the excessive drinking of *someone else* was reported for every 10 or 12 people identified as having drinking problems themselves (Devon Council on Alcoholism 1984). This probably represents a gross neglect of the role of excessive drinking in families. Social workers, followed by GPs, followed by school nurses and medical officers, were the agents most likely to recognise the stressful impact of drinking problems upon other members of the family, while health visitors and district nurses are others who may be particularly well placed to identify such problems.

Alcohol problems in general practice

In Britain, the NHS general practice service, with which nearly all citizens are registered and which the majority use at least once a year, provides probably the single most important opportunity for the early detection of, and for making effective responses to problems associated with excessive alcohol use. There have been a number of British studies of alcohol problems in general practice (e.g. Anderson 1985; Tether 1985; Wallace & Haines 1985), and much thought is being given to the preparation of self-help and advice materials for general practitioners and their patients — one example is the DRAMS (Drinking Reasonably and Moderately Sensibly) pack produced by the Scottish Health Education Group. One of the best surveys of alcohol problems in general practice was carried out by Wilkins (1974) and reported in his book, *The Hidden Alcoholic in General Practice*.

Wilkins was one GP member of a Manchester group practice, serving approximately 12 000 patients. For a period of one year, he and his partners invited any patient between the ages of 15 and 65 years who was considered to be 'at risk' of having a drinking problem to complete a short questionnaire, administered by the doctor at the end of the consultation. If any relatives of a patient considered 'at risk' attended later in the year, they were also given the questionnaire. To be included in the Alcoholic at Risk Register (AARR), a patient had to show at least one of a whole range of possible signs or factors associated with having a drinking problem: these included those which were apparent from the medical history, evident on presentation, or emerging during the consultation. The questionnaire given to all those 'at risk' was disguised as a general Spare Time Activities Questionnaire (STAQ), and took an average of seven minutes. Amongst questions about eating, smoking, and leisure activities, were a number about the frequency of alcohol use, whether this had increased or decreased, whether it had caused health, family or work problems, and whether the patient or anyone else thought his/her drinking was excessive.

During the year, 544 patients received the questionnaire; of these, 87 were considered, as a result of their answers, to be problem drinkers, which was a considerable increase on the 11 who were already 'known' to the practice to be 'alcoholics'. However, Wilkins considered this to be a considerable underestimate, because not all the patients in the practice consulted during the year and questionnaires were not administered on home visits. Paton et al's (1981) estimate was that a general practitioner with 1800–1900 adults on his/her list would have approximately 40 problem drinkers and 10 more who were addicted to alcohol; they would therefore agree that Wilkins' figures probably represent a considerable underestimate.

Nevertheless, Wilkins' simple expedient of drawing up an 'at-risk' register and asking a few definite questions about drinking and its effects dramatically improved these doctors' awareness of the possibility of excessive drinking as a factor in their patients' problems. Wilkins was able to analyse the AARR to find out which factors were most predictive of discovering a drinking problem, when the STAQ was administered. On the basis of this analysis, he drew up a modified Alcoholic at Risk Register (shown as Table 10.7 here). This provides a good indication of a range of factors which are present in the general practice setting and which should at least alert GPs to the possible presence of a drinking problem.

More recently, Wallace & Haines (1985) mailed a Health Survey Questionnaire (HSQ) to patients registered with two general practices serving a public housing estate in North-West London. They defined excessive drinking as more than 42 units a week for men and more than 21 for women (a unit being the equivalent of half a pint of beer, 1 glass of wine, 1 glass of sherry, 1 single measure of spirits, or 8–10g of absolute alcohol). Of those replying (75% of all patients), 11% of men and 5% of women were drinking excessively by these definitions. Of these, 45% expressed concern over their drinking, either by admitting to a 'possible' or 'definite' problem or by answering affirmatively to at least two of four questions which are often used for screening. In one practice, where a disease register was kept, only 18 patients had been recorded as excessive drinkers prior to the study, and the use of the HSQ added 70 further patients to this number.

Alcohol problems in the general hospital

A number of recent studies of general hospital patients in Britain (Table 10.8) confirm the findings of previous work in the USA and Australia; all demonstrate a consistently high rate of problems judged to be related to alcohol intake. These studies also agree that although admissions related to alcohol are over-represented amongst certain diagnostic groups (in particular those with self-poisoning, gastrointestinal, and neurological disorders), problem drinkers and those for whom alcohol use has contributed to admission, span a wide variety of illness categories. Jarman & Kellett (1979), for example, were surprised that problem drinking was almost as common amongst orthopaedic and medical patients as amongst those attending casualty; drug overdose was the only diagnostic group that did contain an excess of problem drinkers.

Table 10.7   Modified alcoholic at–risk register

1. **Physical diseases**
   - (i)   Cirrhosis of the liver
   - (ii)   Peptic ulcer
   - (iii)   Gastritis
   - (iv)   Epilepsy for first time at 25 years or over, from no apparent cause
   - (v)   Obesity (men)

2. **Mental diseases**
   - (i)   Anxiety
   - (ii)   Depression
   - (iii)   Attempted suicide

3. **Alcoholic Symptoms**
   - (i)   The shakes
   - (ii)   Blackouts
   - (iii)   Delirium tremens
   - (iv)   Alcoholic epilepsy

4. **Occupations**
   - (i)   Catering trade
   - (ii)   Publicans and others working in a pub, or the drink industry
   - (iii)   Seamen

5. **Work problems**
   - (i)   Three or more jobs in year preceding consultation
   - (ii)   Three or more spells of absence off work in year preceding consultation for three days or less
   - (iii)   Patient requesting certificate for absence from work for conditions which are possibly not genuine

6. **Accidents**
   - (i)   At work
   - (ii)   At home
   - (iii)   Road traffic

7. **Criminal offences**
   - (i)   Drunk and disorderly/incapable, and/or drunken driving, and/or offence committed while under influence of drink
   - (ii)   Any other

8. **Family problems**
   - (i)   Children suffering from neglect
   - (ii)   Family disharmony
   - (iii)   Children with mental or psychosomatic disease

9. **Help asked for treatment of alcoholism by**
   - (i)   Patient
   - (ii)   Father of suspected alcoholic
   - (iii)   Mother of suspected alcoholic
   - (iv)   Wife of suspected alcoholic
   - (v)   Husband of suspected alcoholic
   - (vi)   Brother of suspected alcoholic
   - (vii)   Sister of suspected alcoholic
   - (viii) Son of suspected alcoholic
   - (ix)   Daughter of suspected alcoholic
   - (x)   Other relative of suspected alcoholic
   - (xi)   Member of ancillary staff or social agency

10. **Patient smelling of drink at consultation**

11. **Marital status**
   - (i)   Single, male, 40 years or over

Table 10.7 (*cont'd*)

(ii)	Married more than once
(iii)	Divorced
(iv)	Separated

12. **Living in a hostel for destitutes**

13. **Known alcoholic (confirmed by psychiatrist)**

14. **Family history of abnormal drinking**

Source: Wilkins 1974.

Jariwalla et al (1979) found an interesting difference between men and women with alcohol-related admissions. Most of the men presented with physical illnesses related wholly or in part to alcohol abuse, which included acute and chronic gastritis, haematemesis or melaena (without peptic ulcer being found), acute pancreatitis, hepatocellular disorders, major convulsions, confusional states, delirium tremens, psychosis, cardiomyopathy, and inhalation pneumonia. Most of these men were regular heavy drinkers, but a large minority, who did not drink large quantities regularly, presented with physical illnesses after spree drinking (mostly with gastrointestinal or respiratory problems), and four teenage males presented in alcoholic stupor after drinking large quantities of spirits. Women, on the other hand, were most likely to be admitted because of self-poisoning, the majority having taken an overdose of drugs with or after consuming large quantities of alcohol. Most men with self-poisoning, but only a minority of women in this group, were regular heavy drinkers.

Holt et al (1980), in their study of attenders at hospital Accident and Emergency (A & E) departments, also found that a very high proportion of patients who had tried to poison themselves had high blood alcohol levels (BAL) on admission. Other groups who were particularly likely to have high BALs were those involved in assaults, those with head injuries, and those with major trauma. One striking finding was the frequency of high BALs in patients who were not fully conscious on admission. Holt et al found a high rate of false-negative clinical judgements about intoxication in those with positive alcohol breath tests, even though the examining doctors were motivated to detect intoxication during the period of the study. They argue that A & E attenders are a suitable population for screening for alcohol problems, and that alcohol treatment facilities should be better integrated with A & E services.

Barrison et al (1980) examined the case notes of over 300 patients admitted to Charing Cross Hospital, London, during a 10-day period, in order to answer their question: do medical housemen take an adequate drinking history? They found that such a history, including a quantitative assessment of consumption, was recorded in only 37% of cases (of whom over half were teetotalers), in 25% there was only a vague descriptive comment (light, heavy, a lot, little, etc.), and in 39% there was no mention of alcohol in the history at all. Barrrison et al consider this to be

Table 10.8   Recent studies of alcohol problems amongst general hospital patients in Britain

	Location	Sample	Rates of alcohol problems
Quinn and Johnston (1976)	Glasgow	Acute male admissions to a general medical unit	19.0% had admissions related to alcohol and 25.6% were thought to have a drinking problem
Jarman and Kellett (1979)	London	Recent admissions to medical and ortho-paedic wards plus attenders at casualty	19.5% found to be problem drinkers (29.2% men, 8.5% women), compared to 3.1% so defined in a London population study
Jariwalla et al (1979)	Manchester	Admissions to a general medical unit	15.4% had physical illnesses related to alcohol (24% men), and 27% of all admissions directly or indirectly related to alcohol (incl overdoses) (28% men, 25% women)
Holt et al (1980)	Edinburgh	Evening and night attenders at accident and emergency	32% had blood alcohol levels in excess of 80 mgs/100 mls (41% men, 18% women), and in 24% attendance was judged directly related to alcohol (30% men, 14% women)
Lloyd et al (1982)	Edinburgh	Recent admissions to medical wards	22.7% men and 3.2% women identified as problem drinkers
Chick et al (1985)	Edinburgh	Recent male admissions to medical wards	21.3% identified as problem drinkers
Lockhart et al (1986)	London	Emergency admissions to a general medical unit	27% of admissions (same for both sexes) and 17% of bed occupancy judged attributable to alcohol consumption
Taylor et al (1986)	London	Acute admissions to all medical, surgical, intensive therapy and casualty wards in one hospital	12% (15% men, 8% women) of admissions judged to be alcohol related

a serious defect, and contrast it with the fact that a detailed smoking history was recorded in 72% of cases.

Chick et al (1985) reported a study in which they allocated male medical patients, who were found to have drinking problems, to *either* up to one hour's counselling from one specific nurse, experienced in the treatment of alcohol problems, who carried out the screening interview, *or* to a control group who received no advice and no feedback from the results of the screening. An independent follow-up at 12 months revealed that significantly more members of the counselled group were considered definitely improved (score on a scale of alcohol-related problems decreased by at least 50%, or if no problems were reported, then consumption had fallen by 50% or more, in either case improvement was supported by blood tests or a relative's report), as well as showing a greater improvement in problem score and a higher frequency of 50% or greater reductions in consumption. Chick et al concluded that screening for alcohol problems should be incorporated routinely into nursing and medical assessments, and that because patients may be particularly receptive to counselling while being treated for a medical illness, more effort should be directed at treating patients so identified in general hospitals.

McIntosh (1982) reviewed the evidence for alcohol problems in general hospital patients internationally; although reported rates were found to be fairly consistently high, he was critical of the research on a number of counts. These included a failure to distinguish between the alcohol dependence syndrome and alcohol-related disabilities (in this writer's view, not as simple a matter as he implies), and a failure to demonstrate that rates in general hospital patients are higher than those in the population at large. Nevertheless, he agreed that because general hospital patients are a captive group, for whom services can be conveniently provided:

Admission is an opportune occasion to provide treatment for the alcohol addiction of a person who may have been admitted for other causes; for the person admitted because of an alcohol-related disorder, it may be the first occasion for him/her to come to grips with the fact that alcohol, at least for this episode, has been a problem — at this point, immediate counselling and other services may make the difference between acceptance or rejection of help. From some of the high estimates of prevalence recorded in these studies, it would seem that it is not particularly difficult to get hospital patients to admit to alcohol problems if an interested and nonjudgmental approach is used.

TRENDS AND RESEARCH IN SERVICE PROVISION

Along with this expanded awareness of the variety and range of alcohol problems and the various points within a local network of services and agencies at which such problems present, have come a number of trends in service provision. All of these are consistent with the general principles of community mental health work, and some have already been the objects of evaluative research. Four of them — detoxification, client treatment, family services, and residential accommodation — may be picked out for more detailed consideration.

Alcohol detoxification services

For many people with drinking problems, especially those whose drinking is heaviest, most continuous, and most dependent, the first step in treatment has to be the complete cessation of all drinking. Mild-to-moderate withdrawal symptoms, including tremor, profuse sweating, restlessness, agitation, and fearfulness, are quite likely and may persist for a few days; there is also a small but uncertain risk of more serious symptoms including delirium, hallucinations, and epileptic-like seizures. Because of this risk, and because many people find it difficult to stop drinking suddenly on their own, hospital admission for a period varying between a few days and a few weeks has often been the treatment of choice (Arroyave et al 1980).

Over the years, concern has been expressed about the lack of suitable detoxification facilities for those problem drinkers who are chronic drunkenness offenders and/or without stable family support. The 'revolving door' of repeated sentencing and incarceration or repeated hospital admission and discharge, was pointed out long ago (e.g. by Pittman & Gordon 1958), and continues to constitute a problem (Out of Court 1982). Following both American example and Eastern European experiments with 'sobering-up stations', the Department of Health in Britain financed two experimental detoxification centres, one in Leeds and one in Manchester. The former aimed exclusively at the decriminalisation of public drunkenness, and police were the sole referral agents (Otto et al 1982, Rose et al 1979), whilst the latter rapidly widened its brief to take other referrals in addition to those from the police (Kessel et al 1984). The Leeds centre is an example of a 'social setting' detoxification centre, managed by a voluntary organisation, sited away from a hospital, and staffed largely by social workers and nurses. Manchester, on the other hand, is an example of a 'medical setting' centre, situated within a hospital, and staffed largely by doctors and nurses.

A comparative study of four British detoxification regimes, including the Leeds and Manchester centres (Otto et al 1982), a comparative study of a range of detoxification centres in Ontario, Canada (Smart 1977), and a review of these and other studies (Orford & Wawman 1986) all demonstrate how varied these forms of residential provision are. Some aim at decriminalisation of public drunkenness and take many police referrals, whilst others take a few or none; some centres are medical, and others in a social setting. In addition, some prescribe medication for the majority or all of their patients or clients, whilst others have a policy of prescribing sparingly or not at all, stressing instead factors such as appropriate lighting and noise levels, and the availability of staff support. These differences are largely a matter of philosophy and policy, but there is also the possibility that patients referred by general practitioners may be at greater risk of serious withdrawal symptoms than are those who are homeless or offenders (Otto et al 1982).

Evaluative studies of detoxification centres are inconclusive. The Canadian group reached rather negative conclusions, finding that centres frequently drifted away from providing a service for police referrals, and did not defeat the revolving door problem. On the other hand, in Scotland, Hamilton (1979), in one of the few well controlled studies, found that an experimental detoxification scheme for homeless problem drinkers (which, incidentally, had to be switched from a general hospital to a psychiatric hospital because of negative staff attitudes towards problem drinkers in the former), was associated with subsequent improved accommodation and social life, although not with significantly reduced drinking.

A relatively recent development has been towards outpatient or home-based alcohol detoxification. A number of reports from the USA have described outpatient detoxification (Feldman et al 1975, Stinnett 1982, Tennant 1979, Whitfield et al 1978), in which typically, patients attend an outpatient centre daily and receive medication for a period of at least a few days. Home-based detoxification is also developing as the preferred alternative to outpatient detoxification in Britain, and has been the object of Department of Health funded research. The Exeter experience has been that this can be satisfactorily carried out in people's own homes, provided the patient's GP is fully aware of the procedure and able to prescribe medication if necessary, and a member of the community alcohol team and/or the GP is able to visit daily for a few days and less frequently for a while thereafter. The potential advantages include the patient remaining in his/her own home, often the full involvement of a close relative or other carer at an early stage in the treatment process, and the involvement of the patient's own GP. An evaluation, based upon detailed monitoring plus 10-day and 60-day follow-up of 41 consecutive referrals to the Exeter Home Detoxification Service (Stockwell et al 1989, 1990), reported that of this number, only 8 failed to complete detoxification at home (of whom 4 were admitted to hospital). The number of non-completers was identical in the comparison sample of people detoxified in psychiatric hospitals in the area in the 12 months prior to the start of the home detoxification project. Only one person in each group (home and hospital) experienced a withdrawal fit. All but three of those who completed home detoxification then engaged in further treatment, and reports from those undergoing detoxification, their close relatives, and their GPs were mostly very positive. Regular home visits by community psychiatric nurses who supervised detoxification — CPNs made an average of 6.9 visits (range 1–12) over an average period of 6.2 days (range 1–13) — were particularly appreciated. So too were the regular breathalyser checks that were carried out. Stockwell et al (1989) conclude that: 'the great majority of problem drinkers can safely stop drinking with social support and no medication, the majority of those who require medication can receive this safely in their own home — only a very small minority require inpatient care if adequately supervised HD (home detoxification) is available'.

Treatment services

There have been equally great changes in the ways in which treatment is delivered, once detoxification, if that is necessary, has taken place. This change can be traced to a number of sources, of which the first is the growing awareness of the scale of the problem and the diversity of types of clients represented. This has meant that small treatment units in psychiatric hospitals (the alcoholism treatment units, or ATUs, favoured by the Department of Health in the late 1950s and 1960s), which may continue to be centres of excellence for the intensive treatment of relatively small numbers of the more severely dependent drinkers, and for research and for training of professional staff, are inappropriate for responding to the whole range of the community's alcohol problems.

Secondly, research has failed to demonstrate clearly that better outcomes are produced either by intensive treatment as opposed to briefer treatment, or by professional treatment as opposed to counselling by non-professionally trained volunteers, or by any one specific type of treatment above all others (Edwards & Grant 1980, Emrick 1975, Orford 1980). This is not to say that treatment does not work, but rather that the experts were wrong in their assumption about *how* treatment works. For example, in the Addiction Research Unit Study of treatment versus advice (Orford & Edwards 1977), it was found that referral to a psychiatric outpatient department for (1) a thorough assessment of drinker and partner, carried out by a team of psychiatrist, social worker, and psychologist; (2) clear, sympathetic, and direct advice to the drinker in the presence of his partner; and (3) brief, monthly, follow-ups of the partner alone for 12 months — produced the same rate of improvement as did a more conventional treatment package. More recent studies have shown a modest improvement in outcome after more intensive treatment, in comparison with minimal treatment, however (Chick et al 1988, Robertson et al 1986).

The effective ingredients of treatment seem to be: active engagement in a process of change (Armor et al 1978, Prochaska & DiClemente 1986); the availability of a range of treatments from which those best suited to the client's needs can be chosen (Costello 1980); vigorous follow-up — particularly for those who drop out of treatment early on (Costello 1980; Potamianos & Papadatos, 1987); the involvement of a family member or other carer or 'buddy' wherever possible (Ewing et al 1961, Smith 1969); and positive therapeutic attitudes towards the treatment of problem drinkers on the part of those who detect, refer, and treat (Cartwright 1980). Many people with drinking problems, particularly those whose level of dependence is mild or moderate rather than severe, overcome their problems with minimal treatment, which might take the form of brief advice or the use of a self-help manual (Heather 1986), or without any expert help at all (e.g. Saunders & Kershaw 1979).

Attitudes towards drinking problems

The need for positive attitudes by staff, towards working with people who have drinking problems is stressed by nearly all those who have written about alcohol detoxification services (Orford & Wawman 1986); at present, such attitudes are often negative. Some years ago, Chafetz et al (1970) demonstrated that US hospital doctors frequently failed to notice excessive drinking amongst their patients, and that this was more likely to be the case when patients were employed, married, and socially stable. In Britain, Cartwright (1980) has developed the Alcohol Problems Perception Questionnaire (AAPPQ) to assess the degree to which medical, social, and other potential treatment agents possess positive or negative therapeutic attitudes towards working with problem drinkers. Its findings have been that many professionals are low on therapeutic commitment to working with this client group, and lack confidence ('role security') in their ability to deal with the problems involved (Shaw et al 1978). The evidence so far is that academic teaching about the subject makes relatively little difference, but that experience of working with a number of people with drinking problems, coupled with the existence of support in this work from colleagues or a case discussion group, produce changes in the direction of more positive attitudes (Cartwright 1980). Thus, attention has shifted away from technical and procedural aspects of treatments, and away from a concern with particular therapeutic theories or schools, and towards therapist variables such as therapeutic commitment and role security.

Investigations by the Community Alcohol Team in Salford — a city in the north-west of England — have revealed information about the attitudes and involvement of different community agents which, if it is representative, will be of great value in planning how to deliver a training and supportive service to these agencies. Samples of social workers, probation officers, community psychiatric nurses (CPNs), health visitors, district nurses, and GPs, were administered the AAPPQ, and sub-samples were interviewed (Clement 1984, 1987). Probation officers and CPNs were most likely to have received some alcohol education, and were more likely than others to have had personal experience in dealing with more than a few people with drinking problems. Probation officers referred problem drinking clients to the widest range of specialist services, and had the most positive attitudes towards working with them. In general, however, attitudes were very negative; even amongst probation officers, only 29% agreed with the statement: 'In general it is rewarding to work with drinkers'. The word most frequently used to describe problem drinking clients was 'frustrating'. Unlike most proba-tion officers, who saw working with problem drinkers as part of their job, the majority of CPNs thought that their role was to identify and refer only.

Social workers displayed ambivalence about working with problem drinkers; most felt that management in their organisations afforded it a low priority. Less than half felt they had the right to ask their clients for information relevant to a drinking problem, and less than half felt it was part of their job. Most of the rest believed in shared responsibility, referring the drinking problem client on to a specialist and retaining responsibility for the family.

Health visitors and district nurses, on the whole, felt lacking in the ability to deal with problem drinkers, and lacked experience; like social workers, less than half felt they had the right to ask relevant questions. Attitudes towards clients who had drinking problems were negative, and satisfaction with the way the agent worked with drinkers was low amongst these two groups, particularly amongst health visitors. When asked whether the agent could easily find someone who would be able to help formulate the best approach to a problem drinker, percentages of those answering in the affirmative varied from a high of 88% amongst CPNs, to lower figures of 56% for health visitors, 54% for district nurses, and 37% for social workers, with GPs and probation officers lying between.

GPs were in a special position; they felt it was legitimate to enquire of their patients about drinking and drinking problems, and nearly all felt they had a working knowledge about alcohol and alcohol-related problems. Most, however, felt they did not know how to counsel problem drinkers, and GPs had the most negative attitudes of all — only 9% thought it was rewarding to work with drinkers, and as many as 74% disagreed with the statement. Recent work by Anderson (1985) has confirmed this general picture of the attitudes and feelings of general practitioners. Amongst GPs in Oxfordshire and West Berkshire, he found a relatively high level of what Cartwright terms 'role legitimacy' (e.g. having a right to ask patients questions about drinking when necessary), but a relatively low level of 'therapeutic commitment' which includes motivation to work with problem drinkers, feel satisfaction in working with them, and self-esteem about one's own ability to work with this group. However, growing awareness of the importance of the GPs's role in the prevention and treatment of alcohol problems has been demonstrated by the publication of a report on the subject by the Royal College of General Practitioners (RCGP 1986).

Non-professional and volunteer counsellors

Consistent with this trend has been an acceptance of the idea that non-professionally trained workers, often working in a voluntary capacity, and sometimes having recovered from drinking problems themselves, can be successfully recruited and trained for the task of counselling (Orford 1980). This move is consistent with the tradition of ex-problem drinkers and ex-addicts contributing in a large way to self-help and treatment services. Alcoholics Anonymous was a forerunner of many modern self-help groups in this and related fields, and has been uniquely successful as an organisation, continuing to expand its membership and to spread to many countries around the world, 50 years after its beginnings (Robinson 1979, 1986). This movement towards the recruitment of non-professionals in the treatment of alcohol problems is also consistent with the emphasis placed on the volunteer and non-professional contribution in community mental health generally, and with existing evidence that non-professionals are often as effective as professionals, and in some cases — particularly with specific client groups — more effective (Durlak 1979).

Alternative drinking goals

Another source of changing ideas about treatment has been a progressive undermining, by a steady accumulation of research findings, of the formerly held idea that 'alcoholism' was incurable, in the sense that no 'alcoholic' could expect to be able to return to drinking that was 'normal', 'controlled', or 'social'. Davies (1962), who followed-up patients treated at the Maudsley Hospital, London, was one of the first to report that a proportion of patients, even though they had been advised to abstain totally, appeared to be able to return to 'normal drinking'. Numerous such reports continue to appear: for example, two independent follow-up studies of people treated at ACCEPT (Alcoholism Community Centres for Education, Prevention and Treatment), London, have shown that the majority of clients who improve over a period of 12 months nevertheless continue to drink (Potamianos & Papadatos 1987, Sierakowski 1984). Amongst the first to treat excessive drinkers with an explicit goal of controlled drinking were Sobell & Sobell (1973). These and later studies, as well as those such as Davies', have been comprehensively reviewed by Heather & Robertson (1983), although Edwards (1985) has carried out an independent, long term follow-up of

Davies' patients, casting some doubt on the reliability of the initial findings and on the long-term stability of his patients' controlled drinking, and although the Sobells' findings have been disputed in the USA (Pendery et al 1982, Sobell & Sobell 1984), there is now little doubt that a comprehensive service in a locality should offer a range of approaches within which either goal (abstinence or limited drinking) can be pursued with hope and commitment on the part of both client and helper.

In the search for client variables which might provide an indication of which treatment goal was the most appropriate in a particular case, there appear to be two leading contenders (Orford & Keddie 1986). The first is level of dependence, for which the SADQ (Severity of Alcohol Dependence Questionnaire: Stockwell et al 1983) has become a popular measure. The second is the client's own orientation towards, and belief in, the possibility of attaining one goal rather than the other. At present, both hypotheses find support (Heather & Robertson 1983), which leaves counsellors in some dilemma when the two factors are in opposition.

Involving families

The argument for involving close family members in alcohol treatment services is a strong one; it rests on the evidence, briefly reviewed above, that considerable stress is experienced by partners and children, and that involvement of partners is associated with better clinical outcome. A number of family treatment models are available, and these are summarised in Table 10.9. Concurrent group treatment for partners was the subject of evaluative studies in the 1950s and 1960s, but since then they have been less popular than conjoint groups and family therapy. Until recently, studies of family therapy had been limited, involving very small numbers or giving few details of procedures and outcome), and conjoint group treatment had been the subject of better evaluation (particularly by Corder et al 1972, and by Cadogan 1973). Some good studies of family therapy are now available, however (Bennun 1986, Zweben et al 1988). The group of treatment programmes which Harwin (1982) termed 'ecological' were aimed at a slightly different target group, including 'multi-problem families', single-parent families with young children, and in the case of the best evaluated of these projects (Hunt & Azrin 1973), some single men for whom one aim was to build up 'synthetic families'. These ecological studies have focussed rather less on family interaction (stressed by those who have used conjoint and family therapy approaches) and much more upon problems of child-care, household management, job seeking, and the law.

A comprehensive service should also make available counselling and advice for those many partners who continue to live with an unresolved drinking problem in the family, and when the excessively drinking family member is unavailable for treatment (Orford 1985a, Kaufman & Pattison 1981, Yates 1988). There has been a disappointing lack of research in this area, although studies have been undertaken of how partners cope naturally (e.g. Orford et al 1975, Schaffer & Tyler 1979), and there is no lack of books and pamphlets advising family members how best to react (e.g. Meyer 1982, Seixas 1980). Al-Anon, a self-help organisation closely associated with Alcoholics Anonymous for family members of people with drinking problems, exists like AA in most areas of Britain and the US, and is a local resource, again like AA, upon which local services should draw. Amongst other things, Al-Anon recommends that family members should distance themselves emotionally, stop carrying the burden of thinking that they are part of the cause of the problem, and should stop making futile attempts to control the drinker and his/her drinking. In one of the very few studies of Al-Anon, Gorman & Rooney (1979) found that the longer a wife had been a member, the less likely she was to use 'negative coping strategies', which included coaxing, nagging, pleading, covering up, and such drink-focussed responses as pouring drink away. On the other hand, a study of coping behaviour of wives of men attending a psychiatric hospital outpatient department (Orford et al 1975) found that the latter, drink-focussed, strategies were associated with a relatively *good* prognosis for the husband's drinking.

The balance of opinion, and what little research has been carried out on the subject, suggests that partners may usefully be helped to *reduce* the level of their criticism of the drinker, any encouragement of his/her drinking which they may have been doing, the level of their enmeshment in attempts to modify the drinker to the exclusion of pursuing their own lives, and also their own level of guilt, whilst at the same time to *increase* their engagement with the drinker in a constructively confronting manner. This includes doing such things as: 'pointing out calmly that

Table 10.9   Models of treatment for families with drinking problems

	Examples
Concurrent groups	Ewing et al 1961 Smith 1969
Conjoint groups	Corder et al 1972 Cadogan 1973
Family therapy	Hedberg & Campbell 1974 Zweben et al 1988 Bennun 1986
Ecological family treatment	Hunt & Azrin 1973 Davis & Hagood 1979
Individual advice or treatment for relatives	Cohen & Krause 1971 Yates 1988
Family therapy and advice for relatives combined	McCrady 1986

his/her behaviour is causing inconvenience or upset', 'making it clear that things cannot go on as they have been', 'making your position about his/her drinking quite clear', 'sitting down together and talking frankly about what can be done', 'taking opportunities to state correct facts about drinking', and 'suggesting that he/she seek outside help' or 'seeking outside help yourself'.

Husbands have proved more difficult to engage in treatment, and special attempts may have to be taken to do so. Similarly, relatively little attempt has yet been made to engage the children of problem-drinking parents, despite the evidence of the stress which they experience, and the likelihood that they constitute a high-risk group for both present and future problems.

Halfway houses

Specialised halfway houses for problem drinkers have become a major form of community provision both in Britain and North America. Most have been established since the mid-1960s, and in Britain, most were set up once the Department of Health made special funds available for this purpose in 1973. By the mid-1970s, the National Institute of Mental Health in the US was able to report the existence of 597 houses, covering every State but one (NIMH, 1975), while Ogborne et al (1978) estimated that there were around 50 such houses in Ontario and more than 150 in the whole of Canada. By the early 1960s, over 60 such houses existed in Britain, offering a total of approximately 800 beds. In their survey of houses in London, Otto & Orford (1978) noted that a number had their origins in a religious mission or society, whilst others derived from modern, secular concerns with treatment or rehabilitation. Many of the latter were set up as a result of the special interest of a professional person working in the psychiatric treatment services, although this was usually in conjunction with a voluntary organisation. Some alcohol halfway house staff have a relevant professional background training, such as probation, social work, clinical psychology, or nursing, but most do not, and many, particularly in North America, have recovered from drinking problems themselves.

Halfway houses differ in size (from as few as 4 places to as many as 30 or 40, although around 12 is a common number), in ratios of care staff to residents (from 1:3 to 1:15/20), in the degree to which they encourage resident autonomy and involvement in decision-making, and in the incorporation of a formal structured programme of treatment activities (Martin & Segal 1977, Ogborne et al 1980).

However, Otto & Orford's (1978) survey, and more detailed study of two houses, revealed a number of difficulties in the operation of alcohol halfway houses. First and foremost was a lack of clarity about organisational goals and means; there was frequent uncertainty and difference of opinion about whether houses should be transitional or non-transitional, treatment-orientated or homely in atmosphere, democratic or paternal. Secondly, leaving a house was very often premature, without planning or staff approval, and associated with drinking. This was confirmed in Ontario by Ogborne et al (1978), who found that half of all new residents in a variety of houses had left within the first 4 to 7 weeks, and that only 22% did so with staff approval. There is some hope for overcoming these problems in Ogborne & Wiggins' (1981) finding that houses with a formal structured programme of therapeutic events, occupying 20 or more hours a week, produced longer median lengths of stay than did other houses. Another problem associated with running halfway houses of this kind is support for staff, who often find themselves isolated; integration of halfway house staff within a multidisciplinary community alcohol team, with other members of the team providing specialised input to the house in exchange, is one way of ensuring that this does not occur.

A DISTRICT COMMUNITY ALCOHOL SERVICE

Starting a service

Because of the legacy of the moral view of excessive drinking and the continued stigma associated with the term 'alcoholism', and because of the low priority afforded to alcohol problems by many agencies, experience suggests that the development of services within a district is dependent on the formation of a core planning group of individuals who are committed to the setting up of those services. Ideally, this group should include members who have experience of working directly with clients with alcohol problems, have knowledge of recent developments and research in the provision of services for people with drinking problems, and who have sufficient seniority and management responsibility to be of influence with local health and social service planners. However, if the group is lacking the necessary direct experience or knowledge at the outset, then it must be willing to acquire these, or to locate and co-opt individuals who can provide them. The exact constitution of the group will vary from place to place; within localities with teaching hospitals, for example, a psychiatrist or gastroenterologist with a special interest in alcohol problems may be an important member.

In areas with a voluntary Council on Alcohol or Alcohol Advisory Service, the director is certain to be an important member, and may indeed provide the principal momentum as well as accommodation for meeting, and it may well be around the voluntary organisation that the emerging community service develops. In any event, the voluntary sector should be well represented, along with the strongest permutation of representatives of Social Services and the Probation Service, a physician, general practitioners, clinical psychologist, occupational therapist, police officer, health promotion officer, and other relevant personnel. The presence in the locality of a university, polytechnic, or teachers training college, may bring in academics, researchers, and teachers with an interest in some aspect of the treatment or prevention of alcohol problems.

It is from this group that the initiative may come to set up a Community Alcohol Team (CAT) or its equivalent such as an alcohol resource team. This parallels the pattern in other areas of health and social care, such as mental handicap teams, community mental health teams, and teams for the development of services for the elderly in the community, and is rapidly becoming the form of provision favoured in those areas in Britain without already well-developed services for alcohol problems. Fennell & Wardle (1982) have given an account of a CAT in Norwich, with a small sample client follow-up study and suggestions for the further development of the service. There has also been a parallel study of the service provided by ACCEPT in West London, which has features in common with a number of CATs (Sierakowski 1984). Other evaluative investigations of CATs in Exeter, Liverpool, Salford, and Derry in Northern Ireland, have been undertaken and the results of several of these are being reviewed by the Department of Health (Stockwell 1988).

Structure of a community service

Table 10.10 indicates some of the structure and functions of a community alcohol service. Although the evolving community services differ one from another in the details of their organisation and in the emphasis they give to different functions, most of the features listed are typical, and serve to distinguish community services from the hospital-based services which often preceded them. The first structural feature is the existence of a base, or centre, situated within a town, away from a hospital, but sometimes, as in Exeter and West London, making use of obsolete former hospital premises. This community base, as foreseen by the UK Department of Health's report on the Pattern and Range of Services for Problem Drinkers (1978), provides the focus for the team's activities, whether these are mainly directly delivered to clients with drinking problems or mainly consultative, educative, and preventive. Whatever the priority given to different functions of the team, the existence of this focal point is generally considered to be essential for purposes of building team cohesion and morale, and for publicising its work within the district. Against the advantages of such an arrangement should be set the possible disadvantage of the perpetuation of work with alcohol problems as a speciality which a central base may appear to imply. Although comparative evaluative studies to prove the point are lacking, the general consensus at the present time is that a centrally-based team is necessary in order to develop services for this large and neglected client group.

Such a centre need not, however, inhibit organisational growth. Indeed, community alcohol services in Exeter, Derry, Norwich, and West London, have all been characterised by the kind of growth which Katz & Kahn (1978) call intra-organisational replication. Both in metropolitan West London and the regional centre of Norwich, for example, smaller replicas of the central organisation have been set up in neighbouring areas, although some of the difficulties of establishing community alcohol services in small market towns are described by Fennell & Wardle (1982). In Exeter, replica CATs have been set up in neighbouring districts, and a policy pursued of attaching CAT members on a sessional basis to community mental health teams in outlying areas of the district. In Derry, the policy has been to set up Alcohol Advice Centres within general practice health centres (Bradley 1983).

The team that is able to deliver a service actively (as opposed to merely set it up and obtain resources for it) is likely to develop by a process of accretion. The pebble around which it grows may well be the voluntary council or its equivalent (ACCEPT is a non-profit making organisation started by a former problem drinker). In the first instance, this may be purely by attracting sessional work from professionals already employed by statutory organisations and from others willing to give sessions free of charge. These may include social workers and probation officers, clinical psychologists, occupational therapists, psychiatrists and other medical specialists, general practitioners, art therapists, and drama therapists. The team can be much augmented and enriched by recruiting, training, and effectively deploying voluntary counsellors, some of whom may have had drinking problems themselves.

Whatever their patterns of growth, community alcohol services mostly involve a partnership of the voluntary and the statutory, the non-professional and the professional. This reflects both the nature of alcohol

---

Table 10.10   Some aspects of the structure and functions of a community alcohol team

Structure
District or locality-based
Multidisciplinary
Voluntary and professional partnership
Leadership shared?

Functions
Home detoxification
Counselling
Day centre
Halfway House
Professional education and consultation
Public education

problems themselves, and the history of the development of services in which the voluntary sector and non-professional worker have played such a large part. The professionals bring their attitudes and values, theories, and techniques for assessment, treatment, education, and evaluation. The non-statutory organisation, on the other hand, brings its tradition for pioneering and innovation, its ability to respond flexibility, and, in the words of the Wolfenden Report on Voluntary Organisations (1978), its capacity for 'spontaneous, speedy and autonomous action'. This combination, although it carries many opportunities for disharmony (e.g. the case example described by Orford (1988)), is generally a winning one.

In hybrid organisations of this kind, often with multiple affiliations and origins, the question of leadership is of particular interest (Katz & Kahn 1978, Yetton 1984). Almost all community alcohol services are delivered by multidisciplinary teams, reflecting the contribution that can be made by a variety of professional disciplines, and by others with a variety of skills and experiences. Sometimes, leadership is vested in the director of the voluntary council or advisory centre, or non-profit making organisation; this person may have had training in a mental health-related discipline or alternatively may have entered the field as a result of recovery from his/her own personal problem. In other cases, the team may be led by one particular professional worker such as a consultant psychiatrist, while in yet others decision-making is vested in the team as a whole, and leadership functions shared as widely as possible.

Functions of a community service

Professional education and consultation

The priority given to different functions of a community alcohol service will vary from place to place, but most services will probably give high priority both to professional education, consultation and liaison, on the one hand, and to direct client treatment services on the other. The confidence and skills required to deliver a professional education and consultation service, however, may well be relatively lacking in an emergent community alcohol team, whose members may feel more comfortable supplying direct client services. Furthermore, without a coherent policy for the provision of educational services, the team may be at the mercy of a random assortment of requests to provide speakers and participants on teaching occasions, many of which may be peripheral to the main course curricula or everyday work of the professions concerned. Links with the Health Promotion Department of the District Health Authority, and with the Health Education Authority, nationally, the seeking out of new education skills, and the formulation of a coherent policy with clear priorities and principal target groups for education, will be useful.

In any event, the expanded awareness of alcohol problems in a community, which was the theme of earlier sections of this chapter, leaves little doubt that education of those professionals and staff of other agencies who may come into contact with drinking problems, as well as of the general public, should be high on the list of priorities. Indeed, the Pattern and Range of Services' Report (DHSS 1978) recommended that the training and support of 'primary level' (non-specialist) agencies should be the first priority of the alcohol service.

Although health professionals in general practice and in general hospitals, social workers, probation officers, magistrates, and others who regularly come into contact with people with drinking problems and/or with members of their families, should be the principal targets of such training and support initiatives, both at basic training and post-basic training levels, there are many other locations in any district where some alcohol education and consultation would be useful. A research team at the Institute for Health Studies at Hull University (Tether & Robinson 1986) has compiled an exhaustive inventory of local sites for alcohol preventive education. In addition to the more obvious ones, they include: Local Authority Housing Departments; supermarkets, which have the option of segregating or desegregating alcohol and other sales; the licencing justices and local authority officers and members responsible for planning, few of whom may be aware of their capacity to influence the availability of alcohol and hence alcohol-related problems within a locality; driving schools and examiners, who could place relatively greater or lesser emphasis upon drinking and driving; insurance brokers, who have the option to vary premiums depending upon drinking habits as much as upon smoking habits; and local press and radio, whose capacity for influencing local opinion may now be very considerable.

In comparison with research on the outcome of treatment of clients, there has been relatively little study of the impact of education and consultation services delivered by community alcohol services. Indeed, the Norwich Report (Fennell & Wardle 1982) suggested that although this was a priority for the team, there was little evidence that education and consultation were noticeably affecting the attitudes of agents such as social workers, and that more effort might be devoted to direct client work. This may only indicate that this type of work, being non-traditional, requires a clearly formulated policy and concerted effort. Despite a background of theory and ideas for practice in the area of mental health consultation (Caplan 1970, Gallessich 1982, Ketterer 1981), it is notoriously difficult to break the pattern of client referral from the 'primary level' (non-specialist) to 'secondary level' (specialist) and to work instead in an educative and consultative fashion (Spector 1984).

A more hopeful outlook is provided by Clement's (1987) evaluation of the impact of the Salford CAT's work on primary care workers. Using an updated version of Cartwright's (1980) AAPPQ, she was able to demonstrate increased therapeutic commitment for working with clients with alcohol problems amongst those workers who had had access to the clinical/support services of the CAT and who had also received education and training. In addition, one of her main conclusions was that continued good practice by primary care workers in this area was dependent upon management support for this kind of work. As Clement put it: 'the problem, then, is not the 'therapeutically uncommitted agent' but rather the 'therapeutically uncommitted agency'. In the absence of support from management in working with drinkers in those cases where alcohol problems are being identified, the consultative role of a CAT will become minimised'.

This conclusion is in keeping with that of Lightfoot & Orford (1986), who added a Situational Constraint scale to the AAPPQ, and found social workers to be much more constrained by the practices and attitude of their work settings than were CPNs, when confronted with the possibility of working with alcohol-related problems.

Client services

Specialist treatment services are likely to remain a priority for some time to come — indeed it is difficult to see that they could ever disappear altogether. Indeed, the major conclusion of Stockwell's (1988) review of CATs in Britain was that their most clearly demonstrated achievement had been the provision of direct client services which were far more accessible than pre-existing services. The backbone of the client treatment service is likely to be counselling, with relatively greater emphasis placed upon individual and family counselling in some localities, and greater weight given to group work elsewhere. Day centre and halfway house provision are relatively costly in terms of staff resources, but they are also important ingredients of a comprehensive service, particularly if the service is to extend to those people with drinking problems who are without families and/or jobs and are candidates for rehabilitation. Some services, such as ACCEPT, place relatively great emphasis on the importance of regular attendance at a day centre, at least for a period of a few weeks (Sierakowski 1984) whilst others such as the CAT in Leicester consider day centre provision to be relatively unimportant in comparison with the development of home-based client services, including 'home detoxification'.

It is probably wrong, in any case, to view treatment and education as separate entities, since they are clearly interwoven (Grant & Ritson 1983). For one thing, principal targets for education are the many groups in a community (listed in Table 10.3), including family and friends, who may be in a position to exert direct therapeutic influence upon those with drinking problems. Secondly, theories of therapeutic change in the field of addictive behaviours are now more frequently being couched in terms such as 'attitude change' and 'decision-making', which make the distinction between education and treatment more difficult to uphold (Janis & Mann 1977, Orford 1985b, Prochaska & DiClemente 1986).

Table 10.11 Dimensions of Community mental health versus Clinically oriented services

	Community mental health	Traditional clinical services
1. Location of intervention	Practice in the community	Practice in institutional mental health settings
2. Level of intervention	Emphasis on a total or defined community (e.g. a catchment area, or population at risk)	Emphasis on individual clients
3. Type of service	Emphasis on preventive services	Emphasis on therapeutic services
4. How service is delivered	Emphasis on indirect services through consultation and education	Emphasis on direct clinical services to clients
5. Strategies of service	Strategies aimed at reaching large numbers of people, including brief psychotherapy and crisis intervention	Emphasis on extended psychotherapy
6. Kind of planning	Rational planning aimed at specification of unmet needs, high-risk populations, and coordinated services	Unplanned, individual services with no overall community coordination, a 'free enterprise' system
7. Source of manpower	Mental health professionals together with new, including non-professional sources of manpower, such as college students and persons indigenous to the target group	Traditional mental health professionals (psychiatrists, psychologists, social workers)
8. Locus of decision-making	Shared responsibility for control and decision-making with regard to mental health programmes between community and professionals	Professional control of all mental health services
9. Aetiological assumptions	Environmental causes of mental disorder	Intrapsychic causes of mental disorder

Source: Rappaport 1977.

Minimal therapeutic interventions often take an explicitly educational approach, and educational materials, such as those contained in the Drinking Choices pack developed by the Health Education Authority, can be used with a range of populations, including clients with drinking problems themselves.

CONCLUSION

How does the approach advocated in this chapter measure up against the principles of community psychiatry and community psychology? Table 10.11 lists nine principles of community psychology, as enunciated by Bloom (1973) and reiterated by Rappaport (1977). The new approach to the development of services to meet alcohol problems, embodied in the concept of the community alcohol team, shares a number of elements with this catalogue of criteria for the practice of community psychology. There is agreement that practice should be in the community rather than in an institution, that services should be aimed at the community's problems or at a catchment area rather than at a stream of individual clients who use the services on a free enterprise basis, and that manpower should include non-professionals as well as professionals. Other criteria are more a matter of emphasis: that environmental determinants of alcohol problems should be better recognised than formerly, that there should be as much emphasis on consultation and education as upon providing a direct client service, and that prevention and low intensity treatments should figure as largely in the services as intensive treatments. Whether there will be a move away from exclusive professional control of services towards the ideal of shared decision-making with lay representatives of the community, is a question for the future.

Acknowledgements

Acknowledgements are due to Dr Ron Wawman and Dr John Shanks, Principal Medical Officers, Department of Health and Social Security, London, who kindly provided the data upon which the information in Table 10.1 is based; and to Mrs Liz Mears who so ably typed the manuscript.

REFERENCES

Anderson P 1985 Managing alcohol problems in general practice. British Medical Journal 290: 1873-1875
Armor D, Polich J, Stambul H 1978 Alcoholism and treatment. Wiley, New York (originally 1976 Santa Monica, Rand Corporation)
Arroyave F, McKeon S, Cooper S E 1980 Detoxification — an approach to developing a comprehensive alcoholism service. British Journal of Addiction 75: 187-195

Bailey M B 1967 Psychophysiological impairment in wives of alcoholics as related to their husband's drinking and sobriety. In: Fox R (ed) Alcoholism: behavioral research, therapeutic approaches. New York, Springer 134-144

Barrison I G, Viola L, Murray-Lyon I M 1980 Do housemen take an adequate drinking history? British Medical Journal 281: 1040

Bennun I 1986 Evaluating family therapy: a comparison of the Milan and problem-solving approaches. Journal of Family Therapy 8: 225- 242

Bloom B 1973 Cited by Rappaport 1977

Bradley D 1983 Alcohol Advice Centres. In: The prevention of alcoholism report of a symposium, Belfast, June. Alcohol Education and Research Council, London

Cadogan D A 1973 Marital group therapy in the treatment of alcoholism. Quarterly Journal of Studies on Alcohol 34: 1187-1194

Cahalan D, Room R 1974 Problem drinking among American men. College & University Press, New Haven

Caplan G 1970 The theory and practice of mental health consultation. Tavistock, London

Cartwright A 1980 The attitudes of helping agents towards the alcoholic client. British Journal of Addiction 75: 413-431

Chafetz M, Blane H, Hill M (eds) 1970 Frontiers of alcoholism. Science House, New York

Chick J, Lloyd G, Crombie E 1985 Counselling problem drinkers in medical wards: a controlled study. British Medical Journal 290: 265-267

Chick J, Ritson B, Connaughton J, Stewart A, Chick Jo 1988 Advice versus extended treatment for alcoholism: a controlled study. British Journal of Addiction 83: 159-170

Clement S 1984 Salford Community Alcohol Team Project. Research Progress Report (October)

Clement S 1987 The Salford Experiment: an account of the community alcohol team approach. In: Stockwell T, Clement S (eds) Helping the problem drinker: new initiatives in community care. Croom Helm, London

Cohen P C, Krause M D 1971 Casework with the wives of alcoholics. Family Service Association of America, New York

Corder B F, Corder R F, Laidlaw N D 1972 An intensive treatment program for alcoholics and their wives. Quarterly Journal of Studies on Alcohol 33: 1144-1146

Costello R 1980 Alcoholism treatment effectiveness. Slicing the outcome variance pie, In: Edwards G, Grant M (eds) Alcoholism treatment in transition. Croom Helm, London

Coventry Probation Service Alcohol Education Group 1982 A constructive programme for working with the offender with an alcohol problem: a report on the first twelve months with a structured course pack. Alcoholism Information Centre, Coventry

Dahlgren L 1979 Female alcoholics IV marital situations and husbands. Acta Psychiatrica Scandinavica 59: 59-69

Davies D L 1962 Normal drinking in recovered alcohol addictions. Quarterly Journal of Studies on Alcohol 23: 94-104

Davis T S, Hagood L 1979 In-home support for recovering alcoholic mothers and their families: the family rehabilitation co-ordination project. Journal of Studies on Alcohol 40: 313-317

Devon Council on Alcoholism 1984 An agency survey of drinking problems. Unpublished Report. Devon Council on Alcoholism, Exeter.

Department of Health & Social Security 1978 The pattern and range of services for problem drinkers. Report of a working party under the chairmanship of Professor N Kessel

Durlak J A 1979 Comparative effectiveness of para-professional and professional helpers. Psychological Bulletin 86: 80-92

Eberle P A 1982 Alcohol abusers and non-users: A discriminant function analysis of differences between two sub-groups of batterers. Journal of Health & Social Behaviour 23: 260-271

Edwards G 1985 A later follow-up of a classic case series: D L Davies's 1962 report and its significance for the present. Journal of Studies on Alcohol 46: 181-190

Edwards G, Grant M 1980 Alcoholism treatment in transition. Croom Helm, London

Edwards G, Gross M 1976 Alcohol dependence: provisional description of a clinical syndrome. British Medical Journal i: 1058-1061

Edwards G, Chandler J, Hensman C 1972 Drinking in a London suburb I: correlates of normal drinking. Quarterly Journal of Studies on Alcohol suppl 6: 59-93

Edwards G, Gross M, Keller M, Moser J, Room R (eds) 1977 Alcohol-related disabilities, World Health Organization Offset Publication No. 32. World Health Organization, Geneva.

el-Guebaly N, Offord D R 1977 The offspring of alcoholics: a critical review. American Journal of Psychiatry 134: 357-365

Emrick C 1975 A review of psychologically oriented treatment of alcoholism II. The relative effectiveness of different treatment approaches and the effectiveness of treatment versus no treatment. Journal of Studies on Alcohol 36: 88-109

Ewing J A, Long V, Wenzel G G 1961 Concurrent group psychotherapy of alcoholic patients and their wives. International Journal of Group Psychotherapy II 3: 329-338

Feldman D J, Pattison E M, Sobell L C, Graham T, Sobell M B 1975 Out-patient alcohol detoxification: initial findings of 564 patients. American Journal of Psychiatry 132: 407-412

Fennell G, Wardle F 1982 The Parsonage Square Centre, Norwich (Day centre for alcoholics) a research report. School of Economic & Social Studies, University of East Anglia

Gallessich J 1982 The profession and practice of consultation. Jossey-Bass, San Francisco.

Gayford J J 1975 Wife battering: a preliminary study of 100 cases. British Medical Journal 1: 194-197

Goodwin D 1976 Is alcoholism hereditary? Oxford University Press, New York

Gorman J M, Rooney J F 1979 The influence of Al-Anon on the coping behaviour of wives of alcoholics. Journal of Studies on Alcohol 40: 1030-1038

Grant M, Ritson B 1983 Alcohol: the prevention debate. Croom Helm, London

Hamilton J R 1979 Evaluation of a detoxification service for habitual drunken offenders. British Journal of Psychiatry 135: 28-34

Harwin J 1982 Alcohol, the family and treatment. In: Orford J, Harwin J (eds) Alcohol and the Family. Croom Helm, London

Heather N 1986 Change without therapists: the use of self-help manuals by problem drinkers. In: Miller W, Heather N (eds) Treating addictive behaviors: processes of change. Plenum, New York

Heather N, Robertson I 1983 Controlled drinking. Methuen, London (Revised edn)

Hedberg A G, Campbell L 1974 A comparison of four behavioural treatments of alcoholism. Journal of Behaviour Therapy & Experimental Psychiatry 5: 251-256

Holt S, Stewart I C, Dixon J M J, Elton R A, Taylor T V, Little K 1980 Alcohol and the emergency service patient. British Medical Journal 281: 638-640

Hore B, Plant M (eds) 1981 Alcohol problems in employment. Croom Helm, London

Hunt G M, Azrin N H 1973 A community reinforcement approach to alcoholism. Behaviour Research & Therapy 11: 91-104

Janis I, Mann L 1977 Decision-making: a psychological analysis of conflict choice and commitment. Free Press, New York

Jariwalla A G, Adams P H, Hore B D 1979 Alcohol and acute general medical admissions to hospital. Health Trends 11: 95-97

Jarman C M B, Kellett J M 1979 Alcoholism in the general hospital. British Medical Journal ii: 469-472

Katz D, Kahn R L 1978 The social psychology of organizations, Second edn. Wiley, New York

Kaufman E, Pattison E M 1981 Differential methods of family therapy in the treatment of alcoholism. Journal of Studies on Alcohol 42: 951-971

Kendell R 1979 Alcoholism: a medical or a political problem? British Medical Journal 367-371

Kessel N, Makanjuola J D A, Rossall C J et al 1984 The Manchester detoxification service: description and evaluation. Lancet i: 839-842

Ketterer R F 1981 Consultation and education in mental health. Sage, New York

Ledermann S 1956 Alcool, alcoolisme, alcoolisation. Presses Universitaires de France, Paris

Levinger G 1965 Marital cohesiveness and dissolution: an integrative review. Journal of Marriage & the Family 27: 19-28

Lightfoot P, Orford J 1986 Helping agents' attitudes towards alcohol-related problems. Situations vacant? A test and elaboration of a model. British Journal of Addiction 81: 749-756

Lloyd G G, Chick J, Crombie E 1982 Screening for problem drinkers among medical inpatients. Drug & Alcohol Dependence 10: 355-359

Lockhart P, Carter T H, Straffen A M, Pang K K, McLoughin J, Baron J H 1986 Detecting alcohol consumption as a cause of emergency general medical admissions. Journal of the Royal Society of Medicine 79: 132-136

Lothian Regional Social Work Department 1981 Alcohol related problems in current social work cases. Unpublished paper. Social Work Department, Edinburgh

McCrady B 1986 The family in the change process. In: Miller W R, Heather N (eds) Treating addictive behaviors, vol. 2, Processes of change. Plenum New York

McDonnell R, Maynard A 1985 The costs of alcohol misuse. British Journal of Addiction 80: 27-35

McIntosh I D 1982 Alcohol-related disabilities in general hospital patients: a critical assessment of the evidence. The International Journal of the Addictions 17: 609-639

Martin P Y, Segal B 1977 Bureaucracy, size and staff expectations for client independence in halfway houses. Journal of Health & Social Behaviour 18: 376-390

Mather B 1988 Child mistreatment and the misuse of alcohol. Unpublished dissertation submitted for the Award of Diploma in Advanced Social Work Studies. University of Exeter

Mayer J, Black R 1977 Child abuse and neglect in families with an alcohol or opiate addicted parent. Child Abuse & Neglect 1: 85-98

Meyer M 1982 Drinking problems equal family problems: practical guidelines for the problem drinker, the partner and all those involved. Momenta, Lancaster

Moser J 1980 Prevention of alcohol-related problems: an international review of preventive measures, policies, and programmes. Alcoholism & Drug Addiction Research Foundation, Toronto

National Institute of Mental Health 1975 Halfway houses serving the mentally ill and alcoholics, United States 1971-1973. Mental Health Statistics Series A (No. 9) Author: Rockville, Md

Office of Health Economics 1981 Alcohol: reducing the harm, Series No. 70 Author: David Taylor. Papers on Current Health Problems, London

Ogborne A C, Wiggins T R I 1981 Person-programme interactions in halfway houses for problem drinkers. British Journal of Addiction. (In press)

Ogborne A C, Annis H M, Sanchez-Craig M 1978 Report of the task force on halfway houses. Addiction Research Foundation, Toronto

Ogborne A C, Wiggins T R, Shain M 1980 Variations in staff characteristics, programmes and recruitment practices among halfway houses for problem drinkers. British Journal of Addiction 75: 393-403

Orford J 1980 The relative costs of deploying specialists, non-specialists and volunteers in alcoholism counselling. In: Christiansen B (ed) Does psychology return its costs? Proceedings of a conference held at Geilo, Norway, Dec 1979. Norwegian Research Council for the Sciences and Humanities, and the Institute of Psychology, University of Bergen

Orford J 1985a Alcohol problems and the family. In: Lishman J (ed) Research highlights in social work 10. Approaches to addiction. Kogan Page, London

Orford J 1985b Excessive appetites: a psychological view of addictions. Wiley, Chichester

Orford J 1987 The need for a community response to alcohol-related problems. In: Stockwell T, Clement S (eds) Helping the problem drinker: new initiatives in community care. Croom Helm, London

Orford J 1988 An enquiry into the closure of the Berkshire Council on alcoholism. Unpublished report prepared for the Association of Directors of Councils on Alcoholism (U K)

Orford J, Edwards G 1977 Alcoholism: a comparison of treatment and advice, with a study of the influence of marriage. Oxford University Press, London

Orford J, Keddie A 1985 Gender differences in the functions and effects of moderate and excessive drinking. British Journal of Clinical Psychology 24: 265-279

Orford J, Keddie A 1986 Abstinence and controlled drinking in clinical practice. A test of the dependence and persuasion hypotheses. British Journal of Addiction 81: 495-504

Orford J, Velleman R 1990 Offspring of parents with drinking problems: drinking and drug-taking as young adults. British Journal of Addiction 85: 779-794

Orford J, Wawman T 1986 Alcohol detoxification services: a review. DHSS, London

Orford J, Guthrie S, Nicholls P, Oppenheimer E, Egert S, Hensman C 1975 Self-reported coping behaviour of wives of alcoholics and its association with drinking outcome. Journal of Studies on Alcohol 36: 1254-1267

Orford J, Oppenheimer E, Egert S, Hensman C, Guthrie S 1976 The cohesiveness of alcoholism-complicated marriages and its influence on treatment outcome. British Journal of Psychiatry 128: 318-339

Otto W, Orford J 1978 Not quite like home: small hostels for alcoholics and others. Wiley, Chichester

Otto S, Shaw S, Hashimi L 1982 Detoxification evaluation project. Final report to the Department of Health & Social Security

Out of Court 1982 Dealing in Drunkenness: a report from the 'Out of court alternatives for drunkenness offenders' Group

Paton A, Potter J F, Saunders J B 1981 ABC of alcohol: nature of the problem. British Medical Journal 283: 1318-1319

Pendery M L, Maltzman I, West L J 1982 Controlled drinking by alcoholics? New findings and a reevaluation of a major affirmative study. Science 217: 169-175

Pittman D J, Gordon C W 1958 Revolving door: a study of the chronic police inebriate. Rutgers Center for Alcohol Studies, New Brunswick, New Jersey

Potamianos G, Papadatos Y 1987 The 'Accept' community programme for problem drinkers: a comparison with general hospital-based care. In: Stockwell T, Clement S (eds) Helping the problem drinker: new initiatives in community care. Croom Helm, London

Prochaska J, DiClemente C 1986 Towards a comprehensive model of change. In: Miller W, Heather N (eds) Treating addictive behaviors: processes of change. Plenum, New York

Quinn M A, Johnston R B 1976 Alcohol problems in acute male medical admissions. Health Bulletin 34: 253-256

Rappaport J 1977 Community psychology: values, action and research. Holt, Rinehart & Winston, New York

Robertson I, Heather N, Dzialdowski A, Crawford J, Winton M 1986 A comparison of minimal versus intensive controlled drinking treatment interventions for problem drinkers. British Journal of Clinical Psychology 25: 185-194

Robinson D 1979 Talking out of alcoholism. The self-help process of Alcoholics Anonymous. Croom Helm, London

Robinson D 1986 Mutual aid in the change process. In: Miller W, Heather N (eds) Treating addictive behaviours: processes of change. Plenum, New York

Rose H, Bluckert R, Hearn J 1979 Getting dry and housed in Leeds: an evaluative study of a detoxification centre. Unpublished manuscript. School of Applied Social Studies, University of Bradford

Royal College of General Practitioners 1986 Alcohol: a balanced view. Royal College of General Practitioners, London

Saunders W, Kershaw P 1979 Spontaneous remission from alcoholism — a community study. British Journal of Addiction 74: 251-266

Schaffer J B, Tyler J D 1979 Degree of sobriety in male alcoholics and coping styles used by their wives. British Journal of Psychiatry 135: 431-437

Seixas J 1980 How to cope with an alcoholic parent. Edinburgh, Canongate

Shaw S, Cartwright A, Spratley T, Harwin J 1978 Responding to drinking problems. Croom Helm, London

Sherwood J (ed) 1987 Alcohol policies and practices on college and university campuses. In: NASPA Monograph Series 7: National Association of Student Personnel Administration, Inc (USA)

Sierakowski M 1984 The ACCEPT evaluation study. Institute of Family and Environmental Research: final report submitted to DHSS

Smart R G 1977 The Ontario detoxification system: an evaluation of its effectiveness. In: Madden J S, Walker R, Kenyon W H (eds) Alcoholism and drug dependence: a multidisciplinary approach. Plenum, New York

Smith C G 1969 Alcoholics: their treatment and their wives. British Journal of Psychiatry 115: 1039-1042

Sobell M B, Sobell L C 1973 Alcoholics treated by individualized behavior therapy: one year treatment outcome. Behavior Research Therapy 11: 599-618

Sobell M B, Sobell L C 1984 The aftermath of Heresy: a response to Pendery et al's 1982 critique of 'individualized behavior therapy for alcoholics'. Behavior Research Therapy 22: 413-440

Spector J 1984 Clinical psychology and primary care: some ongoing dilemmas. Bulletin of The British Psychological Society 37: 73-76

Stinnett J L 1982 Out-patient detoxification of the alcoholic. International Journal of Addictions 17: 1031-1046

Stockwell T 1988 Community alcohol teams: a review. Paper prepared for DHSS, London

Stockwell T, Murphy D, Hodgson R 1983 The severity of alcohol dependence questionnaire: its use, reliability and validity. British Journal of Addiction 78: 145-155

Stockwell T, Bolt L, Milner I, Pugh P, Young I 1989 Home detoxification from alcohol: its safety and efficacy in comparison with in-patient care. British Journal of Addiction 84

Stockwell T, Bolt L, Milner I, Pugh P, Young I 1990 Home detoxification for problem drinkers: acceptability to clients, relatives, general practitioners and outcome after 60 days. British Journal of Addiction 85

Taylor C L, Kilbane P, Passmore N, Davies R 1986 Prospective study of alcohol-related admissions in an inner city hospital. Lancet August 2nd, pp 265-267

Tennant F S 1979 Ambulatory alcohol withdrawal. In: Galanter M (ed) Currents in alcoholism, VI, treatment, rehabilitation and epidemiology. Grune and Stratton, New York, pp 59-62

Tether P 1985 Identifying and responding to problem drinkers in general practice — the results of a British survey. Paper given to the conference 'Alcohol problems — caring and coping' sponsored jointly by the World Health Organisation, the International Council on Alcohol and Addictions, The Royal College of General Practitioners and Charter Medical of England Limited. ESRC Addiction Research Centre, University of Hull

Tether P, Robinson D 1986 Preventing alcohol problems: a guide to local action. Tavistock, London

Velleman R, Orford J 1984 Intergenerational transmission of alcohol problems — hypotheses to be tested. In: Krasner J, Madden J S, Walker R J (eds) Alcohol-related problems: room for manoeuvre. Wiley, Chichester

Velleman R, Orford J 1990 Adult offspring of parents with drinking problems: recollections of parents' drinking and its immediate effects: British Journal of Clinical Psychology (in press)

Wallace P, Haines A 1985 Use of a questoinnaire in general practice to increase the recognition of excessive alcohol consumption. British Medical Journal 290: 1949-53

Whitfield C L, Thompson G, Lanb A, Spencer V, Pfeifer M, Browning-Ferrando M 1978 Detoxification of 1.024 alcoholic patients without psychoactive drugs. Journal of the American Medical Association 239: 1409-1410

Wilkins R 1974 The hidden alcoholic in general practice. Elek, London

Wilson C 1982 The impact on children. In: Orford J, Harwin J (eds) Alcohol and the family. Croom Helm, London

Wolfenden Committee 1978 Report on the future of voluntary organisations. Croom Helm, London

Yates F 1988 The evaluation of a 'cooperative counselling' alcohol service which uses family and affected others to reach and influence problem drinkers. British Journal of Addiction 83: 1309-1319

Yetton P 1984 Leadership and supervision. In: Gruneberg M, Wall T (eds) Social psychology and organisational behaviour. Wiley, Chichester

Zweben A, Pearlman S, Li S 1988 A comparison of brief advice and conjoint therapy in the treatment of alcohol abuse: the results of the marital systems study. British Journal of Addiction 83: 899-916

11. Drug misuse in the community: meeting the need

E. Oppenheimer

'The most serious peacetime threat to our national well being' was the description given by the Home Affairs Committee of the House of Commons (1984–1985) of the scale of drug misuse in Britain. Since then, the threat has become even more acute by the advent of AIDS leading the British Government's Advisory Committee on the Misuse of Drugs (ACMD) to assert that 'the spread of HIV is a greater danger to individual and public health than drug misuse' (ACMD 1988)

The estimated extent of drug misuse worldwide is believed to be on the increase, with a most striking escalation in heroin and cocaine abuse (UN 1989). In Britain, it is estimated that there are between 75 000 to 150 000 misusers of opioid drugs, of whom probably half are injectors. In addition, there may be as many again who are using a variety of other drugs such as tranquillisers, sedatives, hypnotics, stimulants, solvents and hallucinogens (ACMD 1988).

Societal concerns about drug misuse are based on the awareness of the physical, psychological and social damage which may be experienced by the individual drug misuser, the damage to the family, and the cost to the community of wasted human resources. Of major concern too are the health and social care costs and the cost of drug-related crime. Since it was realised that the HIV virus could be transmitted through the sharing of injecting equipment, that concern has been multiplied. In the USA as a whole, a quarter of the 50 000 cases of AIDS have occurred in drug misusers, while in Europe, the proportion of cases of AIDS which occurred in drug misusers has risen from 2% in 1984 to 17% in 1987, with much higher trends in some countries and cities (ACMD 1988). This new dimension to the problem gives an extra emphasis to the Home Office (1985) assertion that 'helping drug misusers to give up drugs is beneficial for society as well as for the individual concerned'. In Britain, although the number of cases of people with AIDS is still small, nevertheless, drug injectors are at highest risk, with 1500 cases of injecting drug misusers known to have the HIV virus and many more infected but untested (ACMD 1988).

'Drug misuse' is a term which requires clarification in view of the range of social attitudes and practices in that field. Thus, the use of some psychoactive substances, notably alcohol, is sanctioned in some societies and prohibited in others, as are the smoking of opium or coca leaf-chewing, which have long been practised in certain traditional societies (Edwards & Arif 1980) but considered as misuse in others. In the same way, the excessive use of drugs such as benzodiazepines, which have a legitimate place in medical practice, went unremarked for a long period (Gabe & Williams 1986) but is now regarded as 'misuse'.

A useful definition was proposed by the Specialist Committee on Drugs & Drug Dependence of the Royal College of Psychiatrists (1987). They saw drug misuse as 'any taking of a drug which harms or threatens to harm the physical or mental or social well-being of an individual, or other individuals, or of society at large or which is illegal'.

TREATMENT OR CONTROL?

Among the problems confronted by health professionals in considering their response to drug misuse, are certain factors which affect their selection of an appropriate response. Drug taking is often secretive and so its extent and severity are unknown. Its consequences are frequently ignored or denied by the drug taker and many of its effects are social, legal or economic, as well as medical or psychiatric.

The illegality of much drug-taking means that most societies combine treatment and care with policing and systems of controls, including legal penalties. The emphasis varies between treatment and legal controls, according to prevailing political, social and economic factors.

For example, in a national statement of policy for Burma, where records of opium growing and use go back to the 16th century, the measures taken by the government today are largely an attempt to control the cultivation, production, sale, supply and use of narcotic and dangerous drugs, so that the law is used against both drug traffickers and drug users. Those who do not voluntarily submit themselves for treatment and rehabilitation can be legally compelled to do so. Likewise in Malaysia, the 1983 Drug Dependence (Treatment and Rehabilitation) Act places a requirement upon addicts to undergo compulsory treatment, and a 'tough and rugged' requirement has been developed for this (Report of the Conference of Ministers of Health 1986).

By contrast, it is the stated belief of the Dutch government that 'drug use should be shorn of its taboo image and its sensational and emotional undertones', and it has rejected the idea of any kind of compulsory treatment. The Dutch government takes the view that drug users should as far as possible be seen as 'normal' people, and that 'drug users or even addicts should not be regarded primarily as criminals nor as dependent helpless patients' (Ministry of Welfare Health & Cultural Affairs, Netherlands, 1985). Despite this diversity, however, the Ministerial Conference (1986) ended with a consensus view on the 'need for a satisfactory balance between control and enforcement on the one hand, and treatment and prevention strategies on the other', adding that 'the health element within the total response deserves greater prominence'.

Treatment and control in Britain

The ACMD (1982) noted that: 'the individual drug misuser's rights as a patient or client are often at conflict with health and legal protection of the community and the wider context of society at large'. Indeed, the presence of legal factors may complicate the response to drug misusers as patients; examples include cases of pregnant drug misusers or addict parents (where a legal responsibility to protect the child may become paramount), or the management of syringe exchange schemes, in which drug misusers who attend are in fact breaking the law because they are injecting illicit drugs.

In Britain, the legal framework for both treatment and control was established in the 1971 Misuse of Drugs Act, which regulates the import and export of drugs, and defines offences in respect of cultivation, importation, and supply of certain specified substances. The Act also restricts the prescribing of specified controlled drugs, and sets out regulations for the notification by doctors of addicts to the Home Office. Controlled drugs are listed in three categories, based on the relative dangers which might result from their misuse. The UK government summarised its long-term strategy on drug misuse (Home Office 1985) as aiming to reduce supplies from abroad, tighten controls on drugs produced and prescribed in Britain, make policies even more effective, strengthen deterrence, and improve prevention, treatment and rehabilitation. In other words, an integration of treatment and control.

There is a strong emphasis in British policy on prevention. The ACMD in 1988 emphasised that 'prevention of drug misuse is now more important than ever before and in the longer run the success or failure of efforts to prevent young people from embarking on a career of drug misuse will have a major effect on our ability to contain the spread of AIDS'.

The main focus of this chapter will be on Britain, and on the evolution and present shape of the community response to drug misuse. This will be followed by a description of a number of options for community responses and finally major concerns and priorities will be examined.

CARING FOR DRUG MISUSERS

Drug-misusers come to the notice of numerous agencies in the community: the police, courts, prisons, the probation service, legal advice centres, hospital accident and emergency departments, specialist drug treatment clinics, specialist and non-specialist voluntary agencies, and the statutory social services. The first observer of a case of drug misuse is often either a general medical practitioner, a psychiatrist, a parent, a friend, a teacher, or a clergyman. The practical response to drug misuse often involves action by several of these concerned and interested parties. Below are some examples, not untypical, of the varied routes into treatment and of varied results.

Adam is 23 years old and unemployed. He has been injecting drugs for seven years and is charged with possession and supplying of heroin. The magistrate, putting him on probation, recommends treatment. The Probation Officer makes an appointment for him at the local Drug Treatment Clinic, but Adam repeatedly fails to attend. Three months later, he presents at an Accident and Emergency Department following an overdose. He is detoxified, offered counselling, an AIDS test, and further help for his drug problem, but takes his own discharge and disappears.

Gillian is a 20-year-old prostitute in the King's Cross area of London. She is noticed by an outreach community worker from a local street-agency which specialises in drug problems. Gillian is urged to consult a GP because she looks ill and thin. An urgent hospital admission is arranged and she undergoes a battery of medical tests. She is found to have the HIV virus. However, one week later, she takes her own discharge and returns to working as a prostitute in the same area of London.

George is a 30-year-old Scot with a 10-year history of heroin addiction and of petty crime to finance his drug-taking. In prison, the Welfare Office suggests that he tries going into a Therapeutic Community when he completes his sentence; this he decides to do. He spends six months in treatment, but leaves against staff's advice. He is, however, believed to have remained drug-free, working for a building firm in the Midlands.

Caroline is a 19-year-old art student from West London who has been sniffing cocaine and smoking cannabis for about a year. Some of her friends have taken heroin. Following the death by overdose of her best friend, she contacts Narcotics Anonymous and attends it regularly for the next six months.

Joanna is a 22-year-old, living with her boyfriend. Both had been using amphetamines and cocaine, generally at weekends only, but lately occasionally during the week. Both were working. When Joanna discovered that she was pregnant, fear about the effect of her drug use on her unborn child, and worries that the child would immediately be taken into care, stopped her from going to see a doctor. She came off all drugs by herself and then went to see her doctor. Nevertheless, she was immediately admitted to hospital and remained under intensive medical supervision until the baby was born. Supportive services from the social services department and from the health visitor were put into place, and she remains under supervision for the time being.

As the above illustrations show, drug-takers find different routes into treatment, make use of both specialist and non-specialist agencies, and in some cases show marked reluctance to engage in treatment when it is offered. Furthermore, the choice of agency depends on what is available at a local level and on the knowledge the drug-taker has about services. As studies of the problem have abundantly shown, drug-takers are a heterogeneous group, coming from different social classes and different ethnic origins, misusing different drugs, and experiencing numerous and diverse problems.

Therefore, no single approach to controlling the drugs problem or to treatment, rehabilitation, or prevention will adequately serve this whole clientele; the need is for a variety of measures, a range of service provisions and flexibility in treatment goals. Those who inject drugs are a particularly high risk group, but in addition, certain users — women, adolescents, the elderly, members of minority ethnic groups — have specific problems and require specialist interventions. Also, different stages in the career of a drug-taker will require different sorts of approaches and varying professional skills. Short-term counselling may be an adequate and appropriate response to a schoolchild experimenting but not yet injecting drugs, but a long-term user and injector may best be helped by a lengthy therapeutic programme. Someone dependent on opioids may first require medical supervision to come off drugs or at the very least learn to use drugs in a less harmful way and subsequently participate in psychological treatment. Someone not physically dependent but experiencing family difficulties might best be served by family therapy.

There are sound theoretical and practical grounds for believing that early treatment is to be preferred and that all efforts should be made to engage drug takers in treatment, more especially if AIDS is to be prevented (ACMD 1988). The aim of care should be to intervene as early as possible in the process of drug-taking in order to prevent 'a career of narrowing options' (Rosenbaum 1981), in which a drug misuser risks entering a chaotic lifestyle: 'hassling' for drugs, ill-health, poverty, incarceration, loss of self-respect, the breakdown of social and family relationships, and possibly early death either through contracting the HIV virus or from the many other drug-related health risks. In response to this progression from experimentation to chaos, a programme for arresting and reducing the harmful effects of drugs, alongside provision of treatment and rehabilitation facilities, is crucial, both for the drug-misusers themselves and in the interests of society.

SERVICE PROVISION IN THE COMMUNITY

Identifying the need

Society's response to the drug problem varies according to its perception of priorities. It can never be a static response because the extent of drug misuse, the patterns of use, and the drugs that are abused are all subject to change.

The ACMD (1982) drew attention to the need to ensure that the extent of problem drug-taking is continuously monitored, and to maximise the number of drug-misusers who make contact with services

(ACMD 1988). However, because of the very nature of the problem, with uneven distribution of drug misuse as well as the changeability of drug-taking patterns, traditional epidemiological techniques (such as population surveys or the analysis of national statistics) are not adequate for identifying service needs and planning community responses.

Numerous alternative methodologies have been proposed (e.g. Hartnoll et al 1985, Brodsky 1985) and employed (e.g. Dorn et al 1987). Much of the emphasis is on developing techniques to monitor local trends; these techniques focus on developing a local database, using information obtained from the local community (e.g. from parents, doctors, teachers, policemen, public houses, social workers, youth workers, clergymen, etc.). Ironically however, even such continuous vigilance may have unexpected consequences. Dorn et al (1987) pointed out that extensive surveillance may cause the drug problem to shift to another neighbourhood thereby altering the distribution of the problem but contributing little to its solution.

In practice, much of the treatment and rehabilitation of drug misusers is initially based on inadequate information about the size of and the needs of the client group, but is subsequently adapted to those who come forward and use these services.

Service options

The ongoing debate about the role of community psychiatry and community care often sets comprehensive planning against selective and ad hoc responses, but there is increasing emphasis on using the strength and resources of the local community whenever possible.

Ch'ien (1981) identified nine types of service elements which he believed to be essential, beginning with community-wide education and primary prevention, and proceeding to outreach and early detection, counselling services for the young who are most 'at risk', the development of self-help groups within the community and the involvement of these groups in neighbourhood activity. He emphasised the need for detoxification facilities for those who become addicted, both ambulatory and inpatient, along with counselling services, residential treatment facilities, methadone maintenance programmes, a range of related social services, and the development of community-based forensic facilities to link the health care and legal systems. Finally, the need for research and evaluation was stressed. Other observers, conscious of the need to make choices in a situation of finite resources, have attempted to identify particular elements in such a programme as having the highest priority.

In Britain, the recommendation of the ACMD (1982) for a community-based service for drug misusers corresponds closely to the prevailing view on Community Care in the UK that 'appropriate care should be provided for individuals in such a way as to enable them to lead as normal an existence as possible... and to minimise disruption of life within the community' (Social Services Committee, 1984–1985), and to the view that a comprehensive service should be provided within a defined community, using the psychiatric hospital as part of a network of integrated local facilities (Freeman 1983). The ACMD's (1982) stated objectives concerned the need for a co-ordinated multidisciplinary approach. They noted that 'for the majority of problem drug-takers treatment by doctors will be an important component of the help they receive' but that 'the prime responsibility for responding to these problems [should be] at local level'.

There is greatest consensus about where services should be available — most leading authorities urge the merits of the organisation of services at a local level. The ACMD (1982) states that: 'the nature and extent of problems from drugs misuse vary from area to area... even if there were to be central funding, the prime responsibility for responding to these problems should be at a local rather than a national level where the needs of both the potential clients and of those caring for them can be assessed'. Thorley (1983) drew attention to the importance of rehabilitation, distinguishing it sharply from treatment, as 'a much more active process in which the patient or client is urged to abandon the passive sick role and to assume responsibility... a clear appeal of rehabilitation in relation to drug misuse is that optimum results may be achieved'.

Strang (1989) discusses services based on the recommendations described above in the north-west of England, which he termed an 'integrated model'. He sees an ongoing partnership between generalist health and social care and specialist medical, drug treatment care as a key element of the community response. The specialist drug services, rather like specialists in other branches of medicine deal with complex problems and then pass clients back to general health care, essential elements being the open lines of communication between the different arms of the services.

The spread of the HIV virus lent urgency to the recommendations about integrated and community-based responses. In reviewing what has happened thus far, the ACMD (1988) noted that although there has been a very significant increase in community-based services, there are variations in the level and range of services available in the country. They noted that in some areas, positive and enthusiasitic attitudes led to a full range of services but that elsewhere, entrenched attitudes have contributed to incompetence and ill co-ordinated facilities. They emphasised that prevention of AIDS is crucial and argue that the most effective way of disseminating knowledge about HIV and changing addicts' behaviour involves, first of all, bringing them in touch with a helping agency. They further acknowledge the importance of accessible and relevant services and the role of G.P's and other generic professions. The report concludes that 'community based services for drug misusers provide the best opportunity for this'.

COMMUNITY CARE FOR DRUG MISUSERS

In this section the various component services which may be available to drug misusers will be examined in detail. It is not possible to assess their relative importance to the user or to the community, except to point out that the services described vary from society to society and from one era to the next and that treatment and care models are continuously undergoing evaluation and change. Medical treatments, therapeutic communities, detoxification programmes and outpatient treatments have all been evaluated separately. However, for both practical and ethical reasons, it has been impossible, as yet, either to conduct a study which randomly assigns clients to one or other treatment or to evaluate scientifically one entire system of care.

Medical care

The medical profession has long held a key role in the treatment of drug misuse and addiction — a role held since the end of the 19th century, when 'morphinism' came to be regarded as a disease. Since then, treatments for addiction have included the prescription of morphine substitutes (including heroin) and of a synthetic longer-acting heroin substitute — methadone, (introduced in the 1960s), the supervision of detoxification (often helped by psychoactive drugs such as benzodiazepines), as well as treatment of withdrawal and relapse prevention programmes using opiate-antagonists such as naltrexone. Treatments are also offered for psychological problems, in which increasingly, the concern is focused on AIDS and on the prevention and treatment of physical complications arising from drug misuse and AIDS.

Up until the mid-1960s opiate addicts in Britain were usually treated by their GPs. The prevailing understanding of addiction 'as a manifestation of disease and not as a mere form of vicious indulgence', (Departmental Committee on Morphine & Heroin Addiction 1926), allowed for the medical provision of prescription heroin at a level that would enable the addict to live a normal and non-criminal life. However, this approach was revised when reports of a drug 'epidemic' began to appear in the press; those involved were young, experimental drug users who began socially and not, as so often before, as a consequence of illness. There was further evidence that some of the drugs used by the new users were obtained from over-prescribing doctors.

Drugs — a problem for experts

Worries about irresponsible and ill-informed doctors led to the treatment of addiction being substantially taken out of the hands of GPs and placed in the hands of specialists. In 1967, following the recommendations of the Second Inter-Departmental Committee on Drug Addiction under the chairmanship of Sir Russell Brain (1965), Specialist Drug Treatment Centres were set up in some large cities on an ad hoc basis in psychiatric hospitals or in psychiatric departments of general hospitals. Only doctors licensed by the Secretary of State were allowed to treat patients by prescribing heroin, cocaine or certain other restricted drugs. GPs were allowed to prescribe some opioids (e.g. methadone), both for the treatment of pain and for the treatment of addiction. Every doctor who saw a patient believed to be addicted to drugs, was legally obliged to notify the Home Office.

The most important change, however, was the new role given to doctors. Brain's conclusion that 'addiction is after all a socially infectious condition' led the committee to give doctors a role in controlling the drug problem — the idea of 'judicious prescribing'. The rationale for this was that if 'the restrictions are so severe as to prevent or seriously discourage the addict from obtaining any supplies from legitimate sources, it may lead to the development of an organised illicit traffic'.

Changes in treatment approaches and technologies

In the decade after the first Treatment Clinics were opened in 1968, there were some important changes in treatment practice, which were the result of advances in knowledge about heroin addiction. The first major change was the widespread introduction of methadone to clinical practice in Britain. This drug had been introduced into the treatment of heroin addiction in the USA in 1965 by Dole & Nyswander who, viewing the condition as a metabolic disorder, used methadone — a synthetic opioid, available in a linctus form — to block the euphoric effects of heroin. This approach provides useful help to addicts in trying to normalise their lives. Soon afterwards, methadone was also used in Britain, both in detoxification programmes and also as a maintenance drug in the long term treatment of addiction. The use of opiate-antagonists such as naltrexone or clonidine is limited in Britain to a few detoxification programmes.

Other changes in treatment approaches emerged slowly, following the opening of the Drug Treatment Centres. At the beginning of the 1970s, it looked as if the drug problem had been controlled in Britain, but with changes in social and economic conditions and a much greater avail-ability of illicit drugs, the idea of containing the drug problem by careful prescribing became increasingly untenable. It was also argued that maintenance prescribing of opioid drugs did not offer a real therapeutic challenge. Soon, most clinicians stopped prescribing injectable drugs or allowing long-term maintenance, and began to insist that clients give up drug use; they were therefore willing to prescribe methadone only in the short term.

The emergence and development of a specialised clinical service for drug-misusers occurred as an expedient measure in response to a change in the 1960s in the size and nature of the addiction problem and to its perceived mis-management by GPs. The new provision allowed the gradual development of specialised knowledge and expertise on drug misuse, which had not existed hitherto. However, as further changes in the drug scene occurred, these specialised facilities were rendered inadequate in their ability to deal with the new problems. It was time for them to lead the way in educating the non-specialists.

The re-emergence of non-specialist provision

The enormous increase in the size of the drug problem since the mid 1970s was not matched by an increase in the available specialist clinical provision, which became under-resourced, overloaded and remained understaffed (Smart 1985). A pragmatic approach reasserted itself with renewed attention given to the role which non-specialist medical services could play — a role which they had abandoned when the specialised clinics were set up.

Some of the overall recommendations for services have already been described above. In order to achieve a broader base for treatment provision, the ACMD (1982), in a major departure from previous policy objectives, recommended that each regional health authority should establish a multi-disciplinary regional drug problem team, each team having a permanent and identifiable base — usually a Drug Dependence Unit (DDU). Apart from providing a specialist service, these teams should have a peripatetic role within the region — giving support and advice, liaising with both specialist and non-specialist agencies and encouraging the development of new services. It was also suggested that, at the health district level, a drug advisory committee should be established to monitor the extent of problem drug-taking there and to assess the efficacy of existing services. The ACMD accepted that doctors working in general practice were increasingly involved in the treatment of addiction, but cautioned that 'while there may be a role for some of these doctors in the treatment of problem drug-takers, there is also a need to ensure that this role is consistent with good medical practice'.

Following these recommendations, a national Medical Working Group on Drug Dependence was set up (1984) which suggested that 'all doctors have a responsibility to provide care for both the general health needs of drug-misusers and their drug-related problems. Indeed, there is evidence that many drug-misusers do turn to GPs for help: it was estimated that between 30 000 – 44 000 new opioid misusers in England and Wales consult their GPs each year (Glanz & Taylor 1986). The Working Group offered wide-ranging advice to family doctors on the best way to treat drug-misusers, urging them to take a full history, test urines, and check with the Home Office as to whether the person is known as an addict.

They were also advised that 'at the first interview it should be made clear that treatment will not necessarily involve the prescribing of opioids or barbiturates, nor will it involve long-term maintenance prescribing'. Identified cases should be referred to the local DDU, where one exists, and to local authority social services or voluntary agencies, where appropriate. Thus, doctors in general practice have been encouraged to consider treating drug-takers themselves, while the specialists in drug clinics undertake a role of support and advice.

Medical interventions in the light of AIDS

Drug treatment has undergone a considerable re-think since the dangers posed by the HIV virus have become known. In general, at the end of the 1980s there was an emerging consensus in Britain about medical treatments for drug misuse. An emphasis on a hierarchy of treatment goals has superseded the conviction held in the 1970s that the goal of treatment should be abstinence. The role of prescribing became important once again, and attitudes to methadone maintenance have reverted to an acceptance of its utility. The ACMD (1988) identified a number of purposes for prescribing, in addition to assisting in withdrawal: these include attracting more drug misusers to services, keeping them in contact and facilitating change away from behaviour which puts the user at risk of contracting HIV. Furthermore, they acknowledge that for some drug misusers 'a move away from injecting will not be achievable at the time they seek help'; for those individuals, some provision of injectable drugs is recommended but the ACMD emphasises that such a course of action should only be undertaken in 'exceptional cases' and in the short term. They recommend that other acceptable treatment goals could be 'switching from injecting to oral use and avoiding sharing equipment'. They assert that drug misusers fit somewhere on a continuum between wanting to change or not and show an ambivalent attitude about drug treatment services. They suggest that services should therefore strongly encourage drug misusers towards a goal of abstinence, but should be willing to accept other realistic goals.

It is reassuring, therefore, that there have been consistent reports, particularly from the USA, to suggest that prescribing methadone is generally beneficial to clients and does no physical harm and that, in general, those who remain in treatment (i.e. are maintained), report a cessation of, or a reduction in, illicit heroin use, as well as increased employment and decreased criminal involvement (NIDA 1981, Dole & Nyswander 1983). This hoped-for movement away from the illicit market and from the dangers of injecting is critical in any AIDS-prevention strategy.

The role of general practitioners has been further extended by the dangers of HIV in the drug-taking population. The ACMD (1989) recommends that 'care for drug-misusers with HIV disease will and should be provided in the community', and assert that as GPs are the key providers of health in the community, ways should be found to increase GP involvement with drug-misusers: GPs should inform drug-misusers of the risks of HIV and should have the facility to provide them with free condoms. They further recommend that, where possible, shared care systems should be developed so that GPs and physicians with experience of treating HIV disease combine to monitor the health of these patients.

In 1987, the UK government established a number of syringe-exchange schemes. These schemes are controversial in many countries because they are seen as enabling drug-takers to continue drug-taking. Indeed, they have limited objectives: they aim to prevent the sharing of needles and syringes amongst injecting drug-users and to discourage behaviour with a high risk of transmission of the HIV virus. These projects have been evaluated and have been found to reach a high number of injectors who are not in touch with other helping agencies (Stimson et al 1989). However, the overall effect of AIDS prevention is less easy to measure.

In theory at least, caring for drug misuse in Britain should now more than ever be a partnership between specialist and non-specialist medical services, alongside a range of non-medical, non-statutory facilities which have developed alternative models of care.

Non-medical provision

In the UK, the reformulation of the drug misuse problem from one of addiction (requiring medical help) to one of 'problem drug-taking' (ACMD 1982), which requires social and economic rehabilitation, set the seal of approval on a concerted development of non-medical provision, including drug-free residential facilities, street agencies, day centres, and a variety of self-help groups. These agencies are non-statutory provisions in that the service they offer is not mandatory under the Misuse of Drugs Act or other legislation. They are established by voluntary efforts, but most of their money comes from the public purse, by a mixture of funds derived from both central and local government.

Residential facilities

The Therapeutic Community (TC) model of treatment was initially developed in the USA; it represented an alternative to the medical model of care, and was based on the self-help principle. The first such community, Synanon, was founded in the USA in 1959 as a treatment facility for alcoholics, gradually expanding to cater for heroin addicts (Yablonsky 1965). This has been followed by a sturdy growth of the movement worldwide; the first Therapeutic Community opened in Britain in 1969.

The Therapeutic Community's underlying philosophy is to view drug misuse as 'deviant behaviour', reflecting impeded personality development and deficits in social, educational, and economic skills. Its antecedents may lie in socio-economic disadvantage and poor family effectiveness, as well as in psychological factors; addiction is seen as a symptom, not the essence of the disorder' (De Leon & Deitch 1985). The programmes, which may last 12–18 months or longer, aim to 'emphasise notions of democracy, order and discipline, personal responsibility, convivial labour, public confession, punishment and a commitment to life within the community' (Brook & Whitehead 1980).

The programmes vary in their detailed application of the therapeutic goals, but underlying the diversity are two key elements which are found in most programmes. The first is the provision of a range of specific therapeutic interactions, e.g. encounter groups, consciousness-raising groups for both men and women, as well as gestalt, bio-energetic and relaxation therapies. This is complemented by a structured and hierarchical work schedule, operating within the community (tasks include cooking, house-maintenance, administration, refurbishing, etc.), designed to represent a microcosm of the outside world, where the higher the work status and the seniority, the greater the responsibility. The work in the house is often supplemented by remedial and skills training and by counselling. The problems of leaving a Therapeutic Community to rejoin society at large are dealt with in the final stage of a resident's stay, when practical help to gain employment and accommodation is coupled with ongoing support both from staff and from peers in the community. In Britain, these Therapeutic Communities are staffed by a mixture of recovered drug-misusers and professional social workers.

It may be concluded from the available evidence that the Therapeutic Community is highly suitable for some drug-misusers, but the high drop-out rate suggests that it is not a useful treatment option for all. Research has not yet been able to identify definitively which clients are most appropriate for this regime, but motivation to stay in treatment is undoubtedly an important element in good outcome (De Leon 1984). De Leon concluded that the 'findings provide convincing evidence for the effectiveness of the Therapeutic Community approach for drug abuse: firstly, there is a striking replication in rates of success and improvement and in the social adjustment profiles; and secondly, the consistent relationship between time in programme and post-treatment success status provides further evidence of programme effectiveness'.

Another major model of residential treatment is based on the Minnesota Model. The cornerstone of that programme's philosophy is the disease concept of alcohol and drug dependency, offering a promise of recovery but not of cure. The over-riding ethos is the belief in the possibility of change: that addicts or alcoholics can change their beliefs and behaviour. It is hypothesised that 'addiction-prone people are vulnerable to many different mood-altering substances'. Furthermore, chemical dependency is seen as 'multiphasic', involving a spiritual component in addition to physical psychological and social factors (Anderson 1981 quoted in Cook 1988a). To effect recovery, the principles of Alcoholics Anonymous (AA) and Narcotics Anonymous (NA) are employed, while treatment goals are abstinence from all mind-altering drugs and an improvement in life style.

The programme is generally 6–8 weeks long and encompasses a whole range of services ranging from referral and detoxification to help with rehabilitation and aftercare. The programme includes lectures, individual and group therapy, family therapy, work assignments, a 12-step programme, daily reading groups, giving of life history by residents, recreation, AA/NA groups, etc. In a review of available evidence on the success of this model Cook (1988b) concludes that 'despite exaggerated claims of success, it appears to have a genuinely impressive 'track record' with as many as two-thirds of its patients achieving a good outcome one year after discharge'. However, he suggests that 'more research is needed upon outcome in patients exposed to this programme'. Furthermore, in Britain, this model is strongly associated with the private sector and is, to date, still a treatment available mostly to those able to pay (Cook 1988).

Social work agencies

Social workers who are involved in helping drug-misusers operate in hospitals and social service departments, and in probation and correctional setting, as well as in front-line, low-threshold street agencies.

Generic social work agencies   In Britain, the Social Service Departments of local authorities are the 'primary local agency, with responsibility not only for children and young people at risk as a result of parental or their own misuse of drugs, but also for some broader issues of social policy on drug abuse' (Association of Metropolitan Authorities 1985). Social workers in such departments most commonly become involved in drug abuse cases where children of drug-takers are thought to be at risk.

Probation officers are frequently called upon to supervise drug-misusers who break the law (not only the drug laws). In evidence to the Social Services Committee hearings on Drug Misuse (1985), one local authority claimed that over half of the children on its 'at risk' register had drug-misusing parents.

Specialised social work agencies   A number of specialised, non-residential social-work agencies which are focused on drug abuse have emerged in Britain; these non-statutory 'street agencies' offer a range of practical, referral, and counselling and information services. They are generally in inner city areas, close to locations where drug-misusers congregate, they operate from simple premises and are staffed by social workers who, as in the case of Therapeutic Communities, are typically a mixture of ex-addicts and professionally trained personnel. The service they offer is directed mainly to the more chaotic, homeless drug misuser, who finds it difficult to use other, more formal facilities. Most of these agencies include a strong outreach component in their service, i.e. making contact with drug misusers or those 'at risk' in the street or in locations where they congregate, and helping them to make use of other services. Increasingly, the emphasis is on harm-reduction and risk-minimisation. Some street agencies run needle-exchange schemes and give help and information to drug-misusers about how to inject drugs safely.

Dorn & South (1985) described three such facilities in London and noted that they 'are best understood not as separate agencies but as complementing pieces in a wider jigsaw of responses to drug-related problems... they operate primarily... in two main ways — services to individual clients and families and friends and to other agencies... services include telephone and face-to-face advice work (sometimes over an extended period of time), referral of users and professional enquirers to other appropriate services, and education and training'. For the drug misuser, the main attractions of street agencies are their informality, accessibility, minimalisation of bureaucratic procedures and non-pressuring, non-threatening atmosphere. The staff often view their work as providing a sort of 'safety net' for drug-takers. As non-statutory organisations, they are dependent on an ad hoc system of funding by both central and local government.

The work of these agencies does not easily lend itself to systematic evaluation, as contact with clients can be erratic and record-keeping is frequently minimal. However, observers see their value as being critical as far as AIDS prevention is concerned, in pioneering new ways of working with chaotic drug-misusers, in providing invaluable assistance in motivating users to seek more intensive help and in linking them in to formal medical and social services.

As part of the trend towards more non-specialist treatment options, a closer partnership has been recommended between generic social workers, community nursing services, and specialists in the drug field (ACMD 1982), though a subsequent report from the DHSS social services inspectorate (DHSS 1987) suggests that, in practice, the development of such integrated help services has been 'sparse'. The ACMD (1988) report urges that 'in the light of HIV, early identification and intervention by these agencies is of heightened importance'.

Self-help groups

The proliferation of self-help groups for people with drug problems and for their relatives has stemmed from a perceived lack of professional resources in the community or from a disenchantment with existing facilities, followed by the desire to take initiatives. Parents' and relatives' groups provide mutual support, counselling, and telephone help-lines for drug-takers and their relatives, and act as pressure groups to stimulate communal action. Narcotics Anonymous (NA), which is an offshoot of Alcoholics Anonymous (AA), has also been growing. It originated in the USA and began to gain momentum in the late 1970s, so that by 1980 there were an estimated 20 000 recovering addicts involved. At that time, over 6500 NA groups were recorded, spanning 36 countries. In the UK, NA started in 1980 and has grown from a single weekly meeting to 60 meetings weekly in the London area. NA provides continued support for those who have undergone treatment, as well as for those who wish to become drug-free. It offers an alternative pathway to recovery by suggesting a 12-step programme (as in AA) of self-discipline and commitment, with the help of other members of the fellowship (Wells 1987).

CONCERNS AND PRIORITIES

The ACMD (1988) concluded that 'in all areas, substantial further expansion will be necessary if services are to reach more drug misusers and play an effective role in combating the spread of AIDS'. A number of areas which have been identified as important for the provision of community services are discussed below: prevention of drug taking, specific treatment needs of young drug-takers and the needs of women drug-misusers and their children. There is also a growing awareness of the special needs of ethnic minorities, but as yet relatively little attention has been paid to this problem in Britain, whereas in the USA this has received considerable attention.

The need for early prevention of drug misuse

'The prevention of substance misuse ought to be everyone's business. First and most importantly, the avoidance of chemical misuse must be seen as essential to every individual's personal responsibility' (Royal College of Psychiatrists 1987). In its 1988 AIDS report, ACMD added its own emphasis — 'prevention of drug misuse is now more important than ever before and in the longer run the success of efforts to prevent young people from embarking on a career of drug misuse will have a major effect on our ability to contain the spread of HIV.'

Educating the community at large

Interrupting a young person's potential career from experimenter to drug-misuser is an obvious way of limiting damage. This often depends on people in the community — teachers, youth-workers, parents — being intelligently observant. The importance of educating parents and other adults who are in positions of responsibility for young people is evident; for them, information should be available covering the nature and danger of drugs and the detectable signs of use. This simple level of adult vigilance, at which prompt observation leads to early intervention, may be more productive of results than costly and lurid public warnings of the dangers of drugs.

Educating the young

Many concerned observers have emphasised the need to educate and warn the young directly. However, how this should be done is a matter of some controversy. In the USA a comprehensive review of the role of the mass-media campaign in preventing adolescent substance abuse (Flay & Sobel 1983) concluded that 'an overwhelming majority of mass-media drug-abuse prevention programmes have failed to change behaviour'. Nevertheless, such campaigns are undertaken from time to time.

In fact, multiple preventive strategies are needed to prevent drug-taking amongst young people. Perry & Jessor (1985) emphasised the importance of approaching prevention from the standpoint of health promotion including physical, psychological, social and personal health. They argued that this can be done by focusing attention on either health-enhancing or on health-compromising behaviours. Bry (1985) suggested an even more comprehensive approach which would include educational measures using the media, social interventions involving the whole environment, modelling the 'saying no' approach, encouraging parental influence, family effectiveness and communication training, emphasising religious commitment and training and formal therapy for troubled young people. Above all, it is argued, prevention must be made relevant to the culture, interest and aspirations of young people. Even so, 'the question of the most useful method for achieving the aim of reducing casualties and increasing health remains open' (ISDD 1984). The Royal College of Psychiatrists (1987) recommended a pragmatic approach: 'methods of prevention directed at drug problems should be sustained, multi-faceted, and usually a matter of small focused remedies rather than grand strategies'.

The special needs of adolescents

Drug-taking generally begins during adolescence or young adulthood and evidence about drug-taking amongst the young is abundant (UN 1989). Much adolescent drug-taking is in the nature of experimentation, and may be seen as part of typical adolescent behaviour patterns. Nevertheless, there is some evidence that those who use drugs tend to be more troubled than those who do not. For instance, research from the USA shows that psychological disturbance may pre-date drug abuse (Beschner & Treasure 1979) and that the severity of the drug problem is significantly related to family factors (Friedman et al 1980). Parents, and especially mothers, provide a powerful modelling influence for their children (Newcombe et al 1983); the excessive use by parents of psychoactive drugs (Smart & Fejer 1972) and the example of other siblings, has also been shown to be significant (Brook et al 1983). Considerably more users report poor relationships with parents, e.g. broken homes (Streit et al 1974), compared with non-users. There is further research evidence that behaviour such as rebelliousness, poor school performance, delinquency and criminal activity have been found to pre-date drug use (Kandel 1982).

Young people thus present a host of problems to community services, many of which are either family- or school-related. These may be coupled with emotional and psychological problems, difficulties in expressing feelings and a general condition of boredom and restlessness (Beschner 1985). Crucially, many young people simply do not identify drugs as being a problem to them.

Treatment needs of adolescents

It is important that adolescent users should be helped to overcome treatment barriers by providing them with services that are relevant to them, but in fact most adolescents either remain untreated, or are treated in facilities which are designed for the older opioid drug-takers. As yet there is scant evidence about programme effectiveness in relation to the young. The Treatment Outcome Prospective Study (TOPS) from the USA (Hubbard et al 1984) concluded that 'early treatment can give a youth a better chance for rehabilitation or, at worst, can interrupt the development of more serious drug-user careers. The results of available studies on drug treatment for youths, however, are only moderately encouraging ... many continue to abuse both alcohol or marijuana'.

It has been suggested (Feldman et al 1985) that programmes for the young should be based firmly on understanding the socio-cultural context in which drug use occurs, using ethnographic methods to build up such understanding, and that treaters should avoid being seen as agents of social control. Furthermore, young people should not feel criminalised by the system of care. They recommend neighbourhood-based community programmes which would offer help within the social context of young people's friendship groups, 'taking counselling services and programme activity out to the natural environment where youth groups tend to congregate, which would include playgrounds, street corners, school yards, beaches and shopping malls'. If such an approach is adopted, drug use would not be the sole focus of the intervention, which would tackle other social problems as well. For example, since many adolescent users are still of school age and many are known to be truants and to have difficulties at school, alternative education and day care programmes might be developed designed to operate during the school day, offering counselling alongside other school activities. Such programmes would have the aim of 'installing the value of education as an explicit socialisation goal of treatment' (De Leon and Deitch 1985).

Family treatments are also crucially important for young people still living in a home environment. Numerous ways of working with drug-misusers and their families have been suggested, mostly using and adapting existing models of family treatments (Kaufman & Kaufman 1979, Stanton 1980) as well as more innovative therapies such as the one-person family therapy developed by Szapocznik et al (1985).

The special needs of women and their children

Both in Britain and elsewhere, the number of women who misuse a wide variety of psychoactive drugs is believed to be on the increase (UN 1989). Home Office Statistics (1985) indicate that in 1974 a quarter of heroin users were women, while in 1984, the proportion of women had risen to a third. In 1988, 29% of new addicts were women and an increase in the number of young women has been particularly noted (Home Office Statistics 1989). Furthermore, in the UK, as in many other countries, injecting drugs has been a principle route of contracting the HIV virus for women, most of whom are of child-bearing age. Consequently, the number of babies born with the HIV antibodies has been increasing (ACMD 1988). Undoubtedly, official statistics under-represent the number of women opioid drug-misusers and totally ignore those not actually addicted to opioids but misusing a variety of other drugs. There is strong evidence (Dorn & South 1985) to suggest that women are particularly reluctant to make themselves known to the authorities and to approach a treatment agency.

The special needs that women experience have thus remained largely ignored until very recently. The ACMD (1984) has summarised the prevailing view on women's needs: 'in the 1960s and 1970s drug misuse amongst women was not considered an area of particular interest' so that 'researchers and policy-makers have often assumed that hypotheses and policies drawn up in response to male drug-misusers are equally applicable to women ... The women's movement has drawn attention to the need to conceptualise 'social problems' (such as the drug problem) from the point of view of women's interest and position in society'.

Reviewing the literature on the characteristics of drug-abusing women, Burt et al (1979) found few sex-specific differences between men and women drug-takers in demographic and drug-use patterns, but research into the family antecedents of such women reveals certain distinct characteristics. Cuskey & Watney (1982) found that a majority of studies on female addiction reported that a significant number of addicted women were raised by a single parent or another relative, that parents of female addicts were more discordant than parents of non-addicts, and that at least one-quarter of female addicts had experienced sex with a member of their family. Burt et al (1979) concluded that female drug-abusers are more psychologically disturbed than male abusers, while De Leon (1984) found greater evidence of depression and anxiety amongst female than male addicts, and Martin & Martin (1980) reported that 'female addicts appear to be somewhat more neurotic and less psychopathic than male addicts'. Low self-esteem is also commonly observed amongst women addicts, and although it is possible that addiction may lead to low self-esteem, it is also possible that those who already have this characteristic may gravitate towards drugs (Nurco et al 1982).

Treatment problems

Women's difficulties in obtaining relevant help from the existing social agencies are numerous, one of the major reasons being that the treatment system is designed for men. Nadeau (1978) comments that 'when conceived, Therapeutic Centres were an answer to an addiction problem that was primarily shared by men: *the needle world is a man's world*, in which three out of four users are male. The answer to the problem was given within the framework of the men's culture'. Research shows that women need most of the same services as men, but that some services are more important for them than for men. Most prominent is the issue of child care; women cannot use available help for their drug problems if they have no facilities for their children. There is a need for day nursery care for children at centres where their mothers attend for treatment, and for accommodation for both mother and child at residential facilities. Pregnant drug-misusers also need special care; the Medical Working Group on Drug Dependence in Britain (1984) gave guidelines to doctors on helping pregnant drug-takers. Despite this, medical witnesses at the Social Services Committee Hearings on Drug Misuse (1985) noted that: 'we have ... had a number of cases in which pregnant addicts were so scared that their babies would be removed from them by social workers that they went right through pregnancy and delivery without mentioning the fact that they were addicted ... their visitors brought in their drugs secretly and no special attention was paid to their babies'. Although it is certainly true that 'motherhood and addiction do not go very well together' (Densen-Gerber & Rohrs 1973), the conclusion that women addicts invariably make bad mothers is not borne out by research (Rosenbaum 1981). However, the need to support women in the mothering role is crucial to the treatment of women addicts.

Furthermore, the particular psychological problems that have been identified as critical for women drug-misusers require sensitive and specialised interventions. Reed (1981) recommended that services should abandon traditional sex-role stereotyping, which does a disservice to women, and concentrate on helping women develop new means of socialisation and a range of new life skills. Women drug misusers need the provision of nursery care for children at places where they attend for treatment, accommodation for themselves and their children at residential facilities, the establishment of all-female therapeutic communities with a predominance of female staff for those who prefer to be in a women-only therapeutic milieu and much greater emphasis on all-female therapy sessions at existing mixed-sex therapeutic communities.

THE WAY FORWARD

The extent and nature of drug misuse vary from year to year and from place to place. Therefore, a flexible response, governed by a willingness to encompass new issues and new complexities, is needed in tackling the drug problem. So for example, the advent of the HIV virus, its spread in the drug-injecting population and the impact it would make on treatment and service needs could not have been predicted. Yet today the prevention of AIDS has superseded all previous concerns and has become the premier drug treatment goal.

As the difficulties presented by drug misusers may be social, psychiatric or medical, numerous skills and professions must play their part in meeting the needs of these clients. Any integrated community-care approach demands a partnership between specialist and non-specialist medical care and between statutory and non-statutory agencies.

It is important that those working with drug-misusers communicate and learn from others in the helping professions. In turn, drug workers have accumulated experiences in helping troubled people and have developed ideas about systems of care that may well be of use to other community-care workers. In the drugs field, many innovative treatment and rehabilitation models have been successfully implemented. For example, the Therapeutic Communities for drug takers, although they have their roots in the Psychiatric hospital and in the self-help Alcholics Anonymous, have nevertheless developed unique and valuable therapeutic features. Likewise, low threshold outreach programmes have been a notable feature of service development for drug takers. It is crucial that the development of ideas in one field of community care is shared by all in the field.

The importance of training cannot be over-emphasised — training both for those wishing to develop specialist skills and training for those undertaking primary care. To date, the time allocated to drug-misuse training both in medical schools and in social work faculties is derisory.

Finally, the often-made plea for research and evaluation to inform policy choices should be re-iterated. There are too few objective and reliable data about the nature and extent of the drug problem and about the most effective ways of dealing with drug misuse.

REFERENCES

Advisory Council on the Misuse of Drugs (ACMD) 1982 Treatment and rehabilitation. Department of Health and Social Security. HMSO, London
Advisory Council on the Misuse of Drugs (ACMD) 1984 Prevention. HMSO, London
Advisory Council on the Misuse of Drugs (ACMD) 1988 AIDS and drug misuse Part 1. HMSO, London
Advisory Council on the Misuse of Drugs (ACMD) 1989 AIDS and drug misuse Part 2. HMSO, London
Association of Metropolitan Authorities (AMA) 1985 Misuse of drugs: a paper of evidence proposed by the association of Metropolitan Authorities to the House of Commons Social Services Committee. 36 Old Queen Street, London
Beschner G 1985 The problem of adolescent drug abuse: an introduction to intervention strategies. In: Friedman A S, Beschner G (eds) Treatment services for substance abusers. National Institute on Drug Abuse. Maryland, USA
Beschner G M, Treasure K 1979 Female adolescent drug use. In: Beschner G M, Friedman A S (eds), Youth drug abuse: problems issues and treatment. Lexington, Mass: 169-212.
Brodsky M D 1985 History of heroin prevalence estimation techniques. In: Self-report methods of estimating drug use; meeting current challenges of validity. National Institute on Drug Abuse, Research Monograph 57
Brook B C, Whitehead P C 1980 Drug free-therapeutic community — an evaluation. Human Sciences Press, New York.
Brook J S, Whiteman M, Gordon A S, Brenden C 1983 Older brother's influence on younger sibling's drug use. The Journal of Psychology 114: 85-89
Bry B H 1985 Empirical foundations of family based approaches to adolescent substance abuse. In: Glynn T J, Leukefeld C G, Ludford J P (eds) Preventing adolescent drug abuse: intervention and strategies. National Institute on Drug Abuse. Maryland, USA
Burt M, Glynn T, Sowder B 1979 Psychosocial characteristics of drug abusing women. National Institute on Drug Abuse. Maryland, USA
Ch'ien J M M 1981 Evaluation of methadone treatment options. Organization of rehabilitation services for different modalities of drug dependence treatment. In: Man, drugs and society — current perspectives. Proceedings of the First Pan-Pacific Conference on Drugs and Alcohol. Australian Foundation on Alcoholism and Drug Dependence. Canberra, Australia
Cook C C H 1988a The Minnesota model in the management of drug and alcohol dependency: miracle, method or myth? Part I The philosophy and the programme. British Journal of Addiction 83: 625-634
Cook C C H 1988b The Minnesota model in the management of drug and alcohol dependency: miracle, method or myth? Part II Evidence and conclusions. British Journal of Addiction 83: 735-748
Cuskey R W, Watney R B 1982 Female addiction. Lexington Books, D C Heath & Co, Lexington, USA
De Leon G 1974 Phoenix House Psychopathological signs among male and female drug free residents. Journal of Addictive Disease 1: 135-151.
De Leon G 1984 The Therapeutic Community: study of effectiveness. Treatment Research Monograph Series. National Institute on Drug Abuse. Maryland, USA
De Leon G, Deitch D 1985 Treatment of the adolescent substance abuser in a Therapeutic Community. In: Treatment Services for Adolescent Substance Abuse. National Institute on Drug Abuse. Maryland, USA
Densen-Gerber J, Rohrs C 1973 Drug addicted parents and child abuse. Contemporary Drug Problems 2: 683-695

Department of Health & Social Services (DHSS) 1987 Social Services Inspectorate: project on drug misuse. (Unpublished)

Departmental Committee on Morphine & Heroin Addiction 1926. Report. HMSO, London

Dole V P, Nyswander M E 1965 A medical treatment for diacetylmorphine (heroin) addiction. Journal of American Medical Association 193: 645-650

Dole V P, Nyswander M E 1983 Behavioural pharmacology and treatment of human drug abuse — methadone maintenance of narcotic addicts. In: Smith J E, Lane J D (eds) The neurobiology of opiate reward processes. Amsterdam (etc). Elsevier Biomedical Press

Dorn N, James E, Jault N 1987 The limits of informal surveillance; four case studies in identifying neighbourhood heroin problems. ISDD, Research and Development Unit, 1 Hatton Place, London

Dorn N, South N 1985 Helping drug users. Gower Press, London

Edwards G, Arif A (eds) 1980 Drug problems in the sociocultural context. Public Health Papers, 73. World Health Organization, Geneva

Feldman H V, Mandel J, Field A 1985 In the neighbourhood: a strategy for delivering early intervention services to young drug users in their natural environment. In: Treatment services for adolescent substance abusers. National Institute on Drug Abuse. Maryland, USA

Flay R B, Sobel J 1983 The role of mass media in preventing adolescent substance abuse. In: National Institute on Drug Abuse Research Monograph No 47. Maryland, USA

Freeman H 1983 Concepts of community psychiatry. Vol 30. British Journal of Hospital Medicine, August, pp 90-96

Friedman A S, Pomerance E, Sanders R, Santo Y, Utada M 1980 The structure and problems of the families of adolescent drug abusers. Contemporary Drug Problems 9: 327-356

Gabe J, Williams P (eds) 1986 Tranquillisers, social, psychological and clinical perspectives. Tavistock, London

Glanz A, Taylor C 1986 Findings of a national survey of the role of general practitioners in the treatment of opiate misuse: extent of contact with opiate misusers. British Medical Journal 293: 427-430

Hartnoll R, Mitcheson M, Lewis R, Bryer S 1985 Estimating the prevalence of opioid dependence. The Lancet Jan 20: 203-205

Home Affairs Committee 1984–1985 5th Report. Misuse of Hard Drugs (Interim Report). HMSO, London

Home Office 1985 Tackling drug misuse. A summary of the government strategy. HMSO, London

Home Office Statistical Bulletin 1985, 1989 HMSO, London

Hubbard R L, Rachal M S, Craddock G S, Cavanaugh B A 1984 Treatment outcome prospective study (TOPS), client characteristics and behaviours before, during and after treatment. In: Tims F M, Ludford J P (eds) Treatment evaluation: strategies, progress and prospects, National Institute of Drug Abuse, Maryland, USA

Institute for the Study of Drug Dependence (ISDD) 1984. Research Monograph 51 Drugs in health education: trends and issues. Institute for the Study of Drug Dependence, 1 Hatton Garden, London

Interdepartmental Committee on Drug Addiction 1965 Second Report, HMSO, London

Kandel D 1982 Epidemiology and psychosocial perspectives on adolescent drug abuse. Journal of the American Academy of Child Psychiatry 21: 328-347

Kaufman E, Kaufman P N 1979 From a psychodynamic orientation to a structural family therapy approach in the treatment of drug dependence. In: Family therapy of drug and alcohol abuse. Gardner Press Inc., New York

Martin C A, Martin W R 1980 Opiate dependence in women. In: Kalant O J (ed) Alcohol and Drug Problems in Women. Plenum, USA.

Medical Working Group on Drug Dependence 1984 Report. Guidelines for good clinical practice in the treatment of drug misuse. DHSS, London.

Ministry of Welfare, Health and Cultural Affairs 1985 Fact sheet on the Netherlands International relations directorate, Sir W Churchillan 368, Postbus 5406, 2280 HK Rijswijk, Netherlands

Misuse of Drugs Act 1971 HMSO, London

Nadeau L 1978 Women's issues in the therapeutic community: patriarchy and male protection as counter-therapeutic The Addiction Therapist 2(3–4) Pt I: 71–3 Maryland, USA

National Institute on Drug Abuse (NIDA) 1981 Effectiveness of drug abuse treatment programmes. National Institute on Drug Abuse. Maryland, USA

National statements. The socialist Republic of the Union of Burma — Drug Abuse in Burma

National Statement — Malaysia; London 18-20 March. Unpublished

Newcombe M, Hula G, Bentler P 1983 Mothers' influence on the drug use of their children. Confirmatory tests of direct modelling and mediational theories. Developmental Psychology 19: 714-726

Nurco D N, Wegner N, Stephenson P 1982 Female narcotic addicts. Changing profiles. Focus on Women 3: 62-69

Perry L L, Jessor R 1985 Doing the cube: preventing drug abuse through adolescent health promotion. In: Preventing adolescent drug abuse intervention strategies. National Institute on Drug Abuse. Maryland, USA

Reed B G 1981 An Introduction. In: Intervention strategies for drug dependent women. Vol 1. National Institute on Drug Abuse. Maryland, USA

Report of the Conference of Ministers of Health on Narcotics and Psychotrapic Drug Misuse. London 18-20 March 1986. British Journal of Addiction 81: 831-838

Rosenbaum M 1981 Women on heroin. Rutgers University Press, USA

Royal College of Psychiatrists 1987 Drug scenes; a report on drugs and drug dependence. Gaskell, London.

Simpson D D, Sells S B 1982 Effectiveness of treatment for drug abuse: an overview of the DARP research programme. Advances Alcohol Substances Abuse 2: 7-29

Smart C 1985 Drug dependence units in England and Wales. The results of a national survey. Drug and Alcohol Dependence 15: 131-144

Smart R G, Fejer D 1972 Drug use among adolescents and their parents: closing the generation gap in mood modification. Journal of Abnormal Psychology 79: 153-160

Social Services Committee. Session 1984-1985 2nd Report. Community Care. HMSO, London.

Social Services Committee. Session 1984-1985 Misuse of drugs with special reference to treatment and rehabilitation of misusers of hard drugs (4th Report). HMSO, London

Stanton Duncan M 1980 A family theory of drug abuse. In: Theories on drug abuse: selected contemporary perspectives. National Institute on Drug Abuse. Research Monograph Series 30

Stimson G V, Dolan K A, Donoghoe M C, Lart R 1989 The pilot syringe exchange project in England and Scotland — a summary of the evaluation. British Journal of Addiction 84: 1283-1284

Strang J S 1989 A model service: turning the generalist onto drugs. In: MacGregor S (ed) Drugs in British society: responses to a social problem in the 1980s. Routledge, London

Streit F, Halsted D L, Pascale P J 1974 Differences among youthful users and non-users of drugs based on their perceptions of parental behaviour. The International Journal of Addiction 9: 749-755

Szapocznik J, Foote F H, Perez-Vidal A, Hervis O, Kurtins W 1985 One person family therapy. Miami World Health Organisation Collaborating Center for Research and Training in Mental Health, Alcohol and Drug Dependence, Miami, USA

Thorley A 1983 Problem drinkers and drug takers. In: Watts F N, Bennett D H (eds) Theory and Practice of Psychiatric Rehabilitation. John Wiley, London, Chapter 5, pp 83-114

United Nation Economic and Science Council 1989 Commission on narcotic drugs: Situation and trends in drug abuse and the illicit traffic. Vienna, Austria.

Wells B 1987 NA and the Minnesota method in Britain: time to build bridges. Drug Link 2, 1 (8-9). Institute for the Study of Drug Dependence, London

Yablonsky L 1965 The Tunnel Back. Macmillan Company, New York

12. Primary medical care

D. Tantam   D. Goldberg

The purpose of this chapter is to describe the primary care of psychiatric disorder by medical practitioners (GPs) in the United Kingdom. It will focus particularly on the general practitioner (GP) since 'In the United Kingdom...primary medical care is virtually synonymous with general practice' (WHO 1973). However, the general principles which emerge should be relevant, in varying degrees, to all industrialised countries.

The chapter progresses from theory to present practice, and from there to future developments, paying particular attention to the current involvement of British psychiatrists in primary care and to the possibilities for more such involvement in the future. Certain types of psychiatric patient are likely to be referred to psychiatrists and, once referred, to be taken over by the hospital services; however, the collaboration of the GP with the psychiatrists in the care of these patients is not considered here. We have concentrated instead on those patients that are unlikely to be referred on. Neither disorders of childhood nor the problems of the mentally handicapped are considered in this chapter; like alcohol abuse, drug abuse, and the special problems of the elderly, they are dealt with more fully elsewhere in the book.

WHO NEEDS PRIMARY PSYCHIATRIC CARE?

Although most patients on a GP's list consult him or her during the year, it would be wrong to assume that everyone who has psychological symptoms does so, or that everyone who consults a GP should be assumed to be ill. Community surveys in the United States (Hughes & Tremblay 1960, Srole 1962) in the 1950s demonstrated that mild symptoms associated with psychiatric disorder were extremely common: up to 69% of adults were affected in the Stirling County Study. Although dysphoria does occur in association with most psychiatric illnesses (hypomania is a conspicuous exception), it would obviously be unreasonable to suppose that over two-thirds of a community were in poor mental health, unless by 'good health' is meant some idealised notion of best-ever functioning. Most people expect to experience mild, transient symptoms of psychological (and physical) dysfunction in reaction to adversity or stress in everyday life, and do not consult their GP about them. Severe, persistent, or inexplicable symptoms are more likely to be attributed to illness (Ingham & Miller 1976) and therefore to lead to consultation, although the readiness to interpret symptoms as illness is also affected by individual tolerance (Mechanic 1986), by gender (Jenkins 1985), by attitude to the medical profession (Kessel & Shepherd 1965), and by culture.

Recent studies have incorporated some means of distinguishing between sub-clinical disturbance and clinical 'caseness', often so constructed that most psychiatric outpatients are assigned to the group of 'cases'. In recent studies estimates of the point-prevalence of cases of psychiatric illness have ranged from 9% to 20% of the population at risk, (see Goldberg & Huxley 1980 for details); most of these cases will only have symptoms related to depression or anxiety. Depression is the single most common psychiatric disorder, both in the community and in the general practitioner's surgery. Anxiety-related symptoms often predominate in new episodes of illness, but if new symptoms persist, it is usual for depressive symptoms to appear in addition to those of anxiety (Goldberg & Bridges 1985). The prevalence of alcoholism, drug abuse, personality disorder, and organic brain syndromes such as dementia are also affected by the cut-off point chosen for clinically significant disorder, but these conditions may be diagnosable in a substantial minority of community cases. The functional psychoses, which form such an important part of the work of psychiatrists, are diagnosable in only a small percentage of community cases.

About two-thirds of depressive illnesses or anxiety states will remit within six months, but the remainder will run a more protracted course, and some will become chronic. These illnesses have been shown to be associated with adverse social circumstances; they have been called 'chronic neuroses' in the United Kingdom and more recently 'dysthymic disorders' in the United States. The likelihood of remission of these conditions becomes progressively reduced as they become more chronic (see Harvey-Smith & Cooper 1970); chronic illnesses have rather different clinical characteristics, tending to be more mixed than acute illnesses in their symptomatology. The frequency of associated social problems and of mixed disorders will therefore be greater if the prevalence (the total number of cases in the population and for the period of study) of diagnosable psychiatric illness is examined than if only inceptions (onsets of new episodes of illness from the population and during the period of study) are considered.

WHO CONSULTS THEIR GENERAL PRACTITIONER?

It was thought at one time that there were substantial numbers of moderately or severely dysphoric individuals who did not seek medical help, but there are now grounds for treating this assertion with reserve (Goldberg & Huxley 1980), at least in the United Kingdom, where medical care is free. Community surveys of depressive illness have shown that the majority of depressed people had been seen by their GP during the illness, although they had often sought help for somatic symptoms or symptoms of an unrelated physical illness, and the depression had not been diagnosed. One reason for this high rate of consultation is that by the time depression is sufficiently severe for a research diagnosis to be made, the patient is likely to be feeling unwell, to be sleeping poorly, and to be experiencing various bodily pains and discomforts.

In addition to these groups of individuals with diagnosable disorders, there are many other patients who consult their GP with psychological complaints, but who fail to reach the criteria for a research diagnosis. Some have sufficient symptoms to do so, but these clinical features have not yet lasted long enough to satisfy research requirements; others have non-specific symptoms such as tiredness, insomnia, or irritability, which do not meet the requirements for a syndromal diagnosis. In short, a psychiatric illness can be 'sub-clinical' either because of transience or because of insufficient severity. Such patients present primary practitioners with an exquisite dilemma, since although most of their disorders are likely to remit, some will last long enough or will deteriorate sufficiently to become diagnosable. In the DSM-III system, depressive symptoms must last two weeks, and anxiety-related symptoms four weeks, before the clinician is allowed to diagnose 'major depressive disorder' or 'generalised anxiety disorder' respectively. Yet a clinician faced with a man who has a one-week history of severe depressive illness accompanied by suicidal ideas is unlikely to want to wait another week before providing antidepressant treatment. In practice, primary practitioners ignore the time requirements for psychiatric diagnoses, and they are right to do so, whereas the research psychiatrist will usually describe severe mood disorders of short duration as 'adjustment disorders', and will only revise this diagnosis if the disorder persists.

THE DETECTION OF PSYCHIATRIC ILLNESS BY FAMILY DOCTORS

There is a case for arguing that the answer one gets to the question 'Is this a disease?' is really a covert answer to the question 'Should this person be under medical care?' (Kendell 1975): that diagnosis is a 'disguised plan of action' (ibid). Similarly, the availability of a particular type of medical care may affect the symptoms which are selected by the doctor for diagnostic consideration (Howie 1972). In a recent study, Jenkins (1985) showed videotapes of general practice consultations to a panel of experienced GPs, many of whom were familiar with the problem of under-detection of psychiatric morbidity in general practice. The authors found an extremely low level of diagnostic agreement, and quoted with approval Marinker's (1967) observation that a GP's classification of disorder is not a record of the morbidity of the practice population. It is a record of the morbidity that the doctor fancies he sees: it represents the way in which the doctor has organised the 'unorganised illness which is presented to him'.

Three considerations may influence how the GP organises the illness presented to him or her: the availability of a treatment likely to be effective, the legitimation of illness, and the inference of disease. Although these different criteria overlap, they are unfortunately neither co-terminous with each other nor with the research-orientated diagnostic categories already mentioned (see Brown et al 1985, for a detailed discussion of this in relation to depression).

If the GP is inclined to ignore the example of mild hypertension, and so restricts diagnosis to those conditions which are associated with symptoms which are clearly abnormal, it is likely that depression will be restricted to melancholia, and that anxiety states will be rarely, if ever diagnosed. If diagnosis is required to legitimate an assumption of the role of an ill person, then only complainers will tend to be diagnosed. Diagnosis by the availability of treatment will result in considerable variations in practice, depending on an individual practitioner's skill and familiarity with suitable therapeutic techniques, and on the development and marketing of new treatments. If the doctor considered that discussion and listening were effective treatments then, since depressed patients often do benefit from both of these, a depressive diagnosis would be given to a very large number of general practice attenders, including some that would be borderline or even sub-clinical cases according to research diagnoses. On the other hand, a more restricted conception of treatment would result in a more restricted conception of the scope of diagnosis.

In these circumstances, it might be argued that there is no good reason to prefer one conception of illness over another. This would be true if GPs were shown to be consistent in their use of diagnoses, and if it could be shown that these diagnoses led to the most effective treatment decisions. We have just considered evidence that agreement between GPs over the same or similar cases is low; below, we shall consider evidence that the cases that GPs miss are just as likely to benefit from treatment as the cases that they diagnose. Although a symptom score may not be the only axis which should be considered in determining illness in general practice — a physical health axis, a personality axis, and a social burden axis all have their proponents — it remains the best guide for psychological or psychotropic treatment, and the standardised methods of deriving diagnoses from symptom scores which are currently used in research, offer the best standard by which to judge the detection of psychiatric illness.

Analysis of video recordings of general practice consultations surprisingly shows that over half of the patients who had reported many symptoms of psychological distress on a screening questionnaire, given before the consultation, neither mentioned these symptoms to the doctor nor appeared obviously distressed to observers. However, approximately a third of the patients who had previously reported distress repeatedly referred to their psychological symptoms in the consultation, or appeared obviously distressed to observers, and yet the GP made no response to these cues of possible psychiatric illness (Davenport et al 1987). This confirms the previous findings of one of us in the United States that doctors who fail to diagnose psychiatric illness when it is present also tend to miss both verbal and non-verbal cues of distress during the medical interviews (for a general account, see Goldberg & Huxley 1980). Other reasons for the failure to detect disorder include the doctor not having an accurate concept of psychiatric illness, and being so pre-occupied with patients' often inexplicable physical symptoms that the accompanying psychological symptoms are overlooked.

Though GPs have usually received little formal instruction from psychiatrists, the difficult task of detecting disorder usually falls to them. Their task is made more difficult by the brevity of most consultations and by the fact that most psychiatrically disturbed patients are consulting for physical symptoms and that, as already noted, many of those with a high score on the screening questionnaire will not strike an independent observer as abnormal.

Family doctors vary widely in their ability to detect such disorders, with some picking up almost all the cases and others missing most of them. Earlier research showed that on average, about 45% of such illnesses were missed by a large group of GPs in Manchester (Marks et al 1979), and that as many as 80% of cases diagnosable by the RDC system in the USA were not picked up by family physicians in Madison, Wisconsin (Hoeper et al 1979). More recently, Sireling et al (1985) have shown that London GPs failed to make a psychiatric diagnosis in 28% of surgery attenders who met RDC criteria for major depression.

THE MANAGEMENT OF PSYCHIATRIC ILLNESS IN PRIMARY CARE SETTINGS

Many — perhaps most — of the diagnosable psychiatric illnesses do not require specific medical or psychological treatment, and therefore probably do not benefit from being 'labelled'. However, some do respond to therapy from the doctor or his staff, and sometimes a diagnosis can lead to a beneficial social intervention. A few patients do not wish any action to be taken, and another group only need recognition of their symptoms and a discussion about them. These categories are a useful basis for a classification of primary care patients.

Group 1. Those requiring specific medical treatments

Patients with major psychotic illnesses such as schizophrenia, hypomania, and melancholia are sometimes seen in primary care settings, but they account for a very small proportion of those with diagnosable psychiatric disorders who attend: less than 5% in one large study (Goldberg 1979). If we confine ourselves to those psychiatric cases recognised by GPs and prepared to be interviewed by a psychiatrist, the proportion with psychotic illnesses rises, but is still only 20.5% (Casey et al 1984).

The most common indications for drug treatment are anxiety and depression, but there has been recent concern about the steady rise in the prescription of both antidepressants and benzodiazepine anxiolytics (Williams 1980), which were used at least once in a fortnight by 1 in 10 people in a general population survey (Murray 1981). GPs differ widely in the freedom with which they prescribe psychotropics (Fleming & Cross 1984), suggesting that there is no consensus about the indications for treatment. This reflects a lack of adequate hard data about the efficacy of these drugs for the bulk of the distressed patients presenting to GPs.

In the case of depression, it is not known how many depressive symptoms have to be present before a significant drug/placebo difference can be demonstrated in primary care settings, but it is unwise to suppose that what is true of depressive illnesses seen by psychiatrists is necessarily true of those seen in general practice. Depressed patients seen by psychiatrists will typically have more abnormal personalities and less advantageous social circumstances than those seen in community settings, and thus be less likely to recover without treatment. The belief that many British GPs have in the efficacy of what psychiatrists would regard as homeopathic doses of antidepressants (Johnson 1973, 1974) may probably be explained by the fact that most depressive illnesses seen in this setting are self-limiting disorders with a high spontaneous remission rate.

Obviously, a depression which is already showing a tendency to remit before the patient consults the GP can be managed expectantly, but the patient who presents so acutely that the effects of time cannot be gauged presents a management difficulty. Two clinical characteristics (neurovegetative symptoms (Bielski & Friedel 1976) and depressive self-attributions) may be helpful in predicting persistence of depression, and one (reactivity of the mood to circumstance) may indicate the likelihood of spontaneous resolution, although we can find no reference in the literature to this. In the absence of more precise information, patients with a depressive illness should be given antidepressants if:

(a) There is a change in their self-concept, characterised by ideas of inferiority, guilt and self-blame, or

(b) There are pronounced neurovegetative symptoms, such as early morning waking, diurnal variation of mood, retardation of thought and movement, and loss of energy, libido, appetite and weight.

Group 1 disorders, including the type of depressive illness just described, require medical treatment because they are not likely to remit in response to social or psychological interventions. It may be that the symptoms of these disorders, like those of physical illnesses, are usually caused by a derangement of the body or brain: they certainly seem more similar in type to physical illnesses than do the other groups of disorders, considered below.

Since the symptoms of a group 1 illness cannot be improved by an effort of will or by exhortation from others, it follows that patients with these disorders may be less responsible for their behaviour, if this behaviour is symptomatic of their illness, than are patients without such an illness. It also follows that it is appropriate to encourage a patient with a group 1 disorder to adopt a sick role, for example in putting off decisions and in relinquishing duties: this advice is not usually given to patients with other types of psychiatric illness.

Many patients with depression, however, do not have the specific features mentioned above, and would not be placed in this first group. For example, many patients who recover in the first week of antidepressant treatment do not belong in the group; they should be considered to be placebo-responders, and the drug cautiously withdrawn.

Anxiety states, which rarely require specific medical treatment, do not belong in group 1, but in group 2, along with other disorders which benefit from specific psychological treatments.

Group 2. Those benefiting from specific psychological treatment

Group 2 disorders, although often associated with anxiety, are typified by their response to psychological treatments directed to the alteration of habitual behaviours or judgements. Anorexia nervosa, bulimia, phobic neuroses, obsessional disorder, substance abuse (excluding its medical consequences), some sexual disorders, some sleep disorders, and many states of anxiety are examples.

Group 2 contains many disorders whose symptoms are temporarily relieved by the sedative action of psychotropic drugs; indeed, these drugs may have a limited part to play as adjuvants to other treatments. However, they should not be the mainstay of treatment: sedation is only a short-term solution, since tolerance and a disappearance of the pharmacological effect occur with long-term use (Committee on the Review of Medicines 1980). Moreover, all benzodiazepines are now known to have the potential to induce both psychological and physical dependence; although for reasons that are not clearly understood, some of them are worse than others in this respect.

Psychological treatment does not have these disadvantages and has been shown to be equally effective (Catalan et al 1984). In that study, brief counselling given by family doctors was as helpful as the prescription of anxiolytics for patients with a recent onset of anxiety symptoms (over 75% of whom were threshold or definite cases, i.e. at level 5 or above on the Index of Definition) in general practice. The length of the consultation and the number of subsequent visits did not differ in the two groups, nor was there any evidence that self-medication was increased in the group not treated with drugs. However, a minority of the non-drug treated group did require psychotropic medication during the follow-up period: these may have been patients who became depressed — an evolution which is common in long-standing anxiety (Goldberg & Bridges 1985).

All patients in groups 1 and 2 can be offered a medical or psychological treatment of proven value. The patient should be told what is wrong with him, what the treatment is, and what can be expected from it. 'Labelling' of the condition makes a positive contribution to the treatment by increasing compliance, although the presentation of the label will differ in groups 1 and 2. We would not hesitate to tell patients in group 1 that they are ill. We would be more likely to tell patients in group 2 that they have a problem, shared by many other people, which they need to master, with the help of various techniques which we can teach them if they wish.

The delineation of the problem is an important part of the treatment of group 2 disorders. For instance, treatment of bulimia can begin when the pattern of binging and vomiting is laid bare to both doctor and patient. Once this step has been taken, the choice of psychological treatment will depend on whether the primary abnormality is: a repeated or persistent feeling, in which case a counselling approach may be indicated; a repetitive thought, which may respond to an approach along cognitive therapy lines (Beck 1976); or a habitual, unwanted behaviour, which may be altered by the various strategies of behavioural treatment.

Group 3. Those requiring supportive therapy and social intervention

Included here are patients with long-standing disabilities, including those with cerebral damage or dementia; some patients with chronic dysphoria should also be included. These patients will often also suffer from chronic ill-health (Eastwood & Trevelyan 1972), a chronically unsatisfactory social situation (Kedward 1969), or a personality disorder.

Drugs are not likely to produce cure in any of these patients, and they should therefore be used sparingly. A major principle of treatment is the encouragement of normal coping strategies, with the avoidance of any treatment which will reduce self-reliance; drugs which induce dependence should be particularly avoided.

The doctor will need to develop a skill which may well have been omitted from his training at medical school; to be able to listen to the expression of distress or pain without impatience, even when to respond with an investigation or a pill would be inappropriate. Social assistance is of particular importance in the management of the patients in this group: this may be provided by a social worker or, in the form of relief admission to hospital, by the doctor himself.

Chronic social stress is often the product of numerous interlocked social problems, but sometimes a specific marital or family disappointment or conflict is the principal contributor, and marital or family therapy may then be helpful.

Personality disorder may be a cause of chronic dysphoria, usually because the individual concerned is unable to make stable and satisfying social relationships. Significant beneficial personality change can sometimes be produced by long-term psychotherapy, but this treatment can rarely, if ever, be carried out by the GP.

Group 4. Those requiring only recognition and discussion of problems

Every psychiatrically ill patient benefits from the recognition of the illness by the GP and from the discussion which follows from that recognition. This discussion may reveal the need for one of the treatments or social interventions appropriate for one of the three groups of patients described above. A fourth group of patients will need no further intervention beyond recognition and discussion.

The substantial proportion of subjects whose illnesses remit on placebo in drug trials carried out in community settings assures us that these patients are numerous. One GP found that the majority of his psychiatrically disordered patients could be effectively treated by recognition, discussion, the prescription of a placebo, and the offer of a return visit (Thomas 1974). Remission of the symptoms of patients in group 4 may be hastened if they are given a psychotropic or minor sedative drug; but this is because of an increase in hope and the expectation of improvement. Since there are negative effects for patients in this group being identified as being psychiatrically ill, it is usually better if they are regarded as being 'distressed'.

Group 5. Those requiring no action from the doctor or his staff

A small group of patients are aware that they are psychologically unwell, and often know all too well why they are distressed, and prefer not to discuss their problems with the doctor. They may be seeking treatment for problems unrelated to their psychiatric illness, or else reassurance that the somatic manifestations of their psychiatric illness are psychological in origin and do not presage serious physical illness. Their privacy should be respected, although an open door should be left, in case they change their minds.

MANAGEMENT

Drugs

The indications for drug treatment have been considered in the previous section.

Some of the new antidepressants have advantages over the old in the general practice setting, since they have less intrinsic anticholinergic effect. They are in consequence safer in overdose, may be less likely to produce the more serious complications of the older tricyclics such as arrhythmia (although they may be responsible for new ones which are only now becoming apparent as the amounts of the drug prescribed increase), and may be more acceptable to the patient because of fewer unwanted effects like a dry mouth. The latter is an important consideration in general practice, since many patients in this setting stop taking their antidepressants before the end of the prescribed course. Trazodone and mianserin have the added property of sedation, which may be capitalised upon in some patients who would otherwise require a hypnotic, but may also cause unacceptable drowsiness in others, even in very low doses. Fluoxetine and lofepramine do not have these sedative properties.

Selective monoamine oxidase inhibitors (MAOIs), with an antidepressant but no tyramine pressor effect, are not yet fully evaluated clinically. MAOIs therefore, continue to have a restricted place in treatment, although they are reported to be especially effective in mixed anxiety and depression and in atypical depression — disorders which are more likely to be found in general practice than in psychiatric practice. The use of MAOIs has been reviewed by Pare (1985) and by Nutt & Glue (1989).

The publication of a restricted list of benzodiazepines prescribable under the National Health Service in the United Kingdom has simplified the selection of a suitable preparation. Those used in the treatment of epilepsy apart, an adequate repertoire consists of a short-acting agent, such as temazepam or triazolam, for the induction of sleep and the short-term relief of anxiety, and one or more longer-acting agents. There is a suggestion that some of these, such as lorazepam, are more likely to lead to dependence than others. There is a place for non-benzodiazepine sedatives, for example in the elderly or during alcohol withdrawal, but they have the disadvantage of being much more dangerous in overdose. Neuroleptics in low doses do have an anxiolytic effect, but carry the risk of tardive dyskinesia if used long-term.

Behaviour therapy and cognitive therapy

Psychological treatments may be indicated for the management of anxiety and depression, as already noted. Cognitive therapy given by trained therapists has been shown to be equally as effective as tricyclics in the treatment of depression in general practice (Blackburn et al 1981), and to increase the response of depressed patients to their GP's usual treatment (Teasdale et al 1984).

Anxiety management techniques such as progressive muscular relaxation and breathing control, which may be guided by a pre-recorded instructional tape, occupy an increasingly important place in the treatment of anxiety, and their emphasis on self-help makes them particularly appropriate to general practice. Cognitive therapy is also applicable to the general practice situation, especially during the early stages of drug treatment of depression, before the antidepressant effect has fully developed, and in the treatment of depression arising in the setting of low self-esteem. Doctors have been reluctant up to now to undertake such treatment themselves, possibly because they have lacked training and experience in it.

Referral to other members of the 'primary health care team'

Although the term 'primary care team' has become popular, patients still consult their GP in the first instance, even if another professional shares the same practice premises. Several possibilities of collaboration with other professionals exists, however, which may affect the GP's work, directly or indirectly. Patients may be referred on for treatment (sometimes termed the annexation model), may be the subject of a consultation but with the GP carrying out the treatment, or may be treated by both the GP and specialist in collaboration.

The social worker

In the study of Catalan et al (1984), the chronicity of symptoms seemed the be a factor in determining whether patients eventually received drugs; it is a factor which has been shown in other studies to increase the likelihood of the identification of psychiatric disorder, the prescription of drugs, and psychiatric referral. Patients with chronic neurotic disorders in general practice tend to have chronic social difficulties (Sylph et al 1969, Cooper 1972), and their disorders tend to persist until the difficulties resolve (Kedward 1969). It has therefore been a logical development that social workers should have become attached to some general practices, and although this arrangement has spread slowly, 50% of local authorities in the United Kingdom already had at least one social worker attached to a general practice in their area by the end of the 1970s (Gilchrist et al 1978).

Social work is discussed in another chapter. It has been shown to be effective in reducing the severity of symptoms and improving the social circumstances of chronically disordered patients (Cooper et al, 1975), but not of the majority of acutely distressed female patients (Corney 1984): those who did benefit had practical problems on which the social worker could make some impact. A particular advantage of social workers being attached to general practices, as against being available for contact at an area office or on a visit (the liaison model), is that they may receive more referrals from health visitors of people who 'may not be physically or mentally ill or disturbed, but may still need help with other types of problems — for example the young mother who cannot cope with her children or who is suffering from social isolation' (Corney & Briscoe 1977).

Clinical psychologists

The attachment of clinical psychologists to general practices has also grown in recent years, but there is inadequate evidence as yet on which to base an evaluation of their impact on the work of family doctors. In one study, 30 GPs were asked to rank health care professionals according to what they offered such a doctor. Professionals with a nursing background, including community psychiatric nurses, received the highest ranks while psychologists achieved equal rankings with psychiatrists and social workers (Eastman & McPherson 1982). Twenty-five of the 30 GPs in the survey were 'sympathetic' to having a clinical psychologist involved in their practice, 88% of them expected the psychologist to provide therapy, but only 12% expected advice on management.

It is unlikely that clinical psychologists in the United Kingdom will ever become primary practitioners unless their numbers greatly increase and unless there is a considerable change of public attitude from the present one that a doctor should be the first professional consulted by anyone who suspects themselves, or is suspected of being ill. However, more and more psychologists are taking direct referrals from GPs. Psychological techniques have a definite place in the management of acute mood disorders, and these techniques have advantages over the use of drugs, particularly in the treatment of anxiety.

The relatively small number of clinical psychologists practising in the United Kingdom could not treat all the patients who would benefit from a specific psychological treatment, and it is uncertain how their skills can best be deployed. Freeman & Button (1984) pessimistically concluded that the wrong patients had been referred: they were mainly chronically dysphoric people. Salmon (1984) suggested that the 'annexation' model of psychologists treating some of the GP's patients was the wrong one, and that psychologists should concentrate on training.

Community psychiatric nurses and nurse-therapists

The nurse-practitioner, who sees patients in parallel with the GP, stands more chance of becoming a routine sight in British general practices than any other non-medical primary care professional. Nurses and health visitors already provide some first-line care to particular groups such as mothers of young children, the elderly, and the disabled — all groups whose circumstances make visits to the doctor more than usually inconvenient. Nurses can undertake regular domiciliary visiting to these groups, whilst their medical colleagues have decreased the amount of time for such work in favour of regular clinics at the health centres.

It has been shown that nurses can successfully treat neurotic disorders (Paykel et al 1982, Marks et al 1977), but the high spontaneous remission rate of such disorders has led some psychiatrists to question whether this is the most valuable use of a health professional's time. Community psychiatric nurses have a particular role to play in the supervision and support of the psychiatrically disabled patient, although their impact on the care of patients with long-standing schizophrenia has been disappointing (Hunter 1978, Wooff et al 1983).

THE VIEW FROM THE SURGERY

Psychiatrists studying primary health care have repeatedly shown that psychiatrically ill patients may go undetected by their family doctor. One important reason for this is that general practice patients rarely complain of psychological symptoms alone: only 7.8% did so in a consecutive series of 553 at one English practice (Goldberg & Blackwell 1970) and, surprisingly, even fewer (3%) from a similar series in the United States (Goldberg et al 1976a).

In a series of 588 new episodes of illness in 15 general practices, Bridges & Goldberg (1985) showed that a psychiatric diagnosis according to DSM-III criteria could be made in 33% of the patients. Patients whose illnesses consisted entirely of psychological symptoms accounted for only 14% of those with a psychiatric diagnosis (4.5% of all those with new illnesses), but such illnesses were understandably well detected by the GPs, who made psychiatric diagnoses in 95% of this group.

The remaining patients with psychiatric illnesses were presenting somatic symptoms to their doctors, and these symptoms were often part of a physical illness which the patients were known to have. Since the psychiatric illness appeared to be unrelated to this other illness in about 24%, the failure of the doctor to detect it was understandable. A further small group of 3% had psychiatric illnesses secondary to physical illnesses: for example, being anxious about possible implications of rectal bleeding, or depressed during a course of radiotherapy for breast cancer.

The largest group — 59% of those with psychiatric diagnoses, or 19.5% of all new illnesses — consisted of patients who were somatising their psychiatric illness, i.e. the patient consulted for somatic symptoms, and did not consider that he or she was psychiatrically ill. However, psychiatric *symptoms* were reported in sufficient numbers and duration for a research diagnosis of psychiatric illness to be made, and the interviewing psychiatrist considered that there was a relationship between this illness and the somatic symptoms for which help was sought. The relationship might be that the somatic symptoms were part of the psychiatric illness, or that they were exacerbated by it: in either case, psychological treatment might be expected to be helpful to them.

There are many reasons why patients are more likely to have complained of somatic, rather than psychological symptoms. Pains have a greater salience than other symptoms, not only because they hurt, but because of their symbolic meaning. Some people are so concerned about the possibility that their somatic symptoms may be caused by physical disease that they regard the doctor's role as being exhausted by the exclusion of organic causes for their pains; many GPs take the same view, and thus confine their interviews to asking many closed questions which related to possible physical causes of their patients' symptoms. Other patients differentially report somatic symptoms because of the stigma of psychological illness, feeling that their physical symptoms will be better received both by their families and by their doctor. It is also common for affective illness to exacerbate the pains of known organic disease: in this case, the patient presents symptoms of the known disease to his/her doctor, knowing that such symptoms are acceptable to him or her, but not always having made the connection of the worsening of these symptoms with the other symptoms of mood disorder.

Family doctors may miss psychiatric disorders for two reasons: either they make very few psychiatric diagnoses, relative to the number of symptomatic patients that they see (low 'bias' towards psychiatric diagnosis), or else they are just poor judges of psychological distress (low 'accuracy'). Each of these is determined by different factors.

Doctors with a low bias often have little interest in psychiatry, and in their interviews, tend to skirt questions about emotional reactions or the patient's home and family. They are not empathic as interviewers, and tend to ignore both verbal and non-verbal indications of distress. In one American survey, low bias was shown to be associated with each of the following factors: high-status doctors, working in leisurely surroundings, seeing patients of the same race as themselves, and being paid out of private health insurance.

Accuracy is determined by factors which partly overlap with those affecting bias. As one might expect, inaccurate doctors share with low-bias doctors a lack of empathy, a low use of psychological questions, and a lack of response to indications of psychological illness. However, they also avoid eye-contact with their patients, fail to clarify the presenting complaint, ask too many closed questions, and are generally poor interviewers. In addition, they tend to be less confident and to be less well-informed about internal medicine than other doctors. (For further details relevant to this section, see Goldberg & Huxley 1980, and Ch. 4).

The value of detection has been demonstrated in two research studies. In both studies (Johnstone & Goldberg 1976, Zung et al 1984), patients were screened after a first medical consultation, and the results fed back to the doctor in half the cases. Improvement in mood was more rapid in those cases to whom the doctor's attention had been drawn than it was in the controls, even if drug treatment was not thought to be indicated.

THE UNDERSERVED AND THE OVERSERVED

It has already been noted that a majority of adults in Britain consult their GP during the course of a year, and that there is thus a considerable likelihood that a consultation will be made about a new episode of psychiatric disorder. Brown & Harris (1978), for example, found in their survey of Camberwell women that 68% of those who had recently developed depression had consulted their GP. These high consultation figures indicate why the family doctor is so important a figure in British community medicine.

However, 32% of depressed women did not attend their GP, citing practical difficulties, e.g. with young children, as one of their reasons (see also Goldberg et al 1976b). Other reasons for non-consultation may be the expectation that the GP is not interested in psychiatric problems (Dunn 1983), or that he/she will be unsympathetic. An aversion to self-assertion may also be a factor for some immigrant groups, and for some of the psychiatrically disabled. Other groups which have a high non-consultation rate include homeless people, some drug- and alcohol-abusers, and some of the elderly.

The primary care of the chronically, psychiatrically disabled used to be the responsibility of the institution in which many of them lived. It is widely feared that the implementation of policies of deinstitutionalisation, at a time when 'the services for the mentally ill outside hospital are totally inadequate in many parts of the country' (Statement Agreed by National Schizophrenia Fellowship and Richmond Fellowship 1984), has resulted in an unacceptably high level of morbidity, and consequent personal and familial distress. Even in an area where local psychiatrists have considerable interest in and expert knowledge of community psychiatry, 17% of patients with chronic schizophrenia had been lost to follow-up in less than two years, and the majority of the remainder had 'neurotic symptoms', often associated with complaints of social isolation (Cheadle et al 1978). Similar results have been obtained in other areas (see for example, Curson et al 1985). The responsibility for such psychiatrically disabled patients falls between the hospital services and primary care as well as social services. Although chronically psychotic patients benefit from the regular assessment provided by a hospital outpatient clinic, the psychiatrist that they see, often a junior doctor on rotation, may be ignorant of those details of their personal lives which are important in assessing social function, quality of life, and burden on others.

There is also a pressure on hospital departments to discharge patients who are stable. Keane & Fahy (1982), for example, bemoan the 'silting-up of a new area service... by patients with a combination of social disadvantage and severe chronic psychosis'. However, too often the catch-phrase 'back to the care of the GP' in the discharge letter takes no account of the reluctance of most family doctors to follow-up patients who do not present to the surgery for treatment. GPs are well-placed to provide a community care service for the chronically, psychiatrically disabled, but this cannot be done adequately on the reactive basis of most of their consultations. There are precedents for regular assessment being made part of the routine of general practice, for example in the 'shared care' of pregnant women, and a similar scheme could be provided for the chronically disabled.

Psychiatrists have, however, often considered that the treatment of psychosis is one of their core activities. A report of the Royal College of Psychiatrists (1980) on psychiatric rehabilitation, which focussed especially on the needs of the chronically psychotic, recommended that each disabled patient in a district should be identified and the progress of his case tracked by a key-worker. The supervision of this system, as well as the planning and development of new resources, would be the responsibility of a rehabilitation group; the recommended core member-ship of this group did not include a GP, but the report itself gives family doctors a role, albeit a subsidiary one, in providing long-term care.

Community psychiatric nurses have been hailed as a solution to this medical demarcation problem (Conway-Nicholls & Elliott 1982) it being originally assumed that their work would mainly be with the psychiatrically disabled. This seems to be the case in at least one area (Wooff et al 1983), but it remains to be seen whether the community psychiatric nurse can be the 'key-worker' that the college report recommends.

EXPERIENCE IN OTHER COUNTRIES AND ALTERNATIVE MODELS OF SERVICE

Although there have been considerable changes in the practice of primary care in the United Kingdom in the last 20 years (Hicks, 1976) and a shift in psychiatry towards reduced inpatient stay, as well as more day- and out-patient treatment, the GP remains the first point of contact for most ordinary people.

Some other countries, however, have developed health care systems in which a greater amount of primary care is provided by specialist mental health workers, such as psychologists and psychiatrists. The greatest range of types of service delivery is probably to be seen in the United States, and in recent, more cost-conscious years, that country has also provided some of the most detailed evaluations of health care. Though these are reviewed in another chapter of this book (Ch.19), some are particularly relevant to future developments of primary care services elsewhere, and will be considered here.

The prevalence of psychiatric disorder in the United States is probably the same as in the United Kingdom, but the much lower proportion of GPs (or 'family physicians') means that a considerable portion of first-line care is provided by specialists (paediatricians, physicians, and psychiatrists). The greater numbers of psychiatrists also mean that about 50% more of the population (3% according to Brown et al 1977) are seeing a psychiatrist at any one time. Although many more patients are referred to psychiatrists than in the United Kingdom, they are still the minority of people with psychiatric disorder: it has been estimated that only 46% of North Americans with a psychiatric disorder are referred to a mental health specialist (Regier et al 1978), and that only 24% are referred to psychiatrists (Brown et al 1977). As in the UK (Shepherd et al 1981, Whitfield & Winter 1980), the most common reason given for non-referral in an American survey was patient resistance, but the scarcity of psychiatric resources was also given as a reason by 25%, and lack of confidence in the services available by a slightly greater proportion (28%) (Orleans et al 1985).

Patients with psychoses are selectively referred to psychiatrists in the United States, as they are in the United Kingdom (Tantam & Burns 1979), but the majority of psychiatrically ill patients are treated by non-psychiatric medical specialists, who can expect 15% of their patients to have a psychiatric disorder (Regier et al 1978), to make a psychiatric diagnosis in 5%, and to give 12% psychotropics (Brown et al 1977).

The greater availability on average, of psychiatrists in the United States has not therefore resulted in a greatly different situation from that in the United Kingdom, in that most patients still consult a doctor identified with the treatment of bodily disorder for the treatment of a psychiatric disorder, and that these doctors make a diagnosis in the minority and use psychotropics in the majority. The increase in the numbers of clinical psychologists may, however, make for a wider range of treatment options for some patients in the future.

The importance of psychological treatment in the prevention of disorder or subsequent disability is a major raison d'etre of the community mental health centre and its satellite clinics. These centres were conceived to be providers of primary psychiatric care. Their evolution has been towards increasingly close links with general hospitals, with a function somewhat analogous to the District General Hospital psychiatric unit in the UK: their intended impact on 'prevention' has never been documented, however, while the long-term care of the psychiatrically disabled often remains the responsibility of the state hospital, if it is accepted as a responsibility of any particular agency at all.

THE CONTRIBUTION OF THE PSYCHIATRIST TO PRIMARY MEDICAL CARE

One version of the GP has him as an obstinate gate-keeper, obstructing patients who wish to see a psychiatrist or who wish to receive more extensive treatment than most family doctors can provide. Such thoughts have lain behind the development of at least one community mental health centre (Bouras & Brough 1982). Though this concept is an alternative of great interest, it has so far been slow to develop in the United Kingdom. Most new attenders at the centres which have published their statistics are referred by their family doctors, and there has been little hard evidence that the service provided, although liked by its consumers, does in fact substantially reduce morbidity, when compared to primary care by the family doctor. Most patients using such services are probably at or below the borderline of diagnosable illness, and are likely to recover without specific treatment. It is perhaps desirable to have an alternative, to which distressed people may turn if they do not gain satisfaction from their GP, and these centres may turn out to be valuable facilities for such secondary referral and treatment. However, mental health professionals attached to primary care teams might provide the same benefit.

Mental health centres are unlikely ever to provide much primary psychiatric care in the United Kingdom, and they do not tackle the problems of primary care that have been identified in this chapter: its lack of provision to the psychiatrically disabled, and the under-detection of distress, especially when it co-exists with physical disorder. It is possible that they might make some contribution to the prevention of chronic neurotic disability, but the antecedents of this disability, and even its prediction in acutely distressed patients, seem to be more social than psychiatric. Whether a professional intervention is likely to be effective in such cases needs some sceptical evaluation.

Rapidly available domiciliary assessment services, to which the GP can make an urgent referral, (one such has also been developed in Lewisham alongside the community mental health centre, but they also exist in many other places) have an immediate attraction as a means of expediting psychiatric treatment for a disturbed patient, as delay in psychiatric assessment may be a significant cause of distress or danger. However, they may not be so effective in actual practice. GPs in one area preferred to use a conventional domiciliary visiting service (Smout et al 1983), perhaps because of initial bad publicity, which resulted from these teams making use of inexperienced staff and having a bias against admitting patients to hospital.

The highly selective nature of referral to psychiatrists (only 5.1% of psychiatric cases identified during the survey year by their GPs were also seen by a psychiatrist in the early 1960s: see Shepherd et al 1981) has focussed attention on the selection of patients, with a view to considering whether GPs make their selection on the most effective basis. Factitious factors such as the patient's sex and social class do influence referral, but particular symptoms are also an important determinant. Brown et at (1985), on the basis of a community study, suggest that although there is little difference in the severity of symptoms between depressed patients who are or are not referred, that referral is more likely if the patients express suicidal ideas. There has been no study in which a high rate of referral was experimentally compared against a low rate, and so evidence on which to base a definite judgement about the value or otherwise of increased referral is lacking.

In Britain, the availability of psychiatrists is not a limiting factor in referral. Outpatient referral rates did not increase, despite a 28% increase in the number of consultant psychiatrists and a 35% increase in the number of non-consultant psychiatric staff in the years 1970–1975 (Williams & Clare 1981). In these circumstances, attitudes are probably more influential. Patients' dislike of referral (Skuse 1975), the GP's wish not to label the patient, and the GP's view that neurosis was his responsibility were the three most common reasons for not referring in one study (Whitfield & Winter 1980).

It has been suggested that the reluctance of patients to attend psychiatric units can be circumvented by holding clinics in health centres: 19% of patients seen in general practices by one group of psychiatrists said that they would not have attended a hospital clinic (Tyrer 1984). The number of psychiatrists running such clinics is increasing rapidly (Strathdee & Williams 1984): this represents one of the few major initiatives taken by psychiatrists in primary care, in a decade when, according to Martin (1984), they have otherwise failed to rise to the challenges of community psychiatry. However, it has yet to be shown that these clinics effect a sustained improvement in the management of psychiatric morbidity in the community. Tyrer et al (1984) found that admissions fell more in those areas of Nottingham where they were running general practice-based clinics than they did in other parts of the city, however, they had started at a higher level in the former areas, and the rate of admissions with the new arrangement did not fall below that of the conventionally served population. At the same time other changes which may have influenced the rates were also taking place in the services to the city.

An often-noted advantage of psychiatric clinics in general practice is the amount of informal discussion about cases that may occur there. Brook (1978), for example, estimated that he saw only a fifth of the patients that he discussed with the practice staff. They may also provide the opportunity of diffusing special skills, such as psychotherapy, into general practice, although this may meet with resistance (Wilson & Wilson 1985). Whether these benefits will carry over into the generality of psychiatrists' clinics in health centres remains to be evaluated.

A further contribution that the psychiatrist can make is in the training of family doctors. GP trainees have different needs from those of trainee psychiatrists, and some GP training programmes have been criticised for not taking this into account, which might be done, e.g. by providing more opportunity to see and treat non-psychotic patients. Training in interviewing techniques which are suitable for general practice conditions is also required (Lesser 1985).

CONCLUSION

The Royal College of Psychiatrists (1980) noted that it is the GP who should be the co-ordinator of services for the psychiatrically disabled, if not their principal provider. However, this is unsatisfactory in present circumstances, since such patients need regular assessment and active pursuit if they default, not the demand-led service which is the normal mode of general practice. Psychiatrists must decide as a matter of some urgency, where their responsibility lies, now that more and sicker patients are being discharged from hospitals, where they were automatically and without question the psychiatrist's responsibility. The reluctance of many psychiatrists to be involved in the development of community services in the past will surely have to change (Martin 1984).

Another important issue in community psychiatry, also involving primary medical care, is posed by the prevalence of emotional distress. Psychiatrists may occasionally agonise over the political significance of re-casting distress as disease (Vlissides & Jenner 1982), but this does not justify a failure to recognise the distress in the first place. Rational evaluation of different approaches to distress, which do not need to be medical, can only be based on representative samples, and this requires accurate detection. Under-detection remains the biggest obstacle to improved management of distress, and psychiatrists can make a positive contribution to the problem through participation in the training of GPs, and by encouraging them to accept the social as well as the medical elements of their work. A surprising number of people consider that their family doctor is the right person with whom to talk about personal problems (Varlaam et al 1972), but the modern family doctor, far from encouraging this, may consider it to be outside his job description.

Psychiatrists have a contribution to make to research in general practice, and need to play their part in overcoming barriers to early and thorough treatment for some psychiatrically ill patients who are presently underserved. However, their main contribution to primary medical care is likely to be in assisting GPs to talk helpfully to their patients about the latters' emotional difficulties. Whether psychiatrists are as competent as they might be in this area, or whether systematic training also needs to be given to them, is outside the scope of this chapter.

'The primary medical care team is the keystone of community psychiatry' and 'The crucial question is not how the GP can fit into the mental health services, but rather how the psychiatrist can collaborate most effectively with primary medical services' concluded the WHO working group on psychiatry and primary medical care (WHO 1973). It went on to recommend more evaluative studies, more training of GPs in psychiatry, more research into diagnosis and classification, the growth of comprehensive primary health care teams and, with special emphasis, 'much closer communication and co-operation between specialist services and primary health care services than at present operates'.

These recommendations are widely accepted today, and many attempts have been made to implement them, not least in the readiness of many psychiatrists to commit to sessions in general practices and health centres. However, there is little evidence for the efficacy of collaboration, in terms of patient care or cost-effectiveness (Mitchell 1985), nor is there a consensus about the form that such collaboration should take. It is especially important that the costs of primary care psychiatry be carefully considered, since there seems to be a danger of time being spent in this way at the expense of psychiatric collaboration with the 'tertiary carers' — the day centre staff, hostel wardens, and families who maintain the viability of patients with chronic disablement outside hospital.

Now that psychiatrists have become more involved with community care, they are going to face difficult decisions about which section of the community has most claim on their limited resources. Should it be the emotionally distressed patient who is asking for psychological help; the emotionally distressed patient who, while not asking for psychological help, may be using up scarce medical resources in the search for physical disease; or the psychiatrically disabled patient whose emotional distress may not lead to a medical consultation at all until there is a further relapse of psychosis? Answers to these questions will depend on the availability of other mental health professionals and on the efficacy of different types of intervention. They will also depend on the willingness of psychiatrists to consider the interests of all their potential patients, and not only those whom the family doctor selects for them.

REFERENCES

Beck A T 1976 Cognitive therapy and the emotional disorders. International Universities Press, New York

Bielski R J, Friedel O 1976 Prediction of tricyclic antidepressant response. Archives of General Psychiatry 33: 147-9.

Blackburn I M, Bishops S, Glen A I M, Whalley L J, Christie J E 1981 The efficacy of cognitive therapy in depression: a treatment trial using cognitive therapy and pharmacotherapy, each alone and in combination. British Journal of Psychiatry 39: 181-189.

Bouras N, Brough I 1982 The development of the NHS advice centre, Lewisham Health District. Health Trends 14: 65-68

Bridges K, Goldberg D P G 1985 Somatic presentation of DSM-III psychiatric disorders in primary care. Journal of Psychosomatic Research 29: 563-569

Brook A 1978 An aspect of community mental health: consultative work with general practice teams. Health Trends 2: 37-39

Brown G W, Harris T O 1978 Social origins of depression: a study of psychiatric disorder in women. Tavistock Press, London

Brown B S, Regier D A, Balter M B 1977 Key interactions among psychiatric disorders, primary care and the use of psychotropic drugs. Paper delivered to Symposium on Clinical Anxiety / Tension in Primary Medicine, New Orleans

Brown G W, Craig T, Harris T 1985 Depression: disease or distress? British Journal of Psychiatry 147: 612-622

Casey P, Dillon S, Tyrer P 1984 The diagnostic status of patients with conspicuous psychiatric morbidity in primary care. Psychological Medicine 14: 673-682

Catalan J, Gath D, Bond A, Martin P 1984 The effects of non-prescribing of anxiolytics in general practice. II. Factors associated with outcome. British Journal of Psychiatry 144: 593-602.

Cheadle A J, Freeman H L, Korer J 1978 Chronic schizophrenic patients in the community. British Journal of Psychiatry 132: 221-227

Committee on the Review of Medicines 1980 Systematic review of the benzodiazepines. British Medical Journal 1: 910-912

Conway-Nicholls K, Elliott A 1982 North Camden community nursing service. British Medical Journal 2: 859

Cooper B 1972 Clinical and social aspects of chronic neurosis. Proceedings of the Royal Society of Medicine 65: 509

Cooper B, Bickel H 1984 Population screening and the detection of dementing disorders in old age: a review. Psychological Medicine 14: 81-96

Cooper B, Harwin B G, Depla C, Shepherd M 1975 Mental health care in the community: an investigation in general practice. Psychological Medicine 3: 421

Corney R 1984 The effectiveness of attached social workers in the management of depressed female patients in general practice. Psychological Medicine Monograph Supplement 6: 1-47

Corney R, Briscoe M 1977 General practice attachments: investigation into two different types of schemes. Social Work Today 9: 10-14

Curson, D A, Barnes T R E, Bamber R W, Platt S D, Hirsch S R, Duffy J C 1985 Long-term depot maintenance of chronic schizophrenic out-patients: the seven year follow-up of the Medical Research Council Fluphenazine/Placebo trial I. Course of illness, stability of diagnosis and the role of a special maintenance clinic. British Journal of Psychiatry 146: 464-480

Davenport S, Goldberg D, Miller T 1987 How psychiatric disorders are missed during medical consultations. Lancet ii: 439-441

Dunn G 1983 Longitudinal records of anxiety and depression in general practice: The Second National Morbidity Survey. Psychological Medicine 13: 897-906

Eastman C, McPherson I 1982 As others see us: general practitioners' perceptions of psychological problems and their relevance to clinical psychology. British Journal of Clinical Psychology 21: 85-92

Eastwood M R, Trevelyan M H 1972 Relationship between physical and psychiatric disorder. Psychological Medicine 2: 363

Fleming D M, Cross K W 1984 Psychotropic drug prescribing. Journal of the Royal College of General Practitioners 34: 216-220

Freeman G K, Button E J 1984 The clinical psychologist in general practice: a six year study of consulting patterns for psychosocial problems. Journal of the Royal College of General Practice 34: 377-380

Gilchrist I, Gough J, Horsfall-Turner Y et al 1978 Social work in general practice. Journal of the Royal College of General Practitioners 28: 675-686

Goldberg D P 1979 Detection and assessment of emotional disorders in a primary care setting. International Journal of Mental Health 8: 30-48

Goldberg D P, Blackwell B 1970 Psychiatric illness in a primary care setting. British Medical Journal 2: 439-443

Goldberg D P, Bridges K 1985 The diagnosis of anxiety in primary care settings. British Journal of Clinical Practice 39: 28-31

Goldberg D P, Huxley P 1980 Mental illness in the community. Tavistock, London

Goldberg D P, Kay C, Thompson L 1976a Psychiatric morbidity in general practice and the community. Psychological Medicine 6: 565-569

Goldberg D P, Rickels K, Downing, R, Hesbacher P 1976b A comparison of two psychiatric screening tests. British Journal of Psychiatry 129: 61-67

Harvey-Smith E A, Cooper B 1970 Patterns of neurotic illness in the community. Journal of the Royal College of General Practitioners 19: 132-139

Hicks D 1976 Primary health care: a review. HMSO, London

Hoeper E W, Nycz G R, Cleary P 1979 The quality of mental health services in an organised primary health care setting. Final Report, NIMH contract DBE-77-0071. Marshfield Medical Foundation, Marshfield, Wisconsin

Howie J G R 1972 Diagnosis — the Achilles heel. Journal of the Royal College of General Practitioners 22: 310-315

Hughes C C, Tremblay M 1960 People of Cove and Woodlot. Basic Books, New York

Hunter P 1978 Schizophrenia in community psychiatric nursing. National Schizophrenia Fellowship, London

Ingham J G, Miller P M 1976 The determinants of illness declaration. Journal of Psychosomatic Research 20: 309-316

Jenkins R 1985 Six differences in minor psychiatric morbidity. Psychological Medicine, Supplement 7: 1-53

Johnson D A W 1973 Treatment of depression in general practice. British Medical Journal 2: 18-20

Johnson D A W 1974 A study of the use of antidepressant medication in general practice. British Journal of Psychiatry 125: 186-192

Johnstone A, Goldberg D P 1976 Psychiatric screening in general practice. Lancet i: 605-608

Keane P, Fahy T J 1982 Who receives the after-care? Utilization of services by discharged inpatients. Psychological Medicine 12: 891-902

Kedward H B 1969 The outcome of neurotic illness in the community. Social Psychiatry 4: 1-4

Kendell R 1975 The concept of disease and its application to psychiatry. British Journal of Psychiatry 127: 305-315

Kessel N, Shepherd M 1965 The health and attitudes of people who seldom consult a doctor Medical care 3: 6

Lesser A 1985 Problem-based interviewing in general practice: a model. Medical Education 19: 299-304

Marinker M 1967 Studies of contact in a general practice. Journal of the Royal College of General Practitioners 14: 59

Marks I M, Allan R S, Philpot R, Covenly J 1977 Nursing in behavioural psychotherapy. Research Series of Royal College of Nursing, London

Marks I M, Goldberg D P, Hillier V F 1979 Determinants of the ability of general practitioners to detect psychiatric illness. Psychological Medicine 9: 337-353

Martin F M 1984 Between the Acts: Community Mental Health Services 1959-1983. Nuffield Provincial Hospitals Trust, London

Mechanic D 1986 The concept of illness behaviour: culture, situation and personal predisposition. Psychological Medicine 16: 1-7

Mitchell A R K 1985 Psychiatrists in primary care settings. British Journal of Psychiatry 147: 371-379

Murray J 1981 Long-term psychotropic drug-taking and the process of withdrawal. Psychological Medicine 11: 853-858

Nutt D, Glue P 1989 Monoamine oxidase inhibitors: rehabilitation from recent research? British Journal of Psychiatry 154: 287-291

Orleans C T, George L K, Houpt J L, Brodie H K 1985 How primary care physicians treat psychiatric disorders: a national survey of family practitioners. American Journal of Psychiatry 142: 52-57

Pare C M B 1985 The present status of monoamine oxidase inhibitors. British Journal of Psychiatry 146: 576-584

Paykel E S Mangen S P, Griffiths P 1982 Community psychiatric nursing for neurotic patients: a controlled trial. British Journal of Psychiatry 140: 573-581

Regier D, Goldberg I D, Taube C 1978 The de facto US mental health services system: a public health perspective. Archives of General Psychiatry 35: 685–693

Royal College of Psychiatrists 1980 Psychiatric rehabilitation in the 1980s. Royal College of Psychiatrists, London

Salmon P 1984 The psychologist's contribution to primary care: a reappraisal. Journal of the Royal College of General Practitioners 34: 190-193

Shepherd M, Cooper B, Brown A C, Kalton G, Clare A 1981 Psychiatric illness in general practice. 2nd edn. Oxford University Press, Oxford

Sireling L I, Paykel E S, Freeling P, Rao B M, Patel S P 1985 Depression in general practice: case thresholds and diagnosis. British Journal of Psychiatry 147: 113-118

Skuse D H 1975 Attitudes to the psychiatric out-patient clinic. British Medical Journal 3: 469-471

Smout S M, Scott M, Fisher P 1983 Psychiatric crisis intervention in Tunbridge Wells. Bulletin of the Royal College of Psychiatrists 7: 46-47

Srole L 1962 Mental health in the Metropolis. McGraw-Hill, New York

Statement agreed by National Schizophrenia Fellowship & Richmond Fellowship 1984. Bulletin of the Royal College of Psychiatrists 8: 113-114

Strathdee G, Williams P 1984 A survey of psychiatrists in primary care: the silent growth of a new service. Journal of the Royal College of General Practitioners 34: 615-618

Sylph J A, Kedward H B, Eastwood M R 1969 Chronic neurotic patients in general practice: a pilot study. Journal of the Royal College of General Practitioners 17: 162-170

Tantam D, Burns B 1979 An international comparison of two systems of community mental health care. Psychological Medicine 9: 541-550

Teasdale J D, Fennell M, Hibbit G A, Amis P L 1984 Cognitive therapy for major depressive disorder in primary care. British Journal of Psychiatry 144: 400-406

Thomas K B 1974 Temporarily dependent patients in general practice. British Medical Journal 1: 625-626

Tyrer P 1984 Psychiatric clinics in general practice. An extension of community care. British Journal of Psychiatry 145: 9-14

Tyrer P, Seivewright N, Wollerton S 1984 General practice psychiatric clinics: impact on psychiatric services. British Journal of Psychiatry 145: 15-90

Varlaam A, Dragoumis M, Jeffrys M 1972 Patients' opinions of their doctors — a comparative study in a central London borough for patients registered with single handed and partnership practices in 1969. Journal of the Royal College of General Practitioners 22: 8-11

Vlissides D N, Jenner F M 1982 The response of endogenously and reactively depressed patients to electroconvulsive therapy. British Journal of Psychiatry 141: 239-242

Whitfield M J, Winter R D 1980 Psychiatry in general practice: results of a survey of Avon general practitioners. Journal of the Royal College of Practitioners 30: 682-686

Williams P 1980 Recent trends in the prescribing of psychotropic drugs. Health Trends 12: 6-7

Williams P, Clare A 1981 Changing patterns of psychiatric care. British Medical Journal 282: 375-377

Wilson S, Wilson K 1985 Close encounters in general practice: experiences of a psychotherapy liaison team. British Journal of Psychiatry 146: 277-281

Wooff K, Freeman H L, Fryers T 1983 Psychiatric service use in Salford: a comparison of point-prevalence ratios 1968 and 1978. British Journal of Psychiatry 142: 588-597

World Health Organization 1973 Psychiatry and primary medical care. Regional Office for Europe, World Health Organisation, Copenhagen
Zung W W K, McGill M, Moore J T, George D T 1984 Recognition of treatment in depression in family medicine practice. Journal of Clinical Psychiatry 45: 3-6

13. Day treatment and care

G. Shepherd

INTRODUCTION

What place does day care have in a community-based system of psychiatric services? Does it, as Bennett (1981a) has suggested, represent the 'cornerstone' of community care? Or, is it simply an ill-assorted collection of facilities, with poorly defined aims, unintelligible organisation, and little or no empirical backing? Theory and practice in psychiatry are often strange bedfellows, but it is the purpose of this chapter to review some of the theory behind day care and to attempt to spell out its possible aims and objectives. I shall start by examining the history of day services in the United Kingdom, discuss some of the underlying concepts, and then review the empirical research bearing on questions of effectiveness, organisation, management practices, and methods of assessment and treatment. I shall also note some examples of good practice, and it is to be hoped that a clarification of the role and functions of day services will help to make such practices more common as services continue to develop.

If one was to be allowed the luxury of designing a psychiatric service without the legacy of 100 years of care based on the mental hospital, one might actually wish to begin by placing day care at the centre of the stage, since the people who are the consumers of psychiatric services generally only require short periods of care in a closely supervised, 24-hour, in-patient setting. Those who need long periods of care in hospital are a tiny minority. In addition, although many psychiatric patients may benefit from inpatient admission from time to time, their long-term problems are essentially *social* in nature (Shepherd 1984). They have difficulties in coping with the everyday tasks of life — looking after themselves, maintaining a home, finding meaningful occupation, establishing networks of social support, etc. Emotional or psychiatric symptoms may interfere with these basic problems of adaptation, but level of functioning can usually be considered quite independent of symptomatology. Help is also best offered as close as possible to the settings in which these problems occur and not in some remote, closed hospital. Such thinking led the World Health Organisation, in 1953, to propose that the modern system of mental health services would be one in which 'inpatient, day care, domiciliary care, hostels and so on, operated as tools in the hands of the community, and the hospital became only one tool at the disposal of the medico-social team' (quoted in Jones 1972). Inpatient admission was, therefore, to be used as the last resort; it was there as a back-up to care in the community, not the other way around. These ideas helped to shape the 1959 Mental Health Act in Britain and to set the scene for the attempts to move towards a more locally-based psychiatric service (Freeman 1983); we have been struggling with their implementation ever since.

The possible advantages of day care, compared with inpatient admission, were admirably expressed in an early paper by Harris (1956), who was one of its pioneers in the UK. He noted that inpatient admission was generally expensive and that it removed the patient from his/her normal environment, so that when the time came for discharge, this could entail a laborious period of trial visits to the home; when discharge did finally occur, it could be such a shock to the patient and family that it precipitated a further relapse. Inpatient admission could also result in a closing of what Harris refers to as patient's social 'niche' — the family might close 'ranks', rearrange itself, and refuse to accept further responsibility for the care of their relative. Separation from the children, spouse, etc. could then add to the patient's anxiety and distress. Finally, the patient him/herself might refuse to enter hospital, either out of fear, or from a desire to avoid the stigma of mental illness, which might then necessitate compulsory admission, with even greater social costs. Harris suggested that day treatment could avoid many of these problems, and illustrated this thesis with a number of case examples. His paper shows clearly the enthusiasm and optimism for a more community-based approach to care which existed within British post-war psychiatry. However, he was also cautious about the possible limitations of day hospital admission, in particular for suicidal or dangerous patients, and noted the possible problems of causing an enhanced burden for families. To what extent has subsequent experience borne out the opinion of Harris and others like him?

HISTORY OF DAY CARE IN GREAT BRITAIN

The Marlborough Day Hospital is generally recognised as the first independent, day treatment centre to have opened in Great Britain; it was established by Joshua Bierer in London in 1946 (Bierer 1951), but previous attempts to set up day care had already been reported in Russia in the 1930s quoted by Craft (1967) and by Cameron (1947) in Montreal. The Marlborough Day Hospital, developed from Bierer's efforts to create social clubs for recently discharged psychiatric patients, was known originally as a 'social psychotherapeutic' centre. There was considerable emphasis in the UK on using group work, peer pressure, and self-help, while clients were encouraged to take responsibility for developing the programmes and determining their own activities. The unit modelled itself along the lines of the newly fashionable 'therapeutic community', and aimed to provide a social and therapeutic milieu which was geographically and administratively separate from any parent hospital. Thus, at a very early stage, the question was raised of *who* day services should primarily be concerned with. Should they aim to offer an alternative for people who would otherwise go into hospital, or, should they be meeting new demands and serving new client groups, who would otherwise only receive support from existing services?

Following on from Bierer's experience, and other developments, both in Europe and the United States, a number of days units were then established in the UK during the 1950s, and this early work was summarised by Farndale (1961), who reported a survey of 65 day hospitals and day centres, mostly for the adult mentally ill, during the period of 1958–1959. There was a considerable variety in the types of patients attending, the treatment offered, the range of staff employed, the frequency of attendance, the location, and the organisation. Farndale attempted to classify the units according to their location and their degree of contact with inpatient psychiatric units. He felt that day hospitals could make their maximum contributions by working in close co-operation with inpatient settings, particularly on a general hospital site, and his general conclusion was that day care offered significant medical, therapeutic, and social advantages over traditional inpatient admission, at least for some patients. It was also noted that day services might cost less, particularly with respect to the initial capital outlay, but he cautioned against wishful thinking that might overstress the advantages, and specifically mentioned the problem of selecting suitable patients. Day care continued to develop in Britain with this somewhat heterogeneous pattern, and it was not until the Hospital Plan for England & Wales (DHSS 1962) that it was given a specific role in the run-down of the large mental hospitals (Vaughan 1983). Since then, the English Department of Health has issued several statements defining the role and function of day services, and has encouraged both Health and Local Authorities to place greater emphasis in their planning (DHSS 1975, 1981, 1985). Traditionally, a distinction has been drawn between day *hospitals*, which were to be provided by Health Authorities, and day *centres*, which were the responsibility of Local Authorities. The former were meant to offer more active treatment, including medication and a range of professional interventions (psychological, social, and occupational); they were to be aimed at people who needed more intensive treatment than could be given on an outpatient basis, or at those for whom day care was a step towards the community, after a period of inpatient admission. On the other hand, day centres were to meet clients' long-term needs for support and social contact, to assist them in adjusting or re-adjusting to the demands of work, and to relieve the strain on the family.

This distinction between 'treatment' (day hospitals) and 'support' (day centres) has never worked out very well in practice. From early on, it has been apparent that the differences between day hospitals and day centres were in fact much less than was originally envisaged (Freeman et al 1972). This was most clearly illustrated in a national survey of day care conducted by Carter & Edwards (Edwards 1978, 1981, Edwards & Carter 1979), who examined all adult day services in England and Wales, and drew a random stratified sample of 150 units for detailed study. These were visited and both staff and users interviewed, to collect a wide range of qualitative and quantitative data: the most striking finding to emerge was the similarity between day hospitals and day centres. There were indeed some differences; for example, the day centres seemed to be dealing with a slightly more 'chronic' clientele — more men and more psychotics — with longer histories of hospital stay, but in terms of activities provided, expressed aims of the staffs, and most client characteristics, the similarities were much more marked than the differences. The only area in which substantial differences emerged was, in fact, in respect of staffing: day hospitals had, on average, more than twice as many staff as day centres (1: 3.5 vs 1:8) and also a higher proportion of qualified staff. These differences in staffing may reflect the different values psychiatry places on 'curing' as opposed to 'caring'; to some extent they are justifiable, but they do tend to reinforce the view that those with the most severe disorders are worth the least therapeutic effort.

On the question of overall scale of provision, Edwards & Carter's study indicated a national shortfall equivalent to about 100 day hospitals and 800 day centres, i.e. about 30000 places overall. The Department of Health guidelines in 'Better services for the mentally ill' (DHSS 1975) has suggested providing day hospital places at a rate of 30 per 100000 (excluding inpatients) and day centre places at a rate of 60 per 100000. Edwards & Carter also found that about three-quarters of the day places were being provided by the Health Authorities and less than a quarter by Local Authorities; this situation has altered very little in the intervening years. A report of the House of Commons Social Services Committee (1985) showed some increase in day hospital places in England and Wales from 1974 to 1982 (9400 to 15300) but very little increase in day centre provision (3600 to 5000). This left day hospitals still around 1200 places short of the 1975 guidelines, and day centre provision approximately 28000 places short. However, the failure up to then of British local authorities to provide day care for the mentally ill is not really very difficult to understand. In the first place, it costs money; and they had been severely restricted by national policy in their ability to raise funds to pay for new services. There had also been little statutory obligation on them to provide for the mentally ill, and this had been compounded by the loss of specialist experience in social work following the introduction of 'generic' training in social work in 1971. Some change in these factors may be expected, however, following the introduction into England and Wales of the 1983 Mental Health Act. The House of Commons Committees were actually 'appalled' by the inadequacy of day care facilities for those suffering from, recovering from, or liable to recurrence of mental illness, and they also noted a confusion about *what* should be provided, as well as *by whom*. Part of this problem undoubtedly stems from the overall shortage of places. Authorities have been forced to provide too many services under one roof, and there has been a lack of clarity regarding the respective responsibilities of health and social services. The Select Committee also commented on the danger that both agencies may have put the provision of day services low on their list of priorities, in the hope that the other would take it up.

Thus, day care has not developed in the UK as was originally hoped. The overall level of provision has remained low, and there has continued to be confusion regarding the roles and functions of day services. Day care has received little emphasis in many health authorities' plans, yet they still provide the bulk of day places. Paradoxically, a service which was meant to herald a more 'social' approach to mental health problems still relies most heavily on health authorities for its funding, while local social services have so far made only a very modest contribution. Of course, this is a national picture and there are some honourable local exceptions, but before much further progress can be made in developing these services, perhaps there is a need for a clearer understanding of the problems of defining different types of day care (Holloway 1988). A similar point is made by Rosie (1987) in a recent review of evaluative studies on partial hospitalisation in North America and Europe.

CURRENT CONCEPTS IN DAY CARE

From the developments described above, it is clear that there are essentially two kinds of psychiatric day service:

(1) an 'acute', shorter-term, assessment and treatment-orientated service (the day hospital); and
(2) a supportive, longer-term, management and maintenance-orientated service (the day centre).

Rather than contrast these along dimensions of 'treatment' vs 'care', or 'medical' vs 'social', they will be examined according to a number of operational criteria, for example: characteristics of the clients served; range and type of facilities offered; lengths of attendance; pattern of referral and discharge; and sources of possible funding. This may provide a more satisfactory definition of the concepts of day 'hospital' and day 'centre', as well as clarification of their respective roles and functions. The classification is shown in Table 13.1.

Table 13.1 Classification criteria for 'acute' vs 'supportive' day services

	Acute	Supportive
Characteristics of clients served	Recent admissions to hospital, or those currently being considered. Unable to manage with out-patient support alone, but not requiring 24-hour treatment and supervision. Likely to be predominantly suffering from schizophrenic or affective psychoses	Symptomatically less active. Long-term social and/or vocational problems. May contain a minority of clients for whom admission to hospital is never likely
Facilities offered	An 'admission ward without beds', i.e. the full range of medical, social, and psychological assessments and treatments, including family interventions	More specialised social and vocational help. Less medical or family intervention, but with access to these services if required. Less comprehensive facilities provided in one place
Lengths of attendance	Time-limited, perhaps up to one year	Unlimited, with options for re-attendance
Patterns of referral and discharge	Referrals mainly from inpatient services and to supportive day care or other community facilities	More varied pattern of referral sources, e.g. long-stay hospital, acute day services, community agencies, self-referral, etc. Referral on mainly to other community facilities
Source of funding	Health	Local authority, voluntary, education, and employment services

Characteristics of clients served

There is clearly a requirement to provide day services for those people who have recently been admitted to hospital, or who are currently being considered for admission. In the UK, the number of beds in psychiatric hospitals has halved over the past 25 years from over 150 000 to less than 70 000, and lengths of stay have dramatically decreased. However, rates of readmission gradually increased, and this produced the familiar phenomenon of 'revolving-door' patients; readmissions now account for roughly two-thirds of all admissions (Mangen & Rao 1985). If this cycle of readmission is to be broken, then either the effectiveness of inpatient services will have to be markedly improved, or better use will have to be made of after-care and community follow-up; an effective 'acute' day service is clearly one way of improving these after-care services. If day hospitals can work in close co-operation with inpatient units, as originally envisaged, then they can operate between the 'back door' of the acute admission wards and the 'front door' of the long-stay wards. Readmissions may therefore be reduced and, perhaps even more importantly, the accumulation of new long-stay in-patients kept to a minimum. How far can this be achieved in practice? The issue has yet to be thoroughly investigated, but there are some grounds at least for optimism (see below).

To maintain this role of secondary prevention, 'acute' day services must retain a close contact with those patients at the greatest risk of admission: in most cases, these will be the ones who have most recently been discharged, so that discharge acts as a convenient risk 'marker'. Alternatively, patients at a high risk of admission may be identified by their clinical characteristics; for example, they are most likely to be diagnosed as schizophrenic, or with major affective psychoses, and be considered a danger to themselves or others, while in social terms, they are most likely to show chronic and pervasive difficulties in self-care, occupation, and social relationships. They may thus be fairly easily discriminated from patients with short-term, acute problems and good social adaptation, who are at a much lower risk of readmission. The first task facing an acute day service is therefore to clarify this question of *who* they should be aiming at and, if they aim to reduce a reliance on hospital admission, to ensure that they focus on those people who are at the greatest risk. The line between those who require day care, as opposed to inpatient care, is sometimes a difficult one to draw (as is the line between day care and outpatient care), but these are distinctions that must be made if day services are to use their resources most effectively.

After the acute symptoms have subsided, a proportion of day patients may then require longer-term social and/or vocational help, and could be referred on to the supportive day services, where their needs may be considered alongside long-stay patients who have already been resettled in the community, as the mental hospitals have reduced in size. It was envisaged in the 1962 National Hospital Plan that day care would have a specific role in the run-down of the mental hospital but, as indicated earlier, supportive day facilities are even now still in very short supply. There may be an important lesson here regarding the process of 'deinstitutionalisation'. It may have seemed logical to start by developing residential services and then move on to the day facilities, but it could be argued that the reverse order is actually preferable, i.e. to start by establishing the day services and then move on to relocating patients' accommodation. The danger with the former strategy is that by the time the development of day services comes to be considered, the resources are no longer available; yet it is then too late, as there are already large numbers of chronic patients in the community without adequate support.

Finally, there are those people who have needs for day services, but whose problems are unlikely to take them to hospital, either in the short- or the long-term; this group has been touched upon earlier. In diagnostic terms, they are most likely to be labelled as suffering from chronic neuroses or personality disorders, and they stand in the difficult 'grey' area between out-patient and day care. Very occasionally, they may be admitted, but in the UK are likely to receive most of their care in the community, from general practitioners. They often put considerable pressure on services since they tend to be more articulate, more demanding, and often more attractive to therapeutically ambitious professionals than the more chronic clients, but it is doubtful whether they are likely to receive much benefit from day attendance. In the USA they form part of what Bachrach (1980) has called 'the healthy, but unhappy' and she, together with Mollica (1983) and others have shown how at one time they dominated the new community mental health centres, at the expense of the more chronic 'deinstitutionalised' patients (see Chs. 19 and 20). Weighing relative human miseries is surely invidious, but where there are finite resources and almost infinite demands, such decisions have to be taken. Day services must aim for a balanced range, including some provision for those who would not usually find their way into hospital, but this should not happen at the expense of the most severely disabled. Whilst decisions about priorities must be a matter for local discussion, the very least we can do is to try to ensure that the criteria used are made explicit. What must be avoided is a situation where the service drifts towards a particular client group, without either noticing this fact or being aware of the pressures that are leading in a particular direction. There is evidence that this process is already occurring in CMHC's set-up in this country (Sayce 1987).

Facilities offered

It should be clear that if acute day services are to cope successfully with acute problems, they will require much of the same facilities commonly associated with inpatient admission units, e.g. medical assessment and treatment, social and psychological assessments and interventions, and help for families and other carers outside the hospital. An 'admission ward without beds' is perhaps the best way to describe such a service, since this emphasises the relatively high input of professional resources which is required. It is a truism that services can only cope with those problems that they have sufficient resources for, and one cannot expect one with little or no professional personnel to be able to deal effectively with hard-core, acute, psychiatric problems. One of the major difficulties in developing alternatives to inpatient admission has therefore been that of persuading planners — as well as some professionals — that moving services into the community also means moving resources, and sometimes on a substantial scale. However, unless this is achieved, care in the community will be seen to fail without ever really having been given a chance. This is particularly true regarding acute day services, where the temptation to move towards more 'social' and less 'psychiatric' kinds of problems is great. Trying to provide a socially-orientated form of care for a psychiatrically 'acute' population would require a new and much more flexible and imaginative use of medical, social, and psychological expertise. Examples do exist in this country (House of Commons Report, 1985) and in the United States (e.g. Gudeman et al 1983) of successful reorganisations of services along these lines, but at the moment these are relatively few and far between.

Acute day services should be built around individually-centred assessment and treatment programmes, which have been described in detail by the author elsewhere (Shepherd 1978, 1981a, 1983a), but it may be helpful to make a few major statements of principle here. In the first place, assessments must be guided by some kind of overall theory of social adaptation: Watts & Bennett (1983a) stress the interaction between skills and expectations which determines successful performance in certain key social roles. Successful role functioning thus depends not only on the possession of certain skills and abilities, but also upon motivation and the exercise of discretion and judgement in deciding which skills are relevant to which specific role situations; assessments which are simply skills-based are therefore not likely to be adequate. An analysis of adaptation in terms of social roles also emphasises the importance of the specific context in which functioning is assessed; for example, no two friends, spouses, or employers, will have exactly the same expectations for what constitutes effective role behaviour. Social expectations are therefore specific to particular role relationships, and to allow for this 'situational specificity', assessments should be carried out by direct observation, either in the setting where the problems occur or in some close approximation to it. If this is not done, then the specificity of behaviour is likely to invalidate the assessment.

Treatment interventions should likewise be applied in the criterion setting, or in some realistic approximation to it; if not, then problems are likely to arise in relation to transfer of treatment gains (stimulus generalisation). This emphasis on direct observation and on working in the settings where problems occur leads to a more critical evaluation of social skills training (Shepherd 1980, 1983b). Instead of training the client in a set of skills and hoping that these will generalise to 'real' social settings, he/she should be assessed in real social settings (homes, workplaces, families, etc), so that the professional can see what social skills the client requires in order to cope. This 'criterion-orientated' approach means that the skills training should come *after* the generalisation problem has been solved, not before it. It also means that much greater attention must be directed towards placing and supporting people 'in vivo', rather than using remote, artificial settings. Day services provide a useful base in the community, from which direct access to these criterion situations can be made. Assessment and treatment of long-term difficulties are therefore aspects of a single process of defining disabilities. As 'symptoms' (psychiatric, social, psychological) reveal themselves to be refractory to treatment, so the pattern of disabilities emerges. These disabilities must be managed and functioning maintained so that assessment and treatment interact in a dynamic process, which is aimed at identifying and monitoring disabilities. This is in contrast to the more static view of assessment and treatment, which sees them as simple, 'one-off' interventions.

The purpose of assessment and treatment in acute day services is to deal with those symptoms that can be treated effectively in a relatively short space of time, and then to set up ongoing management programmes which may persist after the client has left the acute setting (e.g. long-term medication, family, work). Successful long-term management is therefore not simply about the reduction of disabilities (skills deficits); it is also concerned with management of social disadvantages, i.e. handicaps (WHO 1980). Services for the support of the chronically mentally ill should therefore take into account the ideas of 'normalisation' that have been influential in the development of provisions for mentally handicapped people (Wolfensberger 1972, 1980a, O'Brien & Tyne 1981), which emphasise the importance of culturally-valued means as a method of enabling disadvantaged groups to enjoy life conditions that are at least as good as those of the average citizen. 'Normalisation' is concerned with minimising social disadvantage for already disadvantaged groups, and thus it has links with the more familiar concept of 'stigma', but Wolfensberger (1980a) is at pains to stress that it does *not* mean doing what everyone else does. On this basis, interventions are evaluated according to the social value attached to them, not according to their normative significance. Thus, in the support of chronic psychiatric patients in the community, one would try to avoid the provision of socially devalued roles (e.g. that of 'chronic patient'), and instead, aim to provide age-appropriate and culturally-valued social activities (e.g. education classes, social clubs where members can exercise real responsibility and choice) rather than degrading, non-age-appropriate activities, where patients are treated like children or as passive, dependent, consumers of therapy. This emphasis on socially-valued means, has led to some questioning of services which are explicitly labelled as being for those with psychiatric problems. Wolfensberger (1980b) asserts that 'no good can come of any programme, including normalisation, that is not based on intimate, positive one-to-one relationships between ordinary citizens and those who are handicapped and would otherwise be devalued'. Extreme proponents of this view, therefore, argue that all services should be 'normalised' and that there should be no separate, identifiable, psychiatric facilities, although Wolfensberger himself does not appear to share this view: 'I do not recall meeting a single normalisation advocate, or even zealot, who has not recognised the need for at least some type of sheltered work conditions and circumstances for at least some retarded persons' (1980b). Bearing in mind the overall shortage of provision, an extreme position which attempts to deny access to existing services simple because they are segregated would seem foolish. The issue is not a choice between normalised services and no services at all, but we should ask the question to what extent should those with psychiatric disabilities be integrated with non-handicapped users? Maintaining too rigid an ideology may not even be desirable from the client's point of view, since stigma can have some positive connotations: we are all 'stigmatised' by membership of certain social groups, and sometimes we welcome the opportunity of being with people whom we perceive as 'just like us'. Similarly for psychiatric patients, they sometimes welcome being with people who they think will understand their difficulties and sympathise with their problems, which may imply people who have had similar experiences. Of course, this does not mean that the label 'psychiatric patient' should be the *only* social identity that they are offered, but it may be an acceptable one — at least for some of the time: stigmatisation is not an 'all-or-nothing' phenomenon. The aim must be, therefore, to provide chronic patients with a multiplicity of social settings and roles, and not to force them into being either a 'patient' or a 'non-patient' according to some crude, blanket criterion.

Work had traditionally been one of the major routes of social reintegration for the long-term mentally ill and, in spite of, or perhaps because of the current high levels of general unemployment, the psychological value of work is again increasingly recognised (Shepherd 1981b, Herbst 1984). 'Work' — in the sense of structured, purposeful and productive activity — has considerable social value for socially disabled groups, even if paid employment is scarce. The House of Commons Committee (1985) were impressed by the determination to provide real work for mentally disabled people which they saw in parts of North America, and suggested that more should be done to support sheltered work schemes in the UK. Edwards & Carter's survey suggested that where work was offered within day care facilities, it tended to be of a fairly unimaginative kind, e.g. sub-contract packing or assembly (Edwards 1981). Other British surveys have also highlighted the need for much more extensive work-orientated provision for the long-term mentally ill (Gibbons 1983, Pryce et al 1983, McGrath and Tantam 1987) and similar studies have also been reported in the United States (Harding et al 1987). There should be facilities for the assessment of work performance, for training and preparation in work skills, and for placement in permanent sheltered (or open) work settings. With increasing difficulties in obtaining placements in open employment, various other options may need to be considered in addition to the traditional 'sheltered workshop', e.g. schemes for placing disabled people in a sheltered capacity, but in open employment, as in the 'Sheltered Placements Scheme' (SPS) (formerly referred to as 'SIGs', see Wansbrough 1984). Under these schemes, psychiatrically disabled persons can be placed in any kind of work setting, either singly or in groups, and the MSC contributes to the employer the deficit between what is earned and what would normally be paid for the job. Such schemes are similar to the 'Transitional Employment Programmes' which have been run very successfully in the USA by Fountain House for a number of years (Beard et al 1978), but they are relatively new to Britain. Supported placements in open work settings have obvious advantages in terms of reduced stigma, when compared with traditional sheltered workshops. There are also a number of other exciting developments in sheltered work, mostly sponsored by voluntary agencies, which involves a move away from traditional sub-contract packing and assembly, towards the production and marketing of goods and services by small groups of ex-patients and volunteers working together (e.g. Scott 1986, Pilling 1988). There are even some examples of co-operative ventures employing both psychiatrically-disabled and non-disabled people, but these tend to be on a very small scale (Westland 1983).

Of course, not all patients will be suited to work programmes, even if a wide range of levels and opportunities are available: some may have no inclination to develop their work skills, while for others, their work before illness may have consisted of unpaid labour in the home. This is particularly true of some of those women with chronic affective disorders who are often prominent as long-term day attenders (Pryce et al 1983). Not much is known about the factors contributing to the successful social management of such chronic affective disorders (Bennett 1982, Watts & Bennett 1983a, Paykel & Marshall in this volume), but one can speculate that the provision of a stable social environment, with opportunities for confiding and supportive relationships, may be important. It may also be useful to provide some help with domestic living skills, which does not necessarily imply a high input from psychiatric professionals; the need is for a social setting where patients can behave like people: make a cup of tea, talk to one another, and organise whatever activities, leisure, or recreational pursuits they desire. This is similar to the 'Fountain House Model' as described by Beard et al (1982), in which the members co-operate together to provide amenities for the 'clubhouse', although, as indicated earlier, the 'clubhouse' is very closely linked to transitional employment programmes.

The need for long-term social support of a slightly different kind is highlighted in a study by Mitchell & Birley (1983), who looked at a system of ward support, operating from a large psychiatric hospital, which was run mainly by nursing staff and provided round-the-clock informal help for over 70 chronic patients living in the community. They identified two sub-groups: one was described as 'socially engaged', and tended to consist of women, not schizophrenic, with slightly shorter psychiatric histories, and better existing supports from family and friends; they seemed to seek out specific people — mainly other patients — with whom they had particular, close relationships. The second group was the 'socially unengaged': they tended to be men, and were more likely to have a diagnosis of schizophrenia, were more probably single, and had fewer social supports. They seemed to seek 'company-without-intimacy', preferring to be with people, but not making close relationships, though they did receive considerable material assistance, e.g. a bath, a hot meal, help with finances. This kind of non-intrusive, non-demanding social support also seems important, particularly for some of the more chronic schizophrenic men. There is a need, in fact, for a range of supportive day facilities — some work-orientated, some social in a conventional sense (providing opportunities for close relationships), and others providing 'company-without-intimacy', as well as more practical and material assistance. These kinds of long-term day services need less professional input than the acute services, but this is not to imply that patients requiring them do not also have some specialised clinical needs. Wing and his colleagues in their surveys of high-contact, long-term users of psychiatric services in Camberwell, note the need for care of both physical and mental health problems (Wykes et al 1982, Brugha et al 1988, Brewin et al 1988). Long-term day attenders may benefit from a less 'professionalised' service, but their need for some professional input cannot be entirely ignored.

Lengths of attendance

It is clear from what has been said above that admission to an acute day service, with its high levels of professional input, should be reserved for those in the greatest psychiatric need, and some restriction on the length of admission is therefore inevitable. But the ideal length of stay in such a service is a matter for debate; it depends on many factors — not least financial. One obvious factor which often contributes to increasing lengths of attendance is the non-availability of longer-term supportive day services to which the clients can be referred, so that many day services which set out with the aim of functioning as an acute unit thus gradually become 'silted up' with long-term attenders (Hassall et al 1972, Edwards & Carter 1979, Pryce 1982). In Pryce's study, there was a higher proportion of men than women among the long-stay attenders, especially in the middle age-range (25–44 years), and he attributed this directly to the shortage of work-orientated day facilities.

This spectre of a build-up of chronic day patients may be alarming to administrators and planners, but it is predictable. There is really no reason to suppose that people's need for meaningful activities and social support will ever be 'cured' and one day disappear. Most of us make relatively permanent social adaptation in terms of our work, friendships, and personal relationships, and psychiatric patients are no different — especially if they are restricted in their access to many 'open' social roles (e.g. by unemployment or social prejudice). Some services may therefore have to provide sheltered social roles, and these may have to be relatively permanent. Supportive day facilities cannot operate with a simple throughput model, the reality of long-term needs has to be faced, but this involves painful political decisions about resources. The problem is how to continue providing for these needs without 'institutionalising' patients in the community, and this depends on maintaining the contacts with 'normalised' social supports, as well as maintaining a good quality of long-term care (Shepherd 1984).

Patterns of referral and discharge

These distinctions between acute and supportive day services result in a pattern of referral and discharge which is summarised in Figure 13.1.

This figure shows acute day services engaged in a process of 'early' rehabilitation (Bennett 1983): their role is to take long-term patients early from the acute admission wards (1), to prevent readmission where possible (2), and to minimise the accumulation of new referrals to long-stay beds (3). They may also prevent some first-time admissions (4). Their main source of referral is the acute admission wards, with some direct referrals from the community and a small number from long-stay beds (5). Their main placements for discharge are to supportive day services and other facilities in the community (hostels, care by community nurses, etc.) By contrast, the supportive day facilities receive referrals from a much wider variety of sources: these include the acute day services (6), other community agencies (7), and long-stay wards (8). They refer on to specialised supportive day services in the community, e.g. work-orientated provision (9), social clubs (10), and educational classes (11). All these facilities are open to other community agencies (12).

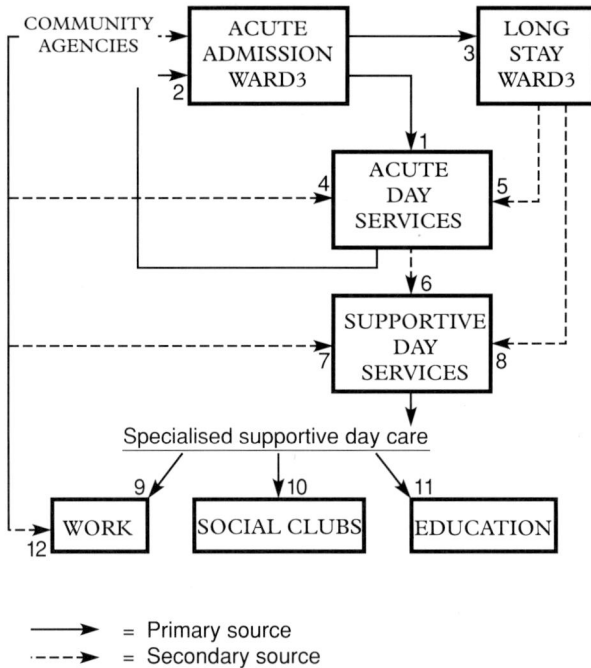

Fig. 13.1   A diagram of acute and supportive day services to show patterns of referral and discharge.

For the physical arrangement of these services, a number of configurations are possible. Clearly, if acute day services are to be effective, then a close working relationship with inpatient units is necessary. The British Department of Health policy (e.g. DHSS 1975) has always envisaged that most day hospital care would be associated with inpatient units on general hospital sites, and there are some good examples of this in the UK, particularly in the north-west region (Freeman 1983). However, other arrangements are possible, and more recent national policy statements have acknowledged the possibility that not all day hospital services are 'preferably' located on the same sites as inpatient facilities (DHSS 1985); the possibility was also noted that day hospital staff may join with local authority staff to provide a combined service linking clinical, social and occupational functions. Such a 'hybrid' service provides a possible resolution of the long-running day hospital/day centre distinction, which has looked increasingly untenable over the years, but the difficulties involved in running such a service have yet to be explored. In particular, will a more 'social' orientation inevitably lead to a drift away from the more acute psychiatric problems?

Other models have placed the day services in the same building as the inpatient beds, e.g. the 'District Services Centre' in Camberwell, South

London (Bennett 1981b), which was designed to enable the individual, whether a day patient, inpatient, or outpatient, to be treated by the same staff team. This arrangement has yet to be formally evaluated, but a disadvantage of having the day places in the same location as beds is the problem of staff in the day areas being diverted from care of the day patients when there are difficult and disruptive patients in the inpatient accommodation. Another possibility has been reported in the USA by Gudeman & Shore (1984) and Gudeman et al (1985) who created two day hospitals, each with a capacity to treat 40–50 patients, linked to a 30 bed intensive-care unit and a 30–35 place 'inn' for temporary residence and transitional support. A basic tenet of this system was that there should be easy movement between hospital and community; thus, the community residence was used as an extension of the centre, and the centre was an extension of the community placements. This attempt to provide different levels of care and easy transitions within a linked system is reminiscent of the original hopes for a district mental health service based on the general hospital unit, which were expressed in Britain almost 20 years ago (Freeman & Mountney 1967).

Sources of funding

In terms of funding, the pattern of services described here is ambitious, but as Bachrach (1978) has pointed out, mental hospitals always provided a complex range of services which can only be replaced by an equally complex network of community-based equivalents. This will certainly not be cheap, and the British Department of Health now formally recognises that a good-quality community service may well be more expensive than a poor quality institutional one (DHSS 1985). So far as specific funding is concerned, it may be expected that Health Authorities will continue to provide the bulk of the acute day services and that the contribution of local Social Services will remain restricted. Long-term day care must therefore be supplemented from other sources, and this means the voluntary sector. There are already examples of organisations like MIND (National Association for Mental Health), NSF (National Schizophrenia Fellowship), the Richmond Fellowship, and the British Institute for Industrial Therapy (BIIT) beginning to take an interest in providing long-term day care in the form of innovative social support and work projects. These projects offer a range of work opportunities, and some are well integrated with non-psychiatric provision. They may therefore have considerable 'normalising' value, and may even be preferable to services offered by the statutory agencies, which tend to be rather less flexible and more stigmatised. The problem with reliance on the voluntary sector is, of course, that these organisations have limited resources, whereas the scale of the demand is enormous (at least 30 000 places in England). Also, funding in the voluntary sector is generally short-term and notoriously insecure. Nevertheless, small scale, local projects sponsored by voluntary agencies, offering work and/or social support, still look the most likely way of providing long-term day services for the future in Britain.

RESEARCH INTO DAY CARE AND OTHER COMMUNITY PROGRAMMES

This section considers research into day care, particularly the evaluation of its effectiveness, and by necessity, will have to draw heavily on the American literature. There have been several substantial reviews in this area, notably Braun et al (1981), Herz (1982), Mason et al (1982) and Rosie (1987), as well as two other important, but more selective reviews by Tantam (1985) and by Wilkinson (1984). All these noted considerable methodological shortcomings in the evidence about outcome, which should not really come as a surprise: an evaluation of outcome in psychiatry is fraught with difficulties, and when one is trying to compare two or more services, the problems involved are almost insuperable. Many studies fail to define their samples adequately and there are often problems with randomisation (sometimes for ethical reasons), difficulties in choosing adequate outcome measures and eliminating observer bias, as well as predictable sample attrition and missing data. Perhaps the biggest problem of all is that of specifying the nature of the independent variables: what is meant by 'standard' inpatient care? What are the crucial elements in a particular day care or community programme? How important is the surrounding social context? These difficulties mean that inductive reviewing, in the strict sense of the word, is virtually impossible. One can only look at the balance of evidence, try to eliminate those studies whose internal validity is clearly flawed, and then come to some cautious general conclusions. Even so, the process can still often feel more like a projective test than a scientific evaluation. The evidence will be examined under a number of headings, viz-

1. Can day care and other community programmes provide an effective alternative to immediate admission?
2. How does day care and/or brief admission compare with 'standard' inpatient care?
3. How cost-effective are day care and community programmes?
4. Is there any evidence of important interactions between day care programmes and client characteristics?
5. What are the outstanding problems with day treatment and care?

Day care and community programmes as an alternative to immediate admission

Braun et al (1981) concluded from their review that 'selected patients managed outside the hospital in experimental programmes do no worse, and by some criteria have psychiatric outcomes superior to those of hospitalised control patients'; they stressed that these results should not be generalised to 'wholly unselected groups of patients'. Similar views were expressed by Herz (1982) and by Tantam (1985). Thus, there seems to be a consensus that some patients can be treated successfully in the community without admission, providing adequate medical and other resources are available, and that this need not lead to any decrement in effectiveness regarding the control of symptoms; in fact, there may be significant advantages for the recovery of social functioning. If such results could be generalised beyond these experimental programmes, then the prospects for more community-based services would seem favourable indeed. But how selective would such services have to be? Are there special categories of patients who can only be safely treated on an inpatient basis?

Most of the experimental programmes included in the reviews mentioned above applied some selection criteria prior to randomisation. For example, Herz et al (1971) excluded 31% of their original sample as being too suicidal, violent, or disorganised, 20% as too 'healthy', 13% because of unfavourable family factors, 7% for reasons of poor physical health, and 6% for other miscellaneous reasons; this left only 22% for assignment to the experimental conditions. Similarly, Fenton et al (1982) excluded 16% as having too high a risk of suicide or violent behaviour, 19% because of a primary diagnosis of alcohol or drug addiction or organic brain syndrome, 19% because they presented at times when the research team were unavailable, 12% because they lived outside the local area, 9% for family reasons, and 6% for other miscellaneous reasons. Dick et al (1985a) screened 242 out of 334 emergency admissions for potential treatment in a new day hospital; of these, 10% were willing to accept day care, while 10% were seen as too disturbed, 6% as too great a suicidal risk, 20% as moderately disturbed, but with complicating factors, e.g. alcohol abuse, aggression, or physical illness, 16% were judged too well, and 5% were rejected for miscellaneous reasons. This left just over 30% of the original sample. These figures from studies in three different countries (USA, Canada, and England) demonstrate the variability — and perhaps the unreliability — of the criteria used to determine suitability for day care. Everyone seems agreed that day care offers an alternative to admission for a proportion of acute patients, but the exact size of this proportion is unclear; on the basis of present research, it seems to vary between 20%–30%. How much this figure could be increased without the restrictions of a research design and with more comprehensive services is open to speculation. One of the challenges for research into day care and community programmes in the future, therefore, is to explore these limits more thoroughly. In particular, we need to determine much more reliable criteria for day treatment, both in terms of inclusion and exclusion.

Hoult et al in Australia have reported on a community-based service which operated with very few restrictions (Hoult & Reynolds 1984, Reynolds & Hoult 1984, Hoult 1986); they accepted all those who presented voluntarily or were taken involuntarily for admission to a State psychiatric hospital, the only exclusion being those not aged between 15 and 65, not resident locally, or having a primary diagnosis of alcohol or drug dependence, organic brain disorder, or mental retardation. It is not reported how many potential subjects these criteria excluded, but the final sample consisted of 120 patients, most with a diagnosis of functional psychosis, and over half suffering from schizophrenia; three-quarters had been previously admitted to hospital on at least one occasion, and two-thirds had been admitted twice or more. The experimental programme was very similar to that of Stein & Test (1978), an attempt was made to treat patients in the community wherever possible, using a range of individually-tailored interventions including medication, help with finding accommodation and work, support for families, etc. The control group received standard hospital care and after-care. Community tenure, clinical status, and family burden were assessed, using standardised measures for both groups, over a 12-month period. The results showed that whereas 96% of the controls were admitted to hospital, only 40% of the experimental group were and, given the overall similarities in outcome, this difference was very striking. Nevertheless, almost half of the 'community treatment' group were admitted to hospital, which underlines the point that day treatment should be seen as complementary to inpatient admission, not as a substitute for it. Admission to hospital on one occasion seemed to predispose to admission on future occasions — a point also made by Tantam (1985). Thus, half the control patients were admitted more than twice, whereas less than 10% of the controls were. The experimental group spent, on average, 8.4 days in hospital over the 12-month period, compared with 53.5 days for the controls. The study also showed, and again this is a common finding, that expressed satisfaction of both patients and relatives was significantly greater with the community-based programme; far from placing additional burdens on carers, if they were properly supported, families (and patients) actually seemed to prefer the treatment to be on a community basis. This may be a function of reduced stigma, or it may simply reflect the greater time and attention given to families in more community-oriented services. Finally, this study — again in common with many others — was dealing with some patients who had long-established psychiatric histories and, despite any advantages of community-based treatments, the authors cannot claim to 'cure' these disabilities. Residual social, occupational, and financial problems often still persisted, and this reinforces the need for long-term support of various kinds.

How does day care and/or brief admission compare with standard inpatient care?

Several studies (e.g. Riesman et al, 1977) suggest that standard lengths of inpatient admissions may be reduced. Hirsch et al (1979) compared 'brief' versus 'standard' care for all admissions to a general psychiatric unit except those with suspected organic brain damage. They found no differences in measures of psychopathology, role functioning, or family burden for a group treated for a median length of admission of nine days, compared with a group which had a median length of 17 days. Although there was also no difference with regard to subsequent readmission rates or use of after-care services, day care was used more as a transitional support for the shorter-admission group. The authors concluded that the major benefits of hospital admission in terms of reduction of symptoms, improvement of social performance, and relief of the stress on families, probably occurs within the first two weeks. A more qualified conclusion, however, emerges from a study by Glick & Hargreaves (1979), who compared short (3–4 weeks) with long admissions (8–16 weeks) for a mixed group of acute psychiatric patients. For schizophrenics, the shorter-admission patients improved rapidly and, by the time of their discharge, were functioning better than their counterparts in the longer admission group, but by the time the latter were ready for discharge, their functioning had improved to a similar extent. They also fared slightly better over the follow-up period, (although this was partly explicable by pre-existing differences favouring the longer admission group, which randomisation had failed to eliminate). For non-schizophrenics, the demands of a limited period of inpatient care rapidly mobilised patients, staff, and relatives alike; the shorter-admission group recovered more quickly, and showed no subsequent differences from the longer-admission group over the rest of the follow-up period. Glick & Hargreaves concluded that longer admissions, e.g. more than four weeks, may be justified for schizophrenic patients with a good prognosis, for whom it may result in a better engagement in after-care services. For the poor prognosis group, however, long inpatient admissions do not seem of particular benefit. Braun et al (1981) concluded that a 'qualified affirmative response' can be given to the feasibility of short-term admission and/or day care as a substitute for conventional hospital stay, but also expressed doubts over the generalisability of some of the findings.

Probably the best study evaluating the effectiveness of day care plus inpatient admission has been reported by Herz et al (1975, 1976, 1977, 1979), who compared brief inpatient admission (average 11 days), with and without transitional day care, with longer-term admission (average 60 days) and standard care. Nearly two-thirds of the sample were schizophrenics, and all lived with a family member or another adult; patients with a primary diagnosis of alcoholism, drug addiction, or personality disorder were excluded. During the first three months, there were no differences between any of the groups regarding resolution of symptoms, and all showed substantial improvements, despite the fact that the shorter-admission day care group received significantly less medication. Social role functioning was generally much less impaired in the shorter-admission/day care group, and they were much more likely to show a rapid return to work. Ratings of family burden also mostly favoured this group, especially after one year, although there was some evidence of increased family burden in the very early stages, i.e. after three weeks; interestingly, 29% of *all* families, irrespective of treatment, felt that the patient had been sent home too soon. Two-year follow-up showed no differences in readmission rates, although the standard group spent 115 days overall in hospital, compared with 47 days for the shorter-admission/day care group. Herz (1982) concluded that although some patients may need a brief period of hospital stay initially, day treatment is 'an effective modality of treatment, especially with regard to enhancing the patient's role functioning'. Mason et al (1982) came to a similar conclusion, but noted that the differences do tend to disappear after two years.

How cost-effective are day care and community programmes?

Evaluating the cost-effectiveness of psychiatric services poses complex problems (Goldberg 1985). In terms of day care and community programmes, it has been shown that they can usually provide a good quality of care for a proportion of acute patients, while avoiding, or at least significantly reducing the time spent in hospital. Given the high cost of inpatient care, direct costs are therefore likely to be lower, but if a long-term commitment to providing supportive services is accepted, then differences may not be so great. Weisbrod et al (1980) attempted a cost-benefit analysis of the Stein & Test community programme, and concluded that it was 10% cheaper; Reynolds & Hoult (1984) found that their programme was 26% cheaper than the standard hospital care. Fenton et al (1982) showed that manpower and operating costs were consistently lower for their home-treated group, compared with those treated in hospital, and that other indirect costs, e.g. time spent out of employment, were also lower. Dick et al (1985b) found that care in their day hospital was approximately 35% cheaper than standard inpatient care, but the magnitude of the difference was dependent on the median length of stay, and they noted that episodes of day care do tend to be longer than inpatient admissions. On the basis of their review, Wilkinson & Pelosi (1987) concluded that services relying wholly or mainly on treatment in the community tend to be more cost-effective and to be preferred by consumers, but also pointed to the hidden contribution often made by general practitioners, and by voluntary and self-help agencies. Thus, while care in the community is certainly not cheap, it may be less expensive than conventional alternatives, at least for some types of patients, and the financial costs have to be set alongside the possible social benefits.

Is there any evidence of important interactions between day care programmes and characteristics of their clients?

Ideally, evaluation of outcome should be concerned with specific questions, not global comparisons (Kiesler 1966): *which* patients, in *which* programmes, according to *which* measures? Unfortunately, however, outcome research in the area of day care has not yet reached such a level of sophistication. Nevertheless, there are some clues as to what may be important interactions between client characteristics and effectiveness of the programmes. It has been shown that some patients may not be managed safely in community settings, although there are doubts regarding the exact criteria defining these individuals, while conversely, some patients may be too 'well' to benefit from day care. For example, Tyrer & Remington (1979) compared day with out-patient treatment for a group of anxious, phobic, or depressive neurotics who had been referred from primary health care teams. They found no difference in terms of ratings of symptoms and social adjustment for the two groups over an 8-month period, while ratings of client satisfaction favoured the out-patient service; it was concluded that out-patient care should be preferred over day-care for the management of many neurotic disorders, on the grounds of economy of time and personnel.

At the other end of the spectrum, Linn et al (1979) attempted to identify those features of day centres which were associated with a favourable outcome for chronic schizophrenics. This was assessed from community tenure, social functioning, and ratings of symptoms: the centres with the poorest outcome tended to have the highest rates of patient turnover, used more intensive treatments (e.g. group psychotherapy), and had greater professional inputs (including more psychologists!). The centres with better outcomes tended to treat schizophrenics more often, offered more recreational time and occupational therapy, and had more part-time staff. Linn et al suggested that for a chronic schizophrenic population, 'it is possible that the less intensively personal and more object focussed activity of occupational therapy produced better outcomes than the intensive interpersonal stimulation often encountered in group therapy'. Thus, there may be an interaction between levels of social stimulation and outcome in day care programmes, at least for chronic schizophrenics, and this would be consistent with other evidence about factors affecting the course and outcome (Wing 1982). It underlines the importance of providing both adequate work-orientated day care and a 'non-threatening' social environment, but the question of what kind of social environment most benefits chronic depressive patients awaits future investigators.

Can we point to any general principles in the organisation and management of day settings? Clearly, the creation of individually-centred care plans is of central importance: without an individualised approach to care, the 'block treatment' and 'depersonalisation' of traditional institutional practice are likely to recur. Shepherd & Richardson (1979) showed how individually-centred management in day settings was correlated with higher and more positive levels of staff-resident interaction. This study also illustrated that changing the location of care is no guarantee that its practices will change; for community services to succeed, both must change. Research by Garety & Morris (1984) and by Raynes et al (1979) also showed that staff involvement in management is crucial. Unless direct care staff are involved in taking some of the decisions about how settings should be organised and run, and unless they receive support from senior managers, we cannot really expect to keep traditional institutional practices from taking over. Combatting 'institutionalisation' is never a battle that is won once and for all; it has to be repeatedly fought, whatever the location or setting. There has been very little direct research into the comparative effectiveness of different kinds of day programmes. Falloon & Talbot (1982) argued for the use of goal-attainment procedures in the context of a behaviourally-orientated, time-limited day programme for 'severely ill' psychiatric patients. One of the interesting features of their approach was the involvement of the clients in setting their own goals; they suggested that interventions directed towards improving interpersonal and vocational functioning tended to be more successful than those which attempted to deal with intrapersonal goals. Milne (1984) has presented a comparative evaluation of two day hospitals, in which he claimed to show that the better outcome was associated with a more directive and behavioural emphasis, but this study has a number of serious methodological flaws (Holloway 1985). A rather better controlled study was reported by Austin et al (1976); this compared a behavioural, goal-orientated day care programme with a more eclectic, therapeutic-community-type programme for groups of chronic patients recently discharged from a nearby state hospital. Although random allocation of subjects was not possible, the data appeared to show few differences in outcome between the patients in the two different programmes. However, significant differences did emerge when a sub-group of clients who had been treated by a 'behaviourally-orientated' social worker at the eclectic centre were dropped from the analysis; the results therefore suggest 'tentative' support for the superiority of the behavioural approach. In summary, there is some weak evidence that more behavioural, goal-orientated day care programmes may produce more effective results than traditional eclectic or milieu approaches. However, as is commonly the case with these kinds of comparative studies, an adequate test has yet to be performed.

What are the outstanding problems with day treatment and care?

The most outstanding problem with day and community-based treatments is probably the reluctance of psychiatric professionals to use them. There are a number of reasons for this: e.g. a lack of knowledge of day care options; difficulties in finding suitable places; and failure to liaise closely between inpatient and community settings. Mosher (1983) also suggests a possible loss of status, inherent in giving up inpatient beds, as well as the inertia based on years of traditional custom and practice. Whatever the reason, it seems likely that a simple review of the evidence will be insufficient to convince the sceptics; established practice is seldom changed by rational argument alone — what is usually required is *demonstration* (Fairweather et al 1974). Professional staff need to experience new ways of working for themselves, and to explore the advantages and limitations of different methods of care, but this can be extremely anxiety-provoking. There is thus a 'chicken-and-egg' situation; more opportunities to work in community-based services need to be offered, but until such opportunities exist, professionals cannot be persuaded to work in them. This dilemma is not easy to resolve, but the anxieties must be confronted. It does *feel* more risky to try and manage acutely ill people without recourse to admission, and good teamwork and staff support are vital. Sometimes, staff can be sustained because of the pioneering nature of a new venture, but sometimes they need education and support (Watts & Bennett 1983b); either way, unless they feel confident in what they are doing, the service is unlikely to make progress.

In addition to the problems of staff support, there are a number of other more practical difficulties. Firstly, day services may be under-used because staff become out of touch with what is on offer; they may misunderstand the function of particular units, expect services which are no longer provided, or simply forget that certain facilities exist. A comprehensive network of day services is likely to be a patchwork of different elements, often involving a number of agencies, and thus there is a need for regular contact and communication between the different units. Ideally, this should be at the level of the direct care staff involved, not the managers, although senior staff may have a role in facilitation. Secondly, nearly all day services suffer from problems of non-attendance by patients, and this has led several authors to stress the need for an 'aggressive' delivery system (Davis et al 1972). However, there may be several reasons for non-attendance: problems of transport and access are often a major issue, particularly in rural areas where public transport may be poor, and this has led to advocacy of the use of 'travelling' day hospitals (Shires 1981); an interesting idea, but one which has not been systematically investigated. Clients may also stop attending because they dislike the activities that are on offer, or because they reject the stigma of attendance at a psychiatrically-labelled facility. Greater client participation in the choice and organisation of activities and greater use of non-segregated community facilities may help to reduce these kinds of problems. One of the few systematic studies of variables associated with under-attendance in day care has been reported by Bender & Pilling (1985), who found that low verbal intelligence, poor premorbid adjustment, and a perception that the patient was unlike most other attenders were the best predictors of poor engagement; they also speculated that these more chronic patients may be more inclined to attend a less verbal and more work-orientated programme. Perhaps the most common reason for poor attendance lies in various family problems: Bennett et al (1976) have stressed the need for a 'family approach' in day care, and the potential benefits in terms of relatives' satisfaction that can result from a real attempt to involve and support families in the community has been described above. Whatever the reasons, poor attendance cannot be ignored. Day services, like other community programmes, thus create a whole new set of problems to do with access, co-ordination, etc. (Holloway 1988). These were not present in the mental hospital, but they lie at the heart of the problems of delivery of community-based services.

CONCLUSIONS

What can be said about the hopes for day care, expressed by Harris and others, more than 30 years ago? The distinction between different kinds of day services are certainly somewhat clearer: in particular, those between 'acute' treatment-orientated services and longer-term support and 'social maintenance' settings. The former demand a simple relocation of professional resources, whereas the latter may be achieved by more 'normalised', less segregated, services with much greater input from voluntary and other non-psychiatric agencies. Care in the community may be cheaper than the equivalent care in hospital, but good-quality care costs money, whatever its location. Nevertheless, the advantages of not admitting to hospital, or of reducing lengths of admission are not simply financial. For many patients, treatment on a daily basis produces the same pattern of symptomatic recovery (provided the same facilities are available as would be available in hospital), and there are significant benefits with respect to the recovery of their social functioning. The likelihood of subsequent readmission may also be significantly reduced. Families (and patients) tend to prefer being treated mainly on a community basis, possibly because this gives them greater access to professional staff. 'Stigma' remains a problem, but an overall shortage of resources is a more urgent issue at present in most countries, while the question of who day services are best suited to deal with remains unresolved. Certainly, some acute patients will still require inpatient admission, but the limits of day treatment have yet to be thoroughly tested. It is clear that day care has an important role to play in the management of chronic conditions like schizophrenia (and possibly chronic affective disorders). It is also clear that day services should *not* be used where outpatient support would suffice. Individual management programmes, with careful and systematic reviews of progress, remain at the heart of a good quality service.

Day care has thus come a long way, but progress depends as much on confidence and willingness to innovate as on a desire to evaluate and learn from the evidence. If that were still the only criterion, then day care would not be the under-used option that it is today. Certainly, there are many unanswered questions, but day services have proved their worth; they provide a tangible alternative base for a psychiatric service which aims to reduce its reliance on the mental hospital. Without them, community services run the danger of 'institutionalising' people in small scattered units, or even in their own homes. Day services can therefore still defend their claim to be at the 'cornerstone' of community care, even if the final size and shape of this edifice remains somewhat obscure.

REFERENCES

Austin N K, Liberman R P, King L W, De Risi W J 1976 A comparative evaluation of two day hospitals. Goal attainment scaling of behaviour therapy vs milieu therapy. Journal of Nervous & Mental Disease 163: 235-262

Bachrach L L 1978 A conceptual approach to deinstitutionalisation. Hospital & Community Psychiatry 29: 573-578

Bachrach L L 1980 Overview: model programs for chronic mental patients. American Journal of Psychiatry 137: 1023-1031

Beard J H, Malamud T J, Rossman E 1978 Psychiatric rehabilitation and rehospitalisation rates. Schizophrenia Bulletin 4: 622-628

Beard J H, Propst R N, Malamud T J 1982 The Fountain House Model of psychiatric rehabilitation Psychosocial Rehabilitation Journal 5: 47-59

Bender M P, Pilling S 1985 A study of variables associated with under-attendance at a Psychiatric day centre. Psychological Medicine 15: 395-401

Bennett D H 1981a Psychiatric day services: a cornerstone of care in New Directions for psychiatric day services. MIND, London

Bennett D H 1981b The Camberwell District Rehabilitation Service. In: Wing J K, Morris B (eds) Handbook of psychiatric rehabilitation practice. Oxford University Press, Oxford

Bennett D H 1982 Management and rehabilitation of affective disorders. In: Wing J K, Wing L (eds) Psychoses of uncertain aetiology, Handbook of psychiatry Vol 3. Cambridge University Press, Cambridge

Bennett D H 1983 The historical development of rehabilitation services. In: Watts F N, Bennett D H (eds) Theory and practice of psychiatric rehabilitation. Wiley's Chichester

Bennett D H, Fox C, Jowell T, Skynner A C R 1976 Towards a family approach in a psychiatric day hospital. British Journal of Psychiatry 129: 73-81

Bierer J 1951 The day hospital. Lewis, London

Braun P, Kochansky G, Shapiro R et al 1981 Overview: Deinstitutionalisation of psychiatric patients, a critical review of outcome studies. American Journal of Psychiatry 138: 736-749

Brewin C R, Wing J K, Maugan S P, Brugha T S, MacCarthy B, Lesage A 1988 Needs for care among the long-term mentally ill: a report from the Camberwell High Contact Survey. Psychological Medicine 18: 457-468

Brugha T S, Wing J K, Brewin C R et al 1988 The problems of people in long-term psychiatric day care: an introduction to the Camberwell High Contact Survey. Psychological Medicine 18: 443-456

Cameron D E 1947 The day hospital. The Modern Hospital 69: 3-23

Craft M 1967 A comparative study of facilities for the retarded in the Soviet Union, United States and United Kingdom. In: Freeman H, Farndale J (eds) New aspects of mental health services. Pergamon Press, Oxford

Davis A E, Dinitz S, Pasamanick B 1972 The prevention of hospitalisation in schizoprenia:

five years after an experimental program. American Journal of Orthopsychiatry 42: 375-388

Department of Health and Social Security 1962 Hospital Plan for England and Wales. Cmnd 1604. HMSO, London

Department of Health and Social Security 1975 Better services for the mentally ill. Cmnd 6233. HMSO, London

Department of Health and Social Security 1981 Care in Action. HMSO, London

Department of Health and Social Security 1985 Government response to the second report from the Social Services Committee 1985-1986 Session Annex 1 Mental illness: policies for prevention, treatment, rehabilitation and care, Cmnd 9674. HMSO, London

Dick P, Cameron L, Cohen D, Barlow H, Ince A 1985a Day and full time psychiatric treatment: a controlled comparison. British Journal of Psychiatry 147: 246-250

Dick P, Ince A, Barlow M 1985b Day treatment: suitability and referral procedure. British Journal of Psychiatry 147: 250-253

Edwards C 1978 A national view of day care services for the mentally ill. In: Report of a seminar on day care for the mentally ill. DHSS, London

Edwards C 1981 Research looks at practice difficulties. In: New directions for psychiatric day services. MIND, London

Edwards C, Carter J 1979 Day services and the mentally ill. In: Wing J K, Olsen R (eds) Community care for the mentally disabled. Oxford University Press, Oxford

Fairweather G W, Sanders D H, Tornatsky L G 1974 Creating change in mental health organisations. Pergamon Press, New York

Falloon I R H, Talbort R E 1982 Achieving the goals of day treatment. Journal of Nervous & Mental Diseases 170: 279-285

Farndale J 1961 The day hospital movement in Great Britain. Pergamon Press, Oxford

Fenton F R, Tessier L, Struening E L, Smith F A, Bendit C 1982 Home and hospital psychiatric treatment. Croom Helm, London

Freeman H L 1983 District psychiatric services: psychiatry for defined populations. In: Bean P (ed) Mental illness: changes and trends. Wiley; Chichester

Freeman H L, Mountney G 1967 Towards a community mental health service 1954-65. In: Freeman H L, Farndale J (eds) New aspects of mental health services. Pergamon Press, Oxford

Freeman H L, Banning B, Richards S 1972 A survey of psychiatric day care in Salford. Community Medicine 26th May

Garety P A, Morris I 1984 A new unit for long-stay psychiatric patients: organisation, attitudes and quality of care. Psychological Medicine 14: 183-192

Gibbons J 1983 Care of schizophrenia patients in the community 1981-3. 3rd Annual Report. Unpublished Paper, Department of Psychiatry, Royal South Hants Hospital, Southampton S09 4PE

Glick I D, Hargreaves W A 1979 Psychiatric hospital treatment for the 1980's. Lexington Books, Lexington Mass

Goldberg D 1985 Cost-effectiveness analysis. In: Helgason T (ed) The long-term treatment of functional psychoses. Cambridge University Press, Cambridge

Gudeman J E, Shore M F 1984 Beyond deinstitutionalisation — a new class of facilities for the mentally ill. New England Journal of Medicine 311: 832-836

Gudeman J E, Shore M F, Dickey B 1983 Day hospitalisation and Inn instead of in-patient care for psychiatric patients. New England Journal of Medicine 308: 749-753

Gudeman J E, Dickey B, Evans A 1985 Four-year assessment of a day hospital-inn program as an alternative to inpatient hospitalisation. American Journal of Psychiatry 142: 1330-1333

Harding C M, Strauss J S, Hafez H, Lieberman P B 1987 Work and mental illness I. Towards an integration of the rehabilitation process. Journal of Nervous & Mental Diseases 175: 317-326

Harris A 1956 Social aspects of psychiatric day hospital treatment. Journal of Social Therapy 2: 1-7

Hassall C, Gath D, Cross K W 1972 Psychiatric day care in Birmingham. British Journal of Preventive & Social Medicine 26: 112-120

Herbst K G 1984 Rehabilitation: the way ahead or the end of the road. Proceedings of the Mental Health Foundation 1983 Conference. Mental Health Foundation, London

Herz M I 1982 Research overview in day treatment. International Journal of Partial Hospitalisation 1: 33-45

Herz M I, Endicott J, Spitzer R L, Mesnikoff A 1971 Day versus in-patient hospitalisation:

a controlled study. American Journal of Psychiatry 127: 1371-1381

Herz M I, Endicott J, Spitzer R L 1975 Brief hospitalisation of patients with families: initial results. American Journal of Psychiatry 132: 413-418

Herz M I, Endicott J, Spitzer R L 1976 Brief versus standard hospitalisation: the families. American Journal of Psychiatry 133: 7-21

Herz M, Endicott J, Spitzer R L 1977 Brief hospitalisation: a two-year follow-up. American Journal of Psychiatry 135: 33–38

Herz M I, Endicott J, Gibbon M 1979 Brief hospitalisation: two-year follow-up. Archives of General Psychiatry 36: 701–705

Hirsch S R , Platt S, Knights A, Weyman A 1979 Shortening hospital stay for psychiatric care: effect on patients and their families. British Medical Journal 1: 442– 446

House of Commons Social Services Committee 1985. Second Report on Community Care. HMSO, London

Holloway F 1985 Evaluation of day hospitals. British Journal of Psychiatry 146: 104

Holloway F 1988 Day care and community support. In: Lavender A, Holloway F (eds) Community care in practice. Wiley, Chichester

Hoult J 1986 Community care of the acutely mentally ill. British Journal of Psychiatry 149: 137-144

Hoult J E, Reynolds I 1984 Schizophrenia — a comparative trial of community orientated and hospital orientated psychiatric care. Acta Psychiatrica Scandinavica 69: 359-372

Jones K 1972 A history of the mental health services. Routledge & Kegan Paul, London

Kiesler D 1966 Some myths of psychotherapy. Psychological Bulletin 65: 110-136

Linn M W, Caffey E M, Klett J, Hogarty G E, Lamb H R 1979 Day treatment and psychotropic drugs in the aftercare of schizophrenic patients. Archives of General Psychiatry 36: 1055-1066

McGrath G, Tantam D 1987 Long-stay patients in a psychiatric day-hospital - a case note study. British Journal of Psychiatry 150: 836-841

Mangen S, Rao B 1985 Mental health services in England. In: Mangen S (ed) Mental health services in the European community. Croom Helm, London

Mason J C, Louks J L, Burmer G C, Scher M 1982 The efficacy of partial hospitalisation: a review of recent literature. International Journal of Partial Hospitalisation 1: 251-271

Milne D 1984 A comparative evaluation of two psychiatric day hospitals. British Journal of Psychiatry 145: 533-537

Mitchell S F, Birley J L T 1983 The use of ward support by psychiatric patients in the community. British Journal of Psychiatry 142: 9-15

Mollica R 1983 From asylum to community — the threatened disintegration of public psychiatry. New England Journal of Medicine 308: 367-373

Mosher L R 1983 Alternatives to psychiatric hospitalisation — why has research failed to be translated into practice? New England Journal of Medicine 309: 1579-1580

O'Brien J, Tyne A 1981 The principle of normalisation: A foundation for effective services. Campaign for Mental Health, London

Pilling S 1988 Work and the continuing care client. In: Lavender A, Holloway F (eds) Community care in practice. Wiley, Chichester

Pryce I G 1982 An expanding 'stage army' of long-stay psychiatric day patients. British Journal of Psychiatry 142: 595-601

Pryce I G, Baughan C A, Jenkins T D O, Venkatesan B 1983 A study of long-attending psychiatric day patients and the services provided for them. Psychological Medicine 13: 875-884

Raynes N, Pratt M, Roses S 1979 Organisational structure and the care of the mentally handicapped. Croom Helm, London

Reynolds I, Hoult J E 1984 The relatives of the mentally ill. A comparative trial of community-orientated and hospital-orientated psychiatric care. Journal of Nervous & Mental Diseases 172: 480-489

Reisman C K, Rabkin J G, Struening E L 1977 Brief versus standard psychiatric hospitalisation: a critical review of the literature. Community Mental Health Review 2: 2-10

Rosie J S 1987 Partial hospitalisation: a review of recent literature. Hospital & Community Psychiatry 38: 1291-1299

Sayce L 1987 Revolution under review. The Health Service Journal 13: 1378-1379

Scott J 1986 Many hands. Kensington and Chelsea. MIND, London

Shepherd G 1978 The contribution of recent research to the creation of non-institutionising environments for the long-term care of chronic disabilities: In Report of a seminar on day care for the mentally ill. DHSS, London

Shepherd G 1980 The treatment of social difficulties in special environments. In: Feldman H P, Orford J (eds) Psychological problems: the social context. Wiley, Chichester

Shepherd 1981a Day care and the chronic patient. In: New directions for psychiatric day services. MIND, London

Shepherd G 1981b Psychological disorder and unemployment. Bulletin of the British Psychological Society 34: 345-348

Shepherd G 1983a Planning the rehabilitation of the individual. In: Watts F N, Bennett D H (eds) Theory and practice of psychiatric rehabilitation. Wiley, Chichester

Shepherd G 1983b Social skills training with adults. In: Spence S, Shepherd G (eds) Developments in social skill training. Academic Press, London

Shepherd G 1984 Institutional care and rehabilitation. Longman, London

Shepherd G, Richardson A 1979 Organisation and interaction in psychiatric day centres Psychological Medicine 9: 573-579

Shires J 1981 From mental hospital to market town — Dorset's travelling day hospital. In: New directions for psychiatric day services. MIND, London

Stein L I, Test M A 1978 An alternative to mental hospital treatment. In: Stein L I, Test M A (eds) Alternative to mental hospital treatment. Plenum Press, New York

Tantam D 1985 Alternatives to psychiatric hospitalisation. British Journal of Psychiatry 146: 1-4

Tyrer P J, Remington M 1979 Controlled comparison of day hospital and outpatient treatment for neurotic disorders. Lancet i: 1014-1016

Vaughan P J 1983 The disordered development of day care in psychiatry. Health Trends 15: 91-94

Wansborough S N 1984 Sheltered industrial groups and other solutions. In: Herbst K G (ed) Rehabilitation: the way ahead or the end of the road. Mental Health Foundation, London

Watts F N, Bennett D H 1983a Theory and practice of psychiatric rehabilitation. Wiley, Chichester

Watts F N, Bennett D H 1983b Management of the staff team. In: Watts F N, Bennett D H (eds) Theory and practice in psychiatric rehabilitation. Wiley, Chichester

Weisbrod B A, Test M A, Stein L I 1980 Alternatives to mental hospital treatment II. Economic cost-benefit analysis. Archives of General Psychiatry 37: 400-405

Westland G 1983 New directions for industrial therapy. British Journal of Occupational Therapy 46: 135-136

Wilkinson G 1984 Day care for patients with psychiatric disorders. British Medical Journal 288: 1710-1711

Wilkinson G, Pelosi A J 1987 The economics of mental health services. British Medical Journal 294: 139-140

Wing J K 1982 Course and prognosis of schizophrenia. In: Wing J K, Wing L (eds) Psychoses of uncertain aetiology. Handbook of psychiatry Vol.3. Cambridge University Press, Cambridge

Wolfensberger W 1972 The principle of normalisation in human services. Toronto National Institute on Mental Retardation, Toronto

Wolfensberger W 1980a A brief overview of the principle of normalisation. In: Flynn R Y, Nitsch K E (eds) Normalisation, social integration and community services. University Park Press, Baltimore

Wolfensberger W 1980b The definition of normalisation: update , problems, disagreements and misunderstandings. In: Flynn R J, Nitsch K E (eds) Normalisation, social integration and community services. University Park Press, Baltimore

World Health Organisation 1980 International classification of impairments, disabilities and handicaps. WHO, Geneva

Wykes T, Creer C, Sturt E 1982 Needs and the deployment of services. In: Wing J K (ed) Long-term community care: experience in a London Borough. Psychological Medicine Monograph Supplement 2.

14. Residential care

I. Morris

Until recent years, residential care for many psychiatric patients with long-term disability in industralised countries was provided by the mental hospitals; as well as shelter and support, those with chronic psychiatric problems received asylum there from the stresses of outside life. However, earlier than is often realised, it was recognized that many patients might benefit from support in smaller residential settings, less detached from the wider community. In the *Journal of Mental Science*, Hawkins (1879) outlined the need for alternative residential facilities for female patients; his observations are no less pertinent today.

Those who are familiar with the inmates of public asylums will probably be able to call to mind cases of female convalescents whose actual dismissal, though warranted by the state of their health, is delayed — postponed from month to month, because they have no friend who can, or will, undertake their charge, on their first return to the world. Some may be literally friendless, others are estranged from their friends or so remote from them as to be beyond reach of their assistance. The friends of others are sometimes so poorly lodged as to be unable to receive, even for a limited period, an additional inmate into their rooms. In some cases, it is to be feared, relatives would be better pleased that the convalescent should find in the asylum a *permanent* abode, than that she should leave it and so possibly become more or less burdensome to themselves.

The efforts of Hawkins led to the foundation in London of the Mental After-Care Association — a society devoted to placing ex-psychiatric patients in settings which would offer accommodation and support. In her history of the British Mental Health Services, Jones (1972) traces the tentative steps taken in the early years of this century to support this type of work; in 1919, sub-committees of the London County Council Asylum and Mental Deficiency Department were authorised to financially support ex-patients placed by the Association, while the Royal Commission of 1924–1926 on mental illness encouraged local authorities to finance after-care facilities. Despite such early developments, though, progress of this kind was slow in Britain and mental hospitals continued their role as the main providers of long-term residential care. However, between 1954, when their population peaked, and 1959, more profound changes in the pattern of services began; Tooth & Brooke (1961) reported a trend of 8000 fewer patients being resident in mental hospitals in England & Wales over the 5-year period. This population decline continued, and between 1971 and 1983, there was a further fall of over 35000 beds (Wilkinson & Freeman 1986).

The reasons underlying this change are complex, but include better methods of treatment and rehabilitation, as well as the development of outpatient facilities, day hospitals, and domiciliary services. Such measures enabled patients who at one time would have become long-stay patients in hospital to remain with their families or in their own homes. Other patients benefited from an expansion in the available range of residential services — mainly hostels — which offer an alternative to hospital care. In 1962, 968 ex-patients were known to be in such facilities in England & Wales — a number which had increased to 2755 by 1970 (Jones 1972) and to 6044 by 1981 (DHSS 1982).

Despite this increase in the provision of residential places outside hospital, their availability in Britain still falls well below the national guidelines of 15–24 places per 100 000 population (DHSS 1975). Some patients, therefore, remain in hospital longer than is necessary, while they await somewhere to live. The problem, however, is not solely a lack of places, but also the issue of whether it is indeed possible to provide *all* residential care within community settings, restricting hospital care to acute admissions, as envisaged by the Hospital Plan for England & Wales in 1962.

As psychiatric hospitals in many countries have pursued more active policies of rehabilitation and community resettlement, their population has in fact steadily declined, but Hailey (1971) drew attention to the curvilinear pattern of this trend. Once patients who were less impaired by psychiatric symptoms and who responded favourably to programmes of rehabilitation had been discharged, an increasingly disabled population was left behind; they have responded less readily to the methods of rehabilitation available, and present staff with problems which would be very difficult to cope with outside hospital. This 'hard core' of patients with formidable difficulties has been described by a number of authors (Baldwin & Hall 1967, Fottrell et al 1975, Early & Nicholas 1981). As well as those long-stay patients from earlier years who have proved difficult to discharge to residential care outside hospital, there are a group referred to in the literature as the 'new' long-stay, who are continuing to remain in hospital, despite the current emphasis on minimising periods of residence. Although a proportion of this group could be discharged, were more residential facilities available (Mann & Cree 1976, McCreedie et al 1983), others are severely impaired by poorly controlled symptomatology and problems of social functioning; they could not have their essential needs easily met by the kinds of provision currently available outside hospital almost anywhere. Although 'new' in the sense of becoming chronic after their most recent admission, most of them have long, but intermittent histories of hospital stay before that.

Comparisons between the 'new' long-stay patients and hostel residents have suggested that those remaining in hospital are considerably more handicapped (Hewett & Ryan 1975, Clifford & Szyndler 1987). Problems which cause particular difficulty and prevent resettlement in the community are those of motivation, under-activity, and behavioural disturbance, including threatening or violent outbursts. In a survey of 'new' chronic patients in 1983, McCreadie et al commented that in the 10 years between their study and that of Mann & Cree, little progress had been made in the development of the type of residential facilities which would meet the needs of the most severely impaired. They suggested that long-term residential care in hospital is appropriate for a proportion of this group, and that, the Health Service, therefore, must continue to provide some residential places. This possibility was also recognised in a government report (DHSS 1975) which acknowledged that some hospital-based hostels might continue to be necessary for those most handicapped and disturbed. Three residential units of this type have been subsequently described — one on a hospital site (Wykes 1982), and two in the community but close to a psychiatric service based in a general hospital (Goldberg et al 1985, Gibbons 1986).

Available research, therefore, indicates that in the three decades since 1960, much progress has been made in providing residential settings for patients as an alternative to admission to a long-stay hospital. However, this type of provision is still in short supply in Britain, as in other countries, and some patients who would be better accommodated in residential care in the community remain resident in hospitals. Others have to wait an excessive time for placement, thus unnecessarily prolonging their hospital stay. The evidence also suggests that the range of residential accommodation outside hospital does not yet provide in a satisfactory way for those most severely handicapped by mental illness. This should not be taken to imply that it is impossible to provide residential care outside hospital for the most disabled, but it does suggest that much more support and professional expertise would have to be made available if the needs of the most severely impaired were to be met, and if the function of the psychiatric hospital in providing long-term residential care was to be comprehensively replaced by community-based facilities.

RESIDENTIAL CARE AND PSYCHIATRIC REHABILITATION

The discharge of patients from long-term care in hospital to alternative homes in the community has been the central focus of psychiatric rehabilitation. So much so that rehabilitation has become synonymous with resettlement outside the hospital (Bennett & Morris 1983), and indices which have been used to measure the effectiveness of psychiatric rehabilitation and the viability of residential care have generally included discharge figures, relapse rates, or the length of community tenure.

Because of this close association between rehabilitation and resettlement in community accommodation, the models of psychiatric rehabilitation which guided the provision of care for people with long-term psychiatric problems greatly influenced the style of residential alternatives to hospital. In the late 1950s and early 1960s, the 'ladder' model (Barton 1959) was influential; this conceptualised rehabilitation as a step-by-step process, resulting in increasing competence and independence, the patient gradually emerging as an independent individual who would be able to cope with the necessary instrumental activities of daily living. This type of thinking permeated approaches to residential care, and was manifest in the development of transitional hostels or half-way houses. Accommodation of this type was designed to provide support for a limited period, leading to the resident's ultimate move to an independent home in the community. The predominance of this approach led Pritlove (1978) to label the 1960s as 'the decade of transitional care', when the residential care provided was 'based on the concept that it was purely transitional between illness and full health'.

Studies published in the 1960s in Britain confirmed the influence of this philosophy. A survey by the Ministry of Health in 1966 of 31 local authority hostels revealed that all but three professed policies of transitional care; the period of residence in hostels was usually restricted to no more than one year, and some stipulated as brief a stay as six months. However, in practice, this type of policy often had to be modified to allow for the fact that most residents needed a longer period of time in that setting.

Admission to transitional hostels was also often based on the expectation that residents should be able to engage in open employment; the ability to hold a job was considered a favourable indication that rehabilitation and eventual discharge would be achieved. This type of concern about eventual departure illustrates the expectation that hostel residents would leave when they were both competent and confident enough to resume an independent life-style. Although the goal of ultimate independence does not appear to have been considered or questioned profoundly, the description of many projects, nevertheless, reflects this underlying assumption. One hostel milieu was described as 'a positive social experience in providing an increasing range of social roles that would enhance the resident's chances of leading an independent life in the community' (Mountney 1965). The Ministry Report itself maintained that, 'following prolonged isolation in a mental hospital or the onset of a personal social crisis in the community, the mentally ill person may derive benefit from a hostel where the support and protection of a sheltered environment can help him back to normal society'.

In retrospect, this pattern of residential services, reflecting the ladder model of rehabilitation, was over-optimistic in assuming that most patients would continue to move up the scale of increasing independence. What was less acknowledged was that many patients plateau during a rehabilitation programme, and that maintaining their functioning at an optimum level might require the continuous support of residential services on a life-long basis. That expectations were too great and unrealistic ultimate goals soon became apparent in the problems which arose in some transitional hostels: 'the experience of several local authorities in regard to hostels for the mentally ill suggests that these are often under-occupied' (May et al 1966).

Many patients did not meet the criteria of being able to hold down outside employment, even when jobs were relatively easy to obtain, or of being able to acquire sufficient independence to move on after a year's residence. In one survey of hostels, carried out in 1973, (Ryan & Hewett 1976) 80% of residents in short-stay hostels were in outside employment, but in a subsequent study in 1976, only 14% of residents were employed (Ryan 1979). Frequently, hostels also failed to adhere to their policy of providing a 'time limited' rehabilitation programme; in a survey of 24 local authority hostels, 23 stated that they had a policy of short-term care (Mann et al 1974), but in only five was this policy adhered to. Most of the hostels had accumulated a group of long-stay residents, comprising 40% to 50% of their total population, who proved difficult to move on. Hostels, it seemed, either maintained a policy of short-stay care and selected their residents accordingly, thereby experiencing unacceptably high levels of vacancy, or by being more flexible in their selection of admissions, ended up with a substantial core of long-stay residents.

Both the idea that rehabilitation is a process of step-by-step improvement and increasing independence, and the policy of transitional after-care were therefore found to have limitations in practice. Many patients who are handicapped by chronic psychiatric illness make only limited progress, and they are likely to require services which provide shelter and support over an indefinite period. Sometimes, as much effort is necessary to enable these patients just to maintain their functioning at an acceptable level as is necessary to help them improve and eventually be able to move on to less supported residential care. There does remain a need for transitional hostels which can provide a more active approach to rehabilitation, but this is likely to be for a relatively small group of patients; yet in the past, a disproportionate amount of accommodation has been provided for them (Hewett & Ryan 1975).

Current approaches to the care of the long-term mentally ill emphasise more flexibility in meeting individual needs. A range of residential and supportive facilities are therefore necessary to place patients in such a way as to enable them to achieve optimal privacy and independence, backed up by adequate support on a long-term or permanent basis, when necessary. Also, resettlement of a patient outside hospital is now not necessarily the central focus of rehabilitation. Increasingly, patients are identified who have not spent lengthy periods in mental hospitals, but who are experiencing difficulty in functioning and in finding somewhere to live in a viable and satisfactory way. They are not a homogeneous group, and their needs for residential support are probably more diverse than were those of the old institutionalised population. The different reasons for which they require residential support must therefore be taken into account, if services are to meet their needs in ways which appreciate each person's unique situation and individuality. Therefore, the various situations in which there is a need for residential support and the spectrum of services required to provide individualised care effectively will now be considered.

Homelessness

Despite the developments described above in the provision of sheltered accommodation and residential care, there is growing concern that policies of deinstitutionalisation have contributed to undermining the social safety net which prevented those with long-term psychiatric problems from drifting towards destitution. Organisations providing shelter to the homeless in Britain have drawn attention to the increasing proportion of their clients who are mentally ill (House of Commons 1985). In a study of destitute men, Leach & Wing (1980) pointed out that the run-down of the large mental hospitals and the inadequate provision made after discharge were substantial contributory factors to the increasing numbers of disabled men then among the homeless. However, the drift towards destitution is a complex social process, and firm evidence is lacking of the role which deinstitutionalisation has played in this trend. The report from the House of Commons Social Services Committee commented that, 'it would be ridiculous to attribute the problems of the homeless mentally ill wholly to the reduction in mental illness beds; the problems of the number of homeless mentally ill and mentally disordered offenders in prisons, long antedate community care policies'.

In the United States, there is stronger evidence that the much more radical process of deinstitutionalisation has contributed to the greatly increasing numbers of homeless people with severe and persistent mental illness. Bachrach (1984) summarised the growing consensus that the numbers of homeless people are steadily increasing, their average age dropping, and the percentage of them who are chronically mentally ill rising. However, even in America where the problem has attracted considerable media attention, it has been argued that, 'the growth of the homeless mentally ill population is not a simple phenomenon, and it should not be concluded that it is entirely an artifact of deinstitutionalisation' (Bachrach 1984). Rather, it is an interaction between the effects of the run-down of the large institutions, a much enlarged population in the age-group at risk for developing schizophrenia, patterns of social deprivation, and other aspects of social policy. Bassuk et al (1984) have commented on these aspects, which include economic recession, increasing unemployment, the unavailability of low-cost housing, and cutbacks in welfare payments which contribute to the social marginalisation of the mentally ill.

It must be acknowledged, however, that those with chronic psychiatric problems are particularly vulnerable to social disengagement and consequent homelessness. Lamb (1984) drew attention to the point that homelessness is not just the lack of a permanent home, but is the wider absence of a 'stable base of caring or supportive individuals whose concern and support help buffer the homeless against the vicissitudes of life'. People with severe psychiatric problems and social handicaps are likely to have particular difficulty making and sustaining close relationships which will serve to bind them more securely to society. Lamb goes on to describe the problems which younger mentally ill people experience in making such relationships: 'a fantasy of finding closeness elsewhere encourages them to move on, yet all too often, if they do stumble into an intimate relationship or find themselves in a residence where there is caring and closeness and sharing, the increased anxiety which they experience creates a need to run'.

Lamb also believes that among the homeless are some of the most severely disabled people, who present major problems in terms of management and have substantial dependency needs. They have not been accommodated successfully in community residential settings, which do not provide the degree of containment and structure which would enable them to live with dignity. Because of their particular difficulty in engaging in supportive services and accepting treatment of any kind, Lamb considers this group to be particularly prone to a 'life filled with intense anxiety, depression and deprivation'.

Developing means of helping those with severe and persistent long-term psychiatric problems who are homeless and rootless is a considerable challenge for community psychiatric services. Bassuk & Lamb (1986) have described the ways in which such people are often difficult to help. They are poorly motivated to participate in treatment and rehabilitation programmes, and sometimes relate to traditional means of service delivery in help-rejecting ways. They are also likely to experience difficulties in finding their way through the range of bureaucracies providing different services. This requires personal organisation and persistence on a scale which is far beyond the capability of those who have motivational problems and who experience difficulty in structuring their lives. They also do not fit easily into services organised around specific geographical or catchment areas, since they often fail to meet the residence requirements which would entitle them to psychiatric and local authority services.

In the UK, the problem of homelessness among the mentally ill has not yet reached the stage of being the focus of much political and media concern. However, the United States' experience, and anecdotal evidence that the problem is increasing in the UK (Audit Commission 1986) have given rise to fears that the current more radical moves towards mental hospital closures will exacerbate this trend. The Audit Commission Report suggested that this process is not simply the result of community resettlement: 'while there is evidence to suggest that long-stay patients are generally discharged only after extensive preparations have been made for their future accommodation ... the same may not be true for short-term patients, and people who have failed to gain admission to long-stay facilities with much tighter admissions entrance now in force'. The difficulty, therefore, is not just the lack of long-stay residential settings, but also the failure to provide medium-term rehabilitation for disaffiliated people with no social supports to sustain them on leaving hospital after a brief admission. These individuals might require a longer period of rehabilitation for staff to assess their potential, determine their need for accommodation, and work with them to build up adequate networks of social support in the community. Minimum follow-up by means of outpatient appointments or occasional visits by a community nurse will not be enough to prevent a decline into destitution.

Other needs for residential support

At the simplest level, the overwhelming need of some psychiatric patients is — like many others in the population for — somewhere permanent to live. Homelessness is an increasing problem in many societies, and disadvantaged groups like the mentally ill suffer more than most: psychiatric patients with a history of chronicity, unemployment, and social disadvantages are in a particularly unfavourable position to compete successfully in the housing market. Compared to physical illness or disability, mental illness has low priority in determining housing need (Lovett 1984). Medical assessments of psychiatric patients on local authority waiting lists for housing in Britain have not always been effective in helping to overcome the disadvantage that results from their prolonged illness. Frequently, the mentally ill do not fall into designated priority groups; in one community sample, 80% of 'high service contact' patients were found to be single (Wing 1982) — a group often perceived as being less needy by housing authorities than those with young families or the elderly. Therefore, even patients who are in a position to cope independently may require some specialised help and accommodation to prevent the problem of homelessness exacerbating their psychiatric difficulties.

Some patients who have had a home with their families find at some stage that this situation is no longer tenable. Most families continue to cope with, and support mentally ill members, even at considerable personal, psychological, and financial expense (Grad & Sainsbury 1968, Johnstone et al 1984), but for some, the relief of the patient's admission to hospital leads them to feel that they can no longer continue the struggle. Scott & Alwyn (1978) hypothesised a process of 'closure' that can occur once a patient has been admitted to hospital, so that some families then close ranks and prevent the patient's return home. Others, however, have interpreted this situation differently — in a study of families coping with schizophrenic patients at home, Creer & Wing (1974) described the difficulties families sometimes experience in getting a relative admitted to hospital when daunting problems arise; this results in them expressing reluctance to accept the patient back, fearing that help and support will not be readily available if further crises ensue. In this type of family breakdown, help will be necessary in finding suitable residential accommodation which will adequately support patients, while encouraging them and their families to maintain close and constructive contact when the previous family accommodation is no longer available.

Other patients continue to be welcomed at home, but in the view of the responsible clinical team, this might not be the optimal placement to minimise the possibility of relapse. The work of Brown et al (1972) has been influential in demonstrating that for some schizophrenic patients, close family relationships are not necessarily the most appropriate social milieu, and that a more emotionally neutral setting is less likely to exacerbate the patient's difficulties. Although work, e.g. by Leff et al (1985) and Falloon & Pederson (1985) has suggested therapeutic approaches which might alleviate this problem, the best solution for some patients and their relatives is to live apart, while retaining close links and interest in each other. Again, this can only be achieved if suitable alternative accommodation is found.

Patients who are more severely handicapped in their social functioning need more than alternative accommodation. They also need support — but how much, and what kind will vary, depending on individual need. For some, this might be minimal, and reflect some degree of social vulnerability; in these cases, a sheltered flat or a supportive neighbour could be adequate. For others, the need will be great, and considerable help and support are required to help them cope with some of the most basic tasks of daily living. A spectrum of residential service is therefore necessary to ensure that the optimum residential support is available to maximise independence, which — when it can be achieved to a reasonable extent — renders community life viable and satisfactory.

RESIDENTIAL SETTINGS PROVIDING MINIMAL SUPPORT

The problems previously described which arose in the transitional hostel led to the realisation that 'for many former patients, the idea of an independent life on their own is not feasible; hence accommodation should be provided for them on a long-term basis, such that it compensates for social handicap' (Pritlove 1978). The function of such settings was recognised to be sustenance rather than growth, and the group home was developed to meet this need. The impetus behind this movement arose from the grass roots; small groups of professional staff and/or volunteers worked to provide supportive accommodation in ordinary houses outside hospital. This was possible because such schemes did not require expensive capital investment, properties being acquired usually from local authority housing departments or from housing associations. Morris (1981) has described different ways of setting up group homes, of which the first was that initiated by staff from psychiatric hospitals, who organised accommodation and provided after-care and long-term support (Leopoldt 1980, Leopoldt & McStay 1980, Morris 1981). Other projects have been initiated by social services departments; for example, Barnes (1973) described a project set up and monitored by a social service department, with support provided by a neighbour who was employed to do some domestic work and cooking. Voluntary agencies have also played a prominent part in enabling patients to leave hospital by the provision of group home places; a MIND Report (1976) indicated that local mental health associations in 41 areas of Britain were then supporting group home schemes, and guidance was given to those wishing to embark on such a project (MIND 1974). Anecdotal accounts reported success, but systematic research was less in evidence to evaluate the achievements of the group home in terms of relapse rates, quality of life, community integration, and consumer satisfaction. Neither has the relative effectiveness of different types of pre-discharge schemes to prepare patients for life outside hospital been examined systematically. However, two studies did attempt to compare the fate of group home residents with those patients in other types of accommodation: Ryan (1979) reported the results of a survey of three group home networks, supporting 39 residents in 11 homes, situated in four North London boroughs, while Collis & Ekdawi (1984) compared the progress of group home residents with ex-patients living in other types of accommodation in the community and with those remaining in the rehabilitation units of a large psychiatric hospital.

Compared with residents of short- and long-stay hostels, Ryan found the group home residents to be older (85% were over 45) and more likely to have experienced a long hospital admission, following a diagnosis of schizophrenia. Two-thirds of Ryan's sample had been living in the group homes for more than two years, and three-quarters expressed a wish to go on living there, but some concern was evident about their lack of integration into the general community. Despite group living, they experienced a rather isolated existence within the homes — only 3 % of residents attended day centres, and contacts with friends and relatives were limited. The aspiration that by resettling ex-patients in small groups, an atmosphere of mutual support would develop appeared to be over-optimistic; Ryan felt that residents were generally withdrawn and tended to be unresponsive to each others' nccds. Despite this, the reported comments of some of the residents suggested that they did appreciate each others' presence; although they did not interact much, they valued having others around. This is similar to the 'social wallpaper effect' described by Mitchell & Birley (1983); despite a lack of interaction and basic knowledge about each other, patients attending a ward for day support expressed appreciation of each others' company.

In a study of the social adjustment of patients with long-term problems, Collis & Ekdawi (1984) assessed their level of social functioning: group home residents, hostel residents, and patients remaining at home with their families were studied, respectively, in the community. The group home residents were found to be the least disabled of the three, functioning best in terms of the performance of instrumental skills such as cooking, domestic tasks, clothes care, household chores, and the use of public services. Use of time did not vary much within the community sample, but the group home residents were found to be less hospital-orientated in their social contacts; in general, these residents felt optimistic, but nevertheless perceived their illness to be a greater burden than did the other groups, and saw the hospital as a refuge. Collis & Ekdawi commented that this might imply their greater independence, and social adjustments were therefore maintained at some cost to the resident's sense of well being.

The group home has therefore been successful in enabling many patients to leave hospital, and has engaged the collaborative efforts of staff working in psychiatric hospitals, social service departments, voluntary agencies, the local community, and various housing agencies. However, research results are equivocal in ascertaining the quality of life experienced, so that the question needs to be asked — how relevant now is the group home as a dimension of community care? The population with long-term problems whose needs for accommodation must be met is changing. Unlike their predecessors, they may not have spent long periods in hospital, though they may have experienced multiple admissions. Pritlove (1978) suggested that they will be younger, far less docile and institutionalised, and in some cases also require more supervision, because their illness is less likely to be dormant or burnt out: 'they will demand more privacy in their living arrangements, being unused to institutional life. The role of the accommodation will be as much to prevent social handicap as to undo it once it has occurred'. Morris (1981) confirmed this view that while group homes had suited patients who were older and had spent many years in hospital but had made good recovery from their illness, younger patients might prefer clustered flats or bedsits. This type of accommodation would be more in keeping with the aspirations of young people leaving home for the first time, who do not yet wish to have a 'substitute family'.

An alternative model of residential care in the community requiring minimal support is the use of sheltered lodgings, referred to as family care, fostering, or boarding out schemes. These projects involve the recruitment of suitable landladies or landlords, who provide accommodation in their own homes and give some degree of support to patients leaving hospital. Olsen (1979) has distinguished between family care or fostering, which implies the provision of a substitute family, and boarding out, which is essentially an economic arrangement.

This method of resettlement is thought to have the normalising features of enabling ex-patients to live in ordinary houses, and — through the integration achieved with their hosts — to become part of the local community. While widespread in Europe (Wing 1957), this approach has not been widely used in the UK; reports suggest that these arrangements have provided accommodation for predominantly middle-aged or elderly patients. Anstee (1978), in a study of 90 patients discharged to sheltered lodgings, reported a mean age of 70, while Smith (1979) stated that most patients in her sample were over 60, and 18% were over 80. Although minimal instances of relapse appear to occur, in a review of the literature, Olsen raises some of the criticisms found in the group home studies. These include the limited degree of independence achieved, lack of real integration, and inadequate supportive staff and facilities to enable patients to make use of the opportunities available in community life. Lodgers may have limited access to their landlady's kitchen, may have their laundry done for them, and might have little scope for decision-making in the day-to-day running of the house. It is possible that in terms of participation and autonomy at a domestic level, boarding out schemes may offer less than either group homes or more permissive hostel environments.

Services which have focussed less on resettling patients from the long-stay wards of large psychiatric hospitals and more on developing a comprehensive spectrum of facilities to prevent long-term admission to hospital have also needed to take account of the needs of younger, less institutionalised people with long-term problems. Birley (1974) described a housing association providing bedsits for discharged patients in which 'the tenant is seen as a resident who is expected to look after himself and is not expected to mix with other residents more than he wants'. Support is provided by a manageress who administers the accommodation, collects rent, and keeps an eye on residents to ensure that they are coping adequately; this post is deliberately not filled by a professional worker trained in one of the mental health disciplines, to try and create, as far as possible, an ordinary relationship between the tenant and those running the project. Psychosocial support is provided through local day centres, outpatient clinics, and social workers. Birley described the accommodation as 'certainly sheltered but not obtrusively so'; the residents had autonomy in ordering their domestic life, and were bound by few rules.

In another service which has evolved along similar lines, Lovett (1984) has described minimal support units, including shared flats and cluster accommodation; 10 two-bedroom flats in one block are supported by four residents living rent-free, who collect rents and 'have a caretaking role'. In the cluster, several flats, dispersed within one housing estate, were offered to people who had been mentally ill. Support was to be provided by neighbours, 'able to provide low-key support through informal social contact', for which they would get a small payment.

In summary, minimally supported accommodation can be said to have the following features: residents require some degree of shelter and support, but social functioning is good enough to ensure that basic needs can be met in an autonomous way; and support is minimal and unobtrusive. It has been maintained that this is more effectively provided in a way which greatly reduces professionalisation — emphasising the normal social exchange between tenant and landlord, and reinforcing the status of an ordinary person, as distinct from that of a psychiatric patient. Where psychological support is needed, this is provided independently from the sheltered accommodation by day centres, outpatient clinics, and social workers. Most of the British schemes described in the literature are financially self-supporting, with state benefits covering the cost of rent, administration, and minimal supervision. Accommodation is therefore provided at minimum cost to health authorities, thus potentially freeing finance to increase the support available to those more severely socially disabled. Finally, there is a growing tendency towards diversification of types of accommodation, to enable more attention to be paid to individual wishes and to promote choice.

SETTINGS PROVIDING A MEDIUM LEVEL OF SUPPORT

For those with continuing difficulties in social functioning, there is a need for domestic and social support as well as for accommodation. Residents who require this level of care might experience some difficulty in carrying out the basic tasks of daily living, so that support might be needed in the areas of personal care, domestic chores, shopping, cooking, and budgeting. Problems might be essentially motivational, when the help needed is prompting and encouragement, but other residents might lack the skills or the confidence to function more independently. For those with poor social skills or excessive withdrawal, stimulation towards social interaction might be important to prevent deterioration in functioning. To overcome such difficulties, the help provided might be conceptualised as either compensatory or developmental. Compensatory help is appropriate when, after a period of assessment and rehabilitation, it is judged that further increments in functioning are as yet unlikely to be successful; such help is therefore necessary to enable a resident to cope with the demands of community life during either a temporary or a prolonged period of time. A developmental or rehabilitative approach assumes that a resident is capable of greater independence; help is given in a carefully structured way to facilitate learning, and is gradually withdrawn as skills and confidence increase. Of course, compensatory and developmental help are not mutually exclusive dimensions of residential care. In compensatory settings, effective staff will be sensitive to any signs of further development, and will promote progress towards greater independence. In more developmentally orientated settings, care must be taken to recognise when expectations are too great, perhaps prompting the experience of failure and consequent crises in confidence. However, the pace of work, level of expectation, and permanence of placement in the setting are likely to be slightly different in those with either a compensatory or developmental emphasis respectively.

Some hostels have provided this combination of residential accommodation and domestic social support. However, the difference between compensatory and developmental settings is reflected in the terminology used about them — the transitional hostels described above in this chapter being developmental. In *Better Services for the Mentally Ill*, the Department of Health & Social Security (1975) distinguished between hostels, which they viewed as being rehabilitative or developmental, and staffed homes, which provide long-term accommodation and a less active approach to further rehabilitation. In his study of hostel accommodation, Ryan (1979) distinguished between short-stay hostels which aimed to 'encourage each resident to achieve maximum independence with a view to final placement in the community' and long-stay hostels, which offered permanent accommodation. The former facilities were more likely to be provided by local authorities and the latter by charitable organisations like the Mental After-Care Association.

What are the characteristics of hostel residents? In the study by Collis & Ekdawi (1984), such residents were found to have more prominent symptomatic behaviour than ex-patients living in group homes or with their families. They scored quite well on measures of their functioning in the work role, but had problems maintaining a good standard of personal hygiene, and in general demonstrated less competence in exercising personal responsibility. Ryan (1979) found differences between those living in short- and long-stay hostels, respectively. Almost all the long-stay residents had a diagnosis of schizophrenia, and had spent long periods in hospital prior to discharge; 50% had experienced a hospital stay of over 20 years. They tended to be elderly, had few existing community contacts, and were rather inactive. Residents in the short-stay hostels were less likely to have a diagnosis of schizophrenia; 57% had experienced personality problems or neurosis. Ryan found that the problem most frequently identified by staff was that of social withdrawal, but poor performance of chores, dependency, lack of involvement, and under-assertion were also characteristic. Falloon & Marshall (1983), in a study of residential care and social behaviour, surveyed the residents in a large residential care setting with a good reputation, situated in central Los Angeles; most of them were unable to take much advantage of community resources without extensive assistance. It was reported that those who in fact took advantage 'appear to have effective social interaction skills and suffer predominantly from affective symptoms'; as this more socially able group improved and moved away from the hostel, the 'proportion of severely withdrawn and handicapped individuals gradually increases and slowly dominates the social structure of the residence'. In a much wider study of sheltered care facilities throughout California, Segal & Aviram (1978) examined the overall disturbance of their sample of residents, using the Overall & Gorham Brief Psychiatric Rating Scale. They found that 16% of residents were severely disturbed, 56% mildly disturbed, and that the remainder lacked any overt psychological disturbance. It was concluded that psychopathology can be a major constraint in promoting community integration, but that the level of psychopathology was significantly handicapping for only a small proportion of those in sheltered care. This conclusion differed somewhat in emphasis from that of Falloon & Marshall — that 'a major factor underlying restricted social behaviour may be the chronicity of schizophrenia'.

There is also some accumulation of evidence to suggest that hostels do not take the most severely impaired patient. Ryan & Wing (1979) commented that the settings which they studied would not be able to deal with the 'new' long-stay, accumulating in mental hospitals — neither the hostels as presently constituted and still less the group homes, would be able (or willing) to deal with these more severely disturbed people'. Pryce (1977) found that patients assessed as suitable for hostels by both hospital and social services staff were less socially withdrawn, less socially embarrassing in their behaviour, and less dependent on nursing staff than those deemed to need continuing care in hospital. Collis & Ekdawi (1984) reported similar differences between their hospital and community samples, while McCreadie et al (1983) considered that only 38% of their hospital patients could be resettled in community settings were places available. Those considered unsuitable for resettlement were functioning at a lower level in terms of dependency, inactivity, alienation, and symptoms, than patients thought to be unnecessarily accommodated in hospital, and waiting for appropriate community placement.

It is difficult to make generalisations concerning the characteristics of hostel residents, which will depend on the type of facility and the range of other residential settings available in a given service. However, trends in the literature indicate that hostel residents are perhaps more socially disabled and less typical of the old institutionalised population than those living in group homes, but less impaired than those remaining on the long-stay or rehabilitation units in mental hospitals, although this picture may be still changing. Hewett et al (1975) pointed out that the community residential facilities tended to be selective — 'hostels are no more likely to tolerate very disruptive behaviour than in a normal home' — but such selectivity is only possible while the large psychiatric hospitals are available to provide a back-up resource. With the now more radical moves towards deinstitutionalisation, the emphasis is on hospital closure, and not just on run-down. A challenge is therefore presented to community residential settings to accept more socially disabled residents and to cope with them by means of better resources, more innovation, and greater expertise.

What kind of care is offered by hostels? In an early evaluation of transitional hostels, Apte (1968) compared the social milieu provided by 25 such hostels with 17 hospital wards, where the majority of hostel residents had lived prior to moving into the community. This study was somewhat discouraging, indicating that some hostels tended to adopt institutional practices which it was hoped community care would eliminate; a few actually provided a more restrictive social milieu than that of the hospital wards from which residents had been discharged, so that there was concern that hostels could easily become mini-institutions in the community, retaining some of the undesirable features of the back wards of mental hospitals. Apte devised a measure — the Hospital-Hostel Practices Profile — to determine the relative restrictiveness/permissiveness of a residential milieu, hypothesising that a permissive milieu was one which would be more rehabilitative, in the sense of promoting the independence of residents. This hypothesis was upheld, in that he found that residents were more likely to move on to a life-style of greater independence from a more permissive environment. In a later study, using a methodology owing much to Apte's, Hewett et al (1975) examined the milieux of a number of hostels, and their results were more encouraging; according to their scores on the Apte Profile, these hostels retained very few characteristics of institutionalism. What restriction did remain, reflected the kind of interest and concern that family members would show to each other. Hewett (1979) pointed out that few of us enjoy absolute freedom; some restrictions are in fact enabling, helping us to achieve a reasonable structure to our lives, and to meet our responsibilities.

Wykes (1982) also used a version of the Hospital-Hostel Practices Profile to study the care practices of residential units used by a community sample of patients in high contact with services. Three hostels in their sample provided relatively restrictive environments, but most had less restrictive settings. Common restrictive practices included staff requiring to know residents' whereabouts at weekends, checking residents were in by 23h and locking the door, and making sure residents were taking prescribed medication: these measures could be seen as caring and supportive. However, other common restrictive practices, such as staff entering residents' rooms without permission and a lack of involvement of residents in helping to plan meals, seem less acceptable. Wykes found no relationship between the level of social handicap and the restrictiveness of the environment, so that there was 'little matching between the levels of handicap and amount of supervision'.

In their study of residential facilities in California, Segal & Aviram (1978) studied the features of residential care which seemed to promote community integration, and found that the optimal type of milieu depended on the degree of psychopathology. For those most impaired by active symptomatology, environments with the following characteristics were helpful: high levels of residents' social involvement within the facility, support, spontaneity, and autonomy. Good residential programmes for this group also included a practical, problem-solving approach, and a clear structure. It was concluded that for those with less severe impairment, a well structured residential programme might be less crucial than a programme which encourages residents to go out and use local facilities.

Falloon & Marshall (1983) also found differences in social integration, depending on the degree of social handicap: the more socially active residents 'appeared to interact freely among themselves, to pursue and achieve, actively and independently rehabilitative goals in the community with minimal support and guidance from the staff'. On the other hand, socially withdrawn residents 'appeared to derive little benefit from the varied opportunities provided and appeared inadequate and uncomfortable in most personal situations'; this was despite a well run programme of psychosocial rehabilitation and supportive attempts by staff to promote greater social participation.

Efforts to elucidate which dimensions of residential care are crucial in providing an optimal social environment that will promote social functioning and community integration have afforded only tentative results. Notions such as the 'least restrictive environment' are perhaps over-simplistic; Bachrach (1980) points out that the concept of restrictiveness 'resides outside the patient and in the environment'. By expressing the concept of restrictiveness as relating to an environment, we reduce the importance of the person — 'it tends to minimise the fact that individual patients vary in their needs and that what is restrictive for one patient may not necessarily be so for another'. In this respect, residents' degrees of social and psychiatric handicap do appear to be important, and further progress may be in the direction of ensuring a flexible, individual approach to each resident, varying accordingly the expectations and need for structure and support in relation to individual need.

HIGH DEPENDENCY AND SPECIALIST SETTINGS

Residential units of a more specialised nature are necessary for some client groups or for residents requiring a more specific therapeutic approach. Groups with special residential needs include those with problems of alcohol or drug abuse, the elderly mentally infirm, those with psychiatric problems accompanied by physical handicap or chronic physical illness, and those presenting with behavioural disturbance or severe regression. Other residential facilities offer a more specialised therapeutic framework, such as a sophisticated approach to group work and social rehabilitation. It is not possible to consider here all types of specialised facility, but two will be examined in more detail — hospital hostels for the most severely impaired by mental illness, and therapeutic communities.

Although not developed specifically for those with long-term psychiatric disability, the principles of the therapeutic community have influenced the style of care provided by some residential settings, and this approach has much in common with the goals of psychiatric rehabilitation. In a therapeutic community, positive measures which involve expectations, limits, constraints, and boundaries are evolved and maintained by its members. Efforts are made to 'reorientate the resident away from the self image of 'patient' and towards a realistic assessment of himself as a participating member of society' (Jansen 1980). However, ideas underlying the therapeutic community have often deviated from Jones' (1953) original exposition, and some are more in keeping with current principles of rehabilitation (Watts & Bennett 1983) than are others. A distinction has been made, for instance, between the more traditional therapeutic community and milieu therapy. The therapeutic community has been described as attempting to treat and rehabilitate by working with the synthetic functions of the ego; by resolving psychological conflicts, the patient is freed to function more effectively. Milieu therapy focuses on the executive function of the ego, directly increasing skills and encouraging adaptive social behaviour. Viewed in this way, rehabilitation has more in common with milieu therapy, attempting as it does to improve functioning directly and being more modest about any more profound psychological change.

Some have criticised the relevance of this approach to psychiatric patients with more severe and long-term difficulties. Lamb (1967) described a day centre in which every effort was made to apply therapeutic community principles; he expressed doubt that given such a democratic process, more severely socially impaired patients would be able to formulate and pursue realistic goals, and concluded that the culture of the setting, including high expectations of the patients' behaviour, must be established — at least initially — by the staff. May et al (1976), in a review of treatment approaches for psychotic patients, commented that group work could be over-stimulating for some patients.

Group therapy which emphasises occupational and social problem-solving was more effective than group or individual therapy which attempted to facilitate psychological insight. They concluded that less intensely personal, more object-focussed activities such as occupational therapy produced better results than the intensive, interpersonal stimulation often encountered in group therapy. Paul & Lentz (1977) compared milieu therapy with a social learning approach; their milieu programme, designed around community and living groups, emphasised group cohesiveness, and hoped to mobilise social pressure as a major source of motivation. They concluded that 'even the most promising reports of milieu therapy with less severely disabled long-stay patients fail to provide support for the principles and procedures characteristic of therapeutic communities'. Van Putten & May (1976), reviewing the value of milieu therapy for patients with schizophrenia, conceded that attention to the social milieu may augment the effectiveness of medication, but warned that some types of group work might have a deleterious effect.

Although the consensus of the evidence therefore questions the value of this type of specialised approach, especially for patients with a diagnosis of schizophrenia, there are nevertheless lessons to be learned from it which are relevant to residential care. Therapeutic communities have engaged residents in decision-making and in the tasks involved in the day-to-day running of the unit; attempts have been made to minimise the social distance between staff and residents; social interaction is encouraged and residents are prompted to face up to the consequences of their actions. All of these features are characteristic of good residential care, and carefully translated, could form a milieu which would be rehabilitative for many people with more severe psychiatric problems. One of the values of specialist settings such as those based on the therapeutic community approach is, therefore, to develop expertise and therapeutic sophistication which will enhance the work of those in less specialised residential units.

In settings which provide for clients with special needs, staff also have to have skills over and above those necessary to provide good residential care. In hospital-hostels, staff need to be able to provide a pleasant domestic atmosphere, but also require the expertise to cope with patients whose psychosis is poorly controlled, who are also at times behaviourally disturbed, and who can be severely regressed. In hospital-hostels designed to care for such patients, the intention is to provide a combination of good social care, skilled psychiatric nursing, and the back-up of full multidisciplinary expertise. Because of the need to have medical support, units of this type are best situated close to the psychiatric services provided by a District General Hospital. Three units of this type have been set up and have fully described their client groups.

Wykes (1982) categorised the problems of the residents living in a 14-bed unit situated on the site of a District Psychiatric Hospital: most showed lack of initiative, reluctance to participate in outside activities, inability to make decisions or take personal responsibility, social withdrawal, and ready acceptance of the patient role. 'Three were very severely affected, nine could be persuaded by staff to follow a routine through the day but needed frequent reminders to keep to it; only two patients could maintain a routine from their own internal motivation'. Added to these negative problems were socially embarrassing or difficult behaviour, including 'hostile attitudes, rudeness, chain smoking, constant tea drinking, frequent mood changes (depression, irritability, hostility) occasional aggression and talking to self'. Gibbons (1986) described the residents in a hospital-hostel in the community, but close to a District General Hospital, as 'suffering severely from the 'clinical poverty syndrome' — underactivity, withdrawal and poor self-care'; this unit rejected some of the patients in the 'new' long-stay group with more severe difficulties of behavioural disturbance. Rejected patients were 'younger and appeared more active and less withdrawn, more aggressive and prone to express and act on odd ideas. They posed more control problems and were felt to be too disturbed for other residents and too much of a risk in a hostel situated off the hospital campus and in the centre of a city'. Goldberg et al (1985) described a similar hospital-hostel population.

These three units differ considerably in certain respects, and it is therefore difficult to make direct comparisons. In the one described by Wykes, most residents were encouraged to go out to day facilities — sheltered workshops, occupational therapy, or local day centres. On the other hand, the unit described by Goldberg et al (1985) emphasised domestic life more: residents spent their day shopping, preparing meals, carrying out household chores, gardening, and decorating. The units were similar, however, in using quite a structured therapeutic approach. For all residents in the units described by Wykes and Gibbons, staff devised a specific plan which listed goals, expectations regarding participation, and management plans to cope with problem behaviour; in the unit described by Goldberg et al, an incentive scheme was used, residents being awarded points for achieving their weekly goals.

All three units have reported success in improving the functioning of residents with more severe difficulties. In two, considerable improvement was described after a 6-month stay, suggesting that residents responded fairly quickly to an environment which offered more opportunities for independence plus high staffing levels to enable residents to make use of the opportunities available. However, with those who are most severely impaired by long-term psychiatric illness, it is not enough to place them in a more normalised setting in the community; therapeutic effort and skills must also be used to increase their capacity to participate more fully in domestic and community life. Specific improvements in functioning which were noted included a decrease in the amount of time doing nothing, together with greater participation in domestic life, organised work, and leisure activity. In one hostel, residents started to increase the use they made of the surrounding locality — independently undertaking trips to shops, cafes, clubs, etc.

It is likely that some of this group of patients will be in need of this type of residential care indefinitely, but it is encouraging to note that some residents do very gradually improve to the extent that less supported accommodation can be considered. Wykes reports that three years after the hospital-hostel opened, it was considered that six residents had improved enough to try and place them in less supervised accommodation; this group had had fewer problems at the outset, and showed marked improvement, being eventually able to move to a supported group home, run as a satellite unit by the hospital-hostel staff. Thus, it is encouraging that even the most severely disabled patients can be helped to live more constructive lives in smaller, domestic units, with adequate staffing levels to give them the structured individual attention which they need to realise their potential. However, these staffing levels — which are comparable to the numbers required for an acute psychiatric ward — are essential to the success of the unit and must be maintained indefinitely — a consideration which the management of health authorities may have difficulty appreciating.

High-dependency and specialist residential settings are characterised by higher direct care staffing levels and greater multidisciplinary support. More specific therapeutic approaches are adopted by the staff, who often gain considerable sophistication and expertise in exercising more specialist skills, and in this way, such units differ from other hostels. Ryan (1979) reported only one hostel in his study where more 'technical skills' were used in its approach to rehabilitation, but even in this unit, 'half the interventions made in response to the problem behaviours they reported, were non-technical in nature and in 17% of instances no intervention was made at all'. In the other hostels he surveyed, even less use was made of more specific interventions, the staff relying mainly on encouragement and support.

CURRENT TRENDS IN RESIDENTIAL CARE

Community care has gradually evolved since the early 1960s, but there is now more pressure in Britain to take this trend to its conclusion, with the actual closure of large psychiatric hospitals (House of Commons 1985). This has resulted in a spurt of growth and innovation in the provision of community-based residential facilities, and several current trends represent a departure from previous notions of good practice.

Previous developments in residential facilities tended to be dominated by a particular approach. For instance, Pritlove (1978) referred to the decade of the transitional hostel and then the decade of the group home, but the emphasis is now more towards a variety of facilities providing a continuum of different levels of residential support, rather than one particular type of unit. Reed (1984) commented that the accommodation needs of patients in his district were much more varied than the facilities which were available — 'clinicians and social workers were constantly hammering 'round' patients into 'square' hostels; not unnaturally the result was a very high readmission rate'. However, the possibilities available in some areas of Britain are now very wide, and amongst facilities which might be considered are 14 options, ranging from special housing schemes to hospital-hostels (MIND 1983, Dick 1983). A comprehensive spectrum of residential facilities enables a more genuine attempt to be made to take account of individual needs, and to give those with continuing psychiatric problems more choice in accommodation and life-style. Unfortunately, such a spectrum so far exists in very few places in the UK or in other countries, and the development of innovative residential projects is hindered by limited resources and complex funding mechanisms.

The trend towards services provided on a multi-agency basis is likely to reinforce diversity and, by moving away from the ward care approach, should enable housing and support to be organised in a more flexible way. All this is to the good. However, in an uncertain political and economic climate, there must be concern that services for the long-term mentally ill could be at the mercy of diverse changes in social policy and public expenditure. The report of the Audit Commission (1986), for instance, comments on the increasing use of supplementary benefit to finance community care; this is not controlled by Health Authorities or Local Authority Social Services and is difficult to target effectively towards the areas of greatest need. The traditional mechanism of funding psychiatric services through the National Health Service, while inappropriate in many respects, does have the advantage of widespread public support and the backing of influential professional bodies.

This move towards diversity is accompanied by an emphasis on flexibility. The ideas of the past about the management of mental illness, expressed as they were in enormous capital investment of bricks and mortar, maintained a rigid hold on the pattern of service for over a century, but the realisation that service provision is a dynamic process has resulted in a move towards settings which can be used flexibly, in the light of changing circumstances. Society continues to evolve, and expectations regarding standards of accommodation and privacy will change. The pattern of family life also changes; people now live in smaller groups and often alone, young people frequently want to move out of the family home earlier, and the increasing elderly population have special residential needs. The aspirations of those handicapped by psychiatric problems will reflect such changes in society; a wide spectrum of residential provision is more likely to be adaptable than services which depend on one particular type of facility.

In keeping with the trend towards more flexibility, there is a tendency to favour smaller residential units rather than large hostels. The use of 'ordinary housing' which blends in with that of the local area is thought to be less stigmatising than readily identifiable units, and the use of such property may be changed fairly easily in the light of changing needs. However, care should be taken to ensure that a new orthodoxy — that a particular size of unit is optimal — does not emerge. Although small units might be preferable for most patients, some who are too handicapped to live alone nevertheless find group living too intimate and stressful, needing space and a degree of anonymity if they are to cope successfully.

There has also been concern expressed that small dispersed residential units will not be adequate to support those who are at times very severely disturbed and may need a degree of containment, or those with multiple handicaps who require skilled nursing care for physical as well as psychiatric disability. Wing & Furlong (1986) elucidated five factors which they argue set limits to the degree of independence that can be achieved. These are: risk of harm to self and others, unpredictability of behaviour and liability to relapse, poor motivation and capacity for self-management or performance of social roles, lack of insight, and low public acceptability. They outline plans for a 'Haven Community' in which a number of small, domestic-style, residential units for the most severely disabled would be grouped. This would offer some of the good aspects of a sheltered community, including specialist facilities for work and leisure, and good opportunities for staff support and training. Some degree of integration could be encouraged by sharing leisure facilities with the local community and by stimulating community interest. While having the advantage of ensuring that it will be possible to meet the needs of the most disabled, the scheme falls short of the ideal of promoting social integration and achieving an 'ordinary life' for even the most disabled. It is to be hoped that further service evaluation will determine the extent to which either a dispersed or a sheltered community model will cater most effectively for the needs of the most handicapped.

Ideas influencing the provision of residential services have also undergone revision. The principle of 'normalisation' is increasingly being used as a conceptual framework in the planning of residential services in the community. Briefly, this approach stresses the extent to which people with severe psychiatric disability are at risk of being devalued and thus marginalised by society (Wolfensberger 1972, 1983). It is argued that hitherto, services provided both by institutions and in the community have colluded with this process by segregation and by emphasising the way in which handicapped people are 'different' from others. By failing to emphasise that handicapped people share the same needs and aspirations as healthy members of the community, residential settings have been developed which may continue to provide a stigmatising, impoverished environment, offering few opportunities for self-development and participation in community life.

Normalisation has articulated in a powerful way the extent to which specialist services may contribute to the cycle whereby, 'the more consistently a person is perceived and treated as being deviant, the more likely it is that she/he will conform to that expectation and will behave in ways that are socially expected of him/her or at least that are not valued by society' (Wolfensberger 1983). Some residential services have added to this process by a combination of low expectations and therapeutic approaches which reinforce the self-concept of 'patient', with the implications of being different and a burden to others. These ideas have resulted in a move away from the concept of residential care towards the provision of ordinary housing, similar in size and style to other housing options available in the community. Support, treatment, and rehabilitation are therefore not provided as an integral part of residential care, but as separate packages, tailored to individual needs (Carling & Ridgway 1989).

These ideas are challenging and optimistic in their aspirations for people with severe, long-term psychiatric problems. There is also some evaluative evidence that the principle of normalisation is effective in improving competence and community integration (Hull & Thompson 1981). However, most of the normalisation literature assumes the approach to be self-evident and it is couched in polemical rather than empirical terms. Furthermore, it is a narrow conceptual framework which, while dealing effectively with the problem of secondary disability, pays scant attention to intrinsic psychiatric impairment. It does not elucidate the approaches to care, treatment, and rehabilitation which will be effective in helping to minimise the impact of distressing abnormal experiences or of behaviour which is disturbed and disturbing.

The absence of any reference to these issues in many current British plans raises some concern that there is an underlying denial of primary psychiatric disability. Well-meaning attempts to minimise the detrimental effects of styles of service provision should not lead us to ignore the need for specialist (sometimes not very 'ordinary') measures which ameliorate the impact of severe and persistent psychiatric problems.

Ideas arising from consumerism are also currently influential and have challenged the notion of the patient as the passive recipient of care. This view seeks to promote users of services to a more central role in determining their future and making informed choices about their needs for accommodation and support. A British review of residential care (Wagner 1988) took this issue as its key theme, stating that it was 'essential that a person entering residential care should do so by positive choice'. This, the report went on to state, has the implication that, 'the choice needs to be a real decision, not simply an expression of personal preference to be accorded limited weight in a judgement to be reached by those in authority'. Evaluation of some projects has indicated that promoting choice is not just a pious hope, but can be achieved with painstaking work which gives long-stay hospital patients more information concerning the options open to them. However, in practice, it seems that few patients feel involved in the choice of accommodation following a stay in hospital (Kay & Legg 1986). Promoting choice also implies that adequate numbers of places in different types of residential setting will be available. Unfortunately, this is not the case in Britain, since even the tentative norms for residential care outlined in 1975 in *Better Services for the Mentally Ill* (DHSS 1975) have not been achieved. In many other countries, the situation is much worse.

The promotion of consumerism has also challenged the concept of a service monopoly. Recent thinking concerning the management of health and social care has advocated that statutory authorities move away from the role of providing services to that of 'buying them in' from a variety of agencies (Griffiths 1988). The role of statutory authorities then becomes one of service co-ordination and monitoring. This monitoring role of the local authorities has been given a statutory basis in England as a result of the Registered Homes Act, 1984. Under this legislation, local authorities have powers to register and inspect residential accommodation which provides board and personal care for those with 'part or present mental disorder', among other groups. While there is obviously a need for this type of monitoring, the implementation of the Act is not without difficulties for those providing residential care for people with long-term mental health problems. The thinking behind this legislation was particularly influenced by consideration of the needs of elderly frail people, and when rigidly interpreted, can result in over-restrictive, sometimes unduly cautious care practices which are inappropriate for the able-bodied.

Also central to the Wagner Report is the criticism that many residential care staff are untrained and have a low status. The committee advocated improved training, supervision, and managerial support, and recommended that more staff obtain formal qualifications in residential social work. This view, however, undermines the role of other disciplines which are of particular importance when working with people who have severe, long-term psychiatric problems. Barr (1988), commenting on these implications, expressed concern that training should be multidisciplinary and in particular, that it should acknowledge the value of nursing skills. Certainly, issues such as training, conditions of service, career opportunities, and status need to be considered if staff are to be attracted to work in dispersed, community residential facilities. This will be a considerable challenge, given the declining number of young people due to enter the labour market in Britain in the next decade, and the ensuing competition for their services.

Finally, there are the issues of co-ordinating residential facilities with other elements in a network of services to support the long-term mentally ill in the community. In the total institution, all aspects of the patients' needs were met by the same facility, but in the community, different needs have to be met by different service elements in a flexible way. By definition, residential services will meet the needs for accommodation, but other needs will be met by the resident himself, by others in his natural social network, or by other agencies in the service network. For instance, a resident in residential accommodation may be able to meet his own personal care needs, rely on family and friends for interpersonal relationships, and attend a day centre for constructive daily activity. All this takes careful co-ordination and integration of services, if needs are to be met in a satisfactory way. Residential services, therefore, have to be closely integrated with the other elements in a comprehensive community care service.

REFERENCES

Anstee B H 1978 An alternative to group homes. British Journal of Psychiatry 132: 356-360
Apte R Z 1968 Half-way houses. Occasional papers on social administration, 27. Bell, London
Audit Commission 1986 Making a reality of community care. HMSO, London
Bachrach L L 1980 Is the least restrictive environment always best? Sociological and semantic implications. Hospital & Community Psychiatry 31: 97-103
Bachrach L L 1984 The homeless mentally ill and Mental Health Services: an analytical review of the literature. In: Lamb R H (ed) The homeless mentally ill. American Psychiatric Association, Washington
Baldwin J A, Hall D J 1967 Estimation of the outcome of a standing mental hospital population. British Journal of Preventive & Social Medicine 21: 56
Barnes R 1973 Helping institutionalised patients back to life outside hospital. Community Medicine 20 October: 566-567
Barr H 1988 Response to the Wagner Report. Community Care 14 April: 26
Barton R 1959 Institutional neurosis. Wright, Bristol
Bassuk E L, Lamb H R 1986 Homelessness and the implementation of deinstitutionalisation. In: Bassuk E L (ed) The mental health needs of homeless persons. New Directions in Mental Health Services, No. 30. Jossey-Bass, San Francisco
Bassuk E L, Rubin L, Lauriat A 1984 Is homelessness a mental health problem? American Journal of Psychiatry 141: 1546-1550
Bennett D, Morris I 1983 Deinstitutionalisation in the United Kingdom. International Journal of Mental Health 11: 5-23
Birley J L T 1974 A housing association for psychiatric patients. The Psychiatric Quarterly 48: 4
Brown G W, Birley J R T, Wing J K 1972 Influence of family life on the course of schizophrenic disorders: a replication. British Journal of Psychiatry 121: 241-258
Carling P J, Ridgway P 1989 A psychiatric rehabilitation approach to housing. In: Anthony W, Farkas M (eds) Psychiatric rehabilitation: programs and practices. Johns Hopkins University Press, Baltimore
Clifford P, Szyndler J 1987 Crossways day centre — a brief evaluation. Report from the National Unit for Psychiatric Research and Development, Lewisham Hospital, Lewisham, London SE13
Collis M, Ekdawi M Y 1984 Social adjustment in rehabilitation. International Journal in Rehabilitation Research 7: 259-279
Creer C, Wing J 1974 Schizophrenia at home. Surrey, National Schizophrenia Fellowship
Department of Health and Social Security 1975 Better services of the mentally ill. Cmnd

6233, HMSO, London

Department of Health and Social Security 1982 Health and Social Services for England. HMSO, London

Dick D 1983 The components of a comprehensive psychiatric service. Creating local psychiatric services. Papers from the long-term and community care team. King's Fund Centre, London

Early D, Nicholas M 1981 Two decades of change: Glenside hospital population surveys 1960-1980. British Medical Journal 282: 1466-1499

Falloon I, Marshall G N 1983 Residential care and social behaviour: a study of rehabilitation needs. Psychological Medicine 13: 341-347

Falloon I R H, Pederson J 1985 Family management in the prevention of morbidity of schizophrenia: the adjustment of the family unit. British Journal of Psychiatry 147: 156-163

Fottrell E, Peermohamed R, Kothari R 1975 Identification and definition of a long-stay mental hospital population. British Medical Journal 4: 175

Gibbons J S 1986 Care of 'new' long-stay patients in a District General Hospital Unit. The first two years of a hospital hostel. Acta Psychiatrica Scandinavica 73: 582-588

Goldberg D, Bridges K, Cooper W, Hyde C, Sterling C, Wyatt R 1985 Douglas House: a new type of hostel ward for chronic psychotic patients. British Journal of Psychiatry 147: 383-388

Grad J, Sainsbury P 1968 The effects patients have on their families in a community care and a control psychiatric service — A two year follow up. British Journal of Psychiatry 114: 265-278

Griffiths R 1988 Community care: agenda for action. A report to the Secretary of State for Social Services. HMSO, London

Hailey A M 1971 Long-stay psychiatric inpatients: a study based on the Camberwell Register. Psychological Medicine 1: 128-142

Hawkins H 1879 After-care. Journal of Mental Science 25: 358-367

Hewett S 1979 Somewhere to live: a pilot study of hostel care. In: Olsen M R (ed) The care of the mentally disordered: an examination of some alternatives to hospital care. BASW, Birmingham

Hewett S, Ryan P 1975 Alternatives to living in psychiatric hospitals — a pilot study. British Journal of Hospital Medicine July: 65-70

Hewett S, Ryan P, Wing J K 1975 Living without the mental hospitals. Journal of Social Policy 4: 391-404

House of Commons (1985) Second report from the Social Services Select Committee. Community care — with special reference to adult mentally ill and mentally handicapped people. HMSO, London

Hull J T, Thompson J C 1981 Predicting adaptive functioning among mentally ill persons in community settings. American Journal of Community Psychology 9: 247-268

Jansen E (ed) 1980 The therapeutic community. Croom Helm, London

Johnstone E C, Owens D G C, Gold A, Crow T J, MacMillan J F 1984 Schizophrenic patients discharged from hospital — a follow-up study. British Journal of Psychiatry 147: 383-388

Jones K 1972 A history of the mental health services. Routledge and Kegan Paul, London

Jones M 1953 The Therapeutic Community. Basic Books, New York

Kay A, Legg C 1986 Discharged to the community: a review of housing and support in London for people leaving psychiatric care. City University, London

Lamb H R 1967 Chronic psychiatric patients in the day hospital. Archives of General Psychiatry 17: 615-621

Lamb H R 1984 Deinstitutionalisation and the homeless mentally ill. Hospital & Community Psychiatry 35: 899-907

Leach J, Wing J K 1980 Helping destitute men. Tavistock, London

Leff J, Kuipers L, Berkowitz R, Sturgeon D 1985 A controlled trial of social intervention in the families of schizophrenic patients: two year follow-up. British Journal of Psychiatry 146: 594-600

Leopoldt H 1980 The psychiatric group home. Nursing Times 76: 829

Leopoldt H, McStay P 1980 The psychiatric group home 2. Nursing Times 76: 866

Lovett A 1984 A house for all reasons. The role of housing associations in community care in psychiatric services. In: Reed J, Lomas G (eds) The community — developments and innovations. Croom Helm, London

McCreadie R G, Wilson O A, Burton L 1983 The Scottish survey of 'new chronic' in-patients. British Journal of Psychiatry 143: 564-571

Mann S, Cree W 1976 The 'new long-stay' in mental hospitals. British Journal of Hospital Medicine July: 56-63

May A R, Gregory E, McQuaker W 1966 A hostel for the mentally ill. A study of outcome. The Medical Officer 301, cxv, 14: 183-185

May P R A, Tuma A H, Dixon W J 1976 Schizophrenia — a follow up study: results of treatment. Archives of General Psychiatry 33: 474-478

MIND (1974) Starting and running a group home. A practical guide. MIND, London

MIND (1976) Home from hospital. MIND, London

MIND (1983) Common concern. MIND, London

Ministry of Health (1962) Hospital plan for England and Wales. Cmnd. 1604. HMSO, London

Mitchell S F, Birley J L T 1983 The use of ward support by psychiatric patients in the community. British Journal of Psychiatry 142: 9-15

Morris B 1981 Residential units. In: Wing J K, Morris B (eds) Handbook of psychiatric rehabilitation practice. Oxford University Press, Oxford

Mountney G H 1965 Local Authority psychiatric hostels. British Journal of Psychiatric Social Work 10: 20-26

Olsen M R 1979 The care of the mentally disordered: an examination of some alternatives to hospital care. BASW, Birmingham

Paul G L, Lentz R J 1977 Psychosocial treatment of chronic mental patients. Milieu versus social learning programmes. University Press, London, Harvard

Pritlove J 1978 What future for the mentally ill? Community Care April 12: 20-21

Pryce I G 1977 The selection of long-stay hospital patients for hostels: a study of patients selected for an experimental hostel and for local authority hostels. Psychological Medicine 7: 331-343

Reed J 1984 The elements of an ideal service: the clinical view. In: Reed J, Lomas G (eds) Psychiatric services in the community — developments and innovations. Croom Helm, London

Ryan P 1979 Residential care for the mentally disabled. In: Wing J K, Olsen M R (eds) Community care for the mentally disabled. Oxford University Press, London

Ryan P, Hewett S 1976 A pilot study of hostels for the mentally ill. Social Work Today 6: 774-778

Ryan P, Wing J K 1979 Patterns of residential care: a study of hostels and group homes used by four local authorities to support mentally ill people in the community. In: Olsen M R (ed) The care of the mentally disordered: an examination of some alternatives to hospital care. BASW, Birmingham

Scott R D, Alwyn S 1978 Patient-parent relationships and the course and outcome of schizophrenia. British Journal of Medical Psychology 51: 343-355

Segal S P, Aviram V 1978 The mentally ill in community based sheltered care. A study of community care and social integration. Wiley, New York

Smith G 1979 Family substitute care in the rehabilitation of the discharged psychiatric patient. In: Olsen M R (ed) The care of the mentally disordered: an examination of some alternatives to hospital care. BASW, Birmingham

Tooth G C, Brooke E M 1961 Trends in the mental hospital population and their effect on future planning. Lancet i: 710-713

Van Putten T, May P R A 1976 Milieu therapy of the schizophrenias. In: Joylon L, Flinn D F (eds) Treatment of schizophrenia, progress and prospects. Grune & Stratton, New York

Wagner G 1988 A positive choice. HMSO, London

Watts F, Bennett D 1983 Theory and practice of psychiatric rehabilitation. Wiley, London

Wilkinson G, Freeman H 1986 The provision of Mental Health Services in Britain. Gaskell, London

Wing J K 1957 Family care systems in Norway and Holland. Lancet ii: 884-886

Wing J K (ed) 1982 Long-term community care: experience in a London borough. Psychological Medicine, Monograph Supplement 2. Cambridge University Press, Cambridge

Wing J K, Furlong R 1986 A haven for the severely disabled within a context of a comprehensive psychiatric community service. British Journal of Psychiatry 149: 449-457

Wolfensberger W 1972 The principles of normalisation in human services. National Institute of Mental Retardation, Toronto

Wolfensberger W 1983 Social role volorization: a proposed new term for the principle of normalization. Mental Retardation 21: 234-239

Wykes T 1982 A hostel ward for 'new' long-stay patients: an evaluative study of a ward in a house. In: Wing J K (ed) Long-term community care: experience in a London borough. Psychological Medicine, Monograph Supplement 2. Cambridge University Press, Cambridge

15. Social work

P. Huxley

INTRODUCTION

It is easy to be negative about social work at a time when, both sides of the Atlantic, the public face of 'welfare' and the actions of social workers in particular are no longer the subject (if indeed they ever were) of positive acclaim and regard. People who are the clients of social workers are frequently the casualties of the materialist society which has grown around us over the past 20 years, and they are an unwelcome reminder of the continued presence of poverty, homelessness, unemployment, and disability. Social workers are expected to protect the rights of these disadvantaged groups, but without infringing the rights of the majority — shades of Catch 22! In the UK, there has been a fundamental shift of government policy in favour of private and informal sources of help, and a reduced level of support for the statutory health and welfare services. The recent review of British community care policies by Griffiths (1988) confirmed the direction of this policy and proposed an enhanced role for the non-statutory sector.

One cannot ignore this context in a discussion of the role of social work in community psychiatry. Indeed, community psychiatry itself must contend with the same context. It must do so by examining the issues and attempting to develop appropriate services, not by retreating to or defending the safe confines of institutional care (in its widest sense).

Changes within social work itself partly mirror changes in the wider society. In most industrialised countries, there was an increase in the use of group and community methods during the 1960s, followed by an emphasis on individual rights, from 'welfare' rights to the rights of minority groups, during the 1970s. In the 1980s, attention turned to the effective and efficient 'delivery' of welfare services, allowing some people to argue that the private and the 'informal' sectors can deliver the 'goods' more efficiently and more effectively. I will consider in more detail below the evidence that informal networks of care can adequately provide care for people suffering from mental illness.

Deinstitutionalisation and a general antipathy to institutional care have been widely supported for many years, 'community care', which is both a policy and a catchword, is less often a reality. In social work, there have been attempts to provide non-institutional services for children, elderly people, and the mentally handicapped. Services which are delivered to people from within their 'local' community are held to be preferable to those delivered from without; the evidence that local services are preferable is also considered in more detail below.

Working in a team in a hospital setting, where nurses, social workers, psychologists, and psychiatrists can share in the care of the psychiatric patient is becoming increasingly rare in Britain. Over the past 15 years, considerable development of professional services has meant that clinical psychologists, social workers, and community psychiatric nurses (CPNs) have become more committed to providing care independently. When these and other professionals, voluntary agencies, and informal networks come together in an attempt to provide care without the structure of an institution, 'teamwork' becomes complicated, if not impossible. The evidence that social workers can make a contribution to the 'community psychiatric team' is not well developed, but the little that is known will be reviewed below. There is considerably more empirical evidence that social workers can make an effective contribution to the direct care of patients. In conclusion, I will look at the growing impression that a 'case management' approach with the social worker in a key role might be relevant in future community psychiatric services. This material is primarily derived from the United Kingdom, but the conclusions are relevant to developed countries in general.

THE ORGANISATION OF MENTAL HEALTH SOCIAL WORK

Overview

Psychiatric social work in the UK has always been a predominantly hospital-based service, but current developments, both positive and negative, are undermining this situation. The positive developments are that large numbers of community mental health teams of variable composition are being established all over the country (NUPRD 1987) and usually include social workers. These teams are sometimes based in a hospital setting, but it is more usual for them to be located 'in the community'. The negative developments concern the financial plight of many local authorities; in many cases, established hospital social work services are threatened with transfer to other duties in community teams. This is partly a question of inadequate resources, but also partly an ideological argument. An antipathy to hospitals, doctors, and in particular the 'medical model' (see Fisher et al 1984 below) reduces the priority which some directors of social services departments give to mental health social work.

There are many arguments for the retention of a strong association between social work and psychiatry, whether the psychiatric service is delivered from the hospital or the community. One, to be mentioned only briefly concerns the educational function of service providers. No matter how 'community orientated' a service becomes, there will always be a need for a number of hospital beds for the most disturbed patients at the height of their disorder. Learning about the nature and effects of major psychiatric disturbance will always be most effective if it can be undertaken in this setting. Although social services may be delivered from another place, it is the hospital which is still the best educational resource in respect of these disorders.

A second argument for a strong association between social work and psychiatry is that patients' problems are invariably complex, and that no one discipline is able to encompass all the necessary perspectives and helping skills.

A third argument is that no matter how social services choose to organise their services, a large number of clients will have problems which are both social and psychological in nature. The following example is not atypical:

Case 1

The W family were referred to a social services office because they had rent and electricity arrears, and were about to have their electricity cut off. When, as in this case, there are young children in the family, the electricity authority automatically refers the case to the local social services, and practical measures are usually taken to alleviate the acute financial difficulties. In this case, the social worker observed that there were several other major contributory factors.

Mr W had recently been made redundant from his job, and was showing symptoms of anxiety and depression. He was becoming increasingly reluctant to leave the house, sensitive about his lack of work role, irritable with his family, and staying in bed for long periods. His wife was having great difficulty managing the behaviour of one of their daughters, who had previously been lively, popular, and well behaved.

The social worker collaborated with the GP, who treated the father with antidepressants and supportive psychotherapy, while the social worker used a casework approach with the mother and daughter. She arranged for the arrears to be paid off in smaller sums, and reduced the overall burden by obtaining a grant from a Charity. The daughter's problem behaviour was eliminated in six months and the father was able to find a part-time job. This work was done by a generic social worker, working in a generic team, but all too often, these cases are offered only practical help, while the mental health and relationship problems are labelled 'low priority' and neglected.

There are now several studies which show that social workers in generic practice are only able to recognise a proportion of the mental health problems in their clients (Huxley et al 1987, Corney 1984, Huxley & Fitzpatrick 1984). On the basis of published work, I estimated the amount of such morbidity which is 'hidden' from the social worker to be about half, compared with 40% for general practioners (Huxley 1985). In one study (Huxley et al 1987), it was found that the cases recognised as such by the social workers were similar to those identified by a psychiatric screening instrument, the General Health Questionnaire (GHQ). The social workers failed to recognise a large proportion of cases where there were clear physical signs of depression; these cases were assigned the diagnosis of depression by the PSE/CATEGO system, and were undoubtedly treatable cases.

In another study (Isaac et al 1986) current child care cases were examined, and the level of parental mental ill-health assessed. Over three-quarters of parents had consulted a psychiatrist, and at the time of interview, over half the mothers had case-positive scores on a psychiatric screening instrument.

Social workers appear to be reluctant to acknowledge these mental health aspects of their existing cases. Fisher et al (1984) refer to ideological, attitudinal, and organisational restrictions on social workers' ability to recognise mental illness in their clients. The social workers they interviewed showed antipathy to the medical approach, preferred environmental explanations of disturbed behaviour, and preferred 'prevention' to institutional care; they regarded the resources devoted to the provision of services for mentally ill people as inadequate, and the priority accorded to them as low. More serious were the perceived inadequacies of supervision of mental health work and the fact that the social workers and their managers lacked the skills necessary to work with people who received psychiatric treatment. The social workers observed by Fisher et al did not have the necessary experience of work with disturbed psychiatric patients to enable them to understand its nature or to develop their relevant social work skills.

In both practice and educational terms, these findings lend weight to the argument for retaining the teaching of social work practice in psychiatric hospital teams. Social workers could be relocated in community teams, but only if they were allowed to retain specialist caseloads, have supervision from experienced and knowledgeable social work managers, and continue to contribute their social perspective to the care of psychiatric inpatients. Without this sort of protection, they would soon be reallocated to work which is considered of greater 'priority'.

An increase in the number of social workers attached to, or working more closely with general practitioners would certainly be likely to increase the number of cases of minor psychiatric morbidity who receive social work help, and it has been recognised for some time that such cases are frequently referred for that purpose. In one study of cases referred to general practice attached workers (Huxley et al 1987), three-quarters of these cases were found to be suffering from psychiatric disorders. None of the cases seen by the attached workers suffered from psychotic disorders, which suggests that the attachment of social workers to general practice is likely to prove useful for certain types of psychiatric problem, while leaving others virtually untouched. A social work service for the most disabled and most floridly disturbed patients needs to have easy access to the specialist health services which are providing care for these categories of patients.

In face of the difficulties of providing a social work service for such disabled and acutely ill patients, some people are prepared to cede this role to the CPN. However, while it is true that there is a good deal of overlap in the activities of many professional groups, particularly when working in the community, it is equally the case that there are substantial differences (Woof 1986). Between social workers and CPNs, these differences in background, training, philosophy, work experience, agency resources, management, and statutory responsibilities are so great that in organisational terms, role-reversal is an impossibility. It seems altogether more appropriate to work towards the development of social work provision in conjunction with other professionals, irrespective of their organisational base, while at the same time trying to enhance the ability of social services staff to recognise psychiatric disorder in their clients and to respond appropriately. It remains to be seen, though, whether the energies devoted to enhancing personal support networks and providing local services actually contribute to or detract from this objective.

Informal support

The case for a more community-orientated style of social work practice — one which relies more heavily on informal caring 'networks' — was made out in the Brown, Hadley & White appendix to the Barclay Report — essentially the same case as in earlier publications (Hadley & McGrath 1984, Clode 1982). However, very little evidence exists that social services will be improved, simply because they are delivered in this way. Furthermore, it remains doubtful whether informal sources of support are readily available for most people with mental health problems. The following case illustration is a fairly typical example of the type of person with such problems who requires professional help, and for whom informal sources of support are lacking.

Case 2

Tom is a 50-year-old man who has had several episodes of mental disorder. He has had a number of different diagnoses during his psychiatric career, but the two main ones are schizophrenia and personality disorder. He was married briefly and has one son whom he never sees. His brother and sister-in-law live about 20 miles away, and they write to Tom a few times each year.

He lived for a time with three other men who had been discharged from the same mental hospital, but his bad behaviour, usually following heavy drinking, resulted in his having to leave. He now lives alone in a damp, poorly furnished, one-room apartment. He has a limited social life and no friends in the neighbourhood.

Tom makes regular visits to the local social services office, sometimes to present the staff with a minor financial problem to solve, but usually to talk about assorted fears and anxieties, and to complain about aspects of his housing and his life in general. He is seen by the duty social worker, who records that 'no further action' is to be taken in his case. In the past 12 months, he has visited his local office 49 times, always with the same outcome.

He continues to visit his old ward in the mental hospital, occasionally taking cigarettes for those patients whom he knows. This and his visits to the local office are his only social contacts.

Hallett (1983) and others (Townsend 1982, NISW 1983) have pointed out that social networks, particularly for handicapped and disadvantaged groups, are not always benign. The prospect of mobilising personal care and social support for Tom and others like him is quite different from the prospect of doing so for an elderly person — even one with few kin or social contacts. Evidence of the existence of a fund of social support in the community comes from studies of mentally healthy client groups. For example, Barclay cited the Equal Opportunities Commission Report on the care of elderly people (1981) in support of the argument for community social work, while in the USA, Gottlieb (1983) also referred primarily to elderly people when he considered the availability of network support.

Bayley et al (1983), in an attempt to investigate the sort of informal care which does exist and how resources could be used to support this, found that community support for the unhealthy 75-year-old-and-over group was much stronger than it was for mentally ill people and for families. The two studies they cited (Hunt 1976, Wenger 1981), which offered evidence that community networks are strong, were both conducted on an elderly population, whereas one of the studies which showed networks to be weak was conducted on an inner city population (Knight & Hayes 1981). There appears to be a differential fund of support related to ethnicity (Guttman 1979), socio-economic status (Hill et al 1970), and health (Rosencrantz et al 1968, Bayley et al 1983).

It is unwise, therefore, to generalise ideas about a fund of informal network support beyond the elderly population, and even in their case, the level of support is obviously also dependent upon a host of socio-demographic variables.

For those mentally ill people who continue to live in their own family, the possibility of mobilising support is more realistic. This is particularly likely to be the case where the patient lives with, or in easy reach of a daughter. In Bayley's study, 39% of visits made to all clients were by daughters, and 88% of the highly personal care was given by daughters. The major criticism of the policy to rely more heavily on informal care networks is that this in effect means increasing the burden on family members, and that the brunt of this care falls upon women. This problem will become increasingly evident in the near future, when the proportion of 'daughters' in the total population reaches an all-time low.

Finally, the mobilisation of support, where this exists, is probably a less skilled job than mobilising support where none is obviously available. Clearly, providing a support network for Tom, who is socially unpopular and behaviourally disturbed from time to time, would be a long-term, taxing undertaking. If social work skills can be profitably employed in 'managing' the drawing together of sources of both formal and informal support for clients, one could argue that the scarce resources of skilled social workers should be reserved for case management or for work with the most difficult cases.

Local services

The desire to provide services from a more 'local' base has become a significant element in both social work and psychiatric provision (Macht 1977, Hadley & McGrath 1984, MIND 1984). Hadley & McGrath, in proposing that services should 'go local', clearly indicated that a major objective was the development of new initiatives which were related to wider issues than 'the clients' problems'. This perspective was partly butressed by use of the familiar argument that evidence of the success of existing methods of intervention is lacking and that there are doubts about the adequacy of the standard of service offered to some client groups, especially the elderly and handicapped (Hadley 1983). The advantages of the 'neighbourhood model' are, it is argued, greater ease of access, contact with a wider range of clients, and enhanced ability to tap natural care-giving networks. It has also been maintained that the model may create pressures for the introduction of more local forms of political representation and control. It is hard to object in principle to these purposes, but as Hey (1983) points out, 'the patch model provides only partial solutions which are better suited to some problems, some aspects of service delivery and some philosophies, than others'.

There certainly are advantages to geographical proximity of services, not just in terms of physical ease of access, but also in the reduced financial burden of travelling costs. Benefits are to be gained from knowledge of local sources of help and support, but also disadvantages, such as the increased difficulty of achieving confidentiality — Case 3 illustrates this problem.

Case 3

Mary suffered an episode of acute depression. She had been looking after her husband, following his stroke, and the burden of caring for him, as well as her difficulty in adjusting to this new style of life, contributed to her problem. She wanted to struggle on, on her own and to avoid using either formal or informal sources of help.

A local community psychiatric service opened in a terraced house in a neighbouring street, and when the workers there found out about Mary's problems, they wanted her to join a small group of women to share the nature of their difficulties. However, she preferred to continue visiting the psychiatric hospital outpatient department for appointments with the psychiatrist. She argued that she was able to discuss her problems with the psychiatrist in confidence, rather than having to face her friends, acquaintances, or neighbours in the small group, or with anyone in the house which had already become known locally as the place where the 'loonies' go.

As well as the fact that clients like Mary choose to take their problems to a distant, but confidential service, local services may be unable to draw on community support if this has already been tried and tested beyond its limits. One respondent in the NISW study found it 'fanciful' that a community should be expected to support those, like Tom (Case 2), whom they had already rejected.

Locally-based workers may gain the advantage of knowledge of local resources, but at the same time lose contact with specialist resources for different client groups. At present, social workers do not recognise much of the psychological disorder presented to them and do not act upon it — either on their own or in concert with others (Corney 1984, Fisher et al 1984). Moving to a local patch system could make this collaboration worse than it is at the moment.

McGrath (1983) suggested that having responsibility for a 'patch' rather than for a 'caseload' offers social workers the chance to undertake more 'one-off' tasks, such as visiting an elderly person who is anxious about an impending hospital admission. In contrast, Judge (1983) doubts whether social workers can offer a service to a geographical area without the recipients of that service each becoming a 'case'. He asks 'where is the evidence identifying the circumstances in which an agency can assume a degree of responsibility for clients without them acquiring case status? It is axiomatic ... that the social care plan should be put into practice at the individual or case level'.

Thus, there is, as yet, no evidence that to adopt a locality-based social work service would lead to a better service for clients with psychiatric illness, and some reasons to suppose that it would lead to both less direct work with mentally ill people and poorer communication within and between services. Hey (1985) wonders whether there is a basic incompatability in the pressures to have in one worker both local knowledge and expertise in mental disorder, and Stevenson (1981) has expressed anxieties about several aspects of local organised services.

RELATIONSHIPS BETWEEN PRACTITIONERS IN THE COMMUNITY

Social workers and doctors

The obstacles facing most social workers and doctors who wish to work together are so great that it seems surprising that any successful joint work is ever achieved (Huntington 1981, Kessel 1986). Huntington, on the basis of a study of the practice of seven doctors and one social worker in South-West Sydney, examined the structural and cultural differences between the occupation of general practitioner and social worker. She observed that although cultural differences exist, there are also similarities: both are sensitive about the type and status of their knowledge and the status of the occupation itself; both are 'vulnerable to recent and continuing identity crises'; and both have similarly 'limitless missions'. She concluded, however, that there are radical structural differences between the professions in age, sex, work setting, income, and type of clientele. She held out little hope that mutual training exercises which are focused on the elucidation and modification of cultural differences will improve the situation, and argued that only modification of the structural differences could have any real impact.

Finding supporting evidence for her thesis is dishearteningly easy. There are anxieties from other professional personnel about the medical profession's desire to exert a prescriptive influence over them (Hill 1978, Webb & Hobdell 1980); psychiatrists continue to assert their position as the 'natural' leader of teams (Zusman & Lamb 1977, Borus 1978, Connell 1980); social workers continue to assume that they are the 'only' defenders of patient/client rights, to the annoyance of other disciplines who argue that they too have this responsibility (Connaway 1975). Also, although team members in psychiatric units may think that they use an eclectic bio-psychosocial model, evidence from hospital ward rounds suggests that the medical model exerts an overriding influence (Sanson-Fisher et al 1979). The struggle for 'primacy' (in which one group takes prime responsibility in work with groups or sub-groups in the same field) is just as likely to be an issue in community-based as in institution-based work. There are many possible organisational arrangements for community psychiatric services, and as recent developments show, social workers and other professional staff may assume the prime responsibility for the development and management of services, in preference to doctors.

Multiprofessional work in the community

Kathleen Jones (1984) identifies structural and cultural obstacles to the achievement of multiprofessional work in community psychiatry — the administrative fragmentation of community services is one of them. Pritchard & King (1980) argue that on some issues, 'there is greater variation within professional groups than between groups, suggesting that personal perspectives may override professional conformity or socialisation'. A number of studies suggest that joint training exercises can be helpful (Loxley 1980, Bruce 1980) — particularly those focussed on the development of the team or on teamwork (Rubin et al 1975, Lowe & Herranen 1981).

Rubin & Beckhard (1971) pointed out that:

It is naive to bring together a highly diverse group of people and expect that by calling them a team they will in fact behave as a team. It is ironic indeed to realise that a football team spends 40 hours per week practising teamwork for two hours on a Sunday afternoon when their teamwork really counts. Teams in organisations seldom spend two hours per year practising, when their ability to function as a team counts 40 hours per week.

Wing (1980) has argued that selection and training of staff and ensuring proper communication between workers in different parts of a service should be given the highest priority, even above the allocation of more resources.

There is in fact little evidence in the social work literature to show that teamwork has many advantages. On the other hand, there is some negative evidence, in that most of the major enquiries into child abuse tragedies in the UK have highlighted the poor communication between disciplines and agencies, and argued for a greater 'sharing' of information and for more joint work.

Studies of social workers' use of time suggests that being part of a team of other disciplines is likely to lead to greater face-to-face contact between the social worker and client. Having a social work member on a team seems to have an indirectly beneficial effect on client 'outcome' — this has been observed in general practice (Cooper et al 1975) and in schools (Rose & Marshall 1974). Client satisfaction with the service received was higher when the social worker was part of a multidisciplinary team (Corney 1983). In Rushton & Briscoe's (1981) view, 'clients with emotional problems appear to benefit most fully from the multidisciplinary approach at the health centre. Problems of this nature were most frequently the subject of detailed discussion between doctor and social worker'. The physical proximity of social worker and GP in the same building obviously provides greater opportunity for collaboration, but one cannot assume that better collaboration will automatically result. Bruce (1980) found that physical proximity only fostered better collaboration if there was positive motivation to do so, while Gilchrist et al (1978) made the same observation on the basis of a survey of GP-attached social workers in Great Britain.

Bruce (1980) reported on two separate studies of teams — the first including GPs, health visitors, and district nurses, and the second also including social workers, voluntary organisations, the police, and day nurseries. The aim of these enquiries was to discover factors which either facilitated or inhibited co-operation between the disciplines. In the first study, 36 teams were examined, and in the second, the names of children under five were sent to all the agencies (177 children in the pilot postal enquiry; 68 cases were the subject of more detailed interviews in the main study). Bruce obtained information from the agencies concerning their knowledge of the child and/or a number of risk factors (such as deprivation and psychiatric disorder) in each case, and whether they considered the child to be 'vulnerable' because of the risk factors.

In the main study, only 20 out of 68 children were mentioned by more than one agency; this confirmed the striking results of the pilot study, in which only one of the 20 particularly vulnerable children was known to more than one agency. Social workers knew very few of the vulnerable children and identified very few of the risk factors in those children whom they did know. One of the two areas selected for study had higher rates of social disadvantage (in terms of alcohol abuse, wife battering, illegitimate births, and high-rise housing); all the agencies involved, except social work, reported higher levels of vulnerability in this area.

Bruce reports examples of the failures of co-operation between the disciplines: for instance, when GPs instituted a fortnightly inter-disciplinary meeting, they and the health visitors attended, but the only social worker who attended regularly was one who worked at the local hospital. Stevenson & Parsloe's descriptive survey of social service teams (DHSS 1978) showed that social workers outside hospitals are reluctant to accept medical referrals, for fear of encouraging the 'medical auxiliary' view of their profession. However, this particular view may become weaker in the future than at present, especially as the establishment of specialist mental health social workers (Approved Social Workers) under the 1983 Mental Health Act gives them a clear responsibility to take medical opinion into account when forming an independent judgement about hospitalisation.

We have already mentioned the unanimity of official reports into child care tragedies in ascribing a central role to a failure to share information and co-operate. In Bruce's study, it was clear that the different agencies involved were identifying different children as being specially vulnerable, and this was because, 'they were working from different information bases, which meant, of course, that they were not sharing the information which was available'. Bruce concludes that there are three patterns of co-operation: 'nominal', in which there is minimal information flow by letter or administrative exchange, e.g. between electricity boards and the social services department (as in Case 1 above); 'convenient co-operation', where there is no substantial barrier to free information exchange, but it only takes place when the benefits outweigh the costs, e.g. health visitor attachment to GPs; and 'committed co-operation', which requires mutual trust or organisational stimulus and the acceptance of 'superordinate goals'. Superordinate goals are those which have a compelling appeal for the members of each group but which neither can achieve without the participation of the other.

Superordinate goals, such as the provision of a comprehensive community psychiatric service, probably cannot be implemented by psychiatrists or the health service without the active collaboration of social workers and social services departments. To attempt to do so will result in an inferior service. It has to be said, however, that the current pattern of working relationships in the community, between psychiatry and social work leaves much to be desired.

COMPETENCE AND EFFECTIVENESS IN MENTAL HEALTH SOCIAL WORK

Following several years of criticism of the standards of social work practice and education, moves, such as the establishment of specialist mental health social workers (Approved Social Workers) and the requirement for ASW training courses to be formally approved may encourage the development of more competent practice in mental health social work in the UK. At the same time, summaries of research into social work interventions (Reid & Hanrahan 1982, Reid 1983, Thomlinson 1984) hold out more promise than earlier, critical summaries (Brewer & Lait 1980). It seems that the use of more specific methods of intervention partly accounts for the greater success in demonstrating a positive effect in studies with randomised, controlled designs. The same point has been made with regard to intervention studies in health settings (Paterson & Anderson 1984, Mumford et al 1982, Westermayer 1982). Simons (1984) argues that a rudimentary empirical base exists for professional approaches which are likely to be effective in the treatment of depression, social anxieties, child behaviour problems, marital distress, and psychosexual dysfunction — a list of problems which constitutes a major portion of the caseload dealt with by social workers in the community. The cases reported in one casebook, (Oliver et al 1988), show a range of methods used by social workers in the mental health field with varying degrees of success.

The existence of some empirical evidence for the effectiveness of social work with people who have mental health problems owes a good deal to work done at the General Practice Research Unit at the Institute of Psychiatry in London. A series of related evaluative studies from there (Cooper et al 1975, Shepherd et al 1979, Corney 1981, 1982) are important because they had sound research designs and concerned clients who were suffering from identified psychiatric disorder. However, the results of intervention were mixed, and in some cases the interventions themselves were not closely specified.

In the first of these (Cooper et al 1975), the clients of an experimental social work attachment to general practice were compared with broadly comparable controls, selected from eight different practices. The clients were those who were suffering from chronic neurotic illness, and were assessed using standardised social and clinical interview schedules. They were followed-up and re-interviewed at 12 months. There were significant differences between the two groups at follow-up: the experimental group had significantly lower clinical and social scores, more of them had been taken off psychotropic drugs, and fewer were considered to be in need of continuing medical care and supervision. However, the element of the social work intervention responsible for the positive result cannot be determined, because its precise nature is not specified.

The mean ratings of change in the psychiatric and social scores of clients were analysed separately for each professional worker: the social worker achieved reductions marginally greater than those of the psychiatrist in the clients' psychiatric scores, but the psychiatrist achieved a change in social score marginally greater than the social worker. When the two worked together, they achieved the greatest reduction in psychiatric score and the lowest reduction in social score. Cooper et al concluded that the effect of the experimental service was to some extent the result of 'group interaction'.

In a later, more detailed analysis of the activities of the social worker (Shepherd et al 1979), those cases referred for social work help (n=61) were compared to those not referred (n=31); the referred group contained fewer married patients, and more had severe or moderately severe psychiatric disturbances. In nearly two-thirds of the cases, practical work only was undertaken, while in the remainder, there was casework, or casework and practical support. Neither the type of work undertaken nor the pattern of contacts with cases were significantly associated with clinical outcome, except in the case of short-term work, which did have an association with 'improved' clinical status. Change in overall score was unrelated to social work activity, and was the same in referred and non-referred cases. While the finding that short-term work may be of benefit confirms previous reports in social work, the study clearly demonstrates the need to study more specific methods of intervention, which are targeted on carefully assessed and circumscribed problems.

One such study was conducted by Corney (1981, 1982, Corney & Clare 1983), who examined the social work interventions of four social workers attached part-time to GPs, with a group of depressed women. The clients were between 18 and 45 years of age, presented 'acute' or 'acute-on-chronic' depression, and were randomly allocated to an experimental or control group. Those in the experimental group were referred to the attached workers, while the controls were referred back to their doctor for routine treatment. There was no difference in clinical or social outcome of the two groups at six months' follow-up, when they were reassessed using the same instruments, although a higher proportion of the experimental group had improved. When all the clients were asked who had helped them, two-thirds of those who saw a social worker mentioned that she had helped them, and when asked who had helped them most, 60% of the 35 clients who had seen a social worker indicated that she had.

Further analysis revealed that a sub-group of the women did benefit from the social worker's intervention; this included women who were initially assessed as having major marital or boyfriend problems and suffering from acute-on-chronic depression. Eighty per cent of this sub-group in the experimental service improved, compared with 31% of the controls. The difference was maintained at one year, and according to the medical notes, 57% were judged by the doctor to be well, compared with only 18% of the controls. Only one-quarter of the clients in the experimental group felt that no-one had helped them, whereas over 70% of the controls felt that.

This study gives a broad indication of the sort of problem which is likely to be helped by the practical and supportive service provided by the social workers, but does little to help specify the 'therapeutic ingredient' in the approach(es) used. In this, as in many other studies reported in the literature, the approaches used by the workers are not described adequately. We are told that the workers were asked to see the clients regularly, to make a 'contract', and to limit the intervention to six months. In addition, the workers used some behavioural techniques and psychosocial interventions. This perhaps is an accurate reflection of work elsewhere in the field, where, according to Fisher et al, workers use individualistic methods indiscriminately.

In future, the evaluation of mental health social work will require us to be more specific about the nature of the intervention, and more rigorous in our approach to the design of evaluative studies. A number of social work writers have called for increasing use of single-case experimental designs in practice and research. Fischer (1978) and Peterson & Anderson (1984) have suggested that this system could be used to try out methods of practice, and thereby generate hypotheses for testing in subsequent experiments.

CASE MANAGEMENT

An alternative approach to the provision of social work for people with psychiatric problems is to employ the social worker as a case manager (Lamb 1980, Davies & Challis 1981, Caro 1981, Lamb 1982, Sherwood & Morris 1983, Ruchlin & Morris 1983). This approach has been advocated for service provision in community settings; it would be suitable for both long- and short-stay discharged psychiatric patients, and is particularly suited for patients who require long-term rather than short-term care in the community.

Care is provided through the individually planned combination of different sources of support, and the whole care-package is overseen by a single 'case manager'. In some instances, the services are paid for or bought in, and a mixture of public and private sector and voluntary help is possible. In some working examples of the approach, the budget which can be spent on each individual client is administered by the case manager, but this is not always the case. Individual assessment is strongly emphasised, and this system is intended to help services meet individual needs, rather than fit the client into a pre-existing network of services. In both the UK and the USA, there are examples of such schemes for elderly people (Davies & Challis 1981, Caro 1981). In Virginia's Service Integration for Deinstitutionalisation, and Florida's Integrated Health and Rehabilitation Services, case managers are responsible for enabling their clients to obtain access to the services to which they are entitled. Case managers undertake assessment, planning, monitoring, and advocacy functions in the NIMH's community support programme. Johnson & Rubin (1983) consider that the mentally ill as a client group are suited to the use of a case management approach, those with long-term problems, in particular, requiring continual reassessment of their needs. A DHSS-funded attempt to introduce elements of this approach for discharged psychiatric patients in Salford (Whitehead 1987) reported only modest success, and the conclusion that case management had to be paid for in addition to all existing services seemed unlikely to be welcomed by service managers.

A skilled case manager working with mentally ill people should be able to recognise early signs of decompensation, motivate clients, ensure that they make use of the available services, and provide them with a stable supportive relationship. The differences between the role of case manager and of case worker in traditional approaches are both of kind and of degree. In the case management approach there is: less reliance on a single mode of helping; a willingness to combine practical and therapeutic forms of help; an increased use of resources in the client's environment and outside the statutory sector; an extended responsibility for aspects of the provision of social services, in particular, a greater responsibility for the expenditure involved in service provision; and therefore a greater emphasis on accountability for the costs as well as the benefits of service.

In an interesting extension of their work in Kent, the Personal Social Services Research Unit established a project in which the case manager had responsibility for staff from both health and social services. This project was concerned with elderly patients. The outcome, in terms of the numbers of people who could be maintained in the community rather than in a hospital bed was so good that the health service decided to continue to fund the whole scheme as part of the normal service provision. This study demonstrates that the services of health and social services can both be managed at the same time by one case manager (Challis et al 1989). However, in order for this approach to work in practice, some fundamental changes in thinking about services and their organisation are needed.

First, the case manager must be able to be responsible for the work of workers in more than one agency. Secondly, the approach seems to work best when the case manager has control, at least nominally, of the budget for the clients served by his team. This may require a joint agency budget. Thirdly, a degree of commitment from all involved to the detailed assessment and regular review of clients is essential, and this is almost certainly more time-consuming than the present system. Fourthly, there must be no reluctance to use private services or voluntary services (where these have to be paid for) if these are essential to the overall plan of care. Fifthly, the support of non-statutory volunteers or carers assumes significance and must not be neglected. Finally, the training implications have to be considered; this may be of particular importance when the client group to be served includes people with behavioural problems.

CONCLUSIONS

If case management services are to be developed for mentally ill people in the UK, then specialist skills will be needed which may not be available at present. Hey (1984) has suggested that the skills involved in planning, implementation, and monitoring of this system may be missing in the middle levels of British social services departments. The (House of Commons) Select Committee Report (1985) confirmed that specialist knowledge and skills in mental health work are not present in middle management. No more than 10 (out of 62 local authorities providing information) had a specialist mental illness senior manager, and in some of these instances, responsibility for mentally ill people was shared with another client group, usually mentally handicapped people. Only 10 of the authorities had an adviser on mental health services, while a mere 14 (out of 75 authorities) had specialist mental health teams (and team leaders) working from area fieldwork offices. However, the Committee noted that developments in community psychiatry were producing 'signs of organisation change and review'. A recent report confirms that there are indications of an improvement in the response of social services departments to services for mentally ill people (Huxley et al 1987). This is partly due to the fact that some authorities have taken the opportunity provided by the 1983 Mental Health Act to develop resources, and to become more involved in the provision of community mental health teams.

A number of further developments in social work will also be required in order to make a sustained and positive contribution to community psychiatric services. Among these is the need to improve social workers' basic understanding of psychiatry. Before the 1983 Mental Health Act, more than half of the trained social workers in the UK had less than five hours' specific training in psychiatry in their basic training course. Approved Social Worker training has improved this position (Huxley et al 1987) to some extent. Another factor will be the extent to which experimental service interventions can be tested in social services, and thoroughly evaluated. Finally, the reorganisation of community care for mentally ill people will not place the sole responsibility with the health service, but allow and encourage social work to play a part. However the services are organised, social workers will have clients, individuals or families, where mental illness is a major factor. To ignore this fact can only diminish the quality of community psychiatry.

REFERENCES

Bayley M, Seyd R, Tennant A, Simons K 1983 What resources does the informal sector need to fulfill its role? In: NISW, the Barclay Report: papers from a consultation day, Paper 15

Borus J 1978 Issues critical to the survival of community mental health. American Journal of Psychiatry 135: 1029-1035

Brewer C, Lait J 1980 Can social work survive? Temple Smith, London

Bruce N 1980 Teamwork for preventive care, research studies press. Wiley, New York

Caro F G 1981 Demonstrating community-based long-term care in the United States: an evaluation research perspective. In: Goldberg E M, Connolly N (eds) Evaluative research in social care. Heinemann Educational Books, London

Challis D Darton R, Johnson L, Stone M Traske K 1989 Supporting frail, elderly people at home: the Darlington Community Care Project. PSSRU, University of Kent, Canterbury

Clode D 1982 The battle of chapter 13. Social Work Today 1338: 8-9

Connaway R S 1975 Teamwork and social worker advocacy: conflicts and possibilities. Community Mental Health Journal 114: 381-388

Connell P H 1980 Multidisciplinary teams - a personal view. Bulletin of the Royal College of Psychiatrists June: 89-90

Cooper B, Harwin C B G, Depla C, Shepherd M 1975 Mental health care in the community: an evaluative study. Psychological Medicine 5: 372-381

Corney R H 1981 Social work effectiveness in the management of depressed women: a clinical trial. Psychological Medicine 112: 417-424

Corney R H 1982 The effectiveness of social work intervention in the management of depressed women in general practice. In: Clare A W, Corney R H (eds) Social work and primary health care. Academic Press, London

Corney R H 1983 The views of clients new to a general practice attachment scheme and to a local authority social work intake team. Social Science & Medicine 17: 1549-1558

Corney R H 1984 The mental and physical health of clients referred to social workers in a local authority department and a general practice attachment scheme. Psychological Medicine 14: 137-144

Corney R H, Clare A W 1983 The effectiveness of attached social workers in the management of depressed women in General practice. British Journal of Social Work 13: 57-74

Davies B, Challis D 1981 A production relations evaluation of the meeting of needs in the community care projects. In: goldberg E M, Connolly N (eds) Evaluation research in social care. Heinemann Educational Books, London

DHSS 1978 Social Service Teams: the practitioners view. HMSO, London

Equal Opportunities Commission 1981 Caring for the elderly and handicapped: community policies and women's lives. EOC, London

Fischer J 1978 Effective casework practice: an eclectic approach. McGraw-Hill, New York

Fisher M, Newton C, Sainsbury E 1984 Mental health social work observed. George Allen Unwin, London

Gilchrist I C, Gough J B, Horsfall-Turner Y R, Ineson E M, Keele G, Scott H J 1978 Social work in general practice. Journal of the Royal College of General Practitioners 28: 675-686

Gottlieb B H 1983 Social support strategies: guidelines for mental health practice. Sage, London

Griffiths 1988 Caring for people: community care in the next decade and beyond. CM849 HMSO (1989), London

Guttman D 1979 Use of informal and formal supports by white ethnic aged. In: Gelfand D E, Kutzik A (eds) Ethnicity and aging. Springer, New York

Hadley R 1983 The philosophy of patchwork and its implementation. In: Sinclair I, Thomas D (eds) Perspectives on Patch. NISW Paper 14: 4-6

Hadley R, McGrath M 1984 When social services are local: the Normanton experience. George Allen Unwin, London

Hallett C 1983 Social workers: their role and tasks 1982. British Journal of Social Work 134: 395-404

Hey A 1983 Not by patch alone. Unpublished

Hey A 1985 The Mental Health Act 1983: practice and organisational implications. In:

Mental health staff development: issues and strategies. Report of a Working Conference, CCETSW, London

Hill M 1978 Relations with other agencies. In: DHSS, Social Service Teams: the practitioners view. HMSO, London

Hill R, Foote N, Aldous J, Carlson R, MacDonald R 1970 Family development in three generations. Schenkman, Cambridge, MA

Hunt A 1976 The elderly at home: a study of people aged 65 and over living in the community in England in 1976. HMSO, London

Huntington J 1981 Social work and general medical practice: collaboration or conflict? George Allen Unwin, London

Huxley P J 1985 Social work practice in mental health. Gower, Aldershot

Huxley P J, Fitzpatrick R 1984 The probable extent of minor mental illness in the adult clients of social workers: a research note. British Journal of Social Work 14: 67-73

Huxley P J, Korer J, Tolley S 1987 The psychiatric caseness of clients referred to an urban social services department. British Journal of Social Work 17: 507-520

Isaac B, Minty E B, Morrison R M 1986 Children in care — the association with mental disorder in the parents. British Journal of Social Work 16: 325-339

Johnson P J, Rubin A 1983 Case management in mental health: a social work domain? Social Work 281: 49-56

Jones K 1984 The mental health professional 2000. Bulletin of the Interdisciplinary Association of Mental Health Workers 1: 2-7

Judge K 1983 From the tyranny of the case to the myth of the community: reflections on the Barclay Report. In: NISW Report 15 The Barclay Report. Papers from a consultation day

Kessel N 1986 Communications between doctors and social workers. In: Partnership or prejudice: communication between doctors and those in other caring professions. The Nuffield Provincial Hospitals Trust

Knight B, Hayes R 1981 Self-help in the inner city. Voluntary Services Council, London

Lamb H R 1980 Therapist case-managers: more than brokers of services. Hospital and Community Psychiatry 31: 14-18

Lamb H R 1982 Treating the long-term mentally ill. Jossey-Bass, London

Lowe J I, Herranen M 1981 Understanding teamwork: another look at the concepts. Social Work in Health Care 72: 1-11

Loxley A 1980 A study of multidisciplinary in-service training in the interests of health care. Social Work Service 24: 39-43

McGrath M 1983 Researching patch teams. In: NISW, Report 15 The Barclay Report. Papers from a consultation day

Macht L B 1977 An introduction to the field. In: Macht L B, Sherl D J, Sharfstein S (eds) Neighborhood psychiatry. Lexington Books, Lexington

MIND 1984 Care in the community: keeping it local. Annual Conference Report. MIND Publications, London

Mumford M, Schlesinger H J, Glass G V 1982 The effect of psychological intervention on recovery from surgery and heart attacks: an analysis of the literature. American Journal of Public Health 722: 141-151

NISW 1983 Responses to the Barclay Report. National Institute for Social Work, Paper 16, London

NUPRD 1987 Community mental health teams: a survey. National Unit for Psychiatric Research and Development, London

Oliver J, Huxley P J, Butler A 1988 Mental health casework: illustrations and reflections. Manchester University Press, Manchester

Paterson K J, Anderson S C 1984 Evaluation of social work practice in health care settings. Social Work in Health Care 101: 1-16

Pritchard C, King R 1980 A study of changes in the mutual perceptions of trainee GPs and social work students. Social Work Service 24: 47-51

Reid W J 1983 Reid and Hanrahan reply. Social Work 281: 79

Reid W J, Hanrahan P 1982 Recent evaluation of social work: grounds for optimism. Social Work 27: 33-38

Rose G, Marshall T F 1974 Counselling and school social work: an experimental study. Wiley, London

Rosencrantz H A, Pihlblad C T, McNevin T E 1968 Social participation of older people in a small town. Unpublished Manuscript. Department of Sociology, University of Missouri, Columbia

Rubin I M, Beckhard M 1971 Factors influencing the effectiveness of health teams. MIT Working Paper 561-571, Massachusetts Institute of Technology, Cambridge

Rubin I M, Plovnick M S, Fry R E 1975 Improving the coordination of care: a program for health team development. Ballinger, Cambridge, Mass

Ruchlin H S, Morris J H 1983 Pennsylvania's domiciliary care experiment II: Cost benefit implications. American Journal of Public Health 736: 654-660

Rushton A, Briscoe M 1981 Social work as an aspect of primary health care: the social workers view. British Journal of Social Work 111: 61-76

Sanson-Fisher R W, Poole D A, Harker J 1979 Behavioural analysis of ward rounds within a general hospital psychiatric unit. Behaviour Research & Therapy 17: 333-348

Select Committee on Social Services 1985 Community care. HMSO, London447

Shepherd M, Harwin B G, Depla C, Cairns V 1979 Social work and the primary care of mental disorder. Psychological medicine 94: 661-670

Sherwood S, Morris J N 1983 The Pennsylvania domiciliary care experiment I: Impact on quality of life. American Journal of Public Health 736: 646-653

Simons R L 1984 Additional findings. Social Work 294: 401-403

Stevenson O 1981 Specialism in social service teams. George Allen Unwin, London

Thomlinson R J 1984 Something works: evidence from practice effectiveness studies. Social Work 291: 51-56

Townsend D 1982 A whole lot of nothing. Social Work Today 1341: 11-13

Webb A, Hobdell M 1980 Coordination and teamwork in the health and personal social services. In: Lonsdale S, Webb A, Briggs T L (eds) Teamwork in the personal social services and health care, Croom Helm, London

Wenger G C 1981 The elderly in the community: family contacts, social integration, and community involvement. Social Services in Rural Areas Research Project, Working Paper, 18

Westermeyer J 1982 Education counselling in hospital care. American Journal of Public Health 722: 126-127

Whitehead C 1987 Care of long-term psychiatric patients. Final report of DHSS Research Project, Salford Health Authority

Wing J K 1980 Innovations in social psychiatry. Psychological Medicine 102: 219-230

Wooff K 1986 A comparison between social workers and CPNs. Unpublished, PhD Thesis, University of Manchester

Zusman J, Lamb H R 1977 In defense of community mental health. American Journal of Psychiatry 1348: 887-890

16. Community psychiatric nursing in Britain

J. W. Rawlinson, A. C. Brown

That this chapter is entitled 'Community Psychiatric Nursing' rather than 'Psychiatric Nursing in the Community' reflects to some extent the problems that the profession in Britain experiences in coping with change. In considering psychiatric nurses who have involvement in the community, we are dealing in the main with that group who are defined and employed exclusively as community psychiatric nurses (CPNs); this contrasts with the way in which some other disciplines have varied their commitment between hospital and community services.

Examining the background, we will consider the historical development and current organisation of community psychiatric nursing, including training, developing ideas which are currently within nursing as a whole, and issues in the field of community mental health which are important for psychiatric nurses in particular.

BACKGROUND

The venture into the community by British psychiatric nurses is a recent phenomenon. The nineteenth century asylum was staffed by keepers and attendants who had no standardised training until 1890, when, under the auspices of the Medico-Psychological Association, a 2 year programme was introduced. In 1908 this became a 3 year training, comparable with that of general nurses, although for many years only a small proportion of mental nurses had completed the course. After the Nurses Registration Act of 1919 and the establishment of the General Nursing Council (GNC) for England and Wales, there was provision from 1921 for nurses trained in the care of people suffering from mental diseases to be registered and certificated separately. In 1926, the Medico-Psychological Association became the Royal Medico-Psychological Association (RMPA) and continued to conduct examinations and award certificates until as recently as 1951; since then, all mental nurses have been dealt with for registration by the GNC on the same basis as other nurses. Training in modern times is discussed in detail below.

Until the 1930s, psychiatric care was mainly custodial, although some therapeutic endeavours were attempted and the first outpatient clinics established. The Mental Treatment Act of 1930 made provision for the admission of voluntary patients to mental hospitals, and from then on, a steady growth occurred in the number of short-term admissions. The introduction of physical methods such as ECT, insulin coma, and pre-frontal leucotomy produced a change in emphasis from containment to treatment; it has been suggested (Baly 1980) that the optimism engendered by this approach initiated an improvement in the status of both nurses and doctors involved in the care of the mentally ill. However, this process re-emphasised the use of the general medical/hospital model for people with psychological problems — an approach that has frequently been challenged (Kennedy 1980) on the grounds that it ignores the importance of moral, social, political, and philosophical aspects of psychiatric illness.

This 'hospitalisation of the asylums' was further encouraged by the introduction in the mid-1950s of another very successful method of physical treatment — antipsychotic drugs — a process accompanied by profound changes in the management of psychiatric patients. At the same time, for a variety of reasons, attitudes towards the need for restriction and supervision of patients were also changing; wards were unlocked and the proportion of discharges increased. The total number of inpatients in British mental hospitals, which had been steadily growing for many years, began to fall and this decline has continued to the present day. The relationship between the introduction of antipsychotic drugs and the 'opening' of hospitals has been much debated, but there can be no reasonable doubt that these treatments allowed for the discharge of many patients who would otherwise have stayed in 'chronic' wards. In the late 1950s, the introduction of antidepressant drugs further decreased the need for inpatient care.

In 1954, the first 'outpatient nurses' in Britain were appointed at Warlingham Park Hospital, Surrey; their work (Moore 1960, 1964) involved supervision of outpatients by visiting those who either failed to attend clinics or were not for admission, attending clinics and therapeutic social groups, providing follow-up support of discharged patients, and helping to find jobs and accommodation for them. Some of these functions might have been seen as the usual province of the psychiatric social worker, and in fact the community nursing service began at a time when there was nationally, a shortage of these workers. For the same reason, in 1957, at Moorhaven Hospital, Devon (Hunter 1974), nurses working with inpatients were given additional roles, which included monitoring patients' progress outside hospital.

However, after some time, it was noted that an extended role was emerging for the nurse working with psychiatric patients in the community (Green 1968). Specified community psychiatric nursing services began to develop, with nurses working entirely outside hospital, though from a variety of bases and with varying referral sources. This coincided with, and may have further accelerated, the continuing decline in the total number of psychiatric inpatients.

The English Mental Health Act of 1959 made both admission and discharge easier and less formal. It encouraged local authorities to develop various forms of sheltered accommodation, sheltered occupation, and other support services for the mentally ill in the community, and also required them to appoint mental welfare officers, who took over the duties carried out by 'duly authorised officers' under the previous legislation. However, the role of the mental welfare officer was intended to be far wider — in fact, that of a specialist mental health social worker. Unfortunately, the reorganisation of social services in 1971 resulted in the disappearance of specialist psychiatric social workers and mental welfare officers in many areas; their work was taken over by 'generic' social workers, who had to divide their time between a number of client groups. These personnel were unable to gain sufficient experience with the mentally ill or mentally handicapped, and lacked any special training in such work. This process further encouraged the development of community psychiatric nursing services because of the gap that had developed in the care of psychiatric patients outside hospital at a time when increasing numbers of the chronically ill were being discharged.

THE PRESENT SITUATION

Psychiatric nursing outside hospital in Britain today is almost entirely performed by those who are full-time CPNs. Since 1969, their overall numbers have increased at a rate probably unrivalled amongst the health professions; the increase between 1954 and 1985 in the UK is shown in Figure 16.1. If that trend continued, the 1985 total would double by 1992, and this would in fact correlate with forecasts of regional health authority strategic plans (CPNA 1985).

This development would appear to suggest that the main way in which health authorities tried to implement the national policy of transferring the psychiatric hospital population into the community, was initially to increase the number of community nursing staff. However, the number of nurses working within hospitals has not declined in line with decreasing bed numbers, since the remaining inpatients are an increasingly elderly, disabled, and dependent group. The CPN/population ratio from the 1985 survey showed a change from 1:50 000 in 1980 to 1:23 800 in 1985, although there were wide regional variations. The 1992 projection (assuming a static, although older population) would give a 1:11 900 ratio — still short of the 1:7500 which the Royal College of Psychiatrists (1980) believed was needed if CPNs were to be effectively based in the primary health care sector. Marks (1985), in a study of nurse therapists (i.e. nurses who had undertaken a special course in behavioural treatments) as distinct from CPNs, suggested that there should be a

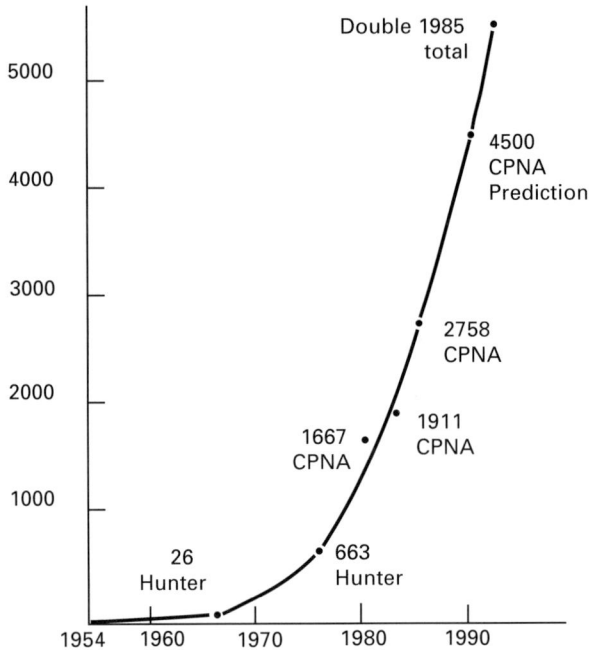

Fig. 16.1 Increase in number of full-time CPNs between 1954 and 1985.

nurse therapist-to-population ratio of 1:10 000. Nurse therapists work both in hospital and community settings, and the overlap of their role with that of the CPN needs to be more clearly defined, but few were then practising in Britain (75 had completed training in 1983).

The Government response to the House of Commons Social Services Committee Report on community care (DHSS 1985b) approached the question of nurse/population ratio by including all psychiatric nurses, whether working in hospital or community. It suggested that although the target of 100 nurses per 100 000 population suggested in *Better Services for the Mentally Ill* (DHSS 1975) has been met, there remained an imbalance both in terms of regional variation, and in the ratio of trained to untrained staff. The 1975 White Paper had suggested this change in approach from previous targets of one nurse per three inpatients, which had penalised community-orientated services.

ORGANISATION OF SERVICES

There are broadly two main groups of CPNs: those working within a specialist multidisciplinary team — often from a psychiatric hospital,

Table 16.1   CPNs by main base

Base	1980*	1985		Change
*	%	%	n	%
Psychiatric hospital	49	37	962	-12
Psychiatric unit (DGH)	28	19	492	-9
Health centre/GP	8	17	442	+9
Day hospital	8	10	252	+2
Other**	3	17	427	+14
Not stated	4	0	0	-4
Total	100	100	2575	

*In the 1980 survey, managers were asked where their CPN service was mainly based.
**The 'other' category for 1985 includes day centres for the elderly, community mental health centres, CPN community bases, drug clinics, rehabilitation centres, and the ESMI units.
Source: ©CPNA 1985. Reproduced with permission

district general hospital unit, or day hospital base — and those working in a primary health care setting. Both are likely to be administered as a separate nursing unit from those nurses working entirely in the hospital or health centre, respectively. The survey of CPNs carried out by the Community Psychiatric Nurses Association (CPNA 1985) revealed that the largest group were still those based in psychiatric hospitals; their numbers had increased between 1980 and 1985, but there had been a far greater increase in the number of community-based CPNs (Table 16.1). The total number of CPNs identified in these surveys increased from 1667 in 1980 to 2575 in 1985.

Differing opinions have been expressed as to the relative desirability of the two situations. According to the CPNA survey, many of the CPNs, as well as the majority of general practitioners, are in favour of continuing the trend towards these nurses being based in primary care. Of those people in the general population presenting with psychological disorders, at least 90% are dealt with in the primary care setting by GPs, and CPNs are seen by them as appropriate professionals with whom to share this burden. The majority (59%) of referrals, however, still come from psychiatrists (CPNA 1985) and there is a much higher proportion of severe disorders among patients seen by them.

A further argument in favour of the health centre/GP-attached CPN is an economic one; many CPN services have been sectorised to geographical areas, which may equate fairly well with GP practices but tend not to correspond with the much larger catchment areas covered by psychiatrists. Not only do the shorter distances travelled save costs, but the time saved can be spent in extra clinical activities.

The argument advanced by many consultants against basing the CPN service in the primary care sector is the concept of the specialist multidisciplinary psychiatric team. Such teams will probably continue to be the basis for the practice of psychiatry in Britain for some time ahead, and nurses are clearly an integral part of them. If the CPN is the only nurse member working in the community, and if CPNs are all attached to primary care services, then direct input to the team by one person from this discipline is lost, and the team must relate to a number of different nurses outside hospital, which adds to communication problems. In addition, if the more serious cases are referred to psychiatrists, attachment to GPs may lead to CPNs being involved mostly with minor cases, at the expense of major ones.

However, proposals made by Griffiths (1988) may lead to a greater division between acute hospital-based services and services provided in the community as part of a 'community care' provision. Wooff et al (1986,1988, Wooff & Goldberg 1988) suggested that the isolation of the CPN from other mental health professionals results in poor clinical supervision and less opportunity for the development of expertise. She has proffered the image of a 'back ward' in the community, with clients making up ever increasing case loads for CPNs, whose managers are unable to offer clinical support. Thus, CPNs may need to be cautious in severing their links with the specialist mental health team and the hospital services.

This division of opinion on the arrangements for nursing services covering the community has led to much criticism of them from both sides. However, the resolution of these problems of nursing organisation probably lies not in changing the nursing structure in isolation, but rather in overall changes of all the specialist psychiatric services into a mental health service with a greater community orientation. This would require some degree of sectorisation of consultant service into smaller areas which relate to particular GPs, health centres, etc. Mental health teams could be established in relation to such sectors within the community, each with the support of its own inpatient and day care facilities, which could either be part of a district general hospital unit or of an existing psychiatric hospital. Some health districts have already changed and others are in the process of changing to such sectorised systems, as part of a re-organisation of their services to give a greater community emphasis. Other facilities required might include small local day care units and drop-in centres, which could be staffed in a variety of ways but would probably include the use of CPN time on a sessional basis; outpatient clinics could be held in any of these locations, in addition to health centres. It then becomes far less important where the nurse members of the team are based, while GPs and other primary health care staff will relate to a single group of mental health workers, who are easily identifiable. Within such a structure, the nurses working with inpatients could also have some community involvement, which would seem to be much more in keeping with nursing theory — i.e. that the primary nurse dealing with the inpatient should remain the nurse involved in the community (see below).

The balance between sectorisation of psychiatric services, to achieve more effective support for primary care services, and specialisation within psychiatry, providing greater sophistication and expertise, may be difficult, but should by no means be impossible to achieve. It is also important to allow some possibility of choice — for both patient and GP — of psychiatrist, CPN, and other specialist staff. The question of specialisation within community psychiatric nursing is further discussed below.

TRAINING AND EDUCATION

Since 1951, basic psychiatric nurse training in Britain has been under the auspices of the General Nursing Councils and their successors, the National Boards. The Councils, however, were not responsible for post-basic, non-statutory training; as a result, a diverse range of nursing courses, of varying standards, came to be offered by individual hospitals and educational institutions. In 1970, the first post-registration pilot course in community psychiatric nursing commenced at Chiswick Polytechnic, London (Rawlings 1970); this consisted only of a 1-week block, followed by five weekly study days, but it was later expanded to a 1-year course. The Joint Board of Clinical Nursing Studies was set up in 1970, and introduced a syllabus, four years later, for a course for psychiatric nurses working in the community. This syllabus was revised in 1979 and five polytechnics offered the 36-week courses (Nursing care of the mentally handicapped in the community and Nursing care of the mentally ill in the community), as well as a short course for enrolled nurses (who are less highly qualified than registered nurses). With the advent of the United Kingdom Central Council (UKCC) and National Boards in 1982, responsibility for both statutory and post-basic training lay with the same body; these courses are now validated and approved by the English, Scottish, and Northern Ireland National Boards, and are specifically designed for community psychiatric nurses. The courses (ENB 810, 811 and 812) include psychology, sociology, research methodology, principles of community medicine and community work, nursing roles and principles, and the structures of other services.

The 1985 CPNA survey, however, indicated that of the total CPN work-force, only 22% had completed a relevant course, and this proportion had not increased since 1980, when it was 24%; there were also wide regional disparities. Not only had the rapid growth of CPN services outstripped the capacity of the training facilities, but District Health Authorities had felt unable to meet the cost of seconding large numbers of staff for training. Proposals have been made by the CPNA that this type of course should become mandatory for all CPNs, but there is no evidence that this could be achieved in the near future.

Skidmore and Friend (1984) found that of their random sample of 120 CPNs, 81% felt that mandatory training was necessary and 64% that it should be a prerequisite to practice. However, it became apparent in this study that there was little difference in the perceived effectiveness of the work of those with an ENB certificate, compared with those without it (a finding confirmed by Wooff et al 1988). Few CPNs felt adequately prepared for their responsibilities, identifying their type of training deficit as being in the area of therapeutic skills, particularly counselling.

A number of other arguments have been advanced against mandatory CPN training. Perhaps the most cogent and the one with the most implications for psychiatric nursing as a whole, is that as a post-basic qualification, CPN training assumes a basic hospital training; this itself is now under major review, both by the national boards, the ENB (1987) and the UKCC (1985). In the context of the generally accepted overall aim to move psychiatric care as far as possible into the community, it would be logical for basic nurse training to be more community orientated. This is not to suggest that all psychiatric nurses should be trained to be CPNs as presently understood, but rather that basic education should be undertaken in community settings, with hospital/residential settings as a form of specialist experience. The traditional situation for nurse training — the large psychiatric hospital — will be disappearing in some areas and reduced in size in others (though generally not in Scotland), and basic experience will have to reflect this. The 1982 (ENB/WNB) syllabus has in fact increased emphasis on individual skills and community care, and is seen as 'a relevant preparation for the mental nurse to enable practice in the hospital or community setting' (ENB 1987). In this context, some of the items dealt with in the CPN courses become basic training issues, and since in a time of constrained resources choices have to be made, the extent and content of mandatory CPN training need to be carefully considered. With the more community-orientated basic training which is now developing, a much shorter post-basic course may be quite adequate. A range of shorter courses for staff moving into the community is evolving — ENB 993: Course for staff working in the community, residential and day care settings; and ENB 945: Principles of rehabilitation, are examples.

Dexter & Wash (1986) have identified general psychiatric nursing skills as: personal, including attributes and self-awareness, counselling, behavioural, creative and management. They also describe skills for specific settings or client groups. Similarly, in her work on basic nurse education, Williams (1986) identified several skills which are required by nurses working in a community setting — observation, listening, communication, counselling, self-awareness, teaching, research and management.

A further point is the closer relevance of other post-basic qualifications to the work done by individual CPNs. These would include courses such as Adult behavioural psychotherapy (ENB 650) — the use of which in a primary care setting has been described by Marks (1985) — and Care of the elderly (ENB 941). A number of other relevant courses are shared with other disciplines, covering such subjects as individual and family therapy, drug and alcohol dependence, and child and adolescent work.

In some hospitals, the separation of community from mainstream psychiatric nursing tends to reinforce the static situation of both inpatient services and nursing attitudes, at a time when resources are shifting from hospitals. The move to community may be perceived then as having been achieved merely by increasing the number of CPNs, and not by a more radical restructuring of the psychiatric services. The reduction in size of inpatient units, and the development of a wide range of alternative forms of residential and day care facilities, all of which will require a nursing input, tend to make the distinction between community and hospital nursing increasingly difficult. Involving hospital nurses in aspects of community as well as inpatient work — a role used in the early therapeutic community models of acute units (e.g. Hunter 1974), but one which receded as the whole-time CPN model gained impetus — could once again be appropriate for developing services.

After discussion of the future of nurse education in its Project 2000 (1985, 1986a, 1986b), the UKCC (1987) proposed a radical change in the whole structure of nurse education, leading to a new type of 'practitioner'. This would involve a 3-year course, the first half of which would be common to all nurses, and the second half specialising in one of four areas: mental illness, mental handicap, nursing of adults and nursing of children. (Midwifery would be a separate course.) During the education process, the learner would be a student (on a non-means-tested grant), and not an employee. The 'practitioner' would be competent to provide care in both institutional and non-institutional settings, while following registration, further specialist training would lead to 'specialist practitioner' status in specific settings, which would include community psychiatric nursing, community mental handicap nursing and district general nursing. Similar far-reaching proposals were made by the Royal College of Nursing in the Judge Report (RCN 1985) and by the English National Board (1985). An evaluation (UKCC 1987) of the cost implications suggests that unless additional funding was made available, Project 2000 would suffer the same fate as the Briggs Report (House of Commons 1972), Platt Report (RCN 1964), and Wood Report (Ministry of Health 1947), all of which were hailed as the new way forward but never implemented. However, the government responded sympathetically (Review Body for Nurses 1988) to nursing by its acceptance of both a salary and grading review, and the first Project 2000 diploma courses began in 1989; however funding for full implementation remains uncertain. The grading review, although implemented with many variations and anomalies, has generally tended to favour nurses working in the community.

NURSING MODELS AND THEORIES

Since the 1960s, the struggle for professional identity and autonomy has led nurses to seek out a field of theory and knowledge which could be perceived as exclusive to their profession. Although this might be interpreted by some as a professional defence mechanism, it has led to rapid change in the theoretical emphasis of nursing, which has not always been in step with grass roots practice. This body of theory can be seen as evolving very neatly from Henderson's (1969) now classic definition: 'the unique function of the nurse is to assist the individual, sick or well, in the performance of those activities contributing to health or its recovery (or to peaceful death) that he would perform unaided if he had the necessary strength, will or knowledge. And to do this in such a way as to help him gain independence as rapidly as possible'. In identifying the uniqueness of the work, nursing theories attempt to encompass all branches of the profession, seeking to find models which have more commonality between a CPN and, say, an intensive care nurse, than between the CPN and a psychiatric social worker. Basic to this evolution has been the concept of the Nursing Process and the proposition of nursing models.

The Nursing Process now forms the basis for changing both practice and training at all levels. It seeks to promote a systematic four stage approach and is defined by WHO (1977) as

'a term applied to a system of characteristic nursing interventions in the health of individuals, families and/or communities. In detail it involves the use of scientific methods for identifying the health needs of the patient/client, family or community and selecting those which can most effectively be met by nursing care; it also includes planning the provision of care and evaluating the outcome. The nurse in collaboration with other members of the health care team and the individual or groups being served, defines objectives, sets priorities, identifies care to be given and mobilises resources. He/she then provides the nursing services either directly or indirectly. Subsequently, he/she evaluates the outcome. The information feedback from evaluation of outcome should initiate desirable changes in subsequent interventions in similar nursing care situations. In this way, nursing becomes a dynamic process lending itself to adaptation and improvement.'

That such an approach, based more on current research than outmoded tradition, is long overdue cannot be disputed. Recognition of the importance of this kind of attitudinal change in nursing is probably the main reason for the acceptance in Britain of the Nursing Process, which has long formed the basis of nursing practice in the USA. The necessary education is now being developed to ensure the implementation of this concept at all levels and in all areas of British nursing.

Unfortunately, a side effect of the Nursing Process for the psychiatric nurse has been the tendency to develop a model of care which is rigidly separate from that of other disciplines, notably medicine. Attempted justification for this can be seen in an emphasis on the inappropriateness of the medical model, i.e. its vision of man as a biological being whose integrity is disturbed by disease, so that the goal of care is to remove the disease entity, by knowledge based on biophysical sciences. Nursing theories seek to differentiate their model from this perception of the medical one, although such a narrow model would be also rejected by many doctors and probably by a majority of psychiatrists. The concepts involved are derived from various perspectives, including behaviourism, system theory, interactional theories, and adaptation. In a proliferation of ideas, some examples are:

1. By assessing the deficiencies in the patient's ability to care for himself, the nurse's intervention is aimed at enabling the patient to make up this deficit, in order to restore a balance between his 'self-care abilities' and his 'self-care demands' (Orem 1980).

2. By assessing the patient in each of 12 'activities of daily living' areas, the nurse can plan with the patient ways of moving towards independence in each (Roper et al 1980).

3. Individuals are subject to stresses (physical, psychological, or social) to which they constantly adapt. Nursing interventions are planned both by the assessment of past responses and by knowledge of the present and future needs (Saxton and Hyland 1979).

Other models have been reviewed by Aggleton and Chalmers (1986), and all have evolved from highly complex theoretical conceptual frameworks, applied to nursing practice; all also share the emphasis of divergence from the medical model.

The implications for the psychiatric nurse of being part of this professional development include both the problems engendered in formulating a nursing diagnosis and in planning action which is demonstrably nursing, and therefore inherently different from the models used by other members of the multidisciplinary team, while at the same time adhering to the ideal of co-ordinated multidisciplinary work. It may be that this is a factor in the favourable perception by nurses of the primary health care option, which is seen by them as more autonomous. Altschul, a well respected nursing theorist, has argued (1984a,1984b) for the need to generate theories of nursing to guide practice which are related to those theories used by medical and other colleagues in a multidisciplinary team in dealing with the same clients. This is not to suggest that nursing contributions are not specific, but that they have to relate to common goals of care and treatment.

The statutory instruments (DHSS 1983) for the 1979 Nurses, Midwives and Health Visitors Act enshrine the role of the nurse in law, by listing the 'competencies' expected of a registered nurse in his/her own field. These are to:

a. Advise on the promotion of health and the prevention of illness.

b. Recognise situations that may be detrimental to the health and well-being of the individual.

c. Carry out those activities involved when conducting the comprehensive assessment of a person's nursing requirements.

    d. Recognise the significance of the observations made and use them to develop an initial nursing assessment.

    e. Devise a plan of nursing care based on the assessment, with the co-operation of the patient, to the extent that this is possible taking into account the medical prescription.

    f. Implement the planned programme of nursing care and, where appropriate, teach and co-ordinate other members of the caring team.

    g. Review the effectiveness of the nursing care provided and, where appropriate, initiate any action that may be required.

    h. Work in a team with other nurses and with medical and paramedical staff and the social workers.

    i. Undertake the management of a group of patients over a period of time and organise the appropriate support services.

This list can be seen as defining the currently conceived role of the nurse in terms of the Nursing Process.

COMMUNITY NURSING PRACTICE

There are wide variations in the work undertaken by nurses, apart from those dictated by their operational base. In practice, despite a loyalty to a 'nursing approach' conceptualised in the model described above, many CPNs could be seen as operating within more socially or medically defined models. Wooff & Goldberg (1988), in comparing the work of CPNs and mental health social workers, noted how the CPNs who were primary care-based were found to apply mainly a biomedical model of care for clients with a diagnosis of schizophrenia, but to provide simple psychotherapeutic support to other clients. This was contrasted by the extensive use of counselling techniques amongst hospital-based mental health social workers. Thus, the work continues to evolve and to diversify, from the original Warlingham Park roles described by Moore (1960).

    In an attempt to analyse the functions of the CPN, Sladden (1979) suggested five different categories: clinical, psychosocial, environmental, internal liaison, and external liaison.

Clinical activities

There are activities to do with psychiatric illness and treatment, observing patients for clinical signs and advising on the nursing management, as well as administering and monitoring prescribed medication, observing side effects, and regulating treatment regimes. Many references to community psychiatric nursing services imply that their main raison d'être is the administration of depot antipsychotic injections, the use of which is the major factor in stabilising some previously quickly relapsing psychotic patients. In her 1979 study of a CPN service in Edinburgh, Sladden reported that 53% of patients in contact with the service were receiving depot medication, but when clinic sessions were excluded, 86% of nurse/patient contacts were not concerned with such injections.

Assessment of the patient's clinical mental state may be undertaken on behalf of the psychiatric team, especially in the case of clients known to them already. The general practitioner may ask for guidance in clinical management of particular patients, as may the health visitor, district nurse, or other primary health care workers. Some physical nursing may be involved in the care of the elderly.

Psychosocial

This area, which includes undertaking psychotherapy and especially behavioural therapies, is one of growth in the role of the CPN. Marks (1985) has described a controlled trial of nurses trained as behaviour therapists working in the primary health care setting, while Paykel and Griffith (1983) have compared the care of neurotic patients by CPNs with outpatient clinic attendance. The results of these and other studies are discussed below. The relationship with the nurse may be a major factor in the support of isolated patients in the community, and many CPNs have undertaken family and conjoint work, often in partnership with members of other disciplines within the psychiatric team; this may also involve probation officers, social workers, health visitors, or other primary health care workers. CPNs have been involved in the establishment of therapeutic groups, away from the hospital setting, especially to help the socially isolated or anxious, or for the teaching of social skills. Crisis intervention is another aspect of work in which the CPN is often the most flexible member of the team, able to respond to a crisis situation early, and so perhaps avoiding the need for hospital admission; however, many services are not yet able to offer 24-hour, 7-day-a-week cover. A significant difference between hospital and community nursing care is that in hospital, nurses give continuous care, which forms an important part of the nursing relationship, whereas in the community, nurses have intermittent contact, in the same way as other professionals, although (up to now) they can refer back to their previous experience of long periods in contact with patients before they became CPNs.

Environmental

Skilled assessment of a home situation may be undertaken by the CPN either on initial referral or, for inpatients, prior to discharge. Domiciliary services such as meals-on-wheels, additional domestic support, home aide or home help, improvement grants, or specific apparatus may make the difference between the patient being able to support himself independently and community care being unsuccessful. Unsatisfactory housing and the shortage of suitable accommodation probably represents one of the most serious shortfalls in the viability of community care schemes. The provision of newer flexible services, such as travelling day hospitals discussed below, increase the opportunity for environmental interventions.

Internal liaison

This refers to communication with other professionals within the team. Where nurses work in a multidisciplinary team, the sharing of information is particularly important; maintaining close contact also means that assessment, admission to hospital, discharge, and follow-up can be quickly and easily facilitated.

External liaison

Wherever CPNs are based, good relationships with other agencies are most important; it is commonly cited by both referring and peripheral agencies which use CPNs, that their most valuable function is to promote liaison between the psychiatric team and primary health care or other community-based services. Sladden also described some of the negative attitudes induced in GPs, who appeared badly informed about the service because of poor communication from hospital-based CPNs. A further important aspect of liaison is as a back-up and advisory service to other organisations; these might include voluntary bodies, self-help groups, and private agencies. Social services 'psychiatric home aide' schemes, which can provide cover within the patient's home, 24 hours a day, seven days a week, for a short period of time, are potentially an exciting development, but require careful co-ordination with the CPN involved.

Skidmore and Friend (1984) identified 11 functions of CPNs, after observing 1000 CPN visits. They found that 35% of visits were for assessment, 22% to administer injections, 11% were to give support, 8% to deliver medication, 7% were made in liaison with other disciplines, 6% were to deliver messages, 6% had no apparent reason (e.g. visiting old clients in the area), 2% were to give other treatment, 1% were to counsel, 1% were to administer physical treatment, and 1% were to advise relatives. These contrasted with the perception of the majority of the CPNs that they had four functions, equally distributed: assessment, treatment, support, and administering medication.

Wooff & Goldberg (1988) compared the work of CPNs with that of mental health social workers (MHSW). Although they found some overlap, significant differences emerged, which also contrasted with the nurse's own perception of her role. CPNs tended to focus more on psychiatric symptoms, treatment, and medication than did the social workers, who dealt with a wider range of topics and looked as much at social interactions and at family and community networks as at individual symptoms. The CPNs spent less time with psychotic than with neurotic clients, compared to the MHSWs, who spent similar periods of time with both. The CPNs had less contact with other members of the mental health team and more with the primary health care team; where CPNs did have contact with the mental health team, this was predominantly with a psychiatrist. However, when working with non-schizophrenic clients, CPNs were more likely to show disapproval; they were also more likely than the MHSWs to be directive, and to undertake physical or behavioural treatments.

This tends to support Skidmore and Friend's (1984) finding, in their sample of 120 CPNs from 12 English bases, that the majority did not feel adequately prepared for the work, and that this deficit lay mainly in the area of skills training. They suggested that community psychiatric nursing seemed to be 'progressing on an ad hoc basis with little evidence of evaluation or intervention assessment'.

EFFECTIVENESS OF SERVICES

Much of the literature on community psychiatric nursing, which has been extensively reviewed by Griffith and Mangen (1980), tends to be descriptive, but several controlled studies have been undertaken since then. Brooker (1984), in attempting to disprove the hypothesis that CPNs are not agents of significant change, described the ethical and other difficulties of evaluating and determining the effectiveness of these services. A study by Mangen & Griffith (1982) used the criterion of patient satisfaction; care in the community by a nurse was compared with outpatient follow-up by a psychiatrist, and a positive outcome in favour of the CPN was revealed. In addition to consumer satisfaction, Paykel & Griffith (1983) used a number of evaluative factors, including a depression scale, social adjustment scale, assessment of the burden on relatives, and treatment received; they did not find large differences in outcome, but where there were differences, these favoured the CPNs. Oyebode et al (1988), in a questionnaire survey of patients being visited by GP-based CPNs, found that the CPN contact was viewed as acceptable and helpful by the majority of the 92 patients referred by GPs.

However, one critical suggestion levelled at measures of the outcome of interventions by CPNs (Sladden 1979) is that nurses are very good at 'maintaining precarious social situations in equilibrium rather than promoting dynamic change'. This should be borne in mind when outcomes such as the amount of inpatient care is used as evaluative criteria. Hunter (1980) pointed out that the avoidance of admission as a criterion for success may be suspect, so that some of the group regarded as 'successful' on this basis might rather be regarded as neglected and perhaps in need of inpatient care. Such perceived neglect has from time to time attracted media concern as being the reality of 'community care'.

In the controlled trial by Marks (1985) of the effectiveness of nurse therapists in primary care, the nurses had been specifically trained in behaviour therapy and the patients selected from specific diagnostic categories, without other psychopathology; the treatment outcomes were compared with that of a control group managed by general practitioners. The group treated by the nurse therapists improved significantly on nearly all the variables considered, compared with the group treated by GPs. This study also included a cost-benefit analysis which demonstrated decreased use of resources on the part of patients treated by the nurse therapists, but increased use by the GP-treated patients.

Wooff et al (1986), using data from the Salford psychiatric case register to study the contributions of CPNs to the work of the mental health service, reported that CPN services were treating the morbidity found at primary care level, rather than reducing the demands made on the traditional mental health services.

SPECIALISATION

Mental handicap nursing is essentially separate in Britain, because of a different basic training and qualification. Communications from the Chief Nursing Officer (DHSS 1985a) and from the ENB (1985), together with the report of an RCN working party (1985), summarise the present situation for the care of the mentally ill, in which field, a number of sub-specialities have established specialist CPN posts. The CPNA Survey (1985), (Table 16.2), showed that those working with the elderly formed the largest specialist group.

Table 16.2 National Analysis of CPNs by specialism

Specialism	n	%
Elderly	505	64.0
Acute/crisis work	100	12.6
Drugs/alcohol	72	9.0
Rehabilitation	42	5.2
Children/adolescents	36	4.5
Behaviour therapy	36	4.5
Family therapy	2	0.2
Total	793	100.0

The regional variation in number of specialist CPNs working with the elderly is significant ($F=1.8026$ sig 0.037). The largest average number per district is in the Wessex Region ($n=5.55$) and the lowest in Northern Ireland ($n=1$).

In total, there were 211 vacancies nationally, ranging from 1 in Northern Ireland to 31 in the North-Western Region. It is possible that the timing of the survey had a large impact on this question; 48.3% of the total vacancies were considered as 'specialist' posts ($n=102$). The largest total number of vacant 'specialist' posts was found in Yorkshire ($n=19$).

Source: CPNA ©1985 Reproduced with permission

Other specialist roles are relatively uncommon for CPNs, but may be very important in the care, rehabilitation, resettlement, and follow-up in the community of particular groups of patients. Some posts which have been developed require very specialised skills, such as helping those with eating disorders or substance abuse, or those requiring specific behavioural approaches. Work with ethnic minorities needs an understanding of cultural differences and may require language skills. The homeless mentally ill, particularly in inner city areas, pose a difficult challenge. With the development of medium secure units, the follow-up by CPNs of potentially dangerous patients is of growing importance.

CPNs based in health centres tend to be generic within psychiatry, but the number of referrals of elderly patients, one in five of total referrals (CPNA 1985), also allows scope for specialist CPNs for the elderly to work from health centres. It is difficult to quantify trends, as the methods of the 1980 and 1985 CPNA surveys were statistically different, but 28% of CPN services offered a specialist service in 1980, while in 1985, 31% of CPNs worked exclusively in one specialty.

It is difficult to assess the relative advantages of a locality-based, generalist CPN service, compared with a series of more specialist multidisciplinary team-based services. Ideally, both should be available in a district, and some highly specialised work may be best organised on a multi-district basis. Similar issues arose in social work following the Seebohm Report (Home Department 1968), which advocated generic training and was then used to argue against specialisation in service delivery. As mentioned earlier, the re-organisation of social services in 1971 and the resulting unavailability of specialist social workers hastened the development of CPN services; a similar pattern could emerge if all CPNs were locality-based and specialist units had to develop their own follow-up services. A related problem is that of balancing the needs of the most disabled with the demands of a larger number of less disabled patients seen in general practice.

RELATED DEVELOPMENTS

The 1983 Mental Health Act made a number of changes which were mainly concerned with the safeguarding of detained or potentially detained patients in England and Wales; a similar Act for Scotland dates from 1984. The Act recognised to some extent the role of the nurse in the inpatient unit by providing the emergency holding power (Section 5.4) (about which there is divided opinion amongst nurses) as well as the requirement to obtain the opinion of a nurse in the confirmation of consent to certain treatments (Section 57) and in the certification of a second psychiatric opinion (Section 58). However, the possibility of a 'community treatment order' was not taken up, and decisions by the courts have confirmed that an on-leave (Section 17) provision should not be used as an alternative. Patients covered by such an order would include some of those who are receiving depot medication from CPNs, who may experience repeated but potentially avoidable compulsory admission to hospital.

The Act makes it incumbent on the district health authority and the local social services authority to provide after-care for detained patients after discharge. This responsibility in the community is in the main shared between approved social workers (ASWs), or other social workers based in psychiatric units, and CPNs, with the back-up of other members of the psychiatric team. However, the First Biennial Report of the Mental Health Act Commission (1985) indicated that plans for the provision of after-care under Section 117 of the Act are 'in general not far advanced'. The overlap in the roles of the CPN and the ASW is considerable, but whereas the latter has been assigned certain statutory duties, the CPN has particular nursing skills, not shared by the ASW, which are not embodied in the law. However, the present situation is part of a continuing process in which much necessary community work has been taken up by the professional staff who were available, rather than divided on any theoretical basis.

At the same time as CPN services have been developing, other members of the specialist psychiatric team have been moving into the community. There has been a very small number of specialist community posts in psychiatry, but a working party of the Royal College of Psychiatrists suggested that work in the community should in fact be part of the role of all general psychiatrists (Freeman 1985). A recent survey revealed that 10% of psychiatrists spend some time in primary care settings (Strathdee & Williams 1984), and the various types of such involvement have been reviewed by Mitchell (1985). Clinical psychologists work both in hospital and in community settings, move freely between the two, and see both types of work as coming within the scope of a district department of clinical psychology; Koch (1986) has described the range of clinical psychologists' work in community settings. Occupational therapists also work in both hospital and community settings, on a sessional basis. Hospital-based social workers have always worked both with inpatients, and in the community, although only some districts have them.

The quality of relationships between the different professionals working in the community is clearly most important, and good communication is essential for the co-ordination of care. However, some thought has to be given as to the most appropriate roles for the different professionals: overlap of functions and role blurring is inevitable to some extent, and does make for a more flexible service, but questions need to be asked as to the best professional training and experience to meet particular patient needs. Since both the ENB and the Central Council for Education and Training in Social Work are exploring ways of co-operating in training for work with the mentally handicapped, there would almost certainly be common areas in respect of mental illness as well. Each profession needs to develop its unique contribution, but also to recognise shared areas of expertise.

Other facilities which are in line with national policy and which involve psychiatric nurses are in varying stages of development. Both psychiatric hospitals and social services departments have established hostels for long-stay patients in the community, and some of these are overseen by hospital nurses from rehabilitation wards; this is similar to the process which occurred in mental handicap hospitals following the Jay Report (DHSS 1979), when large-scale decentralisation of former long-stay mental handicap facilities took place. In other instances, CPNs are also spending increasing amounts of time in resocialisation and support work with patients in group homes and hostels.

Day care facilities are likely to be increased in situations away from district general hospitals or psychiatric units; flexible arrangements such as travelling day hospitals have also been developed and these might provide a further role for nurses currently working with inpatients, as hospitals become smaller. Similarly, less formal arrangements will be needed for drop-in services, although members of local voluntary agencies may staff many of these on a day-to-day basis, with support from nurses and other staff. Such developments are likely to blur the boundary between community nursing and the main body of psychiatric nursing, and raise questions concerning the training needs of nurses in these increasingly varied settings.

For nursing services outside hospitals, a Community Nursing Review (Cumberlege Report, DHSS 1986) has proposed the setting up of neighbourhood nursing services (NNS). Each health authority would then identify localities of 10–25 000 population, within which nursing and related primary care services could be delivered and for each of these, the NNS would co-ordinate, plan, and deliver nursing care. Each health authority would also set up specialist psychiatric multidisciplinary teams, and the report seemed to envisage community psychiatric nurses being members of this team rather than based within the NNS, although working closely with it. All primary care workers in regular contact with people with mental health problems would be expected to understand the role of the specialist team and how and when to make referrals or seek advice. However, implementation of the report has been left to the discretion of local health authorities, and is therefore likely to be patchy.

COMMUNITY PSYCHIATRIC NURSING OUTSIDE THE UK

Surveying community psychiatric nursing practice in other countries is difficult, not least because there are further problems in defining what constitutes psychiatric nursing. Whereas general nursing has been

482   HANDBOOK OF COMMUNITY PSYCHIATRY

sufficiently defined to permit an exchange of nurses between countries, based on an agreed equivalent of training standards and experience, this does not occur for psychiatric nursing. In Europe, separate registers for psychiatric nurses are kept by Belgium, Denmark, Eire, France, Germany, Luxembourg, and the Netherlands, whereas in the majority of other countries, psychiatric nursing is practised by general nurses, who have varying amounts of psychiatric training or experience. In North America, a similar situation exists, although some provinces of Canada maintain separate registers, as do South Africa, Zimbabwe, and Australia. Nurses from other countries who seek psychiatric registration in the UK are therefore dealt with on an individual basis. Thus, in looking at the results of work using community psychiatric nurses in other countries, direct comparisons with experience in the UK should not be made. In most parts of the world, the greater part of the direct care of psychiatric patients is undertaken by untrained staff.

Over differing time periods and from widely differing starting points, a move from hospital-based to community-based psychiatry has taken place in most western countries. The experience in Italy has aroused particular interest and controversy since, unlike the mostly evolutionary deinstitutionalisation of asylums elsewhere, which has been comple- mented by growing community-based services, an attempt was made to set up a completely alternative, community-based service with minimal use of hospital care. This change, which has been reviewed extensively, stems from the work of Basaglia in Gorizia and Trieste, starting in 1968 and leading up to the passage of law 180 in 1978, which stopped first admissions to psychiatric hospitals immediately, and all admissions to psychiatric hospitals from 1981. The effect of such community psychiatry without mental hospitals has been described by Tansella (1986) and its real extent controversially challenged by Jones & Poletti (1985, 1986). Both agree, however, that the general political climate and motivation, rather than professional change alone, make similar radical moves unlikely in the context of most other countries. Emphasis in descriptions of this service tends to focus more on the changed settings and new intent, rather than on specific therapeutic interventions, but where these are described, (e.g. by Muscettola et al 1987), they remain very much medically led. Jones & Poletti (1986) have suggested that the real focus in the new service is on the treatment and containment of the acute psychotic episode, and that relatively less use is made of psycho- therapeutic group or family approaches. In British terms, the role of the nurse appears to be low-key; training, especially of nurses, has been highlighted as a priority need for future spending, particularly in those local services where the psychological approach predominates (see also Ch. 22).

An American comparison (Singer et al 1970) between services in Amsterdam and the Soviet Union describes a role in the latter for a nurse social worker; neither psychiatric nursing nor social work, as we know them, function independently in the Soviet Union, but this approach appears to be much more interventionist than any similar role in either America or the UK, with a greater scope to manipulate either the individual or the environment. As may be expected, though, cultural influences on the system are also profound. In Holland, a profession of 'nurse social worker' exists with a 7-year training and again, more responsibility, than is general in either British or American services.

In the USA, where nurse training varies widely from state to state, Pasamanick et al (1964) described a home care programme for schizophrenics; this included the work of community nurses, but they were 'public health' nurses, with a 6-week training in psychiatry. There were improvements in the home care group over those treated by the state hospitals (and also in those receiving drug treatment over those on placebo). In the follow-up study, Davis (1972) implied that the lack of difference in the groups five years later suggested that a major reason for the success of the home care group was the role of the nurse in bringing medication to the home and in the maintenance of supervision, without the need for initiative by the patient. Home care by nurses had to end for this group of patients at the conclusion of the research project. However, Morgan & Moreno (1973) describe a wider and more blurred role for the psychiatric nurse in the community, indicating some of the role overlap with other disciplines which is becoming known in the UK.

These are, however, isolated examples. It should be emphasised that while comparisons of the outcomes of whole services may be possible, as has been done by ten Horn (1985) in examining mental health services for the elderly in 21 European centres, conclusions about specific influences of those professionals who carry out the tasks broadly described as 'community psychiatric nursing' are so subject to variation in terms of role, training, relationship to other disciplines, etc., that they must be extremely unreliable.

The existence of a well developed primary health care system in Britain, and the tradition of specialist care only being available after referral by a GP, also influence the style of service. In many countries, direct access to specialist services is more usual, although it may be limited on financial grounds. However, the development of community mental health centres accepting self-referrals could change the UK pattern of care.

FUTURE DEVELOPMENT

In the wake of the new British syllabus of basic training, radical proposals for educational change will require equal commitment to the updating and in-service training of the existing staff. Unless this occurs, the credibility of the psychiatric nursing profession may be severely reduced. As Mangen & Griffith (1982) have argued, the expansion of CPN services must be evaluated in the context of the future of psychiatric nursing as a whole, and must be related to overall manpower planning in mental health care. Although further research and evaluation are essential, some stable consensus of a conceptual model of psychiatric nursing needs to be achieved, and it must be one which can co-exist with the models used by other mental health professionals. The range of activities and further training of psychiatric nurses should be flexible, according to the therapeutic environment, rather than being divided into two separate camps, the hospitals and the community — the latter with mandatory specialist training. The sectorisation of hospital-based services into more local community care, and the location of these services in or near to the area served, could create a greater variety of nursing services and roles.

The Griffiths Report on Community Care (1988) suggested a radical reorganisation of the relative roles of the different authorities providing community care. It commended the work of community psychiatric nurses and mental handicap nurses, and saw them as having 'an invaluable role in meeting the needs of both clients and informal carers'. However, the report proposed that the overall management of community care should be the responsibility of local authority social service departments, and implied a separation between the long-term care of chronically ill people on the one hand, and acute services on the other, the latter remaining the responsibility of health authorities. The Royal College of Psychiatrists (1988) criticised this artificial division between acute and chronic health care and suggested that the NHS should have overall responsibility for the care of the mentally ill; Local Authorities should have responsibility for the mentally handicapped, but the NHS must continue to provide for their psychological needs. The passage of the NHS and Community Care Act may significantly affect the role of psychiatric nurses in the care of the chronic mentally ill.

Another factor which may influence the future development of psychiatric nursing, both in the community and other settings, is recruitment. The recent raising of educational standards for entry, and the decreasing numbers of 18-year-olds in the British population, together with uncertainty as to the future of psychiatric nursing as a rewarding career, may undermine many development plans. If the number of trained nurses declines, the role of untrained nursing assistant and homecare aides may have to increase. Some form of basic training for those taking up such posts will be increasingly needed, and working conditions may have to change in order to recruit and retain nursing staff within the NHS.

The relevance of nursing rather than social work or psychology must be established as a background to new professional roles. Psychiatric nurses have the potential to evolve into the key community mental health workers, both because of the numbers required and because of their training and experience, but this can only happen if their profession develops a wider vision of its role.

REFERENCES

Aggleton P, Chalmers H 1986 Nursing models and the nursing process. Macmillan, London

Altschul A 1984a Does good practice need good principles? Nursing Times 80: No. 27 36 - 38

Altschul A 1984b Does good practice need good principles? Nursing Times 80: No. 29 49-51

Baly M 1980 Nursing and social change. Heinemann, London

Brooker C G 1984 Some problems associated with the measurement of community psychiatric nurse intervention. Journal of Advanced Nursing 9: 165 - 174

Community Psychiatric Nurses Association 1985 National Survey Update. CPNA, Bristol

Davis A E 1972 The prevention of hospitalisation in schizophrenia: five years after an experimental program. American Journal of Orthopsychiatry 42: 375 - 388

Department of Health and Social Security 1975 Better services for the mentally ill. HMSO, London

Department of Health and Social Security 1979 Report of the committee of enquiry into mental handicap nursing and care (Jay Report) Cmnd 7468. HMSO, London

Department of Health and Social Security 1983 Statutory Instrument No. 873 HMSO, London

Department of Health and Social Security 1985a Chief Nursing Officer. Letter 18th December. The role of the nurse in caring for people with mental handicap. CNO (85) 5 DHSS, London

Department of Health and Social Security 1985b Community care with special reference to adult mentally ill and mentally handicapped people. Government response to the second report from the Social Services Committee 1984 - 1985 Session Cmnd 9674. HMSO, London

Department of Health and Social Security 1986 Neighbourhood nursing — a focus for care. Report of the community nursing review (Cumberlege). HMSO, London

Dexter G, Wash M 1986 Psychiatric nursing skills. Croom Helm, Beckenham

English National Board for Nursing, Midwifery and Health Visiting 1985 Professional education/training courses for nursing, midwifery and health visitors (consultative paper)

English National Board for Nursing, Midwifery and Health Visiting 1987 Syllabus of training 1982 for the professional register part three. ENB, London

Freeman H 1985 Training for community psychiatry. Bulletin of the Royal College of Psychiatrists 9: 29 - 32

Green J 1968 The psychiatric nurse in the community nursing service. International Journal of Nursing Studies 5: 175 - 184

Griffith J H, Mangen S P 1980 Community psychiatric nursing a literature review. International Journal of Nursing Studies 17: 197-210

Griffiths R 1988 Community care: agenda for action. A report to the Secretary of State for Social Services. HMSO, London

Henderson V 1969 Basic principles of nursing care. International Council of Nurses, Geneva

Home Department 1968 Report of the committee on local authority and allied personal social services (Seebohm Report) Cmnd 3703. HMSO, London

House of Commons 1972 Report of the committee on nursing (Briggs Report) Cmnd 5115. HMSO, London

Hunter P 1974 Community psychiatric nursing in Britain: an historical review. International Journal of Nursing Studies 11: 223-233

Hunter P 1980 Social work and community psychiatric nursing — a review. International Journal of Nursing Studies 17: 131-139

Jones K, Poletti A 1985 Understanding the Italian experience. British Journal of Psychiatry 146: 341 - 347

Jones K, Poletti A 1986 The Italian experience reconsidered. British Journal of Psychiatry 148: 144 - 150

Kennedy I 1980 Unmasking medicine (The Reith Lectures). BBC, London

Koch C H (ed) 1986 Community clinical psychology. Croom Helm, Beckenham

Mangen S P, Griffith J H 1982 Community psychiatric nursing in Britain: the need for policy planning. International Journal of Nursing Studies 19: 157 - 166

Marks I 1985 Psychiatric nurse therapist in primary health care. Royal College of Nursing, London

Mental Health Act Commission 1985 First biennial report. HMSO, London

Ministry of Health, Department of Health for Scotland and Ministry of Labour and National Service 1947 Working party on the recruitment and training of nurses (Majority Report) (Wood Report). HMSO, London

Mitchell A R K 1985 Psychiatrists in primary care settings. British Journal of Psychiatry 147: 371 - 379

Moore S 1960 A psychiatric outpatient nursing service. Mental Health 20: 51 - 54

Moore S 1964 Mental nursing in the community. Nursing Times 467 - 470

Morgan A J, Moreno J W 1973 The practice of mental health nursing: a community approach. J B Lippincott, Philadelphia

Muscettola G, Casiello M, Bolline P, Sebastiani G, Pampallona S, Tagnoni G 1987 Patterns of therapeutic intervention and role of psychiatric settings: a survey of two regions in Italy. Acta Psychiatrica Scandinavica 75: 55-61

Orem D 1980 Nursing: concepts of practice. McGraw-Hill, New York

Oyebode F, Gedd E, Berry D, Lymes M, Lashley P 1988 Community psychiatric nurses in primary care: consumer survey. Bulletin of the Royal College of Psychiatrists 12: 483- 485

Pasamanick B, Scarpitti F R, Lefton M, Dinitz S, Wernert J J, McPheeters H 1964 Home vs hospital care for schizophrenics. Journal of the American Medical Association 187: 177-181

Paykel E S, Griffith J H 1983 Community psychiatric nursing for neurotic patients. Royal College of Nursing, London

Rawlings J A 1970 Course in community psychiatry. Nursing Mirror 130 : (26) 20

Review Body for Nurses, Midwives and Professions Allied to Medicine 1988 5th Report on nursing staff, midwives and health visitors. HMSO, London

Roper N, Logan W, Tierney A 1980 The elements of nursing. Churchill Livingstone, Edinburgh

Royal College of Nursing 1964 A reform of nursing education (Platt Report). Royal College of Nursing, London

Royal College of Nursing 1985 Education of nurses: a new dispensation (Judge Report). Royal College of Nursing, London

Royal College of Psychiatrists 1980 Community psychiatric nursing: a discussion document by a working party of the section for Social and Community Psychiatry. Bulletin of the Royal College of Psychiatrists 4: 114-119

Royal College of Psychiatrists 1988 Comments on the Griffiths Report. Bulletin of the Royal College of Psychiatrists 12: 385-388

Saxton D F, Hyland P A 1979 Planning and implementing nursing intervention: stress and adaptation applied to patient care. 2nd edn. revised. C V Mosby, St Louis

Singer P, Holloway B, Kolb L C 1970 The psychiatrist — nurse team and home care in Soviet Union and Amsterdam. Journal of Psychiatric Nursing & Mental Health Services: 40-44

Skidmore D, Friend W 1984 Community psychiatric nursing. Nursing Times, Community Outlook 80: 179-181, 203-205, 257-261, 299-301, 310-312, 369-371

Sladden S 1979 Psychiatric nursing in the community. Churchill Livingstone, Edinburgh

Strathdee G, Williams P 1984. A survey of psychiatrists in primary care: the silent growth of a new service. Journal of the Royal College of General Practitioners 34: 615-618

Tansella M 1986 Community psychiatry without mental hospitals — the Italian experience: a review. Journal of the Royal Society of Medicine 79: 664-669

Ten Horn G H M M 1985 The elderly in the mental health services of 21 European pilot study areas. Acta Psychiatrica Scandinavica 72: 188-192

United Kingdom Consultative Council for Nursing, Midwifery and Health Visiting 1985 Project 2000 papers 1-6. UKCC, London

United Kingdom Consultative Council for Nursing, Midwifery and Health Visiting 1986a Project 2000 a new preparation for practice. UKCC, London

United Kingdom Consultative Council for Nursing, Midwifery and Health Visiting 1986b Project 2000 paper 8. UKCC, London

United Kingdom Consultative Council for Nursing, Midwifery and Health Visiting 1987 Project 2000 paper 9. UKCC, London

Williams M 1986 Identification of nursing skills, their relevance to patient care and nurse education. Unpublished thesis, Bristol Polytechnic/Frenchay School of Nursing

Wooff K, Goldberg D P 1988 Further observations on the practice of community care in Salford: differences between community psychiatric nurses and mental health social workers. British Journal of Psychiatry 153: 30-37

Wooff K, Goldberg D P, Fryers T 1986 Patients in receipt of community psychiatric nursing care in Salford 1976-1982 Psychological Medicine 16: 407-414

Wooff K, Goldberg D P, Fryers T 1988 The practice of community psychiatric nursing and mental health social work in Salford: some implications for community care. British Journal of Psychiatry 152: 783-792

World Health Organisation 1977 The nursing process: a report on the first meeting of a technical advisory group. Document 0508/77. WHO, Geneva

17. Prevention

J. Newton   T. K. J. Craig

The fundamental principles of prevention are beguilingly simple — define and identify a disease, ascertain its cause, and eliminate this cause or fortify the resilience of the host, so conquering the disease. Implicit in these principles are three assumptions. First, that it is possible to identify a specific disease entity accurately and reliably within a particular population. Secondly, that one or more factors can be isolated which are necessary preconditions for the appearance of the disease. Thirdly, that the effects of these factors can be eliminated through the application of a specific intervention which is itself sufficiently straightforward and clearly specified as to make its utilisation by health care professionals a viable practical undertaking. As will be seen, these assumptions are rarely justified for mental illness.

Elsewhere in this volume, attention has been given to the difficulties surrounding the operational definition of psychiatric disorders and their identification in a non-help-seeking population. In this chapter, we wish to focus on the two remaining principles of prevention — that of the necessity for understanding causal mechanisms, and the development of preventive interventions based on these.

Many medical textbooks subdivide the concept of prevention into three stages: primary, secondary, and tertiary. At the earliest stage, prevention aims to eliminate causal factors prior to any manifestation of symptoms in the 'host' (e.g. purifying sources of drinking water). At the secondary stage, prevention aims to detect the first signs of the disease in affected persons, and to halt or reverse that disease process. Finally, action aimed at minimising the development of disabilities and handicaps which are a natural outcome of unsuccessfully treated disease is seen as tertiary prevention. While such distinctions have gained some popularity in psychiatry (e.g. Caplan 1964), their use is fraught with conceptual problems. They imply rather more understanding of aetiology than we currently possess and require the existence of discrete factors, like bacteria, which are necessary or sufficient preconditions to produce a disorder, and which can therefore become the target of a prevention programme. For instance, it is only possible to define the eradication of smoking as primary prevention of myocardial infarction because it is known that a disproportionately large number of the victims of this disease have been smokers, and because smoking behaviour is clearly not itself an early manifestation of cardiovascular disease. Modifying elevated blood pressure can be classified as secondary prevention only because we have sufficient information to judge that chronic hypertension is itself an indication of cardiovascular pathology of a kind intimately associated with later coronary artery insufficiency and infarction.

In psychiatry, however, despite very considerable advances in understanding, the nature of the relationships between a particular disease and antecedent risk factors is far less clear-cut, and the distinction between primary and secondary prevention can rarely be made with any conviction. To what extent is counselling for the emotionally distressed at times of crisis a primary preventive service, or the secondary prevention of a disorder picked up in its earliest phase? Such distinctions depend entirely on the causal relationship between distressing circumstances, emotional responses to these, and later depression. They also depend on the threshold at which symptoms indicative of depression are deemed marked enough to define the condition as disorder. A low threshold would mean that counselling could only be described as secondary prevention, whereas if a high threshold was used, counselling might often be viewed as a primary preventive strategy (see Newton 1988). Because of these ambiguities, we wish to discuss prevention as a single-stage concept, rather than in the layperson's understanding of the term. Preventive actions, then, are those intended to reduce the incidence of disease — actions aimed at people who are not currently suffering from conspicuous mental disorder, but who may, nonetheless, have some minor or transient symptoms which put them at particularly high risk of developing a disorder of clinical proportions. They may never before have suffered from psychiatric disorder or may have largely recovered from previous illness.

DETERMINANTS OF DISORDER

Essential to the search for effective preventive intervention is a plausible aetiological theory. In order to set up a programme intended to prevent a particular outcome, specific information is needed about the causal chain of antecedent events and circumstances, to enable risk factors to be identified. Intervention can then be planned to eradicate the risk or interrupt the disease process. While it would be convenient were specific psychiatric disorders to have associated single causes, the bulk of available evidence points away from this. Indeed, such a simple model of single pathogen–single outcome is quite inappropriate for almost all illness; even infectious ailments do not occur solely as the result of exposure to a pathogen. The microbiological diseases most prevalent in society are brought about by organisms which are ubiquitous in the environment, can exist in the body without producing symptoms, and are at greatest risk of manifestation as illness when host resistance is impaired.

However, even in the few disorders transmitted through a seemingly straightforward pathway, such as single-gene inheritance or chromosome abnormalities, the prospects for prevention are not in fact as excellent as might be assumed. Genetic counselling against childbearing for relatives of affected individuals, or antenatal screening with termination of affected pregnancies are the primary methods for prevention. Yet given the choices for all the people concerned in deciding to give up a close relationship, the option of having children, or of terminating a pregnancy, it is perhaps not surprising that retrospective counselling concerning the risks to children of affected persons has been found to have a limited effect on the incidence of diseases such as Huntington's Chorea (see Emery 1978). And in Down's syndrome, for example, antenatal screening has so far had a relatively modest impact on the incidence of the disease: it has been found to be cost effective only if restricted to women over the age of 35. If strictly limited to this age-group, and if all cases were identified and pregnancies terminated, it is estimated that the overall incidence of this disorder in the general population would fall by as much as one-third (Stene & Mikkelsen 1984). In practice, however, reductions of only 8% have been achieved, even in areas where intensive efforts have been made. This disappointing result is largely accounted for by the combination of late presentation of pregnancy to the screening service, moral and religious objections to the termination of pregnancy, and failure on the part of obstetricians to offer amniocentesis (Ferguson-Smith 1983).

For most psychiatric disorder, our existing knowledge of causal processes is too limited to allow reduction to final common pathways. It is well established, for example, that schizophrenia has a genetic basis, but manifestation of the disease among people known to be genetically vulnerable is by no means inevitable. Even monozygotic twins have a concordance rate of disorder of less than 50% (Gottesman & Shields 1982). There must therefore be other causal factors, probably of an environmental nature, to account for the emergence of the disease in one genetically predisposed person rather than another. These factors may contribute in an additive fashion as separate causal agents, but more likely, they interact in some way with the genetic factor. In fact, the most widely applicable model is one of multiple causal factors interacting to produce a particular psychiatric outcome, where each individual causal factor also has a number of other possible outcomes in other combinations of circumstances, including other psychiatric disorders and physical pathology.

Identification of all possible antecedent factors in a given disorder, however, is still unlikely to provide sufficient information on which to base preventive proposals, given that in many circumstances, they will each be relatively innocuous. For most psychiatric disorders, the individual's past and present social environments, his/her biological and behavioural characteristics, *and* how each aspect of both person and environment affect each other must be considered (Magnusson 1983). For instance, it is now generally accepted that life events of an adverse nature are implicated in the onset of a range of physical and psychiatric disorders (Paykel 1978, Dohrenwend & Dohrenwend 1974, Craig & Brown 1984). Similar claims have been made for major chronic difficulties in relation to adult depression (Brown & Harris 1978), hypertension, diabetes and peptic ulcer (see Kasl 1984), and childhood psychiatric disorder (Rutter 1979). But while the presence of a number of chronic family adversities, such as poor housing, overcrowding, family discord, and parental mental illness *together* raise the risk of childhood psychiatric disorder, no one of these elevates risk where it occurs in *isolation* (Rutter 1979). While this may be interpreted as evidence for a simple summation of main effects, it is clear from this and other work that much depends on the interaction of the separate deprivations. Two such adversities tend to have a more damaging effect than would be expected from summing their independent effects; four would be more damaging than would be expected from doubling the effect of two (Rutter 1979). One likely explanation for this finding is connected with the perceived meaning of events. In considering the risk of childhood psychiatric disorder following divorce, Hetherington et al (1982) demonstrated that there was an appreciably increased risk of disorder for children with working mothers only when her starting work coincided with the divorce. Having a working mother was not a risk in itself, except where her perceived loss (through starting work for the first time) interacted with the actual loss of the father.

A second feature of the interactional nature of 'risk' factors which is also of considerable importance is the tendency of adversities to multiply. The mother who has hitherto chosen to stay at home with her children may need to seek employment *because* of the loss of her spouse. She may also experience financial hardship, need to move to less expensive accommodation which is away from supportive neighbours, and her children may need to move from their familiar educational system (Hetherington 1979).

When considering the genesis of adult psychiatric disorder, it is clear that a long and often indirect chain of events and circumstances have to be taken into account, and their respective importance becomes increasingly difficult to disentangle. One recent study, which has attempted to explain the relationship between institutional rearing and a high rate of adult adversity and depression, illustrates this kind of link (Quinton & Rutter 1984a & b). In this study, loss of the child's parents and institutional rearing rarely led to childhood psychiatric disorder which then persisted into adulthood. Instead, an indirect link with adult disorder was much more common: girls who were raised in Social Services' care becoming pregnant outside marriage, making bad choices in marriage, experiencing a discordant, unsupportive relationship, as well as a high rate of adverse events and social difficulties. Depression in these circumstances was common. In short, is seemed that the risk for adult depression was modified throughout life, by events in childhood, adolescence, and adulthood, but no single event at one point in time could be identified as having sufficiently damaging effects to make adult psychiatric disorder an inevitable outcome (Rutter 1985). Although each antecedent factor may well be relatively innocuous, however, this does not mean that preventive implications are absent — only that information on other antecedent and related variables also needs to be gained, before a realistic judgement about risk can be made.

The study of such interactional complexities is essential to the development of preventive proposals, as it is to the refinement of the aetiological theory of all multifactorial disorders. We know, for instance, that people who develop schizophrenia in adulthood are more likely than those who do not, to have suffered perinatal complications at birth; to have shown 'difficult' childhood characteristics of temperament (Mednick et al 1981) and to have experienced some unusual patterns of family interaction (see Leff, Ch.6). But it is not clear whether any of these factors plays a causal role, and if so, whether it is direct or indirect, or if (in the latter two cases) the factors are instead a result of an early manifestation of the same characteristics which produce the disorder. While this remains uncertain, there are no clear pointers for prevention.

However, aetiological research has made considerable progress in recent years since the development of more sophisticated tools for measurement, more careful methodology, and the use of longitudinal, prospective enquiry. Several credible interactional models of psychiatric disorder have been formulated (Strauss & Carpenter 1981, Depue 1979, Brown & Harris 1978). These formulations increasingly emphasise the protective or vulnerability factors whose co-existence or prior existence help to explain why any stressor does, and why it sometimes does not, lead to any particular psychiatric outcome. The value of such information is that it both enables 'high-risk' groups to be identified and provides implications for how they might be helped. One constellation of such factors which appears in many aetiological models is stress, social support, coping behaviour, and self-esteem, and these have attractive preventive potential. However, these seemingly straightforward ideas actually represent complex and variable underlying processes. The relationships which are found to be most supportive for the newly divorced woman wanting to make radical changes in her life will be very different from those needed by the mother who has just lost a child. The quality and type of support which is protective will also differ from situation to situation. But the notion that support and coping can be protective has had considerable appeal to those interested in mounting preventive programmes. Unfortunately, as will be discussed in the remainder of this chapter, the subtlety of the ideas (as described in Ch. 4), has not always been appreciated.

SUPPORT AND COPING: SOME POINTERS FOR PREVENTION

Support, coping, and self-esteem are obvious examples of factors which are closely interrelated. Successful coping and control over one's life inevitably contributes to self-esteem, and of course self-esteem may influence the capacity to form intimate and supportive relationships. In turn, these relationships contribute to self-esteem and coping. The separate effects of these variables in causation have been difficult to untangle, and these difficulties are discussed at greater depth elsewhere in this book. We will restrict ourselves here to some of the conclusions drawn by those who have done research in the area, and their practical implications.

Developmental experiences

It has often been assumed that adult coping skills and self-esteem are to a large extent determined in childhood, or even at conception (as inherited characteristics of personality). These in turn have been thought to play an important role in shaping supportive relationships. For instance, Henderson et al (1980) argued that their research shows that enduring personality attributes determine both the social support obtained and the perceived adequacy of that support. Undoubtedly, personality is implicated in some way, but the nature of its contribution is not yet clear. Most investigators would agree, however, that the relationship the young child has with his/her parent is a crucial source of affection, value, and self-esteem, as well as a guide to appropriate behaviour. Where this relationship is damaged through parental mental illness, parental marital discord, or parent–child separation, there is evidence that the child is at increased psychiatric risk (Robins 1966, Hetherington 1979, Douglas 1975, Rutter 1972). Institution-reared children are at an especially high risk, particularly if parent–child separation and subsequent child-care arrangements preclude the development of any affectional bond at all before the age of three years (Bowlby 1951, Rutter 1972).

The importance of the quality of support received by the young child (in determining adult self-esteem, coping, and support) is not only revealed by studying such extreme circumstances as those associated with institutional rearing. In a community survey in Walthamstow, North London, Harris et al (1986) showed that a lack of care in childhood, (sometimes, but not necessarily, following the loss of the mother by separation or death) was associated with a 3-fold increase in the rate of adult depression. By 'lack of care', they meant a marked parental indifference and/or low control, lasting one year or more. A second survey by this team in Islington, North London found more than a 2-fold increase in the rate of depression associated with lack of care (Bifulco et al 1987). The explanation advanced for this link centred on the development of low self-esteem, of a 'helpless' cognitive set, consequent poor coping behaviour, and a raised probability of marrying an unsupportive husband. Early marriage and/or premarital pregnancy was almost invariably a link between childhood lack of care and adult depression (see Ch. 3).

Quinton & Rutter (1984b) have shown large differences in the parenting behaviour of women raised 'in care', compared to similar aged mothers with no such adverse childhood experiences. One-fifth of the children of the former group of mothers had either been taken into local authority Social Services care or were cared for by someone other than their mother, whereas this was true of none of the children of the comparison mothers. Furthermore, the former group had greater problems in child management, showing lower control and sensitivity. Of course, there were also skilled mothers among ex-care girls, and these tended to be the same women who had exercised some foresight and planning and entered into supportive marital relationships. What is apparent, however, is that the poor support in childhood of women raised 'in care' not only raised their own risk of psychiatric disorder, along with a wide range of other psychosocial difficulties (see Quinton & Rutter 1984a & b), but often replicated itself in the next generation.

The results of such investigations lead to the tempting thought that early intervention could go a long way toward averting later disorder. Thus, for example, preparation for parenthood, with training in child management skills for adolescent girls who have experienced poor parenting themselves, and use of educational programmes to teach not only the mechanics of contraception and sources of help and advice, but also the importance of taking a responsibility for one's actions and planning one's life, would appear to offer real hope for effective prevention of later disorder. On a similar basis, foster 'aunties' in the local community may provide valuable support for children in care, and as they reach the age at which local authority responsibility comes to an end, an alternative support system of some kind would seem particularly necessary until such children have established an independent life in the community for themselves, with satisfactory accommodation and friendships. (See Grosskurth 1984 for a disturbing commentary on homelessness among ex-care adolescents; and Rutter et al 1983 for the high rate of premarital pregnancy.)

That such efforts ought to prove effective is indicated by the evidence that good coping behaviours at key points in the causal chain can be protective. For instance, Harris et al (1987) identified premarital pregnancy as a common link in the chain of events between childhood lack of care and adult depression, but noted that coping behaviour at this time appeared to modify the associated future psychiatric risk. Girls who allowed themselves to become trapped into unsatisfactory relationships or single parenthood were found to be considerably more likely to be depressed at the time of the survey. On the other hand, those who coped well, i.e. those who delayed marriage to the father until they were sure of their decision, or arranged termination or adoption, were more likely to find themselves supportive relationships and less problematic life-styles, and had a somewhat smaller risk of depression (Harris et al 1987). Rutter et al (1983) have shown that positive school experiences can be helpful in fostering such planning skills in children without supportive home lives.

Preventive intervention in childhood has proved an appealing idea and many programmes have been developed (see below). However, there have sometimes been over-optimistic views expressed on what can be achieved in terms of wide-scale prevention of adult psychiatric illnesses, given that the ability to form and maintain stable affectional bonds and consequent susceptibility to the impact of later stressors are subject to modification throughout life. The effects of early corrective interventions are only too easily nullified by later hardship and adversity.

Current circumstances

Given the difficulty of creating lasting benefits from interventions made at early points in the causal chain, many practitioners have preferred to focus on more recent antecedents of psychiatric disorder, advocating either the general reduction of adversity or techniques for fostering resilience in the face of adversity.

Reducing adversity directly

Attention has been drawn to the preventive possibilities inherent in reducing stress itself, such as economic and employment policies which minimise the level of unemployment (Smith 1986), housing policies which consider the mental health requirements of residents (Freeman 1985), and adequate child care facilities to enable women to find part-time or full-time employment outside the home (Boulton 1983). Other suggestions include organisational management to maximise individual autonomy in both residential settings and work environments (Rodin 1983, House 1981). Common transitions like retirement or events like hospitalisation might also be made less stressful through gradually cutting down on the working week to phase people into retirement, or having one responsible nurse for a child in hospital rather than several (e.g. Wolfer & Visintainer 1979). Of course, such measures are in any case well justified on moral and humanitarian grounds, independent of their role in reducing the prevalence of serious psychiatric illness.

Enhancing coping skills

Although 'coping' is a widely used term and a familiar concept, it is difficult to discover just what it involves, and to establish whether there are generalisable skills or attributes (i.e. generalisable from one person to another, or one situation to another), that can be taught as part of a prevention programme. It has been suggested that behavioural responses are most important in dealing with everyday problems encountered in marriage and parenthood, whereas psychological resources are more crucial in stressful circumstances which are largely impervious to individual efforts to control them (stressful work conditions, perhaps) (Pearlin & Schooler 1978). In the face of severely threatening and uncontrollable events like discovering a daughter has leukaemia, losing a child at birth, or finding one's life-long employer has become bankrupt, Silver & Wortman's review (1980) revealed at least two factors which have some generalised applicability to effectiveness in psychological coping. The first was the opportunity to talk about feelings and experiences, and the ventilation of anxiety, sadness, anger, or despair; the second was the ability to find some personal meaning for particular experiences. For example, knowing that although death was inevitable for one's own child, that their suffering and treatment may, through contributing to knowledge of the condition, help other children with the same affliction in the future.

Three broad groups of preventive approaches have been advocated for enhancing peoples' capacity to cope with adversity. First, in the absence of any specific imminent crisis, it has been thought possible to teach people a general method for dealing with stress (Meichenbaum 1977). A second approach involves teaching specific coping skills during the weeks and months before predictable crises, while a third method aims to ameliorate the impact of recent stressors by interventions during and immediately after a threatening event. Preventive programmes have been developed, based on each of these principles, and some may offer promise, but before turning to review these efforts, we need to draw attention to the role that close relationships can play in bolstering personal coping skills.

The protective role of social support

Of the various contributions to a satisfactory adjustment to losses and other major life crises, the importance of intimate support has received the most attention. Three aspects of support can be identified: emotional, functional (tangible help), and informational (knowledge, experience, advice) (House 1981). While it might be a relatively straightforward matter for preventive efforts to provide tangible help and information, the extent to which they may create meaningful emotional support when a crisis occurs is less obvious.

Emotional support is provided by relationships which enhance or maintain self-esteem, i.e. enable the person to feel cared for, loved, esteemed and valued, and part of a network of communication and mutual obligation (Cobb 1976). O'Connor & Brown (1984) argued that this comes not so much from feelings of attachment and dependency, but from objectively quantifiable 'support'. Their interviews with women in North London demonstrated that very close relationships, offering regular contact and a high level of confiding, warmth, and positive interaction, were associated both with the woman's psychiatric state and with her evaluation of herself. Dependence on and attachment to the person, however, were not closely related to either.

In other words, it cannot be assumed that the availability of a 'close other' to whom a person might turn for support in the face of a crisis necessarily means that the person actually *receives* help. The spouse or friend may fail to provide the emotional support expected of them, and in the research by Brown et al, women whose husbands 'let them down' fared even less well in adapting to crises than women who had no-one from whom they expected such help (see Ch. 3).

Not only has the absence of (or being let down by) close supportive others been found to increase vulnerability, but so too has the presence of close unsupportive others. For instance, married women with a discordant relationship with their husbands, characterised by a high level of negative interaction, have an increased risk of depression (Brown et al 1986). There is also an increased likelihood that their children will develop psychiatric problems (Rutter 1972). People treated for schizophrenia and living with parents or marital partners who show a highly critical and over-involved communication style toward them are much more liable to relapse than if they were living in a more supportive environment (Brown et al 1962, Leff & Vaughn 1980; other chapters in this volume review this literature in more depth).

Support is therefore a complex concept, since even very close relationships are capable of being either protective or deleterious to mental health. However, the importance of this research for prevention is that it is becoming increasingly possible to identify those people at greatest risk of developing psychiatric disorder following certain kinds of life events. By reducing the numbers in a target population, this should considerably reduce the cost of programmes. But although we may now be able to specify the population most in need of help, do we know how to help them?

WHAT EVIDENCE IS THERE THAT RESILIENCE CAN BE FOSTERED BY PREVENTIVE INTERVENTION?

While on the one hand arguing that programmes based on current interactional causal models should be very valuable, we must also state at the outset that the evidence to demonstrate that they are in fact helpful is far from impressive. This is largely because of the methodological difficulties in conducting research in prevention, but also because of the failure of so many intervention researchers to fully utilise available knowledge and theory in the planning and evaluation of their programmes. In selecting projects to describe, we have chosen a sample which would seem likely to be beneficial, given the multi-factorial models of disorder described elsewhere in this book. Each project focuses on a high-risk group and on attempts to foster their resilience to adversity — either during childhood or in adulthood.

Improving parent–child relationships

There is considerable evidence now that it is not possible to produce long-term changes in children's coping skills and behaviour by training schemes, however elaborate, which do not also involve their parents and teachers. In his impressive review of pre-school educational programmes for disadvantaged American children, Bronfenbrenner (1975) concluded that only if mothers were able to reinforce the training at home and continue to do so after special provision ceased, could such strategies bring about the hoped for changes. Helping parents to be more effective and to find pleasure in their role is also likely to be valuable in enhancing their own self-esteem, with a further potentially beneficial effect on their relationships with their children (see also Pound et al 1985).

The supportive mother–child relationship is often damaged if the mother has a psychiatric disorder. Maternal depression, for instance, has been shown to be associated with poor functioning in her children (Richman et al 1982, Mills et al 1984). Mills et al have shown a poor 'meshing' between depressed mothers and their young children, in terms of verbal and non-verbal 'links', while Richman et al found a poorer cognitive development, higher prevalence of behaviour problems, and even a higher rate of accidents in the children of depressed women. For these reasons, preventive approaches should focus as much on the mother's self-esteem as on the child's social and cognitive skills.

An experimental child development project has been mounted in six disadvantaged areas of England, Wales, and the Republic of Ireland (Child Development Programme 1984). This project used health visitors to help mothers find stimulating and rewarding educational tasks to do with their babies. This intervention differed from normal health visitors' practice in two main ways. First, project health visitors were allocated extra time to spend with project mothers. Secondly, they were trained to modify their usual directive approach, so that they encouraged and supported mothers to develop their own ideas. The health visitor spent an hour or two with mother and child, discussing problems and how they could be resolved, as well as developmental tasks which the child was acquiring which could be encouraged. The health visitor was trained not to make direct suggestions, but to support the mother in her attempts to find strategies and solutions. At the next meeting, some weeks later, she would discuss how the strategies had worked and what aspects of the relationship or of the child's development the mother would work on next. The non-directive method and generous interval between meetings were designed to minimise dependency of mothers on the service, and by seeing themselves as responsible for the child's progress, to maximise their self-esteem, satisfaction, and child management skills.

Over 1000 families took part, randomly allocated to intervention or comparison groups. Some of the mothers and children were also found to be malnourished, so that a strong health and nutritional component was also seen to be important. A research worker in each region conducted lengthy interviews before the intervention began, and 12 and 24 months later. Preliminary evaluation data suggest that the intervention considerably improved the socio-educational and language environments of the children. Subsequent multivariate assessments will reveal any effects on maternal self-esteem, diet, and children's social and activity levels.

This approach is aimed primarily at arming mothers with good coping and management skills, as a way of improving the social and educational development of the child, and with a hoped-for consequence of enhancing the parent–child relationship and the self-esteem of mothers. An alternative approach is to focus instead on supporting mothers within a close friendship, to improve their self-esteem and thence their ability to cope, and to find a more rewarding relationship with their children. Given that many women who might be considered appropriate clients of a preventive service will be overwhelmed by the daily problems associated with low income, poor environment, or child care difficulties, and are unlikely to look favourably on proposals to devote time and energy to their children individually, this approach might hold more promise.

'Homestart' in Leicester, England, developed a mother-to-mother befriending scheme in 1973 which has since spawned numerous other such projects, and been subject to a 4-year evaluative study (Van der Eyken 1982). The project aimed to find volunteer local mothers to befriend women referred by social workers, health visitors, and general practitioners, to help build up their confidence and use of local resources in finding stimulating and enjoyable activities to do with their children. Van der Eyken reports that two-thirds of the 156 families whose befriending had ceased or had been ongoing for at least a year between

1974 and 1978 were judged by the Homestart organiser to have undergone 'considerable change', and only 8% to have shown 'no change'. 'Change' meant different things for different families, but included, for instance, a mother who was under pressure from her environment, children, and poverty being rehoused, or obtaining part-time employment, and pre-school placements for her children, such that she had a noticeably more relaxed and positive attitude towards them.

A similar befriending project in South London has recently been evaluated by Pound et al (1985). 'Newpin' is run by a co-ordinator with a background in health visiting, but the 'befrienders' are all volunteers. Mothers were again referred to the project by social workers, health visitors, or family doctors, usually with some degree of depression, social difficulties, isolation, or problems in parenting. Volunteers used by the project were in many ways similar to client mothers, and in fact had often come to the project originally as clients, but were women who were currently coping more successfully and had wider and more supportive social networks.

After a brief training, volunteers were matched to clients as far as possible in terms of age and personal interests. The volunteer visited the client, often several times a week, offering friendship, support, and practical assistance towards resolving her difficulties. She also aimed to increase the mother's own social network by going with her and her children to the project drop-in centre for training sessions and social meetings with other mothers. The contract terminated when the pair agreed either that the problem had been resolved or that the client had established new supportive friendships.

A pilot evaluation of 12 volunteer–client pairs showed that almost all clients had made new friends, and all now had someone with whom they could confide at a deep level. Very often, volunteers derived as much benefit from the friendship as clients (Pound et al 1985). Although the published report of the service offers no more than a preliminary overview of the progress of participants, the results are encouraging. The majority of women felt they had learned to understand people better, and rated their self-esteem and confidence as improved, while many of the difficulties with families of origin, husbands, or co-habitees had been reduced. Considering the extremely deprived histories of most of the women and their own experience of lack of care, without some kind of help, it would be likely that a poor quality parent–child relationship would be repeated with some of their own children. Among the 11 referrals on whom data were complete, 10 had been separated from one or both parents in childhood, 8 had 3 or more changes of main caretaker in the early years, 9 had been deserted by husbands or co-habitees during pregnancy or shortly after, and finance and housing problems were almost universal. Not surprisingly, most of the women had symptoms of depression. While the project might therefore be argued to be a good treatment programme for mothers, rather than strictly prevention, it can be seen as preventive for the children. This was illustrated by the fact that for seven referrals and six volunteers, relationships with their children was chosen by the co-ordinator as one of the target problems which they aimed to improve, and in all but two families, an improvement was judged to have been achieved.

These projects tackle important problems in a way concordant with a rational, theoretical model, using a high-quality intervention programme. Furthermore, the befriending projects appear to be succeeding with chronically depressed women — a client-group notoriously impervious to outside efforts to help them. For these reasons, they represent some of the more interesting approaches we have uncovered, yet none of the three projects have yet published results which stand up to critical scrutiny. More substantive evidence is expected to be forthcoming, but the fact that such weak evidence is reported here at all is indicative of the poor quality of much of the research in this field.

Supporting people through stressful life events

Common sense suggests that stressful events which come out of the blue are potentially more difficult to deal with and more distressing than events of equal magnitude and significance which are known about in advance. In Caplan's view (1964), people can prepare themselves for impending crises by anticipating the experience and problems involved and working through possible solutions, including mastery of their own negative feelings. In this way, it was claimed, the hazards can be attenuated because they will have become familiar by being anticipated, and the person will have already set out on the path of healthy coping responses.

Some services, such as antenatal care, have for decades been operating on the assumption that it is important to prepare pregnant women with information and advice so that they will know what to expect at childbirth and how to cope with the new baby. There are one or two studies preparing young children for hospital admission for tonsillectomies (e.g. Wolfer & Visintainer 1979, Ferguson 1979) which show that advance information about medical procedures and events and how they should feel, together with continuity of care from one responsible nurse, reduced the child's fears and anxieties and unco-operative behaviour before the operation, as well as problem behaviour after discharge. Similar procedures for adults facing surgical operations have also been evaluated (e.g. gastroendoscopies, Johnson 1984).

That preparation *can* influence people's capacity to deal effectively with specific crises has been demonstrated both in experimental settings and in observations of normal subjects undergoing stress. Studies of how people prepare themselves to jump with a parachute from an aeroplane have found that those successfully overcoming their anxieties do so by mastering progressively greater amounts of stress in the days leading up to a jump. Those who fail to take themselves through a gradual preparation must fall back on an all-or-none mechanism, with attempts to deny all fear. Novice parachutists who tried to block out fear completely were often overwhelmed with anxiety at the last moment and unable to jump, then deciding to give up jumping forever (Epstein 1983). Epstein calls self-preparation 'graded stress inoculation'; he believes it to be the natural healing process of the mind, and one that can be taught to individuals failing to adapt in this way. The techniques include coping strategies to reduce the physiological concomitants of anxiety, self-communications, and 'cognitive restructuring' to promote positive self-statements. These techniques have been advocated in helping people to prepare themselves for specific predictable crises, in treating phobic disorders, and as a broad cognitive approach to everyday stresses of all kinds (Meichenbaum & Jaremko 1983, Janis 1958).

Rodin (1983) used this method to help residents of apartment buildings for the elderly to take greater control over their own lives and to deal with problems as they arose. She observed that older people often have negative attitudes toward themselves and their capabilities, and that these interfere with effective problem-solving.

Forty of the residents of an old peoples' home who were suffering from relatively stable chronic physical diseases, were randomly assigned to one of four groups. There was a no-treatment 'control group', a group encouraged to take responsibility and exercise choice in their daily lives, a third group trained for three weeks in the self-regulation and coping skills described above, and a fourth who spent equal amounts of time with the psychologist, but just chatting. The training course was intended to encourage residents to see themselves as active contributors to their own experiences, and not helpless victims of their thoughts and feelings. They were made aware of their own forms of negative self-statements and taught other self-statements to guide coping behaviour, practising their skills on a number of hypothetical 'helplessness provoking' situations, which might regularly be encountered. A wide range of physical and mental health checks were made before and after the intervention, and a social interview assessed perceived stress, the nature of daily activities, and inter-personal relationships. An activity rating was also made, both from direct observations and from participation in special excursions and activities.

An earlier study (Rodin & Langer 1977) with a more handicapped sample had shown that even regular simple encouragement to take more responsibility for day-to-day decision-making, through the care staff being trained to take this line, was sufficient to produce a change in behaviour. In this study, however, only the self-instructional training was more effective than increased attention. The self-instructional group showed the greatest reduction in perceived stress, in urinary free cortisol (a physiological index of stress), in autonomic symptoms, consumption of tranquillisers, and the largest improvement in the doctors' 'blind' ratings of prognosis. Of the five residents whose illnesses required hospital admission and three who died in the 18 months after the intervention, none were from the self-instructional group.

Usually, preparation for specific known events also includes practical information, as well as psychological self-preparation. Parachutists learn specific skills for landing on the ground, practice in small jumps, and receive detailed information on what hazards to expect and how to deal with them, as well as what the experience in general will be like. Some events of the kinds implicated in depression and anxiety are also amenable to this type of preventive intervention — operations, for instance, relapsing or terminal illness in a close relative, and active military placements. Some attempts to evaluate preparatory programmes have been undertaken. For example, Maguire et al (1980) attempted to reduce the psychiatric morbidity associated with breast cancer and mastectomy by providing counselling by a trained nurse. The nurse saw patients before and after the operation, discussed with the woman her feelings about losing a breast, and demonstrated the use of a range of external breast prostheses. After the patient was discharged from hospital, the nurse visited her every two months to check arm movements, to encourage the woman to do the recommended exercises, to talk about the woman's relationship with her sexual partner and her feelings about breast loss, and to encourage her to return to work and become socially active again.

Over a 24-month period, 152 women who had been randomly allocated for counselling or control groups, took part in the study. The incidence of symptoms of anxiety, depression, and sexual problems was assessed shortly after operation and 3, 12, and 18 months later; the occurrence of any stressful life events was also assessed at each interview. Approximately equal numbers in both groups suffered from an episode of morbid anxiety or depression, or experienced marked sexual problems at some stage following mastectomy. However, episodes of depression and anxiety were of shorter duration in the counselled group, clearing up after an average of six months compared with over 10 months for control women. The counselled group also showed a superior social adjustment, earlier return to work, better adaptation to breast loss, and satisfaction with breast prostheses in the same period (Maguire et al 1983).

No mention was made of the quality of support the woman had in her social relationships, nor the degree to which any of those relationships were providing emotional support at the time of this crisis, and to this extent, the study can be criticised in failing to make full use of current aetiological theory. In terms of improving the women's adjustment to breast loss and preventing prolonged depressive reactions, however, the intervention was clearly successful. Fewer of the counselled group were depressed or anxious at the 12- and 18-month follow-ups. Some of its success in this respect came from early referral for treatment of women showing psychiatric symptoms. It did not prevent the onset of depression or anxiety, and in this sense may be considered a failure. However, both the gravity of the event and the circumstances of some of the women were bound to mean that a period of depression or anxiety would follow, and could be argued as a *normal* reaction. If this is followed by a rapid readjustment, it may be that this is the most which could be hoped for from such an intervention.

There have also been a number of attempts to intervene preventively at the time of bereavement, and here emphasis is inevitably on psychological rather than practical coping. The two best studies identified by Parkes' review of the subject in 1980 offered counselling to a specially selected 'high-risk' group of relatives, and showed more sophisticated methodology than the study described above. Raphael (1977) offered her own services as a psychiatrist in up to nine lengthy interviews, while Parkes (1981) evaluated a pattern of hospice care for the dying in South East London, in which ward staff supported relatives before the death, and which used volunteers in a 'befriending' capacity after bereavement. In an earlier study of psychiatric morbidity among bereaved persons, Parkes (1975) had identified a number of risk indicators to enable him to predict with some accuracy which people would have most problems in adapting to bereavement. These included 'clinging' to the patient before death, angry or self-reproachful behaviour, and an intuitive guess by nursing staff that the relative was likely to cope badly. He therefore had 3 study groups: 57 high-risk persons randomly allocated to a supported or unsupported group, and 85 low-risk controls. Only the first group received the special help, which was that trained volunteers visited relatives in their own homes. It was noted that it took about 12 months before a volunteer became skilled, but after this considerable experience, their competence often rivalled that of many professionals. Twenty months later, the two high-risk groups showed differences in their change of health scores on new or worse autonomic symptoms and on a measure of increased consumption of drugs, alcohol, and tobacco. There was little difference in outcome between the supported high-risk group and the 'low-risk' group, from which Parkes argued that the intervention effectively lowers psychiatric risk among high-risk relatives to the equivalent of a low-risk group.

Preventing recurrent morbidity

Life events and social difficulties have also been implicated in recurrent episodes of psychiatric illness among ex-patients (Paykel 1978, Leff & Vaughn 1980), and the extent to which a person's environment is supportive and he/she is able to cope with the problems which present themselves have been related to risk of relapse. Support does not refer to the provision of goods or services for ex-patients in areas where they are relatively well provided and competent, but to ways of meeting needs that the ex-patient cannot meet himself, to finding emotionally supportive environments, and to ways of helping him become independent rather than dependent (Bennett & Morris 1983, Test & Stein 1978). The level of support in terms of services will therefore need to vary according to the level of disability of the ex-patient. Test & Stein have described some impressive but somewhat costly community programmes, providing the sorts of flexible supports which can enable people who have experienced quite severe mental illnesses to cope with crises arising in their living circumstances, which might otherwise lead to a relapse of symptoms and/or readmission. In this sense, well designed follow-up services can be argued to have an important role to play in prevention.

One area where some level of generalisation can be made about supportive environments likely to reduce psychiatric risk is in the living circumstances of people treated for schizophrenia. It is now widely accepted that these individuals are particularly sensitive to emotional arousal, even when the disorder is in remission, and that high levels of arousal can precipitate relapse. This has been found to have important implications for their life-styles. Over-stimulation, for example, is more likely to arise from living with close relatives with whom the individual has an intense but critical emotional relationship (Brown et al 1962), or after an emotionally arousing event (Leff & Vaughn 1980). These findings have provided clear pointers for preventive intervention, and several studies have been mounted (family programmes are reviewed by Barrowclough & Tarrier 1984).

An important overstimulating variable which has been identified in the home environments of sufferers of schizophrenia is the 'Expressed Emotion' (EE) of family members when talking with the sufferer, including critical comments and emotional over-concern. Neuroleptic medication is protective to some extent in these circumstances, by helping to lower arousal levels, but if the individual's environment is less emotionally arousing *and* he maintains prophylactic medication, then his risk of relapse is substantially lower than with medication alone. EE can be lowered in two ways: either the contact between the individual and relative can be reduced, by finding alternative places to spend much of the day, or relatives can be helped, through participation in educational groups and family therapy to find more supportive ways of relating to the patient.

Furthermore, by meeting in groups, relatives with high EE can pick up from relatives with lower emotional involvement good coping strategies for problem behaviours at home. Leff et al (1982) tried this educational approach, while Falloon et al (1982) broadened it somewhat to encourage families to foster positive skills in the patient.

The study by Leff's team involved educational sessions in the hospital with families of schizophrenic patients, which included information on the nature, course, and treatment of schizophrenia. They learnt that many of the distressing or annoying behaviours were symptoms of the illness, and that the patient was particularly susceptible to new events, criticism, and over-involvement. High-EE families were also given a form of family therapy in their own homes. (The results are described in Ch. 6, this volume, and in Leff et al 1983.)

Together with the work of Falloon, these findings provide important indications for prevention. In particular, they reinforce the evidence from other areas of psychiatric research that the treatment or prevention of psychiatric disorders in individuals cannot expect to have long-term effectiveness if the social environment in which the person lives is not also considered. Many people who have had major psychiatric illness need ongoing support, but even the most flexible of community psychiatric support programmes have time limits, and the risk of relapse may return when this support is removed (Test & Stein 1978). Only more permanent changes to the environment, such as the way key family members relate to the sufferer, can hope to achieve the kind of long-term protective benefits desired; this is the kind of protection which was previously only seen to be possible through maintenance drug treatments. Such approaches are not advocated as alternatives to pharmacological treatments, of course, but as an additional essential element of management.

PAST AND PRESENT INITIATIVES IN PREVENTIVE PSYCHIATRY

The studies reviewed so far offer little more than a general indication of the possible direction that future experimental services might follow, and it is clear that several years of careful extension and replication of the results will be required before the strategies can be developed to a degree which will allow their ready utilisation in routine service provision. Can the caring professions wait for the painfully slow process of theory building and experimental testing to run its course? History suggests they will not.

Interest in prevention and the pressure to implement prophylactic services is not new. It was one of the aims of the mental hygiene movement, toward the beginning of the present century. In the last 25 years, both President Kennedy and President Carter have made strong statements in support of preventive mental health programming in America, which they intended to be a fundamental component in the work of the Community Mental Health Centers (CMHCs) constructed and funded with federal money. However, the allocation of resources for CMHC services, as well as a political shift in ideological response to service planning, has seriously limited the development of relevant services. More important, however, has been the failure to develop realistic priorities for action or to utilise current knowledge and theory to plan programmes and develop cost-effective ways of putting them into practice (Leighton 1982, Newton 1988).

In Britain, the child guidance movement might be considered one of the earliest services with an explicitly preventive aim. The treatment of difficult and neurotic behaviour in children was also intended to prevent more serious mental disturbances in adult life (Sampson 1980). Given the size of the population of children with behavioural, emotional, and educational difficulties (Rutter et al 1975), however, the movement can only be judged a failure in terms of prevention. Child guidance clinics simply see far too few children to be able to make any impact on the problem.

The British primary health care system is perhaps the closest to a preventive service, in which GPs and their allies in the health services aim to intervene 'therapeutically, educationally and preventively' to promote their clients' health (Royal College of General Practitioners 1972). But even in preventing physical disorders, where the benefits of prophylactic action are well established, such as in the regular monitoring of people with type 2 diabetes or hypertension, GPs have been shown to have a disturbingly poor record of preventive care (Lancet editorial 1984).

Caplan's ideas for 'primary prevention' provided an early model for crisis intervention for mental health services, emphasising the need to find widely available means of supporting distressed people, rather than highly specialised ways of helping small numbers of the very disturbed. He saw psychiatrists as providing a consultation service to enable clergymen, teachers, doctors, and other informal care-givers to provide more effective support for people experiencing stressful life events. Some methods of crisis intervention exist in current psychiatric services, but they do not, on the whole, resemble Caplan's model. They involve members of different professional groups working together as a crisis intervention team (CIT) to help resolve acute problems in their clients' own homes with the help of family and friends, in order or avert the need for hospital admission. The kind of crisis Caplan had in mind for primary prevention, however, was a situational one — bereavement, marital conflict, extreme difficulties caused by examinations or work stress, or perhaps the birth of a handicapped baby. The kind of crisis typically referred to a CIT is a psychiatric emergency — very often an ex-psychiatric patient suffering an acute relapse of symptoms (Bouras & Tufnell 1983).

It might be argued, therefore, that Caplan's views have never been given a fair test within psychiatric practice. However, it is hardly a model likely to be adopted with any enthusiasm, given the very high prevalence of such 'crises', and the very small numbers of people likely to develop psychiatric disorder as a direct consequence. In the absence of a simple means of identifying vulnerable people, it is perhaps not surprising that service providers have concentrated their efforts on the acutely ill, with intervention aimed to minimise the escalation of disorder and the emergence of secondary handicaps.

In this regard, suicide has more often been the focus of concern among clinicians attempting to formulate preventive methods. The majority of successful suicide attempts occur in the context of psychiatric illness, commonly an affective disorder (Barraclough et al 1974, Robins 1981) and as many as four-fifths have had medical contact for psychiatric disorder in the year prior to death (Barraclough et al 1974). Furthermore, as most victims have communicated their distress and intent (Robins 1981), these observations have led to the conclusion that suicide ought to be preventable.

Even here, however, there is little evidence that any preventive programme has made a significant general impact. In fact, both the substantial methodological difficulties in the evaluation of preventive work and the weaknesses inherent in many programme designs can all be illustrated from the history of attempts to prevent suicide.

The majority of suicide prevention programmes have been developed in the absence of detailed information about likely causal models. There is undoubtedly considerable heterogeneity in the psychopathological and socio-demographic characteristics of suicide victims, who are affected by widely differing personal and social causal factors (see e.g. Low et al 1981). This would suggest that several high-risk groups may be identifiable, whose separate needs may require quite different preventive approaches. Most efforts at prevention, however, can be accused of attempting to provide a single general solution for all groups, and as a consequence, must fall far short of their potential impact. This, of course, also has implications for the nature of evaluative research into the efficiency of such services. Why should anyone with a serious wish to die want to telephone the Samaritans, for instance? Since so many do, it would be logical for an evaluation of this service to begin by answering this question, and the effectiveness of the service could then be assessed on those distressed persons characterised by those particular needs. Instead, both Bagley (1968) and Jennings et al (1978) looked for general reductions in suicide rates between towns with and without Samaritan telephone counselling services. One recent controlled analysis on the effects of suicide prevention services in the USA which examined the differential effects of telephone counselling services, however, found that there were beneficial effects on one sub-group over a 6-year period (young white females), but these were obscured by overall comparisons (Miller et al 1984).

Similarly Chowdhury et al (1973) and Gibbons et al (1978) have chosen parasuicide cases treated in hospital as target 'high-risk' groups for repeat suicide attempts, and have provided a preventive programme offering social work support. Chowdhury et al used the Samaritans as a 24-hour emergency service, together with domiciliary visits from social workers, while Gibbons provided task-orientated social work support. Both used a randomised experimental treatment versus routine follow-up evaluation; neither found any evidence that the programme prevented repeat suicidal attempts. Nor did either study base the chosen intervention on any adequate model to explain why such a service ought to be beneficial, other than the observation that parasuicides have multiple social problems. Specific social difficulties were not examined in detail, nor is it clear whether the interventions had any significant impact on these social problems.

There are further difficulties beyond those mentioned above, which make the evaluation of suicide prevention programmes so difficult. To begin with, there is the problem of obtaining accurate information on the outcome of interventions, in terms of the number of suicides within the population in which the new service has arisen. Official registers of suicides are notoriously unreliable. Not only is it likely that, in general, official figures provide underestimates of mortality due to suicide, but it seems that in cities which are concerned about suicides, the reported rates may actually be inflated by the over-generous inclusion of ambiguous deaths (Diggory 1976, Bridge 1977). Second, there is the need to rule out alternative explanations for any apparent experimental effects. There may be fluctuations in suicide rates which parallel the introduction of a preventive service, but may have quite independent origins. For example, it has been argued that the fall in suicide rates in England and Wales between 1963 and 1973 (when that of most other countries was rising) was indicative of the efficacy of the newly introduced Samaritan befriending services. In fact, such changes might equally be attributed to the conversion of domestic gas to a non-toxic form (Kreitman 1976) or to the change in prescribing habits of doctors, with the introduction of safer alternatives to barbiturates.

Finally, the majority of studies examining the efficiency of suicide prevention programmes rely on correlations between suicide rates in areas with prevention services, and contrast these with areas without such services. This raises quite serious problems about the comparability between areas and times. In a recent USA investigation, for example, Miller et al noted that the published list of preventive services was grossly inaccurate; at the time of their survey, many centres had moved or were non-existent, while many of the areas for which no agencies were listed did indeed have functioning services (Miller et al 1984).

On balance, if one can make any conclusion, it is that the general case for the Samaritans or other suicide prevention service is 'not proven'. But they are very likely to be effective for specific sub-groups of suicidal individuals, and to provide a service for other human needs, such as the relief of loneliness, for others.

HEALTH SERVICE IMPLICATIONS OF DISEASE MODELS

The perspective adopted in this chapter has been that preventive strategies should be based on a disease rather than a health model, i.e. one which seeks to develop focused interventions which are targeted at a specific illness and which aim to disrupt a discrete causal process. The alternative, health model approach, focuses instead on helping well people to remain free from illness of any kind. In the health model approach, evidence that many different illnesses are associated with social and environmental deprivation is emphasised and disease-specific causal pathways played down. Factors which facilitate growth and well-being are stressed, together with strategies which seek to improve the lot of mankind across a broad front: education, legislation, fiscal measures, organisational change, and community developments (WHO 1984). Typical aims include reducing inequalities in health, improving access to care, and developing environments conducive to health. The two models differ in so far as the former starts from a pragmatic stance (discovering what interventions 'work' for a relatively narrow group of disorders), while the health model often appears to be based on an ideological perspective. Ultimately, the two converge, as the interventions tested in specific disease models are elaborated and applied across larger populations. Often, an intervention designed with a single condition in mind proves valuable for other disorders, and general principles emerge (for example, modern practices of hygiene grew out of quite limited interventions focused on cholera). In the longer term, then, the application of measures based on a health model may well be the most effective means of attaining widespread prevention, but these measures can only be adopted with any conviction once the relevance of specific risk factors is firmly established. In view of the present limits of our knowledge of the aetiology of psychiatric disorder, the disease approach, with its emphasis on limited interventions to both validate causal models and explore preventive possibilities, must take precedence; only once this step is complete can we turn to health promotional recommendations with any fervour.

One consequence of adopting such disease models is to place the onus for developing preventive services largely on traditional health care providers, and this is not without drawbacks — not least the fact that the majority of health service personnel are already over-stretched by the demands of providing treatment, and the responsibility of service administration and supervision. To find yet more time in a busy week to devote to prevention, necessitates both conviction of its value and considerable motivation.

Convincing health service providers of the adequacy and generalisability of experimental preventive interventions is a major obstacle to developing successful preventive programmes. Replication helps, but only partially, since no experiment is ever so free of methodological shortcomings as to escape the critical refutations of the unconvinced. In practice, conviction arises slowly, specific interventions fit in with the general climate of popular clinical opinion, and techniques which are most likely to be adopted are those which are already trusted in other settings. For example, the potential of approaches which modify high EE are particularly attractive because the intervention follows logically from a well-established causal model and is based on family therapy methods which are widely understood.

However, conviction of the potential value of a particular intervention is not enough; service providers have also to be persuaded that the target disorder is one which warrants their concern. While this is not an issue for the severe psychoses, there is in fact little consensus about the need for the health service to be concerned with less severe disorders, such as those which are turned up by surveys in general practice and community settings. That there should be this lack of consensus is surprising, when one considers that population surveys of depression were designed to identify individuals with disorders comparable to those seen by clinicians in outpatient or inpatient settings, in the hope that this would lead to clues about the aetiology, treatment, and prevention of these disorders. As it turns out, these studies have revealed a considerable level of untreated morbidity, and no clear demarcation between disease and distress has emerged. Faced with a demand which easily outstrips any attempt at provision, and having no simple means of identifying which individuals might rightly be considered 'diseased' — short of utilising the criteria of attendance at a treatment setting — the understandable, if lamentable reaction of some health providers has been to deny that they should play any role in designing or administering preventive programmes. But this is too easy a solution. At least a third of valuable psychiatric outpatient resources are committed to the continuing care of patients with these disorders, and effective prevention might go a long way towards easing the burden of congested outpatient services.

This provides the health services with a dilemma: to attempt preventive interventions, knowing that these will necessitate taking on far greater service commitments than hitherto, or finding ways to justify doing nothing at all, and accepting the necessity of providing treatment and care for potentially preventable disorders. There are, of course, solutions which do not mean that health care providers simply wash their hands of any commitment by conveniently redefining the limits of disease; rather, since it is clear that existing resources are inadequate to meet the demand, innovative ways of tackling the problem will have to be developed. Both Caplan (1964) and Gottlieb (1983), considering this dilemma, cast the future role of psychiatrists in prevention not as frontline care givers, but as innovators of novel services, as advocates for their introduction, and as expert consultants and advisers to other workers who would carry out the preventive service.

The task of clinical innovation is perhaps the most exciting and problematic of these roles. Not only do carefully designed experimental interventions need to be set up, but the most successful of these have to be shepherded into a form more akin to rough-and-ready everyday clinical practice. Such translation requires considerable skill, time, and effort. The clinical innovator needs to convince others of the worth of the undertaking; he/she has to tackle the difficult tasks of planning, designing, and implementing the programme. The new service will have to compete with existing service demands for financial and staffing resources, staff have to be trained initially and supervised subsequently, and finally, provision for the evaluation of the efficacy of the service may have to be built in from the outset and managed throughout. At each step along the way, the project leader has to maintain enthusiasm and convey its appropriateness to others who may be less convinced. Throughout the early years of the new service, unanticipated problems will continue to emerge. Small wonder then that such innovations are the exceptions and that for prevention, there remains more talk than practice.

Some of the rhetoric on the subject emphasises an even wider role for the clinician, as advocate of prevention; there are some local social policy issues on which it might be argued that mental health professionals are particularly qualified to comment. For instance, research discussed above has implications for: support programmes for children who have been cared for by local authorities, at the age at which they must establish independent lives for themselves in the community; the management of residential homes for the elderly; and for maintaining in the community people treated for major psychiatric illnesses. There are undoubtedly other practical social implications of psychiatric research.

One of the ways forward is likely to include greater collaboration between psychiatrists and other health care professionals, and the provision of training and supervision for both professional and non-professional workers in the community.

The pursuit of preventive aspirations will inevitably depend on approaches which make the minimum use of highly specialised and expensive resources. Sarason (1972) describes examples where the occasional single doctor, nurse, psychologist, or social worker has responded to the acute absences of other specialists in their hospital or clinic with refreshing and effective, if unco-ordinated solutions. They have taken advantage of a surprisingly heterogeneous pool of local people and employees at the institution to transform the setting to one in which numerous active sub-professionals participate, requiring only modest supervision and a small number of hours of additional training. As this author makes clear, one of the fundamental misassumptions of health service planning is that only certain kinds and quantities of specialists can solve clinical problems — an assumption which often effectively renders the problem insoluble, since the demand for help always outstrips the efforts to match it with numbers of highly qualified personnel.

It has long been recognised, of course, that clinical skills can be shared with other members of multidiciplinary teams, as a cost-effective means of providing more broadly based assessment and treatment facilities. Both nurses and social work members of multidiciplinary teams can accurately assess and manage large numbers of clients across a considerable range of psychiatric disorder. To a large extent, preventive interventions suggested by current research involve adapting techniques which are already widely used by these workers in treatment settings — marital and family counselling, reversing defective coping behaviour, and strengthening social role performances. But collaboration in providing preventive services should also be extended to include non-professional colleagues, volunteers, and family support networks.

Community voluntary preventive initiatives may need a range of support. Many workers will need to turn to professionals for advice and information. Some may require a simple consultative service when faced with disorders with which they feel out of their depth, while others may seek training or personal supervision, and families trying to help a relative with a history of disorder to avoid further relapses need advice and support. Clinicians cannot afford to distance themselves from these efforts: in their role as consultants, they may be able to ensure that interventions follow a theoretical rationale, discourage inappropriate methods, and offer a background referral service for clients whose disorders are clearly beyond the management of project leaders. As trainers, they may be able to help volunteers to support very distressed and vulnerable people in the community, and encourage project managers to collect information which would enable the effectiveness of these innovations to be evaluated. None of these activities need seriously distract the clinician from the core activity of managing illness, and all might well go a long way towards assisting the development of effective preventive services.

REFERENCES

Bagley C 1968 The evaluation of a suicide prevention scheme by an ecological method. Social Science & Medicine 2: 1-14

Barraclough B, Bunch J, Nelson B, Sainsbury P 1974 A hundred cases of suicide: critical aspects. British Journal of Psychiatry 125: 335-373

Barrowclough C, Tarrier N 1984 'Psychosocial' interventions with families and their effects on the course of schizophrenia: a review. Psychological Medicine 14: 629-642

Bennett D, Morris I 1983 Support and rehabilitation. In: Watts F N, Bennett D H (eds) Theory and practice of psychiatric rehabilitation. Wiley, London

Bifulco A, Brown G W, Harris T O 1987 Childhood loss of parent, lack of adequate parental care and adult depression: a replication. Journal of Affective Disorders 12: 115-118

Boulton M G 1983 On being a mother: a study of women with pre-school children. Tavistock, London

Bouras N, Tufnell G 1983 Mental health advice centre: the crisis intervention team.

Lewisham and North Southwark Health Authority. Research Report No 2

Bowlby J 1951 Maternal care and mental health. World Health Organisation, Geneva

Bridge T P 1977 Suicide prevention centres — ecological study of effectiveness. Journal of Nervous Mental Diseases 164: 18-24

Bronfenbrenner U 1975 Is early intervention effective? In: Guttentag M, Strvening E L (eds) Handbook of evaluative research. Sage, Beverley Hills Calif

Brown G W, Harris T O 1978 Social origins of depression. Tavistock, London

Brown G W, Monck E M, Carstairs G M, Wing J K 1962 Influence of family life on the course of schizophrenic illness. British Journal of Preventive & Social Medicine 16: 55-68

Brown G W, Andrews B, Harris T, Adler Z, Bridge L 1986 Social support, self-esteem and depression. Psychological Medicine 16: 813-831

Caplan G 1964 Principles of preventive psychiatry. Basic Books, New York

Child Development Programme 1984 Booklet prepared and published by the Child Development Project. University of Bristol, Bristol

Chowdhury N, Hicks R C, Kreitman N 1973 Evaluation of an aftercare service for parasuicide ('attempted suicide') patients. Social Psychiatry 8: 67-81

Cobb S 1976 Social support as a moderator of life stress. Psychosomatic Medicine 38: 300-314

Craig T K J, Brown G W 1984 Life Events meaning and physical illness: a review. In: Steptoe A, Matthews A (eds) Health care and human behaviour. Academic Press, London

Depue R A 1979 The psychobiology of the depressive disorders. Implications for the effect of stress. Academic Press, New York

Diggory J C 1976 United States suicide rates, 1968-1983 In: Shneidman E S (ed) Suicidology. Grune and Stratton, New York

Dohrenwend B S, Dohrenwend B P (eds) 1974 Stressful life events: their nature and effects. Wiley, New York

Douglas J W B 1975 Early hospital admissions and later disturbances of behaviour and learning. Developmental Medical Childhood Neurology 17: 456-480

Emery A E H 1978 Elements of medical genetics. Churchill Livingstone Edinburgh

Epstein 1983 Natural healing processes of the Mind. In: Meichenbaum D, Jaremko M (eds) Stress reduction and prevention. Plenum Press, New York

Falloon I R H, Boyd J L, McGill C W, Razani J, Moss H, Citerman N 1982 Family management in the prevention of exacerbations of schizophrenia. New England Journal of Medicine 306: 1437-1440

Ferguson B F 1979 Preparing young children for hospitalisation: a comparison of 2 methods. Pediatrics 64: 656-664

Ferguson-Smith M A 1983 Prenatal chromosome analysis and its impact on the birth incidence of chromosome disorders. British Medical Bulletin 39: 355-364

Freeman H L 1985 Housing. In: Freeman H L (ed) Mental health & the environment. Churchill-Livingstone, London: pp 197-225

Gibbons J S, Butler J, Unwin P, Gibbons J L 1978 Evaluation of a social work service for self-poisoning patients. British Journal of Psychiatry 133: 111-118

Gottesman I I, Shields J 1982 Schizophrenia: the epigenetic puzzle. Cambridge University Press, Cambridge

Gottlieb B H 1983 Social support strategies: guidelines for mental health practice. Sage, Beverley Hills

Grosskurth 1984 From care to nowhere. Roof, Shelter's Housing Magazine July/August 11-14

Harris T O, Brown G W, Bifulco A 1986 Loss of parent in childhood and adult psychiatric disorder: the role of lack of adequate parental care. Psychological Medicine 16: 641-659

Harris T O, Brown G W, Bifulco A 1987 Loss of parent in childhood and adult psychiatric disorder: the role of social class position and premarital pregnancies. Psychological Medicine 17: 163-183

Henderson D, Byrne D G, Duncan-Jones P, Scott R, Adcock S 1980 Social relationships, adversity and neuroses: a study of associations in a general population sample. British Journal of Psychiatry 136: 574-583

Hetherington E M 1979 Divorce: a child's perspective. American Psychologist 34: 851-858

Hetherington E M, Cox M, Cox R 1982 Effect of divorce on parents and children. In: Lamb M (ed) Non traditional families. Lawrence Erlbaum, Hillsdale, New Jersey

House J S 1981 Work stress and social support. Addison-Wesley, Reading, Massachusetts

Janis I L 1958 Psychological stress: psychoanalytic and behavioural studies of surgical patients. Wiley, New York

Jennings C, Barrowclough B M, Moss J R 1978 Have the Samaritans lowered the suicide rate? A controlled study. Psychological Medicine 8: 413-422

Johnson J E 1984 Psychological interventions and coping with surgery. In: Baum A, Taylor S E, Singeg J E (eds) Handbook of psychology and health volume IV. Lawrence, Erlbaum New Jersey

Kasl S V 1984 Chronic life stress and health. In: Steptoe A, Matthews A (eds) Health care and human behaviour. Academic Press, London

Kreitman N 1976 The coal gas story. British Journal of Preventative & Social Medicine 30: 86-93

Lancet 1984 Towards better general practice. Lancet ii: 1436-1437

Leff J P, Vaughan C E 1980 The influence of life events and relatives expressed emotion in schizophrenia and depressive neurosis. British Journal of Psychiatry 136: 146-153

Leff J, Kuipers L, Berkowitz R, Eberlein-Vries R, Sturgeon D 1982 A controlled trial of social intervention in the families of schizophrenic patients. British Journal of Psychiatry 141: 121-134

Leff J, Kuipers L, Berkowitz R, Sturgeon D 1985 A controlled trial of social intervention in the families of schizophrenia patients: two year follow-up. British Journal of Psychiatry 146: 594-600

Leighton A 1982 Caring for mentally ill people: psychological and social barriers in a historical context. Cambridge University Press, Cambridge

Low A A, Farmer R D T, Jones D R, Rhode J R 1981 Suicide in England and Wales: an analysis of 100 years 1876-1975. Psychological Medicine 11: 359-368

Magnusson D 1983 Implications of an interactional paradigm for research on human development. Reports from the Department of Psychology, University of Stockholm Supplement 59

Maguire P, Tait A, Brooke M, Thomas C, Sellwood R 1980 The effect of counselling on the psychiatric morbidity associated with mastectomy. British Medical Journal 281: 1454-1456

Maguire P, Brooke M, Tait A, Thomas C, Sellwood R 1983 The effect of counselling on physical disability and social recovery after mastectomy. Clinical Oncology 9: 314-319

Mednick S A, Schulsinger F, Venables P H 1981 A fifteen year follow-up of children with schizophrenic mothers. In: Mednick S A, Baert A W, Bachmann B P (eds) Prospective longitudinal research: an empirical basis for the primary prevention of psychosocial disorders. Oxford University Press on behalf of WHO

Meichenbaum D 1977 Cognitive behaviour modification: an integrative approach. Plenum Press, New York

Meichenbaum D, Jaremko M (eds) 1983 Stress reduction and prevention. Plenum Press, New York

Miller H L, Coombs D W, Leper J D, Marton S N 1984 An analysis of the effects of suicide prevention facilities on suicide rates in the United States. American Journal of Public Health 74: 340-343

Mills M, Puckering C, Pound A, Cox A D 1984 What is it about depressed mothers that influences their children's functioning? In: Stevenson J E (ed) Book supplement to Journal of Child Psychology and Psychiatry No 4

Newton J 1988 Preventing mental illness. Routledge, London

O'Connor P, Brown G W 1984 Supportive relationship: fact or fancy? Journal of Social & Personal Relationships 1: 159-175

Parkes C M 1975 Unexpected and untimely bereavement: a statistical study of young Boston widows and widowers. In: Schoenberg B, Gerber I, Wiener A, Kutscher A H, Peretz D, Carr A C (eds) Bereavement: its psychosocial aspects. Columbia University Press, New York

Parkes C M 1980 Bereavement counselling: does it work? British Medical Journal 281: 3-6

Parkes C M 1981 Evaluation of a bereavement service. Journal of Preventative Psychiatry 2: 179-188

Paykel E S 1978 Contribution of life events to the causation of psychiatric illness. Psychological Medicine 8: 245-253

Pearlin L I, Schooler C 1978 The structure of coping. Journal of Health & Social Behaviour 19: 2-21

Pound A, Mills M 1985 A pilot evaluation of 'Newpin': a home visiting and befriending scheme in South London. The Association of Child Psychology and Psychiatry Newsletter October 1985

Pound A, Mills M, Cox T 1985 A pilot evaluation of 'Newpin': a home visiting and befriending scheme in South London. (Manuscript unpublished)

Quinton D, Rutter M 1984a Family pathology and child psychiatric disorder: a four-year prospective study. In: Nicol R (ed) Longitudinal studies in child psychology and psychiatry: practical lessons from research experience. Wiley, Chichester

Quinton D, Rutter M 1984b Parents with children in care. II. Intergenerational continuities. Journal of Child Psychology & Psychiatry 25: 231-250

Raphael B 1977 Preventive intervention with the recently bereaved. Archives of General Psychiatry 34: 1450-1454

Richman N, Stevenson J, Graham P 1982 Preschool to school: a behavioural study. Academic Press, London

Robins E 1981 The final months. A study of the lives of 134 persons who committed suicide. Oxford University Press, Oxford

Robins L N 1966 Deviant children grown up. William and Wilkins, Baltimore

Rodin J, Langer E 1977 Long-term effects of a control relevant intervention with the institutionalised aged. Journal of Personal & Social Psychology 35: 897-902

Rodin J 1983 Behavioural medicine: beneficial effects of self-control training in aging. International Review of Applied Psychology 32: 153-181

Royal College of General Practitioners 1972 The future general practitioner: learning and teaching. Report of a working party

Rutter M 1972 Maternal deprivation reassessed. Penguin, Harmondsworth

Rutter M 1979 Protective factors in children's responses to stress and disadvantage. In: Kent M W, Rolf J E (eds) Primary prevention of psychopathology. Social competence in children. University Press, New England

Rutter M L 1985 Resilience in the face of adversity: protective factors and resistance to psychiatric disorder. British Journal of Psychiatry 147: 578-611

Rutter M L, Cox A, Tupling C, Berger M, Yule W 1975 Attainment and adjustment in two geographical areas. The prevalence of psychiatric disorder. British Journal of Psychiatry 126: 493-509

Rutter M L, Quinton D, Liddle C 1983 Parenting in two generations: looking backwards and looking forwards. In: Madge N (ed) Families at risk. Heinemann, London: pp 98-111

Sampson O C 1980 Child guidance: its history, provenance and future. British Psychological Society, London

Sarason S B 1972 The creation of settings and the future societies. Jossey-Bass, San Francisco

Silver R L, Wortman C B 1980 Coping with undesirable life events. In: Garber J, Seligman M E P (eds) 'Human helplessness' : theory and applications. Academic Press, New York

Smith R 1986 Occupationless health: what can be done? Responding to unemployment and health. British Medical Journal 292: 263-265

Stene J, Mikkelsen M 1984 Downs syndrome and other chromosome disorders. In: Wald N J (ed) Antenatal and neonatal screening. Oxford University Press, Oxford: 74-105

Strauss J S, Carpenter D T 1981 Schizophrenia. Plenum Press, New York

Test M, Stein L 1978 Training in community living: research design and results. In: Stein L, Test M (eds) Alternatives to mental hospital treatment. Plenum Press, New York

Van der Eyken W 1982 Homestart: a four year evaluation. Homestart Consultancy, Leicester

Wolfer J A, Visintainer M A 1979 Prehospital psychological preparation for tonsillectomy patients: effects on children's and parents' adjustment. Pediatrics 64: 646-655

World Health Organisation 1984 Health promotion: a discussion document on the concept and principles. WHO regional office for Europe, Copenhagen

18. Psychiatric emergency and crisis intervention services

H.Katschnig   J.Cooper

INTRODUCTION

This chapter is largely based on the experiences of the authors while they were conducting an extensive study in European countries of services dealing with psychiatric emergencies and crisis intervention on behalf of the European office of the World Health Organisation (WHO) (Cooper 1979, Katschnig et al 1987). Our purpose is to describe and review the state of development of psychiatric emergency and crisis intervention services in various countries in the European region. The relationship between these two parts of the psychiatric and social services is continually changing as each component develops, and is easily seen to be very different between countries. Such variations depend very largely upon the development and structure of these services in different parts of Europe, but an increase in the demand for such services is common to many, and this is paralleled by a similar increasing demand in the USA (Gerson & Bassuk 1980, Kaskey & Ianzito 1984).

This chapter first gives a brief historical and theoretical introduction, before going on to develop a simple and practical classification of such services. The 34 centres described in the two parts of the WHO study were not intended to constitute a representative selection of European facilities of these types, and many other centres are in existence which were not visited; nevertheless, the sample is sufficient to enable some practical conclusions to be drawn.

Finally, a number of issues of current and future importance are selected for discussion.

The justification for including a discussion of emergency and crisis intervention services under the heading of 'Strategies' is that every type of community psychiatric service needs to have policies, practices, and resources which allow its personnel to cope with at least some aspects of the emergencies and crises occurring in the population served. This becomes clear during the discussion below of specialised versus comprehensive services. However, many of the issues dealt with here could equally well be included under the heading 'Services'.

HISTORICAL AND CONCEPTUAL ISSUES

The origins of emergency psychiatric services

Most European countries had well developed psychiatric institutions during the period between the two World Wars, but these large mental hospitals had comparatively few organisational and functional links with other medical and social agencies. Before the development of special services dealing only with mental health emergencies, patients in urgent need of psychiatric care were first dealt with by whatever service happened to be available for other medical, social, or civil emergencies. General hospital casualty departments ('emergency rooms'), acute medical admission wards, general practitioners, as well as police and ambulance services were all used as a first contact point, before the patient was transferred to the often geographically distant psychiatric unit or large institution. The system of 'observation wards' established in a number of general hospitals in England before the inception of the National Health Service was a development of this 'agency' concept; patients were collected usually in one ward of about 25–30 beds, with minimal facilities and attached specialist staff. The original concept was to provide a safe, convenient, and cheap setting to allow a full examination, but only sufficient space and resources for a stay of a few days, within which time a decision is to be made about disposal of the patient. Most were sent on to the mental hospital dealing with the area in which the patient lived, some were admitted to medical or surgical wards, and a few were kept in the observation ward itself for brief periods of treatment before being allowed home. Similar in function to these British units was the 'observation hospital' in Barcelona — Preventorio Municipal de Psiquitria; this was founded in 1926, and functioned for many years as a centre for psychiatric 'triage' (Katschnig & Konieczna 1986).

However, during the last 20 to 30 years, policies have been developed, particularly in the UK, which provide means of carrying out urgent psychiatric assessments at or near the patient's home, but which specify that admission units should be small and situated in district general hospitals or elsewhere within the local community. These developments depend upon, and also to some extent determine, the threshold of psychiatric contact. When the principal psychiatric treatment facilities are large institutions, often remote and usually with a poor public image, this threshold will be high, but as institutions improve and additional and alternative psychiatric services are provided, both public and professional attitudes change. The psychiatric contact threshold then falls, as does the threshold for inpatient admission.

In many respects, this type of change involves a necessary separation of the psychiatric from the medical services, but there are good reasons for ensuring that the separation does not become complete. A skilled physical examination will always be an essential part of the assessment of psychiatric emergencies, particularly for new contacts (Eastwood et al 1970). Slaby (1981), for instance, has listed 39 medical conditions which can give rise to anxiety states which are superficially undistinguishable from those of purely psychological origin.

Three themes

In the decade since the second World War, it is possible to identify at least three themes or principles that have been important in the development of the general aim of depending less upon large psychiatric institutions, and in the progressive move towards local, easily available, and humanely organised psychiatric services. These themes are:

a. Community psychiatry and the prevention whenever possible of admission to psychiatric hospitals or units.

b. The provision of special 'suicide prevention' services.

c. The development of crisis intervention theory.

The professional activity and service developments that have appeared in many countries on the basis of these themes often seem to have the characteristics of 'movements', whose proponents develop theories and programmes of action stemming from a basic ideology, rather than being based upon systematic planning and data analysis. But whatever these origins and motive forces, there is no doubt about the importance and popularity of these themes amongst the diverse professional groups on whom the psychiatric emergency and crisis intervention services depend.

Community psychiatry and the prevention of admission to mental hospitals

In addition to bringing psychiatric inpatients back into their community, one of the declared aims of the community psychiatric movement is the prevention of admission to mental hospitals. It is often forgotten that the arguments put forward in favour of avoiding psychiatric hospitalisation relate not only to the detrimental effects of institutionalisation (Wing & Brown 1970) and to the social stigma attached to admission itself, but also include economic factors. Historically, the first attempt to reduce psychiatric hospital admission had a mainly financial motivation; in the 1930s, the municipality of Amsterdam asked Querido (1968) to establish a mobile emergency service (alongside several components of rehabilitative service), in order to reduce the heavy costs of a psychiatric inpatient treatment (Gersons 1985).

The US Community Mental Health Centers Act of 1963 offered federal funds for establishing these centres only on condition that a 24-hour, 7 days-a-week emergency service was amongst those provided. These requirements may well have helped to discourage state hospital admissions in the USA, but in Italy, admission to a mental hospital was even forbidden by law in 1978. However, this was not accompanied by any parallel legislation that would make the provision of alternative treatment facilities obligatory.

The extent to which psychiatric hospitalisation can be justifiably avoided, or at least shortened, is still not clear today. There is, however, no doubt that much can be achieved in those cases where admission as an emergency to a psychiatric hospital is chosen simply because of lack of alternative treatment facilities, if such alternatives are developed.

Langsley & Kaplan (1968) demonstrated that a special ambulatory family crisis intervention programme offered to severely ill psychiatric patients was equally as successful as inpatient treatment, while Hirsch et al (1979) and Kennedy & Hird (1980) showed that short-term hospital admission and 'normal' duration of stay were equally effective in terms of outcome. These are valuable research studies, but there is no guarantee that their findings can be generalised to more routine service settings; they were all special projects of limited duration, during which the staff had unusually high levels of interest and motivation.

The use of day hospitals as an alternative to admission as an inpatient for many cases of crisis or emergency is appealing, but it is not yet very widespread and has only recently been subject to detailed studies. Some reports on acute day hospital care in the UK suggest that favourable levels of cost-effectiveness can be achieved with safety, and this type of service development shows great promise (Dick et al 1985). In contrast, most of the specifically labelled 'crisis intervention' wards, as they exist now in many European countries, probably do not contribute much to the general prevention of admissions to psychiatric hospitals, since they are very selective in their admission policies. Notable exceptions to this tendency are the crisis units at the Karolinska Hospital and the Nacka Project, both in Stockholm (Cooper 1979).

One of the paradoxes of an energetic community psychiatric programme is that it may result in an overall increase, rather than a decrease in admissions. This is because of a rise in the number of readmissions of recently discharged patients. The reduction in the total number of occupied psychiatric beds, which can now be observed around the world, is due mainly to reduced length of stay, and not to a reduction in the number of admissions.

The suicide prevention movement

The motive force behind community psychiatry has come mainly from psychiatrists and other mental health professionals, whereas the suicide prevention movement originated largely in the activities of lay workers, often with affiliations to religious organisations. As far back as the beginning of this century, Warren, a clergyman in New York, established a telephone 'hotline' for suicidal persons — the National Save A Life League (Allen 1984). In England, Varah, also a clergyman, founded the Samaritans in 1953 (Varah 1973); this was followed by many similar telephone services in other countries, mainly run by volunteers and frequently organised by the Churches. In 1958, the first American 'Suicide Prevention Centre' was opened in Los Angeles (Farberow & Schneidman 1961), and many others followed (MacGee 1968). The International Association for Suicide Prevention (IASP) was founded in 1960.

By 1970 in the United States of America, some 120 suicide prevention centres existed. However, as Kiev (1970) pointed out, many of these were not providing services themselves but simply re-directed callers by telephone to other services. Kiev suggested that it might have been preferable for the staff of these centres to go in search of individuals at risk, or to set up social and self-help groups, in order to minimise the social isolation of their clients.

The suicide prevention movement now appears to have lost its momentum, and has largely been absorbed into the broader crisis intervention movement. This is partly because the development of community psychiatry has taken over some of its functions, and partly because suicide rates have not fallen (contrary to the hopes and predictions of the prevention enthusiasts).

Thus, the term 'suicide prevention centre', which was popular 10 years ago, is now often replaced by 'crisis intervention centre'. Similarly, the International Association for Suicide Prevention now gives its main biannual conference the title of 'Suicide prevention and crisis intervention', and publishes a journal called simply, CRISIS. Nevertheless, the good work and excellent intentions of the suicide prevention movement should not be forgotten. These resulted in the setting up of services, mainly relying upon telephone hotlines, in many parts of the world. Even if they no longer claim to be able to reduce the suicide rate, they offer valuable help to the distressed and the bereaved.

The development of crisis theory

The contemporary increasing demand for all forms of medical care (Eisenberg 1977) is presumably the result of higher expectations of both physical and mental comfort, which are themselves in turn part of the steady increase in general material standards of life over the last 100 years or so. Demands for psychiatric emergency and crisis services must therefore be seen as only one element in the major social and psychological changes that are part of the 'modern way of life'.

Study of both the immediate and after effects of civilian disasters played a large part in the early development of crisis theory (Lindemann 1944), but military psychiatry also contributed (Tyhurst 1958, Talbott

1969). Both Lindemann and Tyhurst postulated a sequence of symptoms and behaviour that followed acute grief or other severe stress; Tyhurst in particular, emphasised the temporary and changing nature of the stages in the sequence, and suggested the term 'transitional states' to indicate this. In the United States in the 1960s, many others took up these ideas, and there gradually emerged a rather loosely organised set of ideas which became known as 'crisis theory' (Caplan 1961, 1964, Jacobson 1974, 1980). Caplan emphasised that the concept of crisis referred to the brief episode of psychological 'disequilibrium' resulting from being confronted with problems which the person can neither solve nor avoid; the crisis is the state of emotional reaction, not the external problems or events.

Crises fall naturally into two major divisions — one due to unexpected traumatic events, and the other to more predictable life changes such as puberty, marriage, childbirth, and the menopause. Caplan laid great stress on the potentially constructive aspects of professional intervention at a time of crisis, and many of his publications carry a strong implication that the availability of a crisis service can prevent the occurrence of mental illness, both immediately and in the future. Erickson (1959) was responsible for bringing the life-change type of crisis into prominence, and introduced a psychoanalytical dimension with his equally optimistic interpretation of the uses of crisis theory in overcoming 'developmental crises' and assisting in the growth of the personality. However, neither the broadening of the concept of crisis intervention nor these optimistic implications have been justified by subsequent events.

The crisis theory to which these diverse authors contributed is summarised in Figure 18.1.

The periods of impact and recoil are comparatively brief — a few hours and around 12–24 hours respectively. The period of recoil is crucial in this theory, since it is at this time that the patient is in the most malleable state; adaptation rather than failure to adapt may be achieved, it is claimed, if a constructive professional intervention can be interpolated during this phase.

Adoption of this theory led to some important characteristics of crisis practice, which stand in contrast to the practice of analytically orientated psychotherapy. The therapist is much more active in crisis practice than in psychotherapy, and the problems of waiting lists and payment for services that are common with psychotherapy do not intrude into the therapeutic relationship. Indeed, the concepts of transference and counter-transference — so central in most types of psychotherapy — are not prominent, if present at all, in the training and discussions of crisis therapists. Strong relationships, particularly in the form of dependence, must be positively avoided, so that the period of contact with the patient can be brief; the crisis worker must always be available to take on another patient before the crucial but brief period of recoil is past. However, the contrast with psychotherapy is not a complete one, since the emphasis on

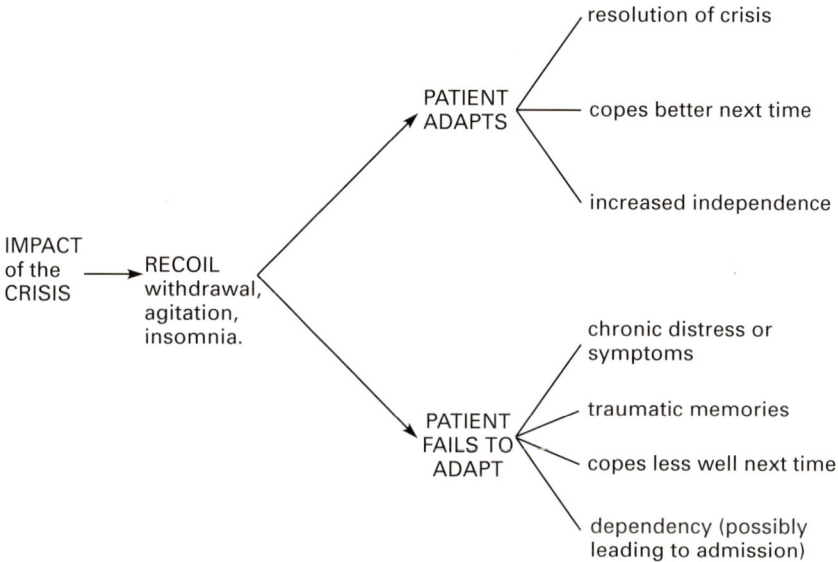

Fig. 18.1   Theoretical stages of crisis

the here and now which is inescapable in crisis intervention work is also common to some forms of brief psychotherapy and family therapy (Malan 1963, Davanloo 1980, Umana et al 1980, Bellak & Siegel 1983).

Crisis intervention theory, as outlined above, is an attractive sequence of concepts, which implies a set of actions (crisis intervention), expected to have a constructive and optimistic outcome; ideas of prevention and personal growth through successful coping with problems abound in the crisis literature. The theory leads potential crisis workers to expect that in such a centre, substantial numbers of patients will be encountered who are passing through identifiable crises of various types, and with whom constructive solutions to these problems can be jointly identified and achieved.

In later sections, it will be necessary to discuss the extent to which crisis theory and the derived expectations about crisis intervention are realistic; it has been suggested that the theory is idealised rather than practically useful, and that patients new to the service with a good prognosis for the crisis constitute only a minority of those who use such services in real life (Cooper 1979).

The unplanned consequences of deinstitutionalisation

The three movements just discussed (community psychiatry, suicide prevention, and crisis intervention) have probably had less effect on psychiatric hospitals and services than was originally expected, but even these limited effects have at least been of benefit to the patients and clients. In contrast, the deinstitutionalisation movement that has been so energetically pursued recently in some countries has had some unplanned and harmful effects on both patients and services. The increased rate of discharge of long-stay patients and shortening of length of stay in acute admission units, which have jointly been responsible to a large extent for the falling numbers of psychiatric beds, started to have their effect about 30 years ago, though it was at first a fairly gentle change. Since the 1950s, bed numbers have fallen steadily in most European countries, but in some the rate has accelerated since the late 1970s, as draconian administrative measures have reinforced the changes in medical attitudes and the use of psychotropic drugs that were the original impetus. In the USA, for instance, the number of psychiatric inpatient beds fell from 559 000 in 1955 to 138 000 in 1980 (Gudeman & Shore 1984) — a fall of 75%, and in England and Wales from 230 464 in 1959 to 158 960 in 1979 — a fall of 30% (HMSO 1981).

Where, as in the USA, this discharge was not paralleled by the development of reasonably adequate community services, the consequence has been an increasing number of poorly supported chronic psychiatric patients in the community who are vulnerable to many types of social, psychiatric, and medical problems. They then naturally turn to, or are brought to the emergency services. In the USA, this has been especially observed in the emergency rooms of the general hospitals, where there has been a steady increase in attendance of patients with psychiatric problems over the years, paralleling the reduction of the psychiatric hospital population (Gerson & Bassuk 1980). For instance, Kaskey & Ianzito (1984) observed, in a catchment area of 500 000 inhabitants in Massachusetts, an increase in referral to the emergency room of a general hospital from 100 in 1972 to 2600 in 1982, while at the same time, the psychiatric hospital responsible for this catchment area was reduced in size from 2500 to 250 inpatients.

Bristol et al (1981) noted, over a 17-year period, an increase in the proportion of emergency room attenders who belonged to the lower social group; social isolation was often an obvious contributor to the attendance. However, in the USA, efforts are now being made to enlarge the holding units, improve the psychiatric staffing levels of emergency rooms, and even create special emergency psychiatric treatment units attached to them.

In the UK, this development is somewhat less marked, partly because, despite many deficiencies, community psychiatric services are better developed than in America and partly because deinstitutionalisation has occurred at a slower speed. In continental Europe, where deinstitutionalisation started later than in these two countries, it has only recently become possible to detect the use of psychiatric emergency services by deinstitutionalised psychiatric patients, but a continued increase of this kind seems very likely (Katschnig et al 1986).

TYPES OF SERVICES

In Europe, including the UK, a variety of institutional settings provide crisis intervention and psychiatric emergency services: the very existence of such a variety presumably reflects a considerable degree of uncertainty as to which organisational structures are the most appropriate for each type of demand for help. The picture is complicated further by a trend away from separate and specialised emergency and crisis intervention units towards comprehensive sectorised psychiatric services which provide emergency and crisis intervention services as an integrated part of the whole service.

In the USA, the development of separate extra-mural services for preventive psychiatry and for crisis intervention (and for the even less clearly specified 'community psychiatry') has a particularly long history compared with other countries. For instance, by the early 1960s, publications had appeared there on the psychiatric patients presenting in the emergency rooms of general hospitals (Coleman & Errera 1963, Atkins 1967). In Europe, however, in spite of a few notable individual exceptions, such as Amsterdam in the 1930s (Querido 1968), and Vienna in the late 1940s (Ringel 1953), most of the developments of specified emergency crisis intervention services have taken place since 1970 (Brandon 1970, Mindham et al 1973, Hafner 1974, Cooper 1979, Lim 1983, Katschnig et al 1988).

A major problem in this field of interest is the extent to which the two closely related concepts of crisis intervention and emergency psychiaric treatment can or should be separated. Whilst it is true that those who set up and provide such services see these two elements as serving different purposes and different persons, it is equally true that the individuals in psychological distress or needing acute psychiatric help (and also those referring them) are not usually so aware of such clear professional distinctions. In practice, the result is that both types of services have to cope with a mixture of persons, showing a wide variety of acute psychological distress or psychiatric illness. For this reason, the discussion of services that follows below is not organised by type of service, but by type of contact, i.e. by how contact is made with the helping agency and where the help is provided. Of the specialised crisis emergency psychiatric services, telephone 'hotlines' are discussed first, followed by ambulatory and mobile services which involve face-to-face contact, and then services with overnight-stay facilities. These different components of service are often available individually, but it is, of course, not uncommon to find that several components are provided by the same organisation. The final section deals with the crisis and emergency service component of general and comprehensive medical emergency services.

SPECIALISED SERVICES

Telephone hotlines (with no initial face-to-face contact)

Telephone hotlines have their origin in the suicide prevention movement, although it is now clear that their actual contribution to suicide prevention is very small. Nevertheless, they have an important comforting and befriending function for the distressed, in providing an easily made contact with someone who, while giving a sympathetic ear, nevertheless stays at a safe distance. The caller can remain anonymous and can break off the contact whenever he wishes. It is probably these qualities, together with the ease of access, that have been responsible for the steadily increasing popularity and use of telephone hotlines. They are also relatively cheap to run, since in most instances they are operated by voluntary helpers, rarely using paid employees. The most widely employed interviewing technique used by hotline workers is the client-centred approach developed by Rogers & Dymond (1954).

The most frequent problems presented by those who use telephone hotlines are partner conflicts or losses and loneliness; persons with obvious psychiatric illness are rarely encountered, and individuals who attempt suicide are not common. The Samaritans, originating in the UK, are a well known example of such a service, which in addition offers direct personal contact after the telephone call (Varah 1973). A number of university campuses, both in the UK and in continental Europe, also possess special 24-hour telephone hotlines specifically for the students. In continental Europe, most telephone services are directly or indirectly run by religious bodies or have at least been founded by them (Telefonseelsorge). They try to give themselves a non-psychiatric image by using names such as Telefono amico (Telephone Friend) in Italy, SOS amitie (SOS friendship) in France, and Die dargebotene Hand (The Offered hand) in Switzerland. In 1960, a number of telephone hotline organisations brought themselves together into the International Federation of Telephone Emergency Services (IFOTES).

Ambulatory (walk-in) and mobile (outreach) services with face-to-face contact

Once a face-to-face contact is made between a client and a helper — either on the premises or the helping institution in the case of ambulatory services, or in the community in the case of mobile services — it is difficult for the client to keep his anonymity. This means that the threshold for making use of such services is much higher than for telephone hotlines. From the point of view of the helper, once a face-to-face contact has been made with a client, the ethical (and possibly legal) responsibilities increase considerably. However, a face-to-face contact makes it more likely that the helper will be able to obtain adequate information and therefore be able to make more rational decisions about possible intervention. One of the most common major problems faced by workers in both ambulatory and mobile services is whether to recommend admission to a psychiatric unit, or whether to risk leaving the distressed client in his environment. In this context, the frequent lack of easy access to short-stay, non-institutional admission facilities for the purposes of a less hurried assessment and a general process of 'gaining time' is one of the most frustrating characteristics of these types of services.

Some other general differences between these two types of emergency service are worth mentioning, since they are not necessarily obvious to those not directly concerned. Time and pressure on the helpers in walk-in and outpatient clinics may be felt as a considerable burden, since groups or queues of waiting clients may be all too obvious. In contrast, although the individual problems of clients may be just as urgent in telephone or outreach services, the time pressure on the helper is far less obvious; this is because only one visit or telephone call can be dealt with at a time, and other clients who are waiting are not exerting pressure simply because of their physical presence. A further difference is derived from the identity of who it is that makes contact with the service. By their nature, walk-in services are usually contacted by the distressed person, even if only as a result of pressure from relatives. There is a different quality about the contacts made with mobile outreach services, which are much more frequently contacted by persons other than the distressed client. For instance, in the mobile service of the city of Zurich, only 15% of all requests for help come from the clients themselves; the large majority of calls come from relatives or other persons or agencies who are unable to cope with a person in distress.

Specific points about ambulatory (walk-in) services

Ambulatory crisis intervention services tend to leave out the word 'psychiatric' from their title, in order to facilitate their psychological image (and therefore their acceptability) to clients in distress. Names like 'crisis intervention centre' or 'walk-in clinic' are examples of this. Others, like the Centre Psychiatrique d'Orientation et d'Accueil (CPOA) (Psychiatric Assessment and Reception Centre) in Paris include the word 'psychiatric', but diluted by several others. Some of these ambulatory services prefer to select clients with psychosocial crises, but others like the CPOA in Paris, declare themselves open to all types of emergencies, including organic psychiatric conditions. The former selective types are more frequently operated by psychologists and social workers rather than by doctors and nurses, while the latter, non-selective types are often manned exclusively by psychiatrists and nursing staff (as in the case of the CPOA).

The name of the centre and the local community's knowledge of the type of help it provides may, of course, act as a powerful selective influence. Centres that are labelled literally as 'crisis intervention centres' do in fact tend to receive mainly persons in crisis rather than those in acute psychotic episodes. It is important to note that ambulatory services which do not have overnight stay available, and do not try to be selective (such as the CPOA) have a high onward referral rate to psychiatric inpatient care; (two-thirds of all callers in the CPOA are referred to a psychiatric hospital). Clearly, the nature of the referrals to a centre itself must determine to a large degree the destination of the client after the contact has been made. In Paris, for instance, with rather poorly developed psychiatric consultation services in general hospitals, there is a tendency for patients presenting themselves to these hospitals with almost any type of psychological or psychiatric problem to be sent to the CPOA; this centre also receives most of the obvious and severely disturbed psychiatric emergency cases.

Another example is the walk-in clinic of the Maudsley Hospital. It has access to overnight 'guest beds' on the wards of the hospital, which is probably why there is a rather low referral rate to ordinary inpatient psychiatric care — only one in eight clients (Lim 1983).

In the USA, the emergency rooms of general hospitals, whose basic purpose is to deal with acute physical emergencies, have been increasingly used by persons in psychological distress, and particularly by chronic psychotic patients living locally in the community. Many of these emergency rooms have responded to this by increasing their psychiatric consultation services and have even, in some instances, organised psychiatric emergency wards which provide inpatient care for a couple of days or so (Kaskey & Ianzito 1984).

In some instances, as in the Vienna Crisis Intervention Centre (Katschnig & Konieczna 1986), outpatient and walk-in services intentionally refrain from having access to overnight beds in order not to be seduced by the early option of removing the patient from his social network. There is then an increased motivation to find some way of coping with the problems by means of other resources in the social network.

Mobile (outreach) services

Specially designated mobile services are rather rare. A typical example is that organised by the Board of Doctors of Zurich, in which emergency help is provided by a single psychiatrist travelling around the city in his private car for a 24-hour spell of duty. He can be contacted via a central telephone hotline, available to those in distress, but this service is responsible not only for psychiatric and psychological but also for physical emergencies; it is operated by experienced nurses, who filter out probable psychiatric cases for referral to the mobile duty psychiatrist. The majority of persons in psychological distress dealt with in this way by the Zurich mobile service have in fact already had contact with other psychosocial or medical institutions earlier in the same crisis, but without obtaining what they consider to be adequate help (Hug 1981). More than one-third of these Zurich patients are finally admitted to inpatient care, and it was probably this high admission rate that was the main cause of a strike by the doctors providing the emergency services in the mid-1980s; demands were made for a crisis intervention unit with a few short-stay beds to act as a transitional unit. It was thought that in many instances, such a facility would allow the emergency doctors to avoid the difficult choice between admission to a mental hospital or simply leaving the patient out in the community.

Examples of special mobile outreach services in the UK are the Crisis Intervention Team (CIT) at the Mental Health Advice Centre in Lewisham, South London (Bouras et al 1986) and the Crisis Intervention Service at Barnet Hospital in North London, where a team consisting of a psychiatrist and either a social worker or a nurse, aim to contact any caller within two hours (Scott 1980).

Mobile services must be prepared to meet all types of problems in the community, including severely psychotic patients who may be suicidal, aggressive, and violent; since requests for help are made more frequently by other persons than by the patient or client, this often implies the presence of complicated interpersonal problems. A common element in these situations is a wish on the part of the person who asks for help to try to delegate the solution of the urgent problem to an outside agency or institution; this may be because sometimes those who constitute the social network around the patient have become intolerant or rejecting.

Crisis intervention centres with overnight facilities

For convenience, these centres will be referred to as Crisis Intervention Wards. Since 1971, when the first such ward in Europe was founded in Amsterdam (De Smit 1972), an impressive number of similar units has been developed throughout Europe. Groningen (1971), Laibach (1974), Reims (1974), Linkoping (1975), Berne (1977), West Berlin (1977), Belgrade (1979), Trieste (1980), Munich (1981) and Budapest (1983) are but a few examples of this generation of crisis intervention and emergency wards.

These centres seem to fall reasonably clearly into two types, according to whether the staff regard themselves as providing 'pure' crisis intervention cover or, in addition, a short-stay admission facility for persons with acute psychiatric illness. Whatever the policies and intentions of the Unit staff, both types tend to perform both functions to some extent, but usually one or the other can be seen to have a clear predominance. The position of a unit on the continuum noted by Cooper (1979) is a result of a balance of policies and professional staff ratios. However, a common purpose is the avoidance, as far as possible, of admissions to a more obviously psychiatric facility, with all the implied stigma and formal processes involved in this. These two types of crisis intervention ward will be discussed separately, with the implicit recognition that some degree of overlap of function is always present.

Crisis intervention wards

Crisis intervention wards have clear therapeutic aims, although on a short-time scale. Persons with psychogenic crises and suicidal feelings are the most frequent type admitted, comprising in many instances of more than 60% of all admissions. It is often found in these wards that their few beds are almost always occupied, and this naturally generates a pressure to discharge patients after a very short stay. However, initial ambitions and policies about very short length of stay are often not fulfilled; for instance, while the Amsterdam Crisis Intervention Centre had as its original aim a maximum length of stay of three days, in practice only 55% of clients can be discharged during that period (Cooper 1979). Such pressures inevitably lead to the setting up of careful selection and screening procedures before a decision to admit is taken; this usually ensures that patients with obvious psychiatric illness are not admitted, even though their illness may be causing manifest crises in interpersonal relationships or at work. As far as possible, admission is usually limited to those with less severe varieties of psychiatric illness, or with acute crises and problems only (who are usually not in an urgent need of medication other than mild hypnotics or sedatives). It is commonly found that the rapid turnover of short-stay patients in a crisis unit causes frustration amongst the staff, because of conflicting desires about whether or not to see the patient after discharge. To provide even a limited number of outpatient contacts with a proportion of patients after discharge would obviously limit the time available for each staff member to deal with urgent admissions, but yet it often seems eminently worthwhile for the crisis worker to complete the episode of care with a patient. There is also the emotional frustration involved from the repeated breaking off of relationships which are inevitably formed during the intensive contacts that occur during the period of admission. The result of these tensions and conflicts has often been that the staff of crisis wards arrange limited and fairly brief periods of after-care, even though such a development was not in the original policy of the unit.

The role of specialised crisis intervention wards is still under discussion, and whether or not a particular town or locality would be well advised to develop such a facility cannot be answered by reference to any universal formula or service development policy. Local needs will depend upon the existing related resources in the psychiatric and social services, and will be particularly affected by the resources available to provide the multidisciplinary team that is necessary for the successful functioning of such a ward.

Psychiatric emergency wards

Psychiatric emergency wards that are clearly labelled as such are usually very different in their staffing and organisational resources from crisis intervention wards. Inevitably they are closely connected, both functionally and physically, with other parts of the psychiatric services. They have usually been set up originally to receive a high proportion of patients under urgent compulsory orders, so as to provide a first port of call while immediate treatment and a process of investigation can occur. Patients with acute states of intoxication due to alcohol or drugs are common in these units, but most cases probably have a diagnosis of schizophrenic, paranoid, or manic-depressive psychosis. A predominantly medical staff and general medical orientation are necessary, and this is usually accompanied by a more hierarchical structure and method of functioning (Cooper 1979).

General comprehensive services

This term is used here to indicate comprehensive health services which are flexible and responsive enough to deal adequately with acute psychiatric emergencies and crises, without having to provide a separately labelled service. The most completely developed form is that of a comprehensive primary medical care (or family doctor/general practitioner system), linked with a comprehensive general hospital service.

The historical development of the way in which psychiatric services have arisen can be divided roughly into three phases, which may still co-exist today within different parts of the same country (and even within the same city). A first phase of one, undifferentiated psychiatric service is followed by the development of specialised services for specified disorders or age-groups, such as children, the elderly, and conditions due to abuse of drugs and alcohol. In addition, some services develop to deal with specific stages of psychiatric disorders, such as the more acute general and short-stay admission wards, and the long-stay rehabilitative and continuing care services. Emergency services have even begun to have sub-specialisations according to specific diagnostic groups, such as drug emergencies being separated from alcoholic emergencies. This second phase of specialisation and differentiation is now being followed by a new type of general service, which in some respects resembles the original comprehensive phase.

It seems therefore that the advantages of specialisation in the field of crisis intervention and emergency psychiatry (such as obtaining extensive experience and developing special knowledges and skills about how to link up with other services), are to some extent outweighed by disadvantages. The principal disadvantages being put forward are first, the lack of continuity of care implicit in a patient being rapidly referred to a specialised agency by the professional who makes the first contact, and secondly, the necessity to travel to a specialised centre. Both of these disadvantages can be avoided if a neighbourhood is served by a well staffed multidisciplinary psychiatric team, which should make it possible for the great majority of contacts to be made quite close to the patient's home or place of work, on the assumption that all the members of the team are sufficiently trained and experienced to be able to make the initial assessments involved in an emergency contact. This balance between local provision and specialisation at a distance highlights another familiar historical point. While emergencies are in a sense a nuisance to the traditionally designed general psychiatric services, dominated by the availability of medically qualified staff, the new varieties of sectorised community services usually have staff who are actually keen to cope with urgent referrals with the minimum of delay. A common motivation of such teams is to try to provide a service in which easy and rapid consultation procedures are available, in the hope of preventing the occurrence of the more serious and dramatic crises and emergencies.

However, new sets of problems inevitably arise, many of which are centered around the difficulty of dealing with comparatively small catchment areas; even with a multidisciplinary team in which expensive psychiatrists are in the minority, it is often not practicable to provide 24-hour cover for the team's locality. In Trieste, for instance, less costly solutions had to be found; whereas in the beginning of the reform period all seven community centres, each serving roughly 40 000 inhabitants, offered emergency help around the clock, crisis intervention and emergency help is now provided by these centres only during the daytime. During the night, all emergencies have to be referred to the crisis intervention ward in a general hospital. This ward is staffed by psychiatrists from all the centres in turn, and patients admitted are referred to the local centres on the next day. Thus, both economic advantage with a centralised service, and also some continuity of care are realised. Something very similar to this has evolved in the UK, where the structure of the National Health Service (NHS) with its comprehensive primary care (general practitioner) coverage, might be expected to promote good crisis and emergency services. If all the components of the NHS are working properly and are correctly integrated, a rapidly responsive and flexible crisis and emergency service should automatically be available. The existence of this integrated NHS since 1948 is probably the main reason why specially identified crisis and emergency services have been comparatively slow to emerge in the UK, compared to other European countries and the USA. However, as expectations and demands from the community have increased, some specified emergency services and additional domiciliary visiting services have developed within comprehensive sector-based general psychiatric services (Scott 1980, Bouras et al 1986, Jones et al 1987). Because of the limitations of team size already mentioned, though, even these most recent developments provide cover by the local team during working hours only, and the night time and weekend cover is provide by duty rotas in the conventional manner.

SPECIAL PROBLEMS

Who needs urgent psychiatric and psychological help?

Only a small proportion of all those in the community who experience acute distress ask for professional help, since other, and often more appropriate options are usually available. 'Distress behaviours' (Kreitman 1977) are diverse and include both constructive and maladaptive varieties, such as rationalisation of the situation, denial, rational coping, reduction of acute stress through medication or alcohol, and indirectly asking for help through attempting suicide and suicide. Little is known about the relationships between these various distress behaviours and the use of the different helping agencies and emergency services that are available, but Kreitman has pointed out substantial socio-demographic differences between those telephoning the Samaritans, those attempting suicide, and those completing suicide.

What is defined by whom as a crisis or as a psychiatric emergency situation needing immediate professional attention differs greatly, depending upon the amount of distress, personal and environmental tolerance, coping capacity, and knowledge and accessibility of crisis and emergency services. Services of a clearly psychiatric nature are less frequently chosen by the distressed persons themselves, whereas relatives or other agencies such as social workers or doctors are usually instrumental when psychiatric contacts are arranged. The site of first contact may depend upon the nature of the problem, but there is also a general tendency for non-medical and non-psychiatric professionals and institutions to be preferred to psychiatric ones (Gurin et al 1960, Regier et al 1978, Satin 1971).

Problems are often caused in both crisis intervention and psychiatric emergency services by the so-called chronic users of 'emergency room repeaters' (Walker 1983), mainly because they tend to produce negative reactions from the staff. Groves (1978) divides them into several sub-groups, such as 'manipulative help rejectors', 'entitled demanders', 'dependent clingers', and 'self-destructive deniers'. However, if they base their work too closely on crisis therapy, the staff of crisis intervention centres and crisis admission units find themselves repeatedly confronted with the problem that in real life, few of their clients correspond to the facility's 'ideal' — a healthy person who is suddenly hit by a trauma or a loss, and who, after going through the different stages of crisis with the help of the professional staff, will finally reach a higher level of functioning.

Keeping in mind the dynamic relationships between availability, demand, and over-use of professional services, three types of persons can be distinguished for whom professional help by means of crisis and emergency services seem appropriate. These are:

1. Patients with acute mental illness, in the narrow sense of the schizophrenic, affective, or organic types.

2. Persons in traumatic crisis after severe disruptive life events, mainly after severe losses.

3. Chronic psychiatric patients living in the community, who are unusually vulnerable to the effects of everyday events and environmental changes.

It is clear that there is no single institution or service which can cope equally well with the diverse demands that these patients represent, and some kind of specialisation seems inevitable if the quality of care is to be of a high standard. The extent to which such specialisation can be provided by different members of the same multidisciplinary team, rather than by different specialist teams, is an important issue that is worthy of investigation for practical, financial, and theoretical reasons. Crisis intervention centres tend to deal mainly with young females with psychosocial problems, seeing few patients with psychotic disorders, whereas medical and psychiatric emergency rooms must be prepared to receive patients with all types of acute illness and problems. These will include acute psychotic episodes, either of organic or psychogenic origin, states of intoxication, states of stress, and adjustment reactions.

Compulsory admissions

A detailed discussion of this complicated subject would be out of place here, but in most countries, the use of compulsory admission or treatment orders occurs largely in connection with emergency admissions. Unfortunately, the degree of urgency surrounding the admission cannot be deduced accurately from the nature of the compulsory order used, even though at first sight, it may seem that this ought to be deducible from the statutory requirements attached to such legal orders. Whatever instructions and guidance are provided to those using the compulsory procedures, there inevitably remains a considerable degree of latitude of interpretation which may result in wide variations in practice, even within the same country. Changes in the formal legislation will also complicate the way in which the official statistics may later be interpreted. For instance, in the UK under the Mental Health Act 1959, it was found in most areas that a significant proportion of emergency admissions took place under Section 29 of the Act, under which a patient could be detained for 72 hours on the authority of only one doctor; this was relatively over-used in preference to Section 25, which required the signatures of two doctors. Under the Mental Health Act of 1983, sections with very similar provisions were again provided, but at the same time much more stringent supervisory measures were introduced, as well as more elaborate appeal procedures for patients. The result was a marked decrease in the use of that Section (now Section 4) requiring the use of only one doctor, for a period of 72 hours detention. For instance, in Nottingham in 1982, 29% of compulsory admissions utilised Section 29, whereas in 1986, only 6% of compulsory admissions utilised the very similar Section 4; there has been compensatory rises in the other Sections of the 1983 Act, which require the signatures of two doctors.

A discussion of problems associated with compulsory admissions highlights the more fundamental question as to whether admission to psychiatric inpatient care is necessary at all. Almost certainly, the great majority of European psychiatrists and primary care doctors with experience of emergency psychiatry believe that, whereas admissions to any type of hospital — particularly psychiatric ones — should be kept to a minimum, it is simply not possible to avoid all admissions. It may well be true that a proportion of admissions become necessary only because there are delays and misunderstandings in the difficult process of recognising and managing acute psychological and psychiatric problems. However, in every community, a small number of unavoidable, acute, and disruptive situations arise which require the prompt intervention of skilled staff, simply because of the potential dangerousness. Subsequently, brief periods of treatment and management must be available, at an intensity and level of sophistication that can be provided only in inpatient units. Nevertheless, a small minority of enthusiasts remain, who ensure a continuation of the debate about the possibility of completely abolishing all psychiatric admission units.

In order to minimise the number of compulsory psychiatric admissions, it seems a reasonable supposition that the number of such admissions will be kept to a minimum if skilled intervention is available promptly and as close to the patient's home or work as possible. Nobody would disagree that this is a desirable aim, since apart from the manifest unpleasantness of the admission processes themselves, there are other subsequent legal penalties in many countries, such as loss of driving licence and refusal of future acceptance as an immigrant. In addition, the motivation of the patient and of the family for fruitful co-operation in the treatment process may be potentially put at hazard by compulsory measures. Although no detailed information on this point is available, there is also a widespread clinical opinion amongst emergency workers that if a patient is known to have been admitted compulsorily in the past, the likelihood of subsequent compulsory admissions is increased.

Some quite simple socio-demographic influences are known to be connected with the likelihood of involuntary hospital admission. For instance, Gerson & Bassuk's (1980) study in a general hospital emergency room in Boston showed that increasing age, male sex, low socio-economic status, and known previous inpatient treatment increased the risk of involuntary admission. The diagnosis itself may not be so important as the severity of the disturbance and perceived danger to self and others (Baxter et al 1968). In California, a comparatively encouraging conclusion emerged from a study by Segal et al (1985): when observing clinicians in general hospital emergency rooms, they concluded that these clinicians were able to make quite consistent decisions about the use of criteria required by the Civil Commitment Law with respect to whether the person concerned suffered from a mental disorder, was dangerous to self or others, or had grave social disability. In contrast, consistency of application of clinical and legal criteria was not a main feature of the findings of the study by Bean (1988) in the UK. This was based upon detailed observations, made by a sociologist working alongside the emergency psychiatrist, as to the style and details of procedures by which the Sections of the Mental Health Act 1959 were applied to a series of 58 compulsory admissions to a fairly typical English mental hospital. The observer was, in general, impressed by the good intentions and practical commonsense of the emergency psychiatrists, but he also noted a wide range of variation between individuals in the interpretation of the Sections of the Act and a surprisingly large number of minor technical infringements of the rules and regulations.

Some social issues have also been shown to be important in determining whether or not compulsory admission is used. Tufnell et al (1985) showed that a poor social network, the degree of disturbance of social environment, and several variables relevant to the professional decision maker are all important. Psychiatrists seem to be more inclined than non-psychiatric professionals to use compulsory orders, and young and inexperienced doctors generally produce higher admission rates than the older and more experienced ones. Patients who are perceived as 'interesting' are less likely than others to be admitted compulsorily, but if, on the other hand, a person induces a feeling of helplessness in the professional, particularly if associated with overt aggression (often evident when dealing with personality disorders and alcohol and drug problems), the risk of compulsory admission increases (Gerson & Bassuk 1980).

Even this brief review of the problems associated with involuntary admission indicates all too clearly that a wide variety of social, professional, and legal issues determine the extent to which compulsory measures are used in any particular situation or in any particular country. To reframe the legal measures alone will not necessarily reduce the frequency of compulsory admissions (Lamb et al 1981), since the basic design of the services and availability of skilled staff must also be of overriding importance. Compulsory admission often carries with it the implication that treatment is available and necessary, but the ethical and legal issues involved in this are outside the scope of this chapter.

Special problems encountered by staff

The rapid turnover of patients, many of whom are in obvious states of distress, inevitably throws a heavy burden on the staff of psychiatric emergency and crisis intervention services. The various types of stress listed by Slaby et al (1981) were clearly in evidence in many of the units visited by the authors. Particularly prominent and common sources of stress are:

(a) The need to interrupt the relationship with the patient and family after a few days of comparatively intense involvement.

(b) Fairly frequent encounters with distressed, occasionally aggressive or potentially dangerous patients.

(c) A need to make many rapid decisions, often on comparatively scanty information.

(d) Critical feed-back coming subsequently from centres and agencies who receive the patients, and who have much more time to do a comparatively leisurely work up of the patient.

(e) Practical problems, such as difficult hours of work and occasional shortage of sleep.

There is little factual information on the frequency of these types of stress and their effects upon the staff, but concepts such as 'burn-out syndrome' and 'overload' are frequent topics of discussion in these units. A general burn-out syndrome has been discussed by Freudenberger (1974), while some authors (e.g. Aguillera & Messick 1982) have gone so far as to describe actual stages of this syndrome in emergency service and crisis intervention workers (enthusiasm — stagnation — frustration — apathy — hopelessness). The comparative lack of experience of some of the members of emergency teams is an additional problem. For instance, in a number of centres in the USA, it is customary for comparatively junior psychiatric residents to spend six months working in the emergency room as part of their training.

How to minimise stress, and if possible avoid its harmful effects on staff have been discussed by Slaby et al (1981) and by Kaskey & Inazito (1984).

A measure which is easy to recommend but difficult to achieve is a good selection process for these personnel, and if at all possible, the duties of the emergency team should be arranged so that each worker sees a wide variety of patients. It is, for instance, frustrating and at times monotonous to work exclusively with self-poisoning cases, day after day. Supervision of all team members, particularly the juniors, by experienced workers of all the disciplines concerned should have a high priority, whilst continuing education by means of seminars and educative case discussions should always be part of a unit's overall programme.

The question of whether or not the members of a crisis and emergency team should keep on a small number of patients for follow-up work is largely an individual matter. Some crisis workers find that having a certain proportion of such work is very satisfying, whereas others prefer a rapid turnover without the implications of the development of a relationship with the patient. One of the most obvious precautions against the development of too much stress and overwork is often the most difficult — the provision of sufficient numbers of staff, particularly at night and at weekends, on those units where 24-hour cover is involved. The many types of stress, however, often combine to produce two problems very familiar to those who work in psychiatric emergency units and crisis centres — a rapid turnover of staff members, and the tendency of some emergency centres to have a short life-span (Kaskey & Ianzito 1984).

The multidisciplinary team that is a particular feature of emergency and crisis centre work has been described by many authors. Its particular style of working, characterised by sharing of responsibility and blurring of professional roles, is usually an interesting and striking feature of the unit when observed by visitors (Cooper 1979). It is likely that this style has evolved as a response to the varieties of stress mentioned above, since the sharing of responsibilities and decisions between the members of the teams probably helps to minimise both the stress and the workload. In spite of this overall beneficial effect, though, the characteristic working methods of the multidisciplinary team also carry with them some potential problems, concerned mainly with potential disagreements and conflicts between staff members about the degree and nature of role-blurring. There is no single discipline out of the several usually involved in a multidisciplinary team whose members are particularly well or poorly suited to the sharing of responsibilities; it is largely a matter of the personality of the team members and their motivation for taking up this type of work. It sometimes becomes clear that one or more staff members are using the meetings of the team to work through their own conflicts with other members, or even to try to solve their own personal relationship problems. One well known sign of trouble is an increasing frequency and length of team meetings at which the programme, staff relationships and general working of the unit are discussed at great length, to the exclusion of the management of patients. This sharing of responsibility for difficult decisions is on the whole a very beneficial effect of multidisciplinary team work, but there can be occasions when it is clearly stressful for all the team if no single person can be held responsible for mistakes or wrong decisions. Even a multidisciplinary team needs to have a recognised leader, though not necessarily a dominant one: one of the advantages of the authoritarian decision processes, often seen in more conventional medical and surgical teams, is that at least somebody is clearly responsible, and therefore can take the blame when something goes wrong.

The presence of doctors (usually psychiatrists in training) in emergency and crisis teams again has both positive and negative aspects. Having someone there with medical knowledge and responsibility is necessary in many respects, but the inevitable differences in outside status, salary, and hours of work can be a source of resentment within the team. Social workers and clinical psychologists may also be accustomed to ordinary working hours, and they may not be so ready as the nursing and medical staff to adopt 24-hour and weekend cover rotas.

Voluntary lay workers can be of great practical value in a crisis unit, and their presence may represent considerable budgetary savings. They are clearly best suited to help with a variety of clerical or administrative tasks, and may be particularly valuable as part-time receptionists. However, there must always be support and supervision available for the lay volunteers on the occasions when particularly difficult or distressed patients are encountered. Most units have a 'running in' period for lay volunteers, during which they work under very close supervision and receive a certain amount of elementary instruction about the nature and purposes of emergency and crisis services. The best guarantee of success is a detailed knowledge of the previous personal and career experiences of the volunteer worker. Once such workers have settled in to the unit, they may also be able to provide invaluable help by keeping the patient and relatives company at times of distress, while professional workers are temporarily otherwise engaged, or by dealing with the enquiries and contacts with the disposal agents that are such a large part of emergency work.

CONCLUSIONS

The number and variety of psychiatric emergency and crisis intervention services in Europe and the USA are large, changing, and perhaps still increasing. This is presumably in response to a demand for such services that is common to modern urban societies. Many different options exist for further developments of these services, and what evolves in any particular place will be the result of this demand interacting with services already existing, and with the political, economic, and medical customs of that community.

It seems wise for planners of medical and social services to consider several options for these developments; some of the main issues concerned are:

1. A choice between developing a specialised psychiatric emergency and crisis intervention service, and not developing one at all. To choose the latter implies that the conventional medical and social services are regarded as appropriate to cope with both urgent and non-urgent types of work.

2. If the choice is for specialised arrangement, then it may be developed as a separate service, or as a special component which is integral with or grafted-on to an existing service.

3. If the choice is for an integrated or grafted-on component, the psychiatric emergency and crisis intervention service may be developed as part of (i) the social services, (ii) the general medical services, or (iii) the specialised psychiatric services.

Solutions are likely to vary widely, even within one country, and urban–rural differences play a large part in determining the most practical arrangements. The experience gained by the authors during the World Health Organisation programme of studies led them to suggest that, if possible, integration of psychiatric emergency and crisis intervention services with the general medical services is likely in the long run to be the most favourable arrangement both for the professionals and for the users. Points in favour of integration with the general medical services are their ready availability, their lack of stigma, and the automatic inclusion of a check on physical health. However, this is a tentative conclusion, subject to many provisos derived from the design of existing services and from the political and medical customs of the community concerned.

REFERENCES

Aguillera D C, Messick J M 1982 Crisis intervention. Theory and methodology. 4th edn. Mosby, St Louis, Toronto, London
Allen N 1984 Suicide prevention. In: Loing Hatton C, McBride Valente S (eds) Suicide. Assessment and intervention. 2nd edn. Appleton-Century-Crofts, Norwalk, Connecticut
Atkins E W 1967 Psychiatric emergency service. Archives of General Psychiatry 17: 176-182
Baxter S, Chodorkoff B, Underhill R 1968 Psychiatric emergencies: dispositional determinants and the decision to admit. American Journal of Psychotherapy 124: 1542-1546
Bean P 1988 Location and stigma. Unwin & Hyman, London
Bellak L, Siegel 1983 Handbook of brief and emergency psychotherapy. CPS, Larchmont
Bouras N, Tufnell G, Brough D I, Watson J P 1986 Model for the integration of community psychiatric and primary care. Journal of the Royal College of General Practitioners 36: 62-66
Brandon S 1970 Crisis theory and possibilities of intervention. British Journal of Psychiatry 117: 627-633
Bristol J, Giller E, Docherty J 1981 Trends in emergency psychiatry in the last two decades. American Journal of Psychiatry 138: 623-826
Caplan G 1961 An approach to community mental health. Grune & Stratton, New York
Caplan G 1964 Principles of preventive psychiatry. Basic Books, New York

Coleman J V, Errera P 1963 The general hospital emergency room and its psychiatric problems. American Journal of Public Health 53: 1294-1301

Cooper J E 1979 Crisis admission units and emergency psychiatric services. Public Health in Europe II, Regional Office for Europe. World Health Organisation, Copenhagen

Davanloo H (ed) 1980 Short-term dynamic psychotherapy. Aronson, New York

De Smit N W 1972 Crisis intervention and crisis centres; their possible relevance for community psychiatry and mental health care. Psychiatrica, neurologica, neurochirurgica (Amsterdam) 75: 299-301

Dick P, Cameron L, Cohen D, Barlow M, Ince A 1985 Day and full-time psychiatric treatment: a comparison. British Journal of Psychiatry 147: 246-250

Eastwood M R, Mindham R H S, Tennant T G 1970 The physical status of psychiatric emergencies. British Journal of Psychiatry 116: 545-550

Eisenberg L 1977 In: Doing better and feeling worse, Daedalus. The search for care. Journal of the American Academy of Arts & Sciences: 235

Erikson E H 1959 Identity and the life cycle. International Universities Press, New York

Farberow N L, Shneidman E S (eds) 1961 The cry for help. McGraw-Hill, New York, London, Sydney, Toronto

Freudenberger H J 1974 Staff burnout. Journal of Social Issues 30: 159-165

Gerson S, Bassuk E 1980 Psychiatric emergencies: an overview. American Journal of Psychiatry 137: 1-11

Gersons B P R 1985 Crisis intervention in the context of social and preventative psychiatry. Vortrag gehalten am X111 International Kongres fur Selbstmordverhutung und Krisenintervention, Wien 1-4 Juli 1985. Unveroffentlichtes Manuskript

Groves J 1978 Taking care of the hateful patient. New England Journal of Medicine 298: 883-887

Gudeman J E, Shore M F 1984 Beyond the institutionalization. A new class of facilities for mentally ill. New England Journal of Medicine Vol. No. 832-836

Gurin G, Veroff J, Feld S 1960 Americans view their mental health. Basic Books, New York, London, Sydney, Toronto

Hafner H 1974 Krisenintervention. Psychiatrische Praxis 1: 139-150

Hirsch S R, Platt S, Knight A, Weiman A 1979 Shortening hospital stay for psychiatric care: effects on patients and families. British Medical Journal 1: 442-446

HMSO 1981 Central Statistical Office, Annual Abstracts of Statistics

Hug H H 1981 Psychiatrische Notfalle und deren Versorgung in der Stadt Zurich. Inaugural-Dissertation. Sozialpsychiatrischer Dienst der Psychiatrischen Universitatsklinik Zurich

Jacobson G F 1974 Programs and techniques of crisis intervention. American handbook of psychiatry. 2nd edn. Basic Books, New York: 2, p 810

Jacobson G F 1980 Crisis intervention in the 1980s. New directions for mental services. Jossey Bass, San Francisco, Washington, London

Jones S J, Turner R J, Grant J E 1987 Assessing patients in their homes. Bulletin of the Royal College of Psychiatrists 11: 117-119

Kaskey G B, Ianzito B 1984 Development of an emergency psychiatric treatment unit. Hospital & Community Psychiatry 35: 1220-1222

Katschnig H, Konieczna T 1986 Part 2 (City reports) of report to WHO on a study of crisis intervention units and psychiatric emergency services in Europe. World Health Organisation, Copenhagen

Katschnig H, Konieczna T, Cooper J E 1986 Final report to WHO on a study of crisis intervention units and psychiatric emergency services in Europe. World Health Organisation, Copenhagen (to be published)

Katschnig H, Konieczna T, Copper J E 1988 Emergency psychiatry and crisis intervention in Europe. World Health Organisation, Copenhagen

Kennedy P, Hird F 1980 Description and evaluation of a short-stay admission ward. British Journal of Psychiatry 136: 205-215

Kiev A 1970 New directions for suicide prevention centres. American Journal of Psychiatry 127: 87-88

Kreitman N 1977 (ed) Parasuicide. Wiley, London

Lamb H R, Sorkin A P, Zusman J 1981 Legislating social control of the mentally ill in California. American Journal of Psychiatry 138: 334-339

Langsley D G, Kaplan D M 1968 The treatment of families in crisis. Grune & Stratton,

New York

Lim Meng Hooi 1983 A psychiatric emergency clinic: a study of attendance over six months. British Journal of Psychiatry 143: 460-466

Lindemann E 1944 Symptomatology and management of acute grief. American Journal of Psychiatry 101: 141-148

MacGee T F 1968 Some basic considerations in crisis intervention. Community Mental Health Journal 4: 319

Malan D H 1963 A study of brief psychotherapy. Tavistock, London

Mindham R H S, Kelleher M J, Birley J L T 1973 A psychiatric casualty department. Lancet i: 1169-1171

Querido A 1968 The shaping of community mental health care. British Journal of Psychiatry 114: 293-302

Regier D A, Goldberg I D, Taube C A 1978 The de facto US mental health services system. Archives of General Psychiatry 35: 685-693

Ringel E 1953 Der Selbstmordl. Maudrich, Vienna, Düsseldorf

Rogers C R, Dymond R F (eds) 1954 Psychotherapy and personality change. University of Chicago Press

Satin D G 1971 Help! Prevalence and disposition of psychosocial problems in the hospital emergency unit. Social Psychiatry 6: 105-113

Scott R D 1980 A family orientated psychiatric service to the London Borough of Barnet. HMSO. Health Trends 12: 65-68

Segal S P, Watson M A, Scott Nelson L 1985 Equity in the application of civil commitment criteria. In: Lipton F R, Goldfinger S M (eds) Emergency psychiatry at the Crossroads. Jossey Bass, San Francisco, London: pp 93-105

Slaby A E, Lieb J, Tancredi L R 1981 Handbook of psychiatric emergencies. 2nd edn. Hans Huber, Bern, Stuttgart, Vienna

Talbott J A 1969 Community psychiatry in the army: history, practice and application to civilian psychiatry. JAMA 210: 1233-1237

Tufnell G, Bouras N, Watson J P, Brough B I 1985 Home assessment and treatment in a community psychiatric service. Acta Psychiatrica Scandinavica 72: 20-28

Tyhurst J S 1958 The role of transitional states — including disaster — in mental illness. In: Symposium on preventive and social psychiatry. Walter Reed Army Institute of Research. US Government Printing Office, Washington DC

Umana R F, Gross S J, McConville M T 1980 Crisis in the family. Gardner, New York

Varah C 1973 The Samaritans in the '70s. To befriend the suicidal and despairing. Constable, London

Wing J K, Brown G W 1970 Institutionalism and schizophrenia. Cambridge University Press, London

19. Community mental health centers in the USA

L.L. Bachrach

It is the special characteristic of all modern societies that we consciously decide on and plan projects designed to improve our social system. It is our universal predicament that our projects do not always have their intended effects. Very probably we all share in the experience that we often cannot tell whether the project had any impact at all, so complex is the flux of historical changes that would have been going on anyway, and so many are the other projects that might be expected to modify the same indicators.

D T Campbell 1979

The United States' federally supported effort in community mental health began with the Community Mental Health Centers Act of 1963. It ended only 18 years later with the Omnibus Budget Reconciliation Act of 1981, popularly known as the 'block grant' legislation. Was this federally funded movement to provide mandated comprehensive mental health services to the American people an aberration? Was it ill-advised? Or was it a necessary step in some greater Hegelian process toward equity in psychiatric service delivery? How may a federal government justify its withdrawal from an experiment that was so short-lived? Were the mental health centres' never-ending problems related to their dependence on regulations, guidelines, and philosophies promulgated in Washington? Or were they merely glitches punctuating a steady stream of progress? Most importantly, how did federally funded community mental health services affect the general quality of mental health care for the nation? What did it do to and for people who were mentally ill?

I shall briefly trace the history of federally funded community mental health services in the United States in an effort to shed some light on these intriguing questions. Following a convention adopted in a report of the Group for the Advancement of Psychiatry (GAP) (1983), the designation CMHC will be used exclusively to refer to federally funded community mental health centres developed in response to the 1963 legislation. Although there have been, and are other community mental health centres in the USA, they are not the subject of this analysis; however, it is safe to say that the findings reported here have great relevance for those other centres (Winslow 1982), many of which are lineal or lateral descendants of the original CMHCs.

HISTORY OF CMHC PROGRAMME

When President John F. Kennedy sent to Congress his famous 1963 message, calling for a 'bold new approach' in the delivery of services for the mentally ill and the mentally retarded, his action represented an important landmark in an ongoing struggle in the United States to gain federal support for mental health care. As early as 1854, on the premise that he could find no constitutional authority for the federal government to become the 'great almoner of public charity', President Franklin Pierce had vetoed legislation to make federal land grants available for the development of public mental hospitals (Task Panel on Community Mental Health Centers Assessment 1978: hereinafter cited as Task Panel A).

Prior to the 1960s, programmes for the mentally ill in the US had largely come under the control of the individual states, but several circumstances contributed to federal participation during the 1960s. The 1930s had witnessed an increasingly positive attitude on the part of the federal government toward its own involvement in issues of social responsibility, and the availability of increasing funds after the end of World War II enabled a variety of interests to capitalise on that shift. Mental health causes were particularly enhanced by the development of brief treatment methods and consultation techniques during the 1940s and 1950s (Goldman & Morrissey 1985): returning military clinicians had reported that immediate and rapid intervention could often diminish psychiatric symptoms, restore patients' functioning, and even prevent their admission to hospital (Langsley 1980b, Smith & Hart 1975). In fact, the stimulus afforded by these reports was largely responsible for the creation of the National Institute of Mental Health in 1949 and of the Joint Commission on Mental Illness and Health in 1955 (Task Panel A 1978).

There was indeed, in the post-War era, a 'can do' attitude dominating American thought (Freedman 1967); it was an era during which the civil rights of various disfranchised populations were being acknowledged and encouraged. Mass media reports documenting inhumane conditions inside state mental hospitals had begun to fuel public concern over the rights of the mentally ill, while the ability of the states to provide humane care, particularly in oversized, isolated, and under-staffed treatment settings was being questioned. Simultaneously, public health, with its emphasis on the prevention of illness, was enjoying widespread popularity. There was, in short, beginning to be a hope that with certain changes in the time of intervention and the locus of care, psychiatric illness might even be eliminated altogether.

As originally conceived, the CMHC programme sought to divide the US into precisely defined service areas, so that all Americans might have ready access to mental health care. There were to be 1500 such 'catchment areas', each serving a population of between 75 000 and 200 000 local residents. Within each catchment area a community mental health centre, 'seeded' by federal funds, would be the core service delivery agency, but federal monies were to be made available for only a limited time. Eventually, communities would 'graduate' to provide community-based mental health services under their own administration and through funding mechanisms of their own determination.

The original CMHC legislation in 1963 had two major priorities: treatment and rehabilitation of mentally ill individuals in community-based settings away from state mental hospitals, and overall promotion of mental health throughout the nation (Larsen & Jerell 1983). Amendments to that legislation, passed in 1965, mandated the provision of five essential services to accomplish those ends: inpatient care, outpatient care, emergency care, partial hospitalisation services such as day care, and consultation and education services. On the other hand, specialised diagnostic services for state hospital patients, and research and evaluation programmes were recommended but not required (Task Panel A).

The 1970s: expansion and problems

The 1960s legislation underwent substantial revision in amendments passed during the 1970s (Ochberg 1976). These served to expand the base of mandated services, so that CMHCs were now required to supplement the original five basic offerings with: services for children and the elderly; assistance to courts and other public agencies in screening individuals being considered for admission to state mental hospitals; follow-up care and halfway house services for patients discharged from state hospitals; and programmes for alcoholism and drug abuse. Under the amendments, centres were also required to conduct evaluative research on the services they offered.

To facilitate implementation of these changes, revisions in the legislation allowed for several new federally supported grant initiatives. Supplementing earlier grant programmes for construction and staffing, additional funding — earmarked for operations — was now available to assist CMHCs during their initial eight years of operation. Moreover, CMHCs could seek further assistance at the end of that period through financial distress grants that would ease the transition to alternative sources of funding. In addition, they could apply for grants for the acquisition, remodelling, leasing, or construction of buildings needed for services.

By the 1970s, it was clear that CMHCs had achieved widespread support; the programme was now a fully legitimated federal endeavour, and the government was backing its activist philosophy with tangible material support. By mid-decade, however, certain difficulties began to emerge, and several forces converged to threaten the future of the programme (GAP 1983); while the initial federal grants were progressively being terminated, the nation was undergoing a period of increasing inflation and unemployment. Many CMHCs were experiencing financial problems, and the prospects for local takeover of facilities seeded by federal monies were, in many places, quite poor. In a growing tide of fiscal conservatism, voters in communities throughout the country expressed their unwillingness to increase local taxes, at the very time when such revenues would be required to continue CMHC operations.

Nor were financial problems the sole source of difficulty (Task Panel A 1978). Despite reports of successful functioning in a number of places, serious problems affecting the efficient delivery of services within CMHCs were becoming apparent. There was increasing evidence that the federal guidelines and regulations for service delivery were, at the same time, both too rigid and too vague. On the one hand, they prescribed a blueprint for the geographical distribution of mental health services for a country with diverse and changing demographic patterns; they also mandated specific services even when the need for those services could not be documented.

On the other hand, the guidelines and regulations were not drafted clearly enough to identify which specific individuals living in any catchment area were entitled to treatment in the CMHC, and how their needs might be assigned priority, in a system of care that was global in its mission. Although services for such groups as children, the elderly, and patients discharged from state hospitals had been required, they were not ranked relative to one another, nor to the other non-mandated services that CMHCs were also expected to offer.

Boundary issues

There was also considerable confusion over who specifically — i.e. which patients — should be served in CMHC settings (Fink & Weinstein 1979). Many planners and service providers felt certain that the primary intent of the 1963 legislation had been to serve seriously and chronically mentally ill individuals first, but other experts were persuaded that assigning such priority to the chronically ill was inappropriate. Subscribing to the notion that their facilities were basically intended for 'mental health' and not for 'mental illness', they argued that selecting such people for care would effectively preempt resources, and leave nothing for other groups of patients. Furthermore, in the absence of clear direction about who was entitled to care, new categories of people who had been previously unserved in the mental health system — described as the 'worried well' (Task Panel A 1978) or the 'healthy but unhappy' (Zusman & Lamb 1977) — sought and received treatments in CMHCs, while the chronically ill often went unserved. Federally funded CMHCs were said to have 'drifted away from their original purpose as defined by Kennedy — the treatment of the mentally ill' — and 'moved into a social service model', and were promoting preventive services that had 'not yet been proven successful' (Langsley 1980a).

In a classic sociological analysis, Dinitz & Beran (1971) contrasted the federally funded community mental health movement with other more traditional treatment initiatives in the United States. Because the CMHC programme was focussing its efforts on populations not usually perceived as the legitimate recipients of mental health services, it had fashioned itself into a 'boundary-less and boundary-busting system'. The federal programme, they wrote, 'seems to have set for itself a boundary-less goal; the improvement of the quality of life of the whole man, and every man, in his total environment'.

The issue of fuzzy boundaries was attacked on both humanitarian and pragmatic grounds. Borus (1978) identified this problem as one of several critical ones threatening the very survival of community mental health services in the United States. Similarly, the American Medical Association (AMA 1979), in a position statement on the CMHC programme, stated that '*The primary goal of any community mental health centre or system should be to treat persons who are sick.* Scarce dollars and scarce manpower should not be diverted to those persons with social maladjustment problems at the expense of persons with demonstrable mental illness who may go untreated because services are being directed elsewhere'.

Nowhere was the potential for loss of boundaries more effectively demonstrated than in a Kansas CMHC which offered a course designed specifically to teach people how to drink.

With that goal in mind, [it] has taken to conducting cocktail parties and using them as forums to discuss alcohol abuse. The program, called 'A new taste of wine', is not a treatment effort. Instead, it focuses on people who drink but have not developed drinking problems. It is also set up to assist party hosts by demonstrating ways to minimise overindulgence by guests and to handle those guests who drink too much (Sheppard 1981).

It should be noted that the National Institute of Mental Health effectively acknowledged both the basic entitlement of chronic psychiatric patients to care in the community, and the general failure of the CMHC movement to provide that care, when it initiated its Community Support Program (CSP) in 1977. That initiative did not begin to approach the CMHC effort in scale or in scope. It is, in fact, only a time-limited demonstration effort providing services for a relatively small percentage of the nation's chronically mentally ill population (Goldman et al 1981). However, in specifically selecting these patients for care in community-based settings, the CSP programme tacitly acknowledges that it is these individuals who are most in need of comprehensive services but who, since the time of the CMHC movement, have been largely overlooked.

The programme's demise

In 1978, the President's Commission on Mental Health, appointed by President Carter, issued a report summarizing a year's intensive study of mental health services in the United States. Noting that local communities had largely failed to assume responsibility for providing adequate and accessible mental health care, this document asserted that the CMHC programme had neglected the mental health needs of the nation. It especially criticized the programme's failure to provide incentives and guidelines to ensure treatment of high-risk populations. The Mental Health Systems Act of 1980, passed shortly before President Carter left office, responded to those concerns by establishing priorities in cases of unserved and under-served populations, and by proposing new funding mechanisms to support such efforts.

But this Act was not destined to change the course of service delivery in the United States: it was repealed in the first year of President Reagan's administration by passage of the block grant legislation. With the advent of this new federal approach to mental health service delivery, the CMHC programme was terminated, and the federal role in mental health service delivery materially altered (Okin 1984).

CMHCs lost their unique identity, as funds for 10 federally funded alcohol, drug abuse, and mental health initiatives were consolidated into single block grants to each of the 50 states. At the same time, authority for administering, distributing, and monitoring the block grant funds was similarly transferred from a centralised federal authority to the states themselves.

However, these changes in the administration and control of federal monies were accompanied by reductions in the total level of federal funding for mental health services (Comptroller General 1984). States now had considerable flexibility in deciding how to spend federal mental health dollars, but there were fewer dollars to spend.

A recent federal document (Redick et al 1985) defines a CMHC as a legal entity receiving funds for the provision of comprehensive mental health services under the original CMHC legislation or amendments thereto. By that definition, there are no remaining federally funded CMHCs in the United States today, although there are still agencies descended from the CMHCs which identify with the original goals of that movement. There are also other agencies that have never received federal funding but nonetheless perceive themselves as comprehensive community mental health centres. However, none of these facilities is under federal mandate to provide 'essential services' to patients, nor must it respond to the federal requirement that the service needs of residents of a bounded catchment area be met. Indeed, Humpty Dumpty would be quite comfortable with the words 'community mental health centre' today, for they mean precisely whatever one chooses them to mean — neither more nor less.

When the block grant legislation terminated the CMHC programme, 18 years after passage of the original Act, the federal government had provided funding to a total of 758 CMHCs at a cost of 2.9 billion dollars (Comptroller General 1984). In less than two decades, CMHCs had become the third largest organised component of the mental health service delivery system in the United States (Thompson et al 1982).

How well had they achieved their aim of providing comprehensive mental health services to the American population in community settings? The reviews are mixed, and relatively little may be concluded from the limited amount of evaluative research that has been published. Indeed, the movement is now generally seen as having been negligent in its general failure to encourage and conduct sophisticated and relevant evaluations of services (Cook & Shadish 1982, Langsley 1980a, Nash & Argyle 1984, Windle & Woy 1983), even though such a deficiency is hardly surprising in view of the boundary-busting nature of the effort. The general absence of precisely defined objectives necessarily confounds the formulation of valid research questions.

The evaluation research that does exist, however, points to several broad findings (Naierman et al 1978, Weiner et al 1979, Woy et al 1981) — primarily that the established CMHCs are diverse and difficult to characterise. Some services in those centres, e.g. outpatient care, seem to have survived graduation from federal funding better than others, e.g. consultation and education, although virtually all facilities have been experiencing financial problems since the withdrawal of federal monies. Many have had to change the services they offer, to conform to their new financial realities.

Some CMHCs have continued to attempt to provide comprehensive services, but others have become increasingly specialised and concentrated on particular groups of patients. Structurally, some resemble the medical service agencies in which they are housed, and serve 'patients', while others pride themselves on avoiding the medical model and serve 'clients'. Some perceive the chronically mentally ill to be a part of their charge; others continue to argue against the presence of these patients — although very recent research points to the possibility that even centres that have resisted treating chronic patients in the past are acquiescing in that task today. Increasingly, state and local governments, finding themselves confronted with a growing and under-served population of 'new long-term' patients (Bachrach 1987, Shepherd 1984, Wing & Morris 1981), are assigning them higher priority in the services that they finance (Jerrell & Larsen 1983, 1985, 1986). However, at the present time, this group's need for care far exceeds what present funding levels are able to support (Lamb 1984).

Such generalisations about the outcomes of the CMHC programme tell only part of the story, though. In the remainder of this chapter, I shall assess the adequacy of some of the assumptions that guided the architects of the CMHC movement, and discuss the programme's overall effects on mental health service delivery in the United States.

CONCEPTS AND PROMISES

When it came into being in the early 1960s, the federal CMHC programme represented far more than a shift in the primary locus of care for psychiatric patients: it aimed to revolutionise the entire service delivery system with new ideas and new treatment philosophies. Central to this approach was the notion of local control of mental health services. There was an implicit belief that many roads might potentially lead to effective care, and that each of the 1500 catchment areas could and would evolve a service system that was consistent with its local needs and resources.

Thus, from the very beginning, and despite the existence of federal guidelines and regulations governing the granting of funds, there was wide structural diversity among CMHCs (AMA 1979, Thompson & Bass 1984). By intent, facilities varied along so many dimensions that there seemed to be an almost infinite number of permutations; there was 'no single existing model' that could adequately describe the 'potential variety of organisation and operation modes' (Person 1969).

CMHCs also differed widely, both within states and among states, in the services that they offered and the personnel that they employed, as well as their financial arrangements. Aggregate statistics reveal that rural CMHCs were distinguished from urban ones not only in their funding, expenditure, and staffing patterns (Bachrach 1974a, National Institute of Mental Health 1977a, 1977b), but also in the socio-economic circumstances and diagnostic distributions of the patients that they served (Bachrach 1974b). Some CMHCs, both urban and rural, operated almost entirely with the funds granted to them by the federal government, whereas others were able to supplement these with state or local government funds, commercial insurance payments, or direct fee-for-service revenues.

There were also substantial administrative and structural variations. CMHCs might be administered wholly by state or local governmental authorities, be located in the private sector, or combine both through contractual arrangements. They might offer all their services at a single site, or be spread out under many roofs. They might be under single administrative sponsorship, or be consortia of several participating service delivery agencies. Finally, they might be physically located — in whole or in part — on the grounds of a general or state mental hospital, be freestanding, or exist as part of some social service agency.

However, despite these extensive variations, CMHCs were united by their affiliation with the federal government under whose auspices they were created. In order to qualify for federal funding, they had to make certain basic mental health services available to populations residing within geographically bounded catchment areas. Moreover, in delivering those services, centres had to observe certain regulations and guidelines that were promulgated at the National Institute of Mental Health. The rationale for these requirements lay in a consensus concerning the basic purposes and goals of federally funded community mental health services which was held by its early planners and advocates.

Guiding principles and goals

In 1978, the Task Panel on Community Mental Health Centers Assessment reported its findings to its parent organisation — the President's Commission on Mental Health — and identified nine basic goals that had stood as cornerstones of the CMHC movement from the time of its inception.

First, the federally funded CMHC movement sought to increase the range and the number of mental health services throughout the United States. Enhancing the availability of outpatient and partial hospitalisation services in preference to hospital-based inpatient care was deemed to be particularly important, and the design of catchment areas was perceived as a device for operationalising this fundamental goal. By dividing the country into segments with manageable population bases, local services could be organised in such a way that every community in the United States could respond to the mental health needs of its residents. In addition, CMHCs would have multidisciplinary staffs, whose combined expertise could be used as needed to enhance the mental health of catchment area residents.

Second, the CMHC programme aimed to eliminate class distinctions in mental health service delivery in the United States. Prior to the 1960s, an essentially two-class system of care had existed, in which those individuals who had sufficient resources to do so received primarily private outpatient treatment, while the economically disadvantaged either received custodial state mental hospital inpatient services or else went unserved. Implicit in these differentials were serious inequities in the availability of adequate services to members of ethnic and racial minorities, but the new legislation promised what Mollica (1983) has called 'unlimited access and universal entitlement'. All Americans would now have access to high quality mental health services, irrespective of their socio-economic, racial, or ethnic backgrounds.

Third, services offered in federally funded community mental health centres were intended to be responsive to the particular service needs of local populations. State administered systems of care had failed to reach all the citizens needing mental health services, and those people who were reached often received only inferior care. However, under the CMHC programme, a federal-local partnership would be effected; states would be bypassed, and the federal government would deal directly with local communities. Local participation in decision-making and in the setting of priorities would be assured through direct grants to communities, and would be enhanced in future years when the federal seed money could be totally replaced with locally generated funds — a time when the community could assume complete ownership of the mental health services offered to its residents (Weiner et al 1979).

Fourth and fifth, two closely related goals of the federal initiative involved reduced utilisation of state mental hospitals and the humanisation of mental health services. In an era emphasising the rights of the disfranchised, state mental hospitals were widely viewed as inhumane, custodial warehouses. There was great confidence that eliminating those service sites and replacing them with community-based alternatives would result in a more humane system of care.

A sixth goal of the federally funded CMHC movement was to improve the fiscal efficiency of mental health service delivery. There was a popular belief that moving the primary locus of care from the state hospital to the community would result in extensive cost savings to tax payers. Indeed, it was this strong belief in the cost-effectiveness of community-based care that permitted social reformers to ally themselves with fiscal reformers in promoting deinstitutionalisation and community mental health care. Ordinarily mutually antagonistic, these two constituencies were now united in the hope of promoting extensive changes in mental health service delivery, though for different reasons.

Seventh, assuming that communities could be, and wished to be involved in decisions concerning the mental health of their residents, the federal CMHC programme sought to increase citizen participation in delivery of services. There were to be citizen advisory boards, directing formulation of policy and implementation of services in all catchment areas. These boards, which were mandated by law, would serve two essential purposes: ensuring that local concerns were influencing service policy, and checking the potential insensitivity that unilateral professional judgements might promote (Langsley 1980a).

Eighth, the federally funded CMHC movement began with a strong hope for, if not a belief in the preventability of psychiatric disorder. Hence, a major goal of the programme, which was essentially derived from public health concepts, was to reduce both the incidence and the prevalence of such illness in the United States, primarily through consultative and educational efforts. This in turn, would result in a diminished need for conventional treatments, and would eventually narrow the tasks of the CMHC (Zusman & Lamb 1977).

Finally, there was a basic belief that CMHCs could and should respond to all the mental health needs of a community's residents; toward that end, there was a ninth goal of providing comprehensive mental health services and ensuring continuity of patients' care. Indeed, the co-ordination of diverse service efforts was one of the most fundamental concepts in the CMHC philosophy — one that symbolised confidence that patients' needs would best be served when all the mental health services required by any one individual could be provided under local auspices. 'No longer', proclaimed a federal document, 'will a patient face the choice between hospitalisation and no treatment at all'. Instead, the patient in a comprehensive community-based system of care would now 'be able to enter or leave the centre from any service component or be able to move from any service to any other service within the centre' (Person 1969), without interrupting the flow of his/her care.

IMPLEMENTATION AND ISSUES

One cannot doubt that these goals were humane and well intentioned, and that their proponents felt assured of their practicability, but hindsight permits us the luxury of assessing their feasibility. The concepts implicit in those goals were in fact often too naive, and the goals themselves frequently too unfocussed to make their implementation possible on any widespread basis. In addition, a variety of serious problems affecting service delivery in CMHCs came to the fore during the years of the programme's operation. Several analytical reports describing those issues in detail pointed out the conceptual and operational limits of the federally funded CMHC programme (AMA 1979, Bachrach 1976, Borus 1978, Comptroller General 1977, GAP 1983, Langsley 1980b, Musto 1975, Task Panel A 1978), and their major conclusions are discussed below.

Increasing services and decreasing inequities

There is no question that the CMHC movement did in fact substantially expand the volume of available services in many catchment areas. With the advent of these new facilities and federal funds to support them, many communities were now able to offer mental health services for the first time, while other communities could, and did expand existing offerings, as well as broadening the base of their target populations. At the same time, however, there is evidence that a full range of essential services, as defined in the CMHC legislation and its amendments, was often not provided for catchment area residents. Many CMHCs, particularly those of small size located in remote communities, could offer only what their limited staffs knew how to do (Task Panel on Rural Mental Health 1978: hereinafter cited as Task Panel B). In larger CMHCs with diversified staffs, on the other hand, competition and guild interests among professional groups often inhibited the provision of diversified services (Langsley 1980b, Leong 1982). Many CMHCs, instead of offering diversified services, thus became identified with a particular treatment philosophy or group of patients.

Success in eliminating the two-class system of care was also mixed. In some parts of the country, CMHCs did in fact reach racial, ethnic, and other minority populations that had previously been virtually unserved, except perhaps in state hospitals (Vaccaro 1988). However, other kinds of barriers often precluded large portions of those groups from actually receiving the kind of comprehensive care that was originally envisioned by the architects of the CMHC movement. For example, professional personnel employed in high-income catchment areas tended to have had more intensive training and better academic preparation than staff in low-income catchment areas (National Institute of Mental Health 1978).

Because many rural catchment areas were designated as areas with high concentrations of populations in poverty (Bachrach 1982, Task Panel B 1978), problems in implementing the CMHC effort in those places may be used to illustrate wider issues encountered in the attempt to eliminate social class distinctions in mental health service delivery. Perhaps because they often lacked expertise in 'grantsmanship' (Task Panel B 1978), rural catchment areas were relatively unsuccessful in the competition for federal funds (Task Panel A 1978). Many were still totally unfinanced when the CMHC programme came to an end, and those that did receive funding usually did not get enough to employ the variety of staff that would be needed to provide comprehensive care to a small population.

Mollica (1983) has presented persuasive arguments that a two-class system of mental health care prevails in the United States, despite the CMHC movement's objective of eliminating financial and geographical barriers to care. It is a system of care in which the state hospital, despite its decline over the past several decades, 'continues to be the principal facility for the acute inpatient care of the lower-class patient'. In fact, there has been a 'pooling of the poorest patients at state facilities, as middle-class and working-class patients have achieved financial access to private institutions' — a situation that is alarming because state hospitals 'continue to bear the brunt of fiscal cutbacks and professional neglect' throughout the United States. But what is even more troubling, according to Mollica, is that the poor tend to receive different treatment even *within* community mental health centres. They are likely to receive such services as psychosocial support from non-professional workers, in place of psychotherapy from psychiatric professionals even though psychotherapy, at least broadly defined, may be regarded as essential even in the care of chronic mental patients (Lamb 1982). For patients of higher socio-economic status, according to Mollica, these likelihoods are reversed.

Local direction

Were the federally funded CMHCs more successful in their effort to respond to the idiosyncratic service needs of local communities? The extensive structural diversity among centres provides a strong indication that efforts were indeed being made by some at least of these facilities to cater to local realities: in many places, CMHCs experimented with and implemented creative solutions to the service needs that they perceived. Yet the federal guidelines and regulations often homogenised programmes and compromised their autonomy; many local planning authorities complained that natural and social boundaries had to be ignored in order to meet catchment area population minima. Although exceptions to the regulations were sometimes granted from Washington, procedures for obtaining them could be complicated, time-consuming, and costly to local communities.

Once again, the situation faced in many rural communities is instructive. Most rural catchment areas exceeded 5000 square miles in land area — a situation fostered by the necessity to serve a base population of at least 75 000 individuals (Bachrach 1983b). The largest catchment area in the United States, in Northern Arizona, consisted of more than 60 000 square miles, and travel from one end to the other meant crossing the Grand Canyon, while another rural catchment area covered more than a third of the land area of the state of Oregon.

Sparsely settled communities were often unable to support the full range of legally required services, and in any case, those services were sometimes unnecessary (Task Panel B 1978). Rural boomtowns with predominantly youthful populations, for example, had little need for geriatric services, and the necessity to provide them deflected resources away from other target groups. At the other extreme, metropolitan areas often found it necessary to create catchment areas with artificial boundaries — to fabricate and sometimes to gerrymander — in order that districts should not exceed the 200 000 population maximum (Marcos & Gil 1984). In short, there was a growing realisation that 'catchment area' and 'community' were not synonymous terms, and that a community mental health system could not be created merely by drawing boundaries and calling the space within them a mental health catchment area.

Further difficulty arose with the use of federal seed money. The notion of a declining formula in federal subsidies was based on the assumption that if CMHCs could be awarded 'start up' funds, they could eventually obtain matching funds from other sources, so that the federal government would ultimately be able to pull out of the business of funding community mental health. In actual practice, however, local communities were often unable to replace the federal monies at the time of 'graduation'. This meant that CMHCs might abandon poor patients who had patterns of high service utilisation, such as the chronically mentally ill, in favour of commercially insured patients who could pay their own way and respond to briefer, less costly treatment interventions (Morrissey & Goldman 1984).

In 1979, Weiner et al re-examined the concept of seed money, and concluded that the federal government should expand, not lessen its financial commitment to community mental health: 'perhaps the time is now for the federal government to re-think the premises of the seed money approach and make available some form of 'floor funding' to help preserve the investment in organised community mental health systems'. With so many dollars invested in the CMHC effort to date, these authors asked, 'should we risk a loss in the investment?'.

Reducing state hospital admissions and humanising care

There seemed, however, to be little difficulty in meeting the goal of reducing state hospital utilisation — at least according to the statistical criterion of patients in residence in those facilities. Deinstitutionalisation was proceeding apace, both through the discharge of resident patients and the diversion of new admissions from the nation's state mental hospitals (Bachrach 1985). In 1962, immediately before passage of the Community Mental Health Centers Act, there had been some 515 000 patients residing in those facilities; twenty years later, in 1982, the count was 121 000, a drop of about three-quarters (National Institute of Mental Health, undated). However, during the same time period, admissions to state hospitals rose by over one-fifth. The nation's state hospitals had become busy places, where many patients stayed for short periods of time (Bachrach 1986) — a situation that gave rise to the notion of a' revolving door'. Whether state hospital utilisation had truly decreased was a matter of which criterion one chose to use.

Moreover, there was some real question about the extent to which the increasing utilisation of CMHCs and the decreasing resident populations within state mental hospitals were paired events. Despite co-ordinated efforts in some communities, there was little evidence on a nationwide basis that the individuals who were no longer being served in state hospitals were the same ones who were enrolling in CMHCs. On the contrary, there was good reason to believe that the two kinds of facilities were serving entirely different patient populations, and that the chronically mentally ill were widely under-served in CMHCs (Comptroller General 1977, Goldman et al 1983, Gronfein 1985, Windle & Scully 1976). Even though some of the CMHC amendments had acknowledged the need to provide care to patients discharged from state hospitals, no co-ordination between the two kinds of facilities had been required (Morrissey & Goldman 1984). Thus, chronic mental patients often had nowhere to go. Caught between emasculated state mental hospitals that were forced by public outcry and diminished funding to reduce their services, and CMHCs that acknowledged little responsibility to them, these patients became the casualties of the CMHC effort.

Those who would assign culpability to the federally funded CMHC movement for this unfortunate situation must however acknowledge that in many instances, CMHCs grew up in virtual isolation from state hospitals, and that ignorance of each other was rife. Many administrators probably failed to appreciate the prevalence of chronic mental illness and the special treatment needs of chronic mental patients. Thus, while the treatment efforts of CMHCs were being developed and implemented for other groups of patients, they often ignored the requirements of the chronically mentally ill. Other community-based facilities such as general hospitals assumed much of the burden of care for these patients, often by default, but the problems they encountered exceeded their ability, or their willingness to step in where the CMHCs had failed (Bachrach 1985). Quite predictably, the tremendous hiatus in services for chronic patients led to homelessness and indigency for many such individuals (Lamb 1984).

Needless to say, these circumstances had a major impact on the adequacy of the mental health service system in the United States; they had the *de facto* effect of negating the CMHC movement's major aim of humanising mental health care.

Reducing costs

If CMHCs largely failed in their efforts to humanise mental health care, did they achieve any greater success in reducing the costs of that care? A report by the Group for the Advancement of Psychiatry (GAP)(1983) reviewed the evidence on this point, and concluded that data available for responding to this question lack comprehensiveness and validity. Although some communities reported cost savings through the implementation of CMHC efforts, it is difficult to evaluate the meaning of their reports because of serious methodological problems.

A retrospective view, however, suggests that no major overall cost savings were likely to occur in the delivery of mental health services unless, and until, state mental hospitals could be totally eliminated. The *per capita* costs of operating and staffing those large physical plants, and of maintaining them in order to ensure their accreditation, are generally very high, and although these are costs that did not show up in CMHC financial statements, they were nonetheless borne by the tax payers.

There were other, even less apparent, hidden costs that accompanied the shift in the major locus of care from state mental hospital to community. One that is very difficult to assess is in the area of family finances. In a decentralised and fragmented system of care, for example, there may be extensive transportation costs associated with delivering patients to treatment sites, and these usually come out of families' pockets. Frequently, too, relatives of mentally ill individuals must themselves remain unemployed in order to perform the custodial functions once provided in state mental hospitals, with an attendant loss of income. This and other burdens — not monetary, but social and psychological expenses (GAP 1986) — are often disproportionately assumed by female relatives of the mentally ill, so that Thurer (1983) has noted that deinstitutionalisation is in many respects a women's issue.

In summary, in the matter of cost-savings, it appears that high-quality mental health care is expensive, wherever it is provided. There is a growing consensus today that the goal of reducing costs through the CMHC effort was naive and premature. We do not even know whether the total elimination of state mental hospitals could materially reduce costs. It is entirely possible that even under such circumstances, the administrative and personnel costs connected with delivering comprehensive care in a fragmented service system would effectively neutralise any dollar savings that might accrue from deinstitutionalisation.

Citizen participation and prevention of illness

There were also major problems associated with realising the goal of citizen participation in CMHCs (GAP 1983, Task Panel A 1978). Although the original CMHC legislation had included requirements for citizen advisory boards to govern centres, productive involvement of that kind lagged in most parts of the country. Members of community boards in some places did in fact succeed in educating themselves about service delivery issues, and became effective agents in policy implementation, but most such advisory oganisations failed to be the creative bodies that had been envisioned.

Quite apart from the issue of citizen involvement and its efficacy, attempts to encourage lay participation in CMHC operations had a serious — and probably largely unintended — byproduct in many places: the frequent deprofessionalisation of service in centres. The notion of community control, coupled with a post-World War II enthusiasm for egalitarianism (Langsley 1980b), fostered a milieu in which the importance of professional judgement was often minimised. Hopkin (1985) ably describes such an atmosphere as one in which greater value is placed on intuitive interpersonal skills than on professional training and experience in the care of patients.

Deprofessionalisation of services was particularly felt by the psychiatrists practising in CMHCs: the frankly anti-professional attitude that some administrators and boards adopted, coupled with a constant need for psychiatrists to protect their area of authority, often rendered CMHCs unattractive as places in which to work (Berlin et al 1981, Donovan 1982). The boundary-less nature of the entire CMHC movement also played a major role in psychiatrists' increasing disaffection. Instead of being able to provide care in primarily medical settings, where they might apply their specialised training, psychiatrists found that they were frequently needed only to 'prescribe medication where large numbers of chronically mentally ill patients were treated, thereby limiting their programme involvement' (Fink & Weinstein 1979).

In 1971, 55% of all CMHCs had been headed by psychiatrists; in 1980, their representation had decreased to 16% (American Psychiatric Association 1985). As with numerous other circumstances that characterised the CMHC effort, problems associated with the recruitment and retention of psychiatrists to work in CMHCs reflected a kind of circularity. The decease of psychiatrists resulted largely from the movement's lack of boundaries, but also served in turn to encourage further boundary-busting.

If the goal of citizen participation is now deemed to have been naive — if it is seen as having resulted from an excessive preoccupation with the role of social factors, as against medical, in psychiatric illness — that was nothing compared with views that emerged on the goal of preventing psychiatric disorder. Assuming basically that inadequate social environments produce psychiatric illness, this goal generated consultative and educative efforts to inform and engage the public in the basics of 'mental health'. However, with the passage of years, it has become increasingly evident that the theoretical foundation for this view is extremely shaky (Langsley 1980a, 1980b, Zusman & Lamb 1977). Certainly, environmental manipulation may be expected to better the life circumstances of the mentally ill, and even to eliminate some varieties of personal unhappiness and stress, but one may hardly expect it to alter the biology and chemistry of illness *per se*. Yet such an expectation, or something very like it, was a focal point of the CMHC movement; it both motivated service planners and unrealistically raised the hopes of the nation (Lyons 1984). However, to understand the appeal of such an expectation, one must remember the strength of the 'can do' spirit in post-War America, and the prevailing wish to better people's lives through social intervention.

Undoubtedly, faith that psychiatric illness could be eliminated largely, if indirectly, contributed to the frequent neglect of chronic patients in CMHCs. There was obviously little need for facilities to be preoccupied with planning and organising treatments for a service population that, through the humane efforts of the CMHC movement, was soon to vanish. The naiveté of this reasoning — so apparent today with the growing population of homeless mentally ill individuals throughout the United States (Bachrach 1984b) — largely eluded the early proponents of the federal community mental health effort. It also had profound consequences for the fundability of CMHCs: 'if one says that mental disorder is not truly an illness but rather a response to social problems, and if one proposes that treatment programmes abandon traditional health care settings and health services leadership, then why should the budgets of the health programme be expected to fund social services and social systems?' (Langsley 1980a).

Comprehensiveness and continuity of care

As much of the foregoing discussion demonstrates, CMHCs regularly and continually encountered major difficulties in their attempts to provide comprehensive services for catchment area residents, and to ensure continuity in their care — the ninth identified goal of the movement. With their predominant emphasis on outpatient care and short-term interventions (Hansell 1978), CMHCs often relied on patients themselves to have sufficient motivation and mobility to present themselves for treatment. Fashioned for an essentially ambulatory and compliant population, CMHC services often overlooked the fact that many patients, particularly those with chronic illnesses, would be forced to traverse considerable physical and psychological distance in order to receive care — major barriers for most individuals with severe disorders.

In addition, comprehensiveness for chronic patients necessarily entails a wide array of psychiatric, medical, social, rehabilitative, vocational, and quasi-vocational services (Bachrach 1981, 1983b, Peterson 1985). It further requires that agencies ensure the availability of the elusive function of asylum for those patients who need it for either a limited or an extended period of time (Bachrach 1984a). Unlike the relative ease with which these varied functions could be fulfilled in state mental hospitals, where all services were concentrated in a single physical setting, CMHCs had to contend with fragmentation of services and authority and with the fact that patients typically encountered severe and unremitting geographical, economic, sociological, and psychological barriers in their efforts to receive mental health care.

Thus, although CMHCs were to have been for all the residents of the catchment area, and although they were to have responded to the global and life-long mental health service needs of the entire population, they frequently failed to make contact with other facilities serving the mentally ill, including state mental hospitals. Episodes of patient care became disjointed , as individuals were often admitted to, and discharged from, a variety of service sites, with no central authority to co-ordinate their treatment plans (Bachrach 1981). Many patients were totally 'lost' to CMHCs that often did not know where or even who they were, even though these were the very agencies charged with serving, or at least co-ordinating all their mental health needs.

Comprehensiveness and continuity proved to be difficult to achieve, even when patients did not have problems of geographical fragmentation, and used CMHCs for all their service needs. Within those facilities there were often serious communication difficulties — boundary problems arising from guild interests among staff members, and inadequate information systems — that prevented them from reaching patients effectively, despite the development early in the movement of sophisticated data collection techniques (Bass 1972, Person 1969).

ACCOMPLISHMENTS

What conclusions may we draw from this discussion of the life and times of the federally funded CMHC movement in the United States? Opinions concerning impacts and effects vary greatly (Panzetta 1985, Pardes & Stockdill 1984), and assessments range from enthusiastic reports of model practices which ought to be diffused in this post-CMHC era (Rieman et al 1985) to negative reports of the movement's 'noble failure' (Smith & Hart 1975). Goldman & Morrissey (1985), on the other hand, see the CMHC programme as the 'third cycle of reform' in the history of mental health services in the United States — the dialectical issue of earlier approaches that had run their course.

Indeed, we probably lack the historical perspective at this time to offer a definitive judgement of the federally funded CMHC programme. However, since the foregoing pages have devoted themselves largely to documenting the movement's inability to realise its several goals, it seems only reasonable and fair to present positive evidence also; for, despite the difficulties in goal attainment, it had an unmistakably salubrious effect on the delivery of mental health services in the United States. The positive aspects of the CMHC initiative lend themselves to briefer discussion than do the problems, but that does not mean that they were any the less remarkable.

The fact is that many Americans have benefited and continue to profit from the new emphases in service delivery that were proposed and promoted by the CMHC legislation. More than a few local services met with considerable success in achieving at least most of the goals described above; and if they did not succeed in preventing and eliminating psychiatric illness, they did at least provide a level of humane care for their patients that probably could not have been imagined in the days before the community mental health initiative (Talbott 1981). It is those successful efforts that continue to encourage planners and providers of services in the US today, to work for the wider distribution of effective and relevant community-based mental health care and to attempt to inject change into a system that often appears to seek its equilibrium in inflexibility and unresponsiveness.

The major accomplishment of the federally funded CMHC effort was its fostering of a basic change in the ways in which these planners and providers — and even the public — now think about services and service priorities for psychiatric patients, particularly the chronically mentally ill (James 1987). This is a lasting and important contribution, albeit a subtle one. Professionals are far more responsive today to the plight of the mentally ill than they were before the CMHC effort began. James (1987), reporting on the results of a survey of the 50 states commissioners of mental health, finds that policy makers at the state level, despite their limited resources, are now indicating a clear preference for serving the unserved and under-served, including the chronically mentally ill, in humane, non-institutional facilities. Similar findings are reported by Jerrell & Larsen (1986). Indeed, as the result of ideologies and priorities adopted during the CMHC era, even state mental hospitals have today become less isolated and have substantially altered the formats of their programmes (GAP 1983). Smaller residential clusters and programmes specifically directed toward patients' psychosocial rehabilitation are increasingly in evidence in state hospitals today (Bachrach 1989).

In fact, there seems to be substantial agreement within the American mental health community that the federally funded CMHC effort gene-rated a variety of tested technologies that may generally be adopted with success in providing non-institutional services for psychiatric patients. Some of these technologies are related to progress in psycho-pharmacology, but many are more closely related to the process of service delivery. For example, Gaylin & Rosenfeld (1978) summarise both positive steps to pursue and caveats to observe in developing community-based mental health programmes. They caution against wholesale placements of large numbers of patients in any particular neighbourhood — a caveat curiously overlooked in much of the early deinsti-tutionalisation literature. They also point out the counter-productivity of 'sneaking' programmes into communities surreptitiously. On a more positive note, Gaylin & Rosenfeld encourage the pursuit of programmes that evolve out of the expressed needs of the community, not out of stipulated state or federal regulations. They also urge the promotion of services that are administratively linked to programmes already in existence and 'perceived positively by the residents of the community'.

Indeed, a corpus of highly specific programme planning literature has emerged, and it emphasises several inter-related principles of planning whose importance has been established over the past several decades (Bachrach 1983a). One such principle revolves around the need for precise identification of the patient population to be treated in community-based service settings, as well as the precise delineation of programme goals (Hagedorn 1977, Rossi 1978). It is no longer considered sufficient to 'reduce the role of the state hospital' — a vague but oft-stated programme goal in the early years of deinstitutionalisation; instead, it is now considered necessary to indicate which particular patients may best be served in the community and what specific interventions they require. Another planning principle involves the individual tailoring of treatments for psychiatric patients and the placement of these people in facilities and programmes that correspond to their needs. The locus of a programme is now widely regarded as less important than its relevance for the individuals it serves — another apparently simple notion that was frequently overlooked in an era when major emphasis was placed on eliminating state hospital activities. Still another planning principle underscores the need to proceed with caution in programme development and to guard against being seduced by the 'quick fix' — an understandable tendency when public policy evolves from strongly held ideals. It is now acknowledged widely that deinstitutionalisation is far too complex a phenomenon to be amenable to 'quick-and-easy' solutions, and that the latent functions of revamping service systems must be anticipated as much as possible (Bachrach 1976).

It is important to note these principles, for they have the potential for surviving the current political climate in the US, and thus may serve as the foundation for future planning. James (1987) appropriately points out that even though the past 20 years have witnessed one 'passive' and two 'frankly hostile' federal administrations, commitment to improving the care of the mentally ill has survived in state and local planning agencies. Moreover, we may anticipate more supportive federal administrations in the future, for attitudes regarding social responsibility in the US clearly undergo major swings. If federal concern peaked during the 1960s, it is assuredly at a low ebb in the late 1980s. Ironically, the federal commitment and dedication of the CMHC era existed in the absence of well-defined principles of planning and service delivery. The reverse is true today, and the implementation of many tested and established procedures awaits the re-emergence of an enabling political climate.

The contributions of the CMHC movement to patient care are manifold. Through its emphasis on local options and citizen participation, the movement demonstrated the importance of mental health systems' responsiveness to the concerns of patients and their families. The publication of a series of eloquent first-hand accounts written by patients for professional audiences (Leete 1987, Leighton 1988, Lovejoy 1982, Sharpe 1987) suggests that service planners and providers have indeed learned to listen to the concerns of those who are most deeply affected by mental illness. Similarly, the growth of family advocacy in the United States, particularly through the organised efforts of the National Alliance for the Mentally Ill (NAMI) (Howe & Howe 1987), continues to promote sensitivity among mental health professionals — a sensitivity largely lacking in the past — to the sociological and economic realities that often divide service providers and service recipients. NAMI, which was founded in 1979 and today consists of more than 700 affiliated chapters in communities throughout the US, reports that during 1987, a new affiliate group was formed every 36 hours. In response, many service agencies today are offering family support programmes which 'appear to provide a unique natural linkage ... and promote a strong alliance among families, citizens, advocacy groups, and service providers' (Craig et al 1987). Even the language describing these programmes is a clear reminder of, and survival from, the 1960s. It is difficult to imagine their existence today without the groundwork laid in the CMHC era.

The CMHC's programme's determination to place psychiatric patients in the mainstream of life and to restore their civil rights has also had a profound and positive influence on American psychiatric services in the 1980s — an influence that may be expected to continue. Although the glamour of 'normalisation' has begun to wear thin (Bachrach 1987), it is likely that mental health professionals will continue to conceptualize clinical care in a rehabilitative framework (James 1987). It is commonplace now — and it was not, prior to the CMHC effort — for service providers to plan programmes responsive to patients' functional and adaptive deficits, even as they look for ways to deal with the underlying illnesses (Anthony et al 1983). Thus, although it may not totally have humanised the mental health system, the CMHC movement did succeed in reinforcing a humane approach to patient care.

A testimony to the strength of these accomplishments lies in contemporary efforts on the part of psychiatrists to preserve the positive values of the CMHC movement by renewing and expanding their involvement in today's community mental health centres, the descendants of the CMHCs (Beigel 1984, Clark & Vaccaro 1987). In 1984, the American Association of Community Mental Health Psychiatrists was formed with the objectives of providing mutual support and developing cohesive and politically effective policies to 'stem the tide of psychiatrists leaving community mental health centers' (Problems 1985). In the following year, a Joint Steering Committee of the American Psychiatric Association and the National Council of Community Mental Health Centers was organised to consider issues in the recruitment and retention of psychiatrists in community mental health centres (American Psychiatric Association 1985), while these centres are being used as training sites for psychiatric residents (Stein 1985). These efforts are clearly directed toward reversing the negative effects of boundary-busting by renewing medical and psychiatric involvement in community mental health.

CONCLUSIONS

Although it will probably be some time before definitive conclusions about the federally funded CMHC programme in the US may be reached, it is not too soon to make some general observations about its basic impact. A first observation is that American mental health policy, lacking as it does a long-term federal and popular commitment to care for those in need, vacillates with the political winds. The United States and South Africa are at present the only two developed countries in the world that lack universal health insurance (Nadelson 1986). The effects of this situation on general access to mental health care in the US are profound. To the extent that the federally funded CMHC programme may be regarded as a 'failure', some of the responsibility rests with a national ethos that idealises independence and individual ingenuity and so minimises the needs of severely disabled persons (Freedman 1967).

Given this reality, it seems that inequities in service delivery in the US are inevitable. Those least able to advocate on their own behalf — the chronically mentally ill — are likely to experience the greatest barriers to care, whatever the political climate, for they represent a patient population that is often devalued by mental health professionals and the public alike (Stern & Minkoff 1979). Future planning efforts certainly ought to be directed toward reducing the effects of these inevitabilities to a minimum; total success is unlikely, but awareness of reality may help to stem the kind of expansiveness that characterised the CMHC era.

A second observation is that, when mental health policy is formulated in an imprecise manner, implementation is not practicable even in a political climate that supports it. If ever federally funded community mental health services could have worked in the United States, it should have been in the days of the Great Society, but with no clear statement of mission, local policy makers were able to project their own priorities onto the federally funded effort. A boundary-less initiative is destined to encounter failure, for in its unbounded enthusiasm to provide everything for everyone, it cannot satisfactorily justify selecting one priority over another.

A third observation is that post mortems often raise more questions than they answer, but may shed light on apparent paradoxes. Dr Bertram Brown, a former Director of the National Institute of Mental Health, who is widely identified with the CMHC effort, has stated that the movement's architects engaged in a political game when they oversold community mental health — 'the bureaucrat-psychiatrists realised that there was political and financial overpromise... doctors were overpromising for the politicians. [They] did not believe that community care would cure schizophrenia, and did allow [themselves] to be somewhat misrepresented'. He continued, 'We [even] knew that there were not enough resources in the community to do the whole job, so that some people would be in the streets facing society head-on and questions would be raised about the necessity to send them back to the state hospital ... [but] it happened faster than we foresaw' (Lyons 1984).

Fourth and finally, in spite of the lack of boundaries, the absence of defined purpose, and inattention to the needs of the chronically mentally ill; in spite of the movement's difficulty in fulfilling its own basic goals, and Brown's statement notwithstanding, it is important to stress the positive legacy of the federal government's involvement in community mental health. The foregoing brief discussion of successes does not do justice to the legitimating influence that the CMHC initiative had. Any policy which generates so much hope and which, through that hope, effects such far-reaching changes in service planning must be viewed positively. At the very least, it provides a source of vital energy for future development. A policy's success may be assessed in a number of ways, and not only on the basis of goal attainment; it may also be measured, for instance, in terms of its potential for future change. More than any other major mental health initiative in the US, the short-lived federally sponsored CMHC movement managed to provide experimental formats for changing the delivery of services and to alter national attitudes about expectations of, and entitlements for psychiatric patients (Talbott 1981). We shall probably never fully return to the wholesale thoughtlessness and cruelty that were standard practice in many service settings in the first half of the twentieth century.

The CMHC movement has, through both its problems and its successes, taught the American people a great deal about how to design — and coincidentally how not to design — mental health services. It remains for future generations of policy makers to carry on from there.

REFERENCES

American Medical Association Council on Scientific Affairs 1979 Evaluation of community mental health centers. Association, Chicago

American Psychiatric Association and National Council of Community Mental Health Centers 1985 Community mental health centers and psychiatrists. Association, Washington

Anthony W A, Cohen M R, Cohen B F 1983 Philosophy, treatment process, and principles of the psychiatric rehabilitation approach. In: Bachrach L L (ed) Deinstitutionalization. New Directions for Mental Health Services 17. Jossey-Bass, San Francisco: pp 67-79

Bachrach L L 1974a Characteristics of federally funded rural community mental health centers in 1971. Mental Health Statistical Notes 101: 1-34

Bachrach L L 1974b Patients at federally funded rural community mental health centers in 1971. Mental Health Statistical Notes 102: 1-22

Bachrach L L 1976 Deinstitutionalization: an analytical review and sociological perspective. National Institute of Mental Health, Rockville, Maryland

Bachrach L L 1981 Continuity of care for chronic mental patients: a conceptual analysis. American Journal of Psychiatry 138: 1449-1456

Bachrach L L 1982 The process of deinstitutionalisation in rural areas. In: Keller P A, Murray J D (eds) Handbook of rural community mental health. Human Sciences, New York: pp 110-121

Bachrach L L 1983a Planning services for chronically mentally ill patients. Bulletin of the Menninger Clinic 47: 163-188

Bachrach L L 1983b Psychiatric services in rural areas: a sociological overview. Hospital & Community Psychiatry 34: 215-226

Bachrach L L 1984a Asylum and chronically ill psychiatric patients. American Journal of Psychiatry 141: 975-978

Bachrach L L 1984b The homeless mentally ill and mental health services: an analytical review of the literature. In: Lamb H R (ed) The homeless mentally ill. American Psychiatric Association, Washington: pp 11-53

Bachrach L L 1985 General hospital psychiatry and deinstitutionalisation: a systems view. General Hospital Psychiatry 7: 239-248

Bachrach L L 1986 Deinstitutionalisation: what do the numbers mean? Hospital & Community Psychiatry 37: 118-119, 121

Bachrach L L 1987 The context of care for the chronic mental patient with substance abuse problems. Psychiatric Quarterly 58: 3-14

Bachrach L L 1989 The state mental hospital and public psychiatry. In: Beels C C Bachrach L L (eds) Survival strategies for public psychiatry. Jossey-Bass, San Francisco

Bass R D 1972 Method for measuring continuity of care in a community mental health center. National Institute of Mental Health, Rockville, Maryland

Beigel A 1984 The remedicalization of community mental health. Hospital & Community

Psychiatry 35: 1114-1117

Berlin R M, Kales J D, Humphrey F J, Kales A 1981 The patient care crisis in community mental health centers: a need for more psychiatric involvement. American Journal of Psychiatry 138

Borus J F 1978 Issues critical to the survival of community mental health. American Journal of Psychiatry 135: 1029-1035

Campbell D T 1979 Assessing the impact of planned social change. Evaluation & Program Planning 2: 67-90

Clark G H, Vaccaro J V 1987 Burnout among CMHC psychiatrists and the struggle to survive. Hospital & Community Psychiatry 38: 843-847

Comptroller General of the United States 1977 Returning the mentally disabled to the community: government needs to do more. General Accounting Office, Washington

Comptroller General of the United States 1984 States have made few changes in implementing the Alcohol, Drug Abuse, and Mental Health Services Block Grant. General Accounting Office, Washington

Cook T D, Shadish W R 1982 Metaevaluation: an assessment of the congressionally mandated evaluation system for community mental health centers. In: Stahler G J, Tash W R (eds) Innovative approaches to mental health evaluation. Academic Press, New York: pp 221-253

Craig T J H, Hussey P A, Kaye D A et al 1987 Family support programs in a regional mental health system. Hospital & Community Psychiatry 38: 459-460

Dinitz S, Beran N 1971 Community mental health as a boundaryless and boundary-busting system. Journal of Health & Social Behavior 12: 99-108

Donovan C M 1982 Problems of psychiatric practice in community mental health centers. American Journal of Psychiatry 139: 456-460

Fink P J, Weinstein S P 1979 Whatever happened to psychiatry: the deprofessionalization of community mental health centers. American Journal of Psychiatry 136: 406-409

Freedman A M 1967 Historical and political roots of the Community Mental Health Centers Act. American Journal of Orthopsychiatry 37: 487-494

Gaylin S, Rosenfeld P 1978 Establishing community services for the mentally ill: a summary of lessons learned. Psychiatric Quarterly 50: 295-298

Goldman H H, Morrissey J P 1985 The alchemy of mental health policy: homelessness and the fourth cycle of reform. American Journal of Public Health 75: 727-731

Goldman H H, Gattozzi A A, Taube C A 1981 Defining and counting the chronically mentally ill. Hospital & Community Psychiatry 32: 21-27

Goldman H H, Adams N H, Taube C A 1983 Deinstitutionalization: the data demythologized. Hospital & Community Psychiatry 34: 129-134

Grofein W 1985 Incentives and intentions in mental health policy: a comparison of the Medicaid and Community Mental Health Programs. Journal of Health & Social Behavior 26: 192-206

Group for the Advancement of Psychiatry 1983 Community psychiatry: a reappraisal. Mental Health Materials Center, New York

Group for the Advancement of Psychiatry 1986 A family affair: helping families cope with mental illness: a guide for the professions. Brunner/Mazel, New York

Hagedorn H 1977 A manual on state mental health planning. National Institute of Mental Health, Rockville, Maryland

Hansell N 1978 Services for schizophrenics: a lifelong approach to treatment. Hospital & Community Psychiatry 29: 105-109

Hopkin J T 1985 Psychiatry and medicine in the emergency room. In: Lipton F R, Goldfinger S M (eds) Emergency psychiatry at the crossroads. New Directions for Mental Health Services 28. Jossey-Bass, San Francisco: pp 47-53

Howe C W, Howe J W 1987 The National Alliance for the Mentally Ill: history and ideology. In: Hatfield A B (ed) Families of the mentally ill: meeting the challenges. New Directions for Mental Health Services 34. Jossey-Bass, San Francisco: pp 23-33

James J F 1987 Does the community mental health movement have the momentum needed to survive? American Journal of Orthopsychiatry 57: 447-451

Jerrell J M, Larsen J K 1983 The mental health system in transition: a summary of changes reported 1980-1982. Technical Report 83-10. Cognos Associates, Los Altos, California

Jerrell J M, Larsen J K 1985 How community mental health centers deal with cutbacks and competition. Hospital & Community Psychiatry 36: 1169-1174

Jerrell J M, Larsen J K 1986 Community mental health services in transition: who is benefiting? American Journal of Orthopsychiatry 56: 78-88

Kennedy J F 1963 (5 February) Message from the President of the United States relative to mental illness and mental retardation. 88th Congress, First session, House of Representatives document 58, Washington

Lamb H R 1982 Treating the long-term mentally ill: beyond deinstitutionalization. Jossey-Bass, San Francisco

Lamb H R (ed) 1984 The homeless mentally ill. American Psychiatry Association, Washington

Langsley D G 1980a The community mental health center: does it treat patients? Hospital & Community Psychiatry 31: 815-819

Langsley D G 1980b Community psychiatry. In: Kaplan H I, Freedman A M (eds) Comprehensive textbook of psychiatry. Williams & Wilkins, Baltimore: pp 2836-2854

Larsen J K, Jerrell J M 1983 Mental health services in transition. Technical Report 83-84. Cognos Associates, Los Altos, California

Leete E 1987 The treatment of schizophrenia: a patient's perspective. Hospital & Community Psychiatry 38: 486-491

Leighton D C 1988 Being mentally ill in America: one female's experience. In: Bachrach L, Nadelson C C (eds) Treating chronically mentally ill women. American Psychiatric Press, Washington: pp 65-73

Leong G B 1982 Psychiatrists and community mental health centers: can their relationship be salvaged? Hospital & Community Psychiatry 33: 309-310

Lovejoy M 1982 Expectations and the recovery process. Schizophrenia Bulletin 8: 605-609

Lyons R D 1984 (10 October) How release of mental patients began. New York Times, p C1, C4

Marcos L R, Gil R M 1984 Psychiatric catchment areas in an urban center: a policy in disarray. American Journal of Psychiatry 141: 875-878

Mollica R F 1983 From asylum to community: the threatened disintegration of public psychiatry. New England Journal of Medicine 308: 367-373

Morrissey J P, Goldman H H 1984 Cycles of reform in the care of the chronically mentally ill. Hospital & Community Psychiatry 35: 785-793

Musto D A 1975 Whatever happened to 'community mental health'? Public Interest 39: 52-79

Nadelson C C 1986 Psychiatry across borders. Hospital & Community Psychiatry 37: 142-147

Naierman N, Haskins B, Robinson G 1978 Community mental health centers — a decade later. Abt Associates, Cambridge, Massachusetts

Nash M D, Argyle N J 1984 Services for the mentally ill: a reversal in federal policy. Administration in Mental Health 11: 263-276

National Institute of Mental Health (undated) Data sheet on number of resident patients, total admissions, net releases, and deaths, state and county mental hospitals: United States, 1950-1982. Rockville, Maryland

National Institute of Mental Health 1977a (21 October) Staffing differences between federally funded CHMCs located in metropolitan and nonmetropolitan catchment areas 1976. Division of Biometry & Epidemiology Memorandum 21. Rockville, Maryland

National Institute of Mental Health 1977b (25 November) A comparison of federally funded community mental health centers in metropolitan and non-metropolitan catchment areas: sources of funds. Division of Biometry & Epidemiology Memorandum 25. Rockville, Maryland

National Institute of Mental Health 1978 (27 January) Staffing differences between federally funded CMHCs located in low income and high income catchment areas, 1976. Division of Biometry & Epidemiology Memorandum 30. Rockville, Maryland

Ochberg F M 1976 Community mental health center legislation: flight of the phoenix. American Journal of Psychiatry 133: 56-61

Okin R L 1984 How community mental health centers are coping. Hospital & Community Psychiatry 35: 1118-1125

Panzetta A F 1985 Whatever happened to community mental health: portents for corporate medicine. Hospital & Community Psychiatry 36: 1174-1179

Pardes H, Stockdill J W 1984 Survival strategies for community mental health services in the 1980s. Hospital & Community Psychiatry 35: 127-132

Person P H 1969 A statistical information system for community mental health centers. National Institute of Mental Health, Rockville, Maryland

Peterson C L 1985 Regulation and consultation in community care facilities. Hospital & Community Psychiatry 36: 383-388

President's Commission on Mental Health 1978 Report to the President. The White House, Washington

Problems in CMHCs spur formation of support group 1985 (1 March). Psychiatric News: 1-16

Redick R W, Witkin M J, Bethel H E, Manderscheid R W 1985 Staffing of specialty mental health organisations, United States, 1978-80. Mental Health Statistical Notes 172: 1-14

Rieman D W, Cravens R B, Stroul B A 1985 Notable solutions to problems in mental health service delivery. National Institute of Mental Health, Rockville, Maryland

Rossi P H 1978 Issues in the evaluation of human services delivery. Evaluation Quarterly 2: 573-599

Sharpe M L 1987 Out of the streets and into the subculture: psychiatry's problem from a patient's perspective. In: Meyerson A T (ed) Barriers to treating the chronic mentally ill. New Directions for Mental Health Services 33. Jossey-Bass, San Francisco: pp 63-74

Shepherd G 1984 Institutional care and rehabilitation. Longman, London

Sheppard N 1981 (1 January) Cocktail parties combating alcoholism. New York Times p 5

Smith W G, Hart D W 1975 Community mental health: a noble failure? Hospital & Community Psychiatry 26: 581-583

Stein L I 1985 (May) Psychiatric residency training and the community mental health center. Community Psychiatrist: Newsletter of the American Association of Community Mental Health Centers 1: 9

Stern R, Minkoff K 1979 Paradoxes in programming for chronic patients in a community clinic. Hospital & Community Psychiatry 30: 613-617

Talbott J A (ed) 1981 The chronic mentally ill: treatment, programs, systems. Human Sciences Press, New York

Task Panel on Community Mental Health Centers Assessment 1978 (A) Reports submitted to the President's Commission on Mental Health vol 2. The White House, Washington: 312-338

Task Panel on Rural Mental Health 1978 (B) Reports submitted to the President's Commission on Mental Health vol 3. The White House, Washington: 1155-1190

Thompson J W, Bass R D 1984 Changing staffing patterns in community mental health centers. Hospital & Community Psychiatry 35: 1107-1114

Thompson J W, Bass R D, Witkin M J 1982 Fifty years of psychiatric services: 1940-1990. Hospital & Community Psychiatry 33: 711-717

Thurer S 1983 Deinstitutionalization and women: where the buck stops. Hospital & Community Psychiatry 34: 1162-1163

Vaccaro J V 1988 (January) Psychiatry in the community. National Council of Community Mental Health Centers News: 2, 5

Weiner R S, Woy J R, Sharfstein S S, Bass R D 1979 Community mental health centers and the 'seed money concept': effects of terminating federal funds. Community Mental Health Journal 15: 129-138

Windle C, Scully D 1976 Community mental health centers and the decreasing use of state mental hospitals. Community Mental Health Journal 12: 239-243

Windle C, Woy J R 1983 From programs to systems: implications for program evaluation illustrated by the community mental health center experience. Evaluation & Program Planning 6: 53-68

Wing J K, Morris B 1981 Clinical basis of rehabilitation. In: Wing J K, Morris B (eds) Handbook of psychiatric rehabilitation. Oxford University Press, Oxford: 3-16

Winslow W W 1982 Changing trends in CMHCs: keys to survival in the eighties. Hospital & Community Psychiatry 33: 273-277

Woy J R, Wasserman D B, Weiner-Pomerants R 1981 Community mental health centers: movement away from the model? Community Mental Health Journal 17: 265-276

Zusman J, Lamb H R 1977 In defense of community mental health. American Journal of Psychiatry 134: 887-890

20. Equity, effectiveness and equality in the mental health services

R.F. Mollica   B.M. Astrachan

INTRODUCTION

The following three vignettes quoted from a doctor concerned about the plight of a homeless woman, a Wall Street investment firm, and the report of a state psychiatric hospital association, respectively, reveal the differing orientations, goals and aims (often contradictory) that exist in modern American mental health policy.

Vignette A

On cold Mondays in February, the victims of winter cluster at Bellevue: infarction and pneumonia, exposure and gangrene, drive the inhabitants of streets and parks to its doors. It was, therefore, a routine event when police brought Mrs Kahaner to the emergency room. Suffering from apparent frostbite, she had been found at the entrance of Lord and Taylor's department store early on Sunday morning, and was admitted with a temperature of 93°F.

The nurse's notes described her belongings. She was evidently the prototypic bag lady; her rags, pots, and jumbled impediments overflowed five shopping bags crammed into a wire cart. An unkempt appointment slip found in her purse identified her as a former inpatient of one of the New York State mental hospitals, from which she had last been discharged three years before. A telephone call to that hospital yielded her provisional diagnosis (chronic schizophrenia), her medication on discharge (the usual phenothiazine derivatives), and her age, 56; there is little chance that the poor mad people (like Mrs Kahaner) will find in American society even the glint of a golden age. In the cities of the US, where the Mrs Kahaners wander outside the asylums in solitary danger, where danger is unchecked, and where the aggressive roam in quest of drugs and easy victims, people have, instead, partly reverted to the Hobbesian state of nature (Weissman 1982).

Vignette B

Because of the nature of psychiatric care, the psychiatric hospital industry is an attractive sub-segment of the hospital industry for investors.

Inpatient care is widely insured against, occurs with predictable and increasing incidence, and is complex enough to render cost control efforts difficult. In addition, psychiatric hospitals enjoy a number of advantages over general hospitals. These include the widespread acceptance of two classes of psychiatric care (high-quality care in private psychiatric hospitals or in psychiatric units of general hospitals versus lower quality care in government-owned mental health centres), the ability of the industries services to be marketed, and certain cost advantages (Sherlock 1984).

Vignette C

In 1966, the Commonwealth of Massachusetts enacted a law (Ch. 735) establishing regional boundaries for mental health services, and encouraging regional programming. In the mid-1970s, under the leadership of Dr Okun, the State Department of Mental Health began a vigorous programme for the development of community-based resources for community care and deinstitutionalisation of the disabledly mentally ill. During the 1970s, Massachusetts also participated in the nationwide growth of psychiatric services (Astrachan 1991, in press). State hospital beds continued to be reduced, as private hospital and general hospital beds opened, while in all settings lengths of stay significantly decreased. However, there is a growing consensus that what is needed is a state-wide policy, clarifying the responsibilities of both private and public sectors, and how they can together shape a greatly needed co-ordinated system of care (Lind et al 1984).

Vignette A decries the discontinuity of care in the public sector for the chronically mentally ill, including lack of co-ordination of psychiatric services, housing, social welfare, and medical care. Vignette B emphasises the opportunity for profit in the delivery of mental health care to the more affluent members of society. The private sector, in contrast to the public one, is not driven by need but by the economics of the market place. Vignette C stresses the perceived lack of co-ordination that exists between the public and private sectors of psychiatry. Yet, many in the private sector view this desire for co-ordination as a 'need' which they want little to do with, especially if it means the use of state authority to restrain or direct private interests.

These three examples reveal only superficially the general lack of consensus that exists between various interests that influence American mental health policy. The present mental health system in the United States (as well as in Europe) is so complex and the terms used to describe it by economists and planners (e.g. Diagnosis Related Groups (DRGs)) are so arcane, that they defy understanding by patients, practitioners, and the general public alike. This chapter, therefore, will use the American psychiatric experience of the past three decades as a model for elucidating what the authors consider to be the three most essential dimensions of modern mental health policy. These dimensions called *equity, effectiveness (efficiency)*, and *equality* will be defined and clarified. They will be used to provide a systematic framework for evaluating the existing organisational structure and priorities of the American mental health system.

Additionally, the major dimensions of psychiatric care describe the psychiatric field's major goals and clinical outcomes. Psychiatric care is both an applied scientific discipline and a social practice. As part of medical science, psychiatric treatments are developed to be utilised in our care-giving systems in order to produce cures for or limit the progression of illness, and to minimise associated psychological distress and social disabilities. Unfortunately, the gap between the scientific study of human behaviours and psychopathology on the one hand, and a practical societal response to mental disorders on the other remains wide (Mollica 1986). The mental health field, and especially its public sector, remains troubled by its continued inability to transform modern psychiatric theories and technical advances into effective clinical and social programmes. For example, in spite of the enormous advances that have occurred in the scientific study of psychiatric disorders over the past 25 years, public mental health services to the poor and seriously disabled remain extremely limited and often ineffective (Mollica 1983). Since mental health services in the United States are not integrated into a coherent social service system, the problems of poverty, of lack of resources, and of failure to co-ordinate social and rehabilitative resources into the overall care of the mentally ill confound the clinical expertise that is available. In addition, new problems have emerged such as the 'homeless', as housing for the poor becomes less possible. Policy planners therefore have a complex and extremely difficult challenge, i.e. to transform psychiatric knowledge into socially useful programmes. That this is no easy task will be revealed by this chapter's review of the essential features of American mental health policy.

THE GOALS OF MENTAL HEALTH POLICY

No simple response exists to the question: what are the major goals of American mental health policy? Hypothetically, such a policy exists to enhance the positive mental health of its citizens (Astrachan & Tischler 1984). It might be assumed (as it is by most Americans) that this can be accomplished by increasing access to mental health services, maintaining quality of care and reducing costs. Yet, behind generalised hypothetical statements of purpose are major disagreements in political values and real policy conflicts that generate fierce political struggles, pitting one vested interest against another. For example, mental health care is not generally seen as an American's intrinsic political 'right': federal, state, and local governments continually shift the degree of commitment that they have on the one hand to providing mental health services to 'highly disabled' groups such as the chronically mentally ill or the alcoholically disabled, or on the other to preventive and educative services that benefit the entire society. Secondly, it is unclear how much the state can influence the direction of both public and private sectors through governmental activities, such as allocation of resources, taxes, licensing, etc. The major issue is a social lack of consensus on the extent to which a state can extend its direct control over a sector of the economy (i.e. mental health care) and define policy, and if so, by using what mechanisms.

Furthermore, a simple statement of mental health goals is further confounded by the different value systems and social interests of the various groups affected by mental health care.

Consumers

The consumers of mental health services are extremely heterogeneous: many individuals who reflect the greatest demand and need for care often have the least amount of money to pay for these services. By struggling to do good for all of its citizens, American society is more often than not confronted with the problem of shifting resources from the 'haves' to the 'have-nots'. Mental Health policy in the United States has traditionally been defined on a state-by-state basis, but the Federal government's first attempts to influence state policy began in the 1960s (see page 543). Additionally, Federal policy initiatives designed to help provide care for the aged, the disabled, and the poor have influenced the continuing development of state policy (Katz 1984). Yet in spite of these initiatives, the poor in America are still mistrusted, and consequently receive limited social welfare support because of the general conception that poverty is caused by moral inadequacies and the lack of initiative (Williams et al 1980, Foucault 1965). Also those bureaucracies which have arisen to serve the mentally ill are usually so large and complex they are difficult for patients to negotiate, and in addition, they only poorly co-ordinate their services with each other. For many recipients of service, questions of liberty versus society's definition of care are also crucially important. Do patients have the right to remain unserved? Do the poor more frequently receive coercive treatments, and even more coercive forms of care? Finally, one citizen's enhanced mental health is another citizen's dilemma — communities have persistently resisted the introduction of mentally ill individuals into half-way houses and day-treatment settings into their communities.

Professional providers

Professionals generally seek to work in conditions in which both their needs for autonomy over practice and their desires for financial recompense are satisfied. In an economic environment in which both regulation and competition are stressed, many organisations attempt to recruit professionals by emphasising both economic and professional practice advantages. The academic world has been particularly successful in meeting these needs, while public sector psychiatric practice has tended to pay poorly — and to dramatically limit professional autonomy. It is not surprising that academic positions remain desirous, while public sector positions have tended to recruit psychiatrists who often view themselves as second-class. Some limited attempts to combine academic and public sector roles have improved psychiatric services in a few states, yet this strategy cannot conceivably answer more than a fraction of the need of public systems for qualified psychiatrists. The challenge to public psychiatry is how to develop systems with clear direction, competent senior level medical leadership, and adequate peer review, so that medical autonomy can be fostered in an accountable manner.

Institutional employees

Publically supported mental health hospitals and community mental health centres provide jobs in large numbers: in many small American towns, the state mental hospital is that town's major industry. These institutionally-based and often highly unionised employees, therefore, have a major vested interest in maintaining the status quo, as well as in resisting wage controls and changes in the management of clinical programmes.

Government units

Government units have a strong interest in pursuing their legislated public policies, and in America, these policies can dramatically change in direction between one political election year and another. For example, many state governments are increasingly emphasising a mental health policy that integrates inpatient, outpatient, and community services for disabled patient groups. Unfortunately, however, government units are often ineffective in accomplishing their goals at reduced costs because of their large bureaucratic structures. These large bureaucracies are usually unable to assess and monitor the quality of care and the effectiveness of literally hundreds of state-supported institutions, programmes, contracts, etc. (Dorwart et al 1986).

Private enterprise

The Salomon Brothers statement (Sherlock 1984) reveals that mental health can be a lucrative profit market. Private enterprise capitalises both on the expansion of the two-tier system of care, and on the allocation of resources to mental health practitioners and procedures that can generate the highest profit margins. These decisions are not necessarily in the best interest of patients, nor do they ensure cost control.

Insurance companies

Similarly, insurance companies and Health Maintenance Organisations (HMOs) attempt to control the mental health market that they dominate by limiting costs and services. In particular, they may attempt to eliminate from their programme those individuals with serious mental handicaps who are in need of long-term mental health care (Wolfe et al, in press). This represents sound policy to the private insurers, because they assume it is the state's responsibility to provide mental health care to the uninsured.

Academic psychiatry

The attention of academic psychiatry has never been strongly focused on the social aetiology of mental disorders or on the social rehabilitation of the mentally ill. Increasingly, the psychiatric academy is directing its interests to 'pure' as opposed to 'applied' research; in emphasising the search for ultimate causes and diminishing attention to social (and even at times biological) contexts, it is diminishing its commitment to the evaluation of mental health services, and is reducing its contribution to mental health policy debates, except as they affect the public funding of the basic sciences.

Finally, although many academic departments have a substantial connection with public practice, only very few have responsibility for the total management of patients. Thus, the service emphasis of most academic departments has been on acute, short-term care and on neurophysiological management. Rehabilitation is rarely stressed, and teaching about rehabilitation even more rarely considered seriously.

THE EVOLUTION OF AMERICAN MENTAL HEALTH POLICY: A 40-YEAR OVERVIEW

Institutions, patients and practitioners

Historically, psychiatric and mental health services within the United States have been separate from the general health care system. In the mid-1950s, when Hollingshead & Redlich (1958) examined the utilisation of psychiatric services in the New Haven, Connecticut area, more inpatient than outpatient treatment episodes were identified, and the single largest provider of care was the state hospital, which assumed sole responsibility for the state's impoverished mentally ill. Outpatient care primarily served the more affluent and/or less disturbed patients: in 1955, only limited outpatient and almost no rehabilitative services were available for the community care of the chronically mentally ill. Relatively few practitioners continued to treat those outpatients who had required inpatient care, so that in general, there was a wide gap between inpatient and outpatient practice, practitioners, and patients; most inpatient care was provided in the isolated, poorly staffed, devalued state hospitals. In contrast, outpatient care was delivered by psychiatrists and some few other professionals in private offices, or in multidisciplinary clinics. The latter treatment was largely orientated to the use of psychological intervention strategies, and little responsibility was assumed for the care of the severely mentally ill.

While it is difficult to discern a coherent attempt to formulate Federal mental health policy in the 1950s (Musto 1975), the National Mental Health Act of 1946 had already set forces into motion which would help establish conditions for change. That Act established the National Institute of Mental Health and thus it further defined a major Federal commitment to the stimulation of research and to manpower training.

In 1955, the United States Congress passed the Mental Health Study Act, authorising 'an objective, thorough and nationwide analysis and re-evaluation of the human and economic problems of mental illness' (Public Law 182 1955). A Joint Commission on Mental Health and Illness was established and this made recommendations for the development of community outpatient clinics, inpatient units in general hospitals, state research and training institutes, the development of rehabilitative services at state hospitals, and increased support for research (Action For Mental Health 1962). Musto (1975) has detailed the tortuous path these recommendations travelled, as attempts were made within the Federal bureaucracy to establish mental health policy. In 1963, following a stirring call to action by President John F. Kennedy, the Community Mental Health Centers (CMHC) Act was passed (Public 88-164 1963), establishing a Federal presence in the delivery of public services to the mentally ill and largely ignoring state government and the role of the state in the delivery of services (Wolfe & Astrachan 1985). In later amendments, the Federal Government, provided grant monies for the staffing of community-based centres.

During that same period of time, the Federal Government made a major commitment for the first time to the health care of its citizens — the elderly and (after 1972) the disabled through Medicare (Public Law 89-97 1965), and the poor through Medicaid (Public Law 89-97 1965) were also provided with access to general health care and to some psychiatric services. However, the Federal Government elected to establish these initiatives within the context of the overall health care system, so that unlike the CMHC Act, which established new institutions for the delivery of services, Medicare and Medicaid paid hospital and practitioner fees for services rendered (Wolfe & Astrachan 1985). The Federal Government, though, was concerned lest payment for services provided in state hospitals should substitute federal support for state support, so that psychiatric benefits for services in state and private hospitals were limited. The care of acutely ill psychiatric patients in general hospitals was supported in a manner similar to other acute in-patient care, but all outpatient psychiatric benefits were markedly limited.

The Medicaid legislation required substantial state matching of federal funds; while many general Medicaid benefits were mandated, states were permitted much leeway in the design of mental health benefit packages. Some states provided liberal psychiatric benefits, but others only limited services. Medicaid also supported nursing home care for the disabled: again, some states provided for extensive services, whereas others carefully restricted entry into care. However, the availability of such support was crucial in spurring deinstitutionalisation efforts in many states (Rose 1979): poor patients who had been treated in inpatient psychiatric units at the expense of the state could be transferred to less costly nursing home settings, where state and Federal Government shared expenses.

These policies initiated a massive change in the delivery of services within the United States (Pardes 1979). First, the number of episodes of care dramatically increased, from 1.7 million in 1955 to 6.9 million in 1977. Secondly, the locus of care shifted: outpatient care, which accounted for 23% of 1.7 million episodes, rose to 70% of 6.9 million episodes. CMHCs, which did not exist in 1955, provided 32% of services (including inpatient, outpatient, and rehabilitative) in 1975. State and county hospitals, which provided 49% of episodes of care in 1955 — over 800000 episodes — provided 9% of episodes in 1977 — less than 600000 episodes — and lengths of stay dramatically decreased (Witkin 1980). Between 1970 and 1980, the number of state and county psychiatric beds decreased from 413000 to 156000 (Katzper & Manderscheid 1984).

Regier et al (1978) studied the location of patients with mental illness by treatment setting in a point-prevalence study, and noted that over 54% were located in the primary care/outpatient medical sector. About 6% were located in both the specialty mental health and primary care/outpatient medical sector and 15% in the specialty mental health sector; 21.5% were not in treatment or were in the human services sector, and 3.4% were in the general hospital/nursing home sector. The vast majority of specialised mental health services were provided through relatively brief, ambulatory treatment in practitioners' offices, CMHCs, clinics, HMOs, etc. The much smaller numbers of patients with prolonged disorders utilised far more resources and services.

Regier et al identified 3.1% of the US 1975 general population (6.7 million persons) as receiving specialised mental health services. Of these, 1.5 million (0.7%) received specialised hospital services, while an additional 1.1 million received treatment in general hospitals without specialised psychiatric units (where length of stay is much less and the

Table 20.1   Growth in the number and rate of mental health professionals: United States, 1955-1980

Group of professionals	1955	1980	Change
Psychiatrists [1]			
Number	10 600	30 023	183% more
Rate per 100 000 population[2]	6.4	13.7	114% more
Psychologists [3]			
Number	13 500	56 933	322% more
Rate per 100 000 population[2]	8.1	25.9	220% more
Social Workers [4]			
Number	20 000	83 000	315% more
Rate per 100 000 population[2]	12.1	37.8	212% more

[1] Data until 1960 included American Psychiatric Association membership plus filled psychiatric residency positions. 1960–1980 data also included non-members of APA who reported their specialty as psychiatry to the American Medical Association. Approximately 10% of all psychiatrists in 1980 were child psychiatrists.

[2] Source for civilian population of the United States: US Bureau of Census: Current Population Reports, Series P–25, nos. 802 and 888.

[3] Data based on membership in the American Psychological Association. Until 1983, 37% of all psychologists were in clinical counseling or guidance psychology (approximately 5400). In 1980, between 26 000 and 28 000 (52%) were licensed or certified health science provider psychologists (approximately 28 933).

[4] Data based on membership in the National Association of Social Workers. Approximately 20% to 25% of all social workers were in mental health practice. In 1980, 11 000 were on the register of 'certified clinical social workers'.

case mix less serious than in special units) and in nursing homes (where length of stay is greater). It is, of course, difficult to obtain more than an impressionistic view from these data: for example, point-prevalence data and data about episodes of care will equate a brief outpatient treatment episode with years of care in a nursing home.

A rapid growth also occurred in the various types of professionals, numbers of practising psychiatrists, and size of departments of psychiatry (Castel et al 1982, Langsley & Robinowitz 1979). Funds for clinical psychology, psychiatric social work, and later for graduate nursing education resulted in a marked growth of these professions. While the number of psychiatrists nearly tripled between 1955 and 1980, the number of psychologists and social workers more than quadrupled (see Table 20.1) (American Psychiatric Association 1983). Additionally, a wide range of innovative programmes to train mental health para-professionals were spawned in the 1960s and 1970s (Rioch et al 1963).

Yet in spite of substantial increases in the number of psychiatrists, their concentration varied greatly from state to state, with greater numbers located near academic centres and in urban areas; psychiatric manpower continued to be limited in public mental hospitals. Knepser (1978) reported that in 32 states, there was an average of two or less psychiatrists per 100 state mental hospital inpatients; only seven states averaged four or more psychiatrists per 100 inpatients. In 1979, Pardes noted that the average number of psychiatrists per mental health centre had decreased. Public practice continues to have difficulty recruiting psychiatrists, whereas practice and employment opportunities in general hospitals, private hospitals, academic settings, HMOs, etc have so far afforded acceptable career paths to practitioners.

Economics and mental health expenditures

It is hard to compile an accurate comprehensive overview of mental health expenditures, though the direct costs were estimated to be between 17.1 and 19.7 billion in 1980. Klerman (1984) estimated that 15% of the health care budget was devoted to mental health care, representing over 150 million dollars a day for direct costs, transfer costs (welfare payments, etc.), and indirect costs related to loss of employment activities and associated productivity.

Table 20.2 reveals that the speciality mental health sector utilises the majority of resources available for mental health care (53%) (Frank & Kamlet 1980).

Perhaps of even greater importance is the need to identify the extent to which public funds support mental health services, but this information is difficult to obtain because states define and pay for their treatment systems differently. In 1983, the National Association of State Mental Health Program Directors undertook a study of funding sources and expenditures of State Mental Health Agencies (SMHA) (Mazach et al 1985a, b). Total direct State expenditure was about 7.1 billion dollars, but additional, non-duplicated state and federal expenditure for direct care on behalf of the mentally ill was conservatively estimated as exceeding 1.8 billion dollars; some relevant expenditures contained in the budgets of other state agencies could not be captured and reported.

Furthermore, these data were only obtained for 36 states and do not include New York and Pennsylvania, which expend substantial amounts for public psychiatric care; nor do they include governmental expenditures for care of psychiatric patients in residential facilities. In addition, more than three billion dollars of Federal funds were expended as transfer costs for the care of the mentally ill (e.g. through disability payments, housing supports, etc.). These expenditures, welfare costs, and costs to other government bodies such as the police are usually not included in estimates of direct costs, but obviously they are not inconsiderable. Direct state mental health expenditures accounted for only 2% of overall state budgets (range 0.4% to 3.8%); direct SMHA expenditures averaged $30.19 per capita (range $8.09 to $74.06).

In the fiscal year 1983, most governmental dollars for direct care (7.1

Table 20.2   The direct cost of mental illness: United States 1980

Locale of care	Cost 1980
Specialty mental health sector	
Community Mental Health Centers	1 514 950 470
General Hospitals Psychiatric Units	463 101 963
Private Psychiatric Hospitals	760 126 200
State Mental Hospitals	3 495 780 534
Outpatient Psychiatric Clinics	602 481 700
Psychiatrist's Offices	785 066 010
Psychologist's Offices	750 374 220
Social Worker's Offices	110 359 845
VA Psychiatric Services	866 456 000
Psychotropic drugs	513 000 000
Residential Treatment Centers	446 279 650
Halfway Houses	43 129 680
Other	191 762 130
Total	10 543 667 590
General medical sector	
General Hospitals	3 188 134 600
VA General Hospitals	649 842 000
Nursing Homes	1 791 005 772
Non-Psychiatric Physician	461 465 070
Total	6 090 447 442
Human services sector	
Schools	2 759 902 301
Criminal Justice System	155 522 290
Total	2 915 424 591

billion dollars) were expended on institutional services: 64% was on in-patient care, 4% on residential care, 16% on ambulatory services, 11% could not be allocated to any specific area, and a further 5% were allocated to prevention, research, training, and other activities.

In examining the additional funds expended by other state and federal sources (1.8 billion), about one-third is spent on special education, rehabilitative and social services, another third on Medicaid (reported differently for each state — but heavily institutionally focused), and the remainder on fringe benefits, capital projects, etc. We would conservatively estimate that about 70% of the 9 billion dollars spent on direct care by state and federal sources go on institutional care (in patient, nursing home). However, in addition to those nine billion dollars, almost one billion more are spent for the mental health of the elderly through the Medicare programme.

No discussion of mental health policy would be complete without some discussion of the development of insurance benefits in the United States. By not taxing corporate contributions to employee insurance plans, and by limiting taxation of dollars expended on health care, the Federal government encouraged expenditure of dollars in the health care arena. In 1940, only about 10% of the population had any private insurance, but by 1970 almost 80% had some inpatient coverage and over 40% some outpatient coverage (Sharfstein et al 1984). The growth of insurance benefits for psychiatric disorder has, however, been less impressive; the way in which services are paid for in the areas of general health and mental health differ significantly. While the proportion of Federal and private dollars expended for health and mental health care are approximately equal, far fewer insurance dollars (12% versus 26%) and far more state dollars (28% versus 9%) are expended on mental health than on general health care. Thus, the poorest and sickest patients have historically received care from government supported services (American Psychiatric Association 1983).

EQUITY OF ACCESS AND MENTAL HEALTH POLICY

The equity concept and psychiatric services

In 1965, the US Congress stated that, 'The fulfillment of our national purpose depends on promoting and assuring the highest level of health attainable for every person, in an environment which contributes positively to healthful individual and family living... To assure comprehensive health services of high quality for every person' (Public Law 89-749 1966). This concept of equity had been a major objective of the US Community Health Center Movement (National Institute of Mental Health 1971). Unfortunately, in spite of a generalised sense within both Western Europe and America that all citizens should have equal access to mental health care, there has not been a clear elucidation of the underlying principles of equity to guide mental health planning.

The term 'equity' is the quality of 'being equal or fair'. Its social meaning is derived from the tradition in Anglo-American law in which rule or procedures constituted by law may be judged 'unfair', allowing them under special circumstances to be remedied by an appeal to the equity concept. Although X may be the legal solution, Y in fact may be the 'fair' and 'equitable' solution. Over the past 30 years, the concept of equity has been primarily applied to the problems of service accessibility and utilisation (Mollica & Redlich 1980). Equity of access to mental health care has had considerable public appeal in the United States, in spite of the fact that the country has no law guaranteeing its citizens a comprehensive right to health and mental health care; Gostin (1983) reviewed the dissimilarities in this regard between the UK and the United States. Notwithstanding this lack of constitutional guarantees of access to health care, the equity concept has been an important factor in all mental health planning in the United States over the past 40 years. Principles of distributive justice characterise mental health policy, even if they are not explicitly stated, because modern societies need to determine the means by which scarce health/ mental health resources are to be allocated. Equity of access is therefore a paramount question for policy planners, whether or not they enforce a 'market'-based approach (e.g. US) or a 'social-welfare' approach (e.g. the UK).

Daniels (1982) has reviewed and clarified the complex and confusing literature on equity of access to health care, which shows that mental health planning is confronted by many perplexing questions. How should society determine who gets mental health services? What are the types and qualities of these services? Should everyone get equal provision? What inequalities in service can a society tolerate? Anderson et al (1975) attempted to answer these questions by providing an operational definition of equity. An 'equitable distribution' does not imply that everyone should receive the same amount of health services; such a distribution occurs when illness or need — and not demographic characteristics, income, or availability of resources — is the determining factor. Daniels states that one common argument used to defend the latter approach has been the moral claim that 'if the main function of health care services is to prevent and cure illness, i.e. to meet health care needs, a distribution of health care services that is not determined by the distribution of health care needs is, therefore, unreasonable in some important sense'. Of course, Anderson et al's (1975) concept of equity of access is disputed by those who believe that individuals should compete for services within a free market system. For only a very limited period in US history, which began in the mid- to late-1960s and ended in the late 1970s, the former approach to access had also supported providing even the poorest members of society with an opportunity to obtain decent, basic minimum standards of treatment. Recently, however, these guarantees have been eroded by policy planners who do not hold that health, and especially mental health services, are basic social goods that must be made available to all citizens. These social attitudes raise such fundamental challenges to the equity concept, as originally stated by Congress in 1965 and re-stated by the President's Commission on Mental Health in 1978, that other associated concerns such as equality of care have become secondary issues.

The economic mechanisms that drive the mental health system

For over 50 years, the cost of health care in the United States has grown at a faster rate than the Gross National Product (GNP) (Kramer 1983). The passage of Medicare and Medicaid legislation gave added impetus to the growth of a health care industry. As the percentage of the GNP devoted to health care approached 10%, significant attempts were made to restrain expenditures and limit costs. However, whilst the health care environment substantially changed, the percentage of the GNP devoted to health care increased to 10.8% in 1988. The approaches used to restrain costs include: the development of capitated systems like Health Maintenance Organisations (HMOs) which contract to provide an agreed upon set of medical services for a fixed fee per enrollee; the growth of multi-institutional corporations which can provide a range of vertically integrated services (inpatient care, ambulatory care, pharmacy, home care, etc.), develop large-scale purchasing arrangements to get services and products at discount, and which actively market services; and changed benefit structures. First payers, including the government, have begun defining how they will pay for episodes of care, e.g. the DRG payment mechanism for inpatient care paid for by Medicare. Secondly, the development of large self-insured programmes by major corporations, which use pre-admission certification before permitting payment for hospital-level care, and active case management, requiring practitioners to first try less expensive forms of care (e.g. very short-term inpatient care, followed by day hospital care).

A strategy used by some providers of care, in responding to these initiatives, is the selection of patient populations who will not be very expensive to treat. Thus, services are geared to a reasonably young, employed, fit population; some HMOs even give new enrolees free membership in health clubs. The development of what is euphemistically described as 'patient acquisition strategies' permits providers to be able to function at a profit in a competitive market place. Not only do providers seek to select-in certain populations for care, but they seek to select-out those patients who cost more to treat than can be recovered from payers.

In this process, increased pressure is placed on the public sector. If the Medicare coverage of an elderly patient is not adequate to support care in the private sector, then transfer to a public hospital is likely. If the patient is discharged home rapidly, then resources of municipal visiting nurses may need to be diverted from other preventive activities to care for a seriously ill person in the home.

Without clear identification of how equity is to be managed, each sector of the health care enterprise seeks to off-load its low pay–high cost patients on to government facilities, subjecting those services to further stress, and permitting their own generation of profit. (Profits are needed, even in the private sector, for the development of new services, including the purchase of new technology.) In this process, the poor and the uninsured have diminished access to services for mild to moderate illness, and the institutions serving them incrementally work with more and more limited resources to serve a more and more disabled population. Not only do the poor and sick and the chronically ill have fewer economic resources, they often have less available family and social support systems, so that problems become compounded as cut-backs in supporting medical care services for the poor are intensified by cuts in social welfare services.

These processes are now evident in many states of the US. Psychiatric emergency room services in general hospitals largely serve a public sector population. Patients often wait for extended periods of time for entry into hospital-level care, sleeping in corridors on stretchers, as entry into state facilities becomes more and more difficult to accomplish. Attempts to develop state–private programmes are frustrated by the almost universal experience that state funding levels do not keep up with inflationary costs. Thus, state contracting mechanisms, which were established to stimulate competition, too often deal with a single contractor, as other potential providers cease to participate in the process, and the original contractor delivers less service, as his dollar support diminishes (Dorwart et al 1986).

THE EFFECTIVENESS (AND EFFICIENCY) OF MENTAL HEALTH SERVICES

Two steps are essential for evaluating the effectiveness of mental health policy. The first is to measure the concrete effects of specific psychiatric procedures on altering the psychological and social impairments associated with psychiatric disorders (Schwartz et al 1973). Effectiveness relates more directly to the primary clinical goal of psychiatric treatment, programmes, and institutions — i.e. to make the patient better. Since the increasing utilisation of case-control studies and scientific methodologies in mental health evaluation, our knowledge in this sphere has increased dramatically. Yet, as will be seen, a strict 'biomedical' model isolates the individual not only from his/her social context, but also from those cultural and historically derived social structures which comprise the existing psychiatric system (Mollica 1987). The second step in evaluating effectiveness is to determine the efficiency of the system. Efficiency is a measure of a community or institution's resourcefulness in achieving optimum use of the manpower and resources that have been allocated to its mental health system; this includes an assessment of everything from evaluation and treatment, through the various organisational levels of care that have been developed in order to achieve good treatment outcome.

Measuring the effectiveness of mental health services

Any policy planner looking at the relative success of social expenditures on a mental health system might initially proceed with an above-down view of the system's outcome. In medicine, this level of description is usually accomplished by comparing changes in mortality rates over time. It is legitimate for a society to ask initially whether its medical expenditures have improved the life expectancy of its members. Although this approach is only a crude measure of effectiveness, its utility to mental health policy has been almost inconsequential, for a wide range of reasons. Mortality data currently are not very useful to policy planners in the mental health arena. While much study has been devoted to suicide, it remains difficult to obtain clear rates of successful suicide by diagnosis. Other premature deaths that occur primarily from mental disorders are difficult to determine, because they are usually associated with the terminal states of underlying medical diseases (such as alcoholic cirrhosis), homicides, and automobile accidents. Yet in spite of limited information, little doubt exists that both the acute and chronic phases of schizophrenia, depression, and alcoholism carry increased mortality risks. Recent evidence, however, suggests that these rates for depression and suicide have been gradually decreasing in the United States over the past 25 years, especially for depression (Tsuang & Simpson 1985). Currently, attempts are also being made to use mortality rates as an index of the effectiveness of various psychiatric treatments (e.g. ECT, psycho-pharmacology), but in spite of these, mortality rates continue to provide little useful information on the overall effectiveness of mental health programmes.

Furthermore, the above-down view is even more opaque when policy planners attempt to assess the quality of care and effectiveness of individual programmes and practitioners. Indeed, in chronic illness, where the impact of an intervention may at best be to limit the progression of disability, adequate baselines for measuring both maintenance of function and decrements in function are difficult to establish.

Cochrane (1971), in his reflections on the effectiveness of the British National Health Service (NHS), ironically stated that, 'I once asked a worker at a crematorium, who had a curiously contented look on his face, what he found so satisfying about his work. He replied that what fascinated him was the way in which so much went in and so little came out. I thought of advising him to get a job in the NHS, it might have increased his job satisfaction'. In spite of Cochrane's cynical view of the NHS' effectiveness (he is even tougher in his evaluation of psychiatry), many studies exploring the relationship of treatment to its outcome have had considerable usefulness and success in describing the effectiveness of psychiatric interventions. This might be described as the down-up view of mental health evaluation. Not surprisingly, the greatest success in demonstrating 'good' outcome has occurred in drug trials (Bollini et al 1984). Yet the implications of these drug trials are usually limited, because they primarily evaluate symptom relief over short-term periods and usually avoid assessing the large number of risk factors (e.g. genetic, social, personality) which may influence both the natural history and the treatment of the disease. Neither do they usually investigate outcome in the social context, where most services actually receive their psychiatric care.

The shift from drug trials to outcome research in non-experimental settings demands a degree of methodological sophistication which is not commonly found in psychiatric research. For example, a recent review of the published outcome research on discharged psychiatric patients concludes that little theoretical or methodological progress has been made over the past 10 years in identifying those factors that are conducive to the successful rehabilitation of these patients on their return to the community (Braun et al 1981). Additionally, few studies have been able to evaluate successfully the complex relationship between psychiatric symptomatology and social functioning. A number of epidemological investigations, in fact, have demonstrated a poor correlation between the level and intensity of symptoms on the one hand and social role performance on the other (Astrachan et al 1974, Strauss & Carpenter 1972, 1974). Furthermore, psychiatric diagnoses remain unable to predict accurately either prognosis or the psychological reality of the condition in a particular patient. Individuals with similar psychiatric diagnoses may have dramatically different interpretations and/or subjective experiences of their symptoms and their causes. The down-up view of the effectiveness of mental health services is therefore extremely complex and difficult to achieve, if the goal of outcome research is to evaluate all three major outcome areas of clinical care — psychiatric symptoms, social functioning, and the individual's subjective experience of psychological distress. Of course, few outcome studies have in fact achieved this goal.

Social handicap and disability

Over the past 20 years, there has been an unprecedented interest by policy planners in one of the three major outcome areas discussed above — the social and community adjustment of psychiatric patients. Weissman (1975), in her extensive review of social adjustment rating scales, broadly defines social adjustment as 'the interplay between the individual and the social environment. Specific ways of behaving, referred to as roles, are commonly accepted as appropriate and the individual is perceived in terms of the way his role performance conforms to the norms of his referrant group'. Social adjustment is based on a summation of specific social role performances. The major social roles a person assumes are a function of his/her age, sex, marital status, education, etc., as well as of the degree of psychopathology, where relevant. Most studies have suggested, however, that psychiatric symptoms are poor predictors of social functioning. Anthony & Jansen (1984), in their overview of the scientific literature of rehabilitation which explored the relationship between work performance and psychiatric symptoms, concluded that:

(a) Diagnostic categories are poor predictors of work performance.

(b) No symptoms or symptom patterns are routinely related to individual work performance.

(c) There is little or no correlation between symptomatology and functional skills.

(d) The best demographic predictor of future work performance is ability to 'get along' and prior employment history.

These results dramatically reveal that psychiatry's traditional emphasis on evaluating and treating psychiatric symptoms may not contribute significantly to the patient's social rehabilitation. The theory and practice of psychiatric rehabilitation is in its infancy (Redlich 1983), and this lack of knowledge and emphasis on rehabilitation is especially troublesome to policy planners because they must confront (and attempt to ameliorate) the negative social impact of debilitating psychiatric illness. Determining the degree to which different treatment approaches improve the social adjustment and economic self-sufficiency of psychiatric patients is crucial to public planning. Disability policy at times provides disincentives to effective rehabilitation, either through the structures of service, or through the definition of entry characteristics of those eligible for rehabilitative programmes. Though attempts to aid disabled psychiatric patients to return to work are often limited, much attention is currently being focused on supervised work experiences as a strategy for social and vocational rehabilitation. Unfortunately, Cochrane's (1971) ironic caveat on the NHS is especially valid in this area. Except for a few case-control studies (Stein & Test 1980) which demonstrate the social effectiveness of their treatment approach (Stein & Test 1980, Weisbrod et al 1980), the utility of treatment strategies in enhancing role performance among the seriously disabled is not well demonstrated.

Efficiency

The problems of measuring effectiveness, though difficult as these may be, are massively compounded when issues of efficiency are considered. For example, when considering the community adjustment of disabled psychiatric patients, current knowledge allows us to identify a host of variables which may be related to adaptation. These include the severity of the underlying disorders, the symptomatic state, social stressors, and the availability of social service supports, rehabilitation resources, adequate housing, family support, etc. Some patients require very intensive intervention for long periods of time in order to preserve community tenure, while others are more likely to decompensate if they receive intensive attention. Too many programmes equate efficiency with a generalised substitution of lower-level employees for professionals and with the maximisation of contact hours and numbers of patients seen. Measures of efficiency, therefore, must consider the special needs of discrete groups of patients, in programmes which are designed to deal with their special needs and to produce agreed results.

EQUALITY OF CARE AND MENTAL HEALTH POLICY

In planning mental health services the use of the term 'equality' usually refers to minimising differences in treatment between individuals who have similar psychiatric problems. Of course, those factors which are known to contribute to differences in treatment include race, gender, social class (including occupation, education, and income) and severity of disability. As already indicated, 'equality of care' and 'equity of access' are not equivalent concepts. In fact, a 'fair' or 'equitable' mental health system need not provide equal care. The community mental health centre movement, for example, attempted to achieve equity by establishing a public alternative (and quite possibly a better one) than the existing private system.

In spite of the distinctions between 'equity of access' and 'equality of care', major social class differences in the prevalence rates of psychiatric illness and the types of treatment received by the lower social classes continue to raise major challenges to the mental health system. For example, is it possible to reduce psychiatric morbidity in poor communities? Should working-class and poor citizens receive different forms of care than higher socio-economic groups simply because of their limited financial resources? Are these differences in care acceptable because of the efficacy of the treatment, or are they disguising ineffective and discriminatory practices? Should delivery of care explicably recognise significant cultural differences among groups, and attempt to meet the needs of patients within acceptable cultural contexts, or are such issues merely icing on the treatment cake? It has repeatedly been demonstrated that attention to cultural dimensions of care increases the acceptance of care, but does it also increase effectiveness? Finally, discussions of 'equality of care' also extend beyond social-class inequalities to those inequalities that are related to the amenities and to the equality of experience received by psychiatric patients, regardless of their social background. These are issues of dignity, patients' rights, and autonomy.

The increased risk for psychiatric disorders among persons of low socio-economic status

Social-class differences in the prevalence of psychiatric disorders have influenced discussions of 'equality' over the past half-century. Since Faris & Dunham's (1939) pioneering work in the late 1930s, American psychiatry — like that of some other countries — has investigated the important relationship between social status and mental illness. As Dohrenwend & Dohrenwend (1969) argued in their comprehensive review of the empirical research up to that time, the relationship between social class and mental illness is one of the most substantiated empirical findings in psychiatric research. In a review of the results of the Epidemiologic Catchment Area Program (ECA), Holzer et al (1986) confirmed this relationship. The ECA programme elicited DSM-III diagnoses in over 18 000 community respondents from five geographical locations, re-establishing the finding that the highest rates of disorders occurred in the lowest socio-economic groups (e.g. the risk for schizophrenia in the lowest social class was 7.85, relative to the highest class).

The dramatic findings of the ECA confirm a class bias in the prevalence of serious psychiatric disorder within the United States: the lower classes are more afflicted by mental illness. Over and above the serious moral implications of these findings to general social policies related to housing, nutrition, education, etc., what do they imply for mental health policy? In an utopian world where health inequality did not exist, every social group would have exactly the same prevalence rates of psychiatric disorder, while types of care and outcome results would also be equal. As we move away from this ideal model of equality, however, concrete realities emerge. Tudor-Hart (1971) once cynically summarised these by stating that 'the availability of good medical care tends to vary inversely with the need for it in the population served'.

The relationship between social class and treatment

In 1958, Hollingshead & Redlich elucidated the influence of social characteristics on the type and quality of care that was assigned to patients. For example, for outpatients, the lower the social class of the patient, the greater the degree of organic therapies as opposed to psychotherapy, the fewer the number of clinic visits, and the shorter the length of the therapy session. Lower-class patients were also found to receive therapists with less training and experience. For inpatients, lower-class patients exclusively used the state mental hospital; the relationship between social class and inpatient treatment was probably the most startling and impressive finding of the study. For psychotic patients, the lower the class of the patient, the longer the period of hospital admission; in fact, the average length of stay of upper-class schizophrenic patients was five years less than for corresponding lower-class patients. In addition, while upper-class patients tended to move in and out of the hospital, the lower-class ones tended to have long, continuous and uninterrupted stays. The lower-class patient — organic treatment/custodial care — inexperienced therapist triad, appears to be a fixed societal relationship in that community, as members of Redlich's team re-demonstrated over 25 years later, in spite of the CMHC reform movement.

These differences in care also appear to be influenced by race, gender, and severity of diagnosis. Even in a relatively resource-rich community, such as New Haven, Connecticut, studies continue to reveal inequality in treatment received by lower-class patients (Mollica & Milic 1986). These results can be summarised thus:

1. The service network has dramatically increased in size and scope. Large numbers of patients of all social classes receive ambulatory psychiatric services.

2. However, treatment assignment remains substantially related to socio-economic status; lower-class patients are generally perceived by staff as 'sicker' and as having a worse prognosis than patients of higher social class.

3. Lower-class patients are less likely to be assigned to individual psychotherapy than are patients of higher social class. They are more likely to be offered organic treatment (e.g. ECT, drugs) and to be placed in medically orientated clinics. To some extent, this reflects assignments which are based on diagnosis, but the resources devoted to management

of care, rehabilitation services, etc. for the chronically ill have been limited.

4. When accepted for psychotherapy, lower-class patients generally receive less experienced therapists, briefer treatment sessions, and shorter lengths of treatment, and have a higher attrition rate than patients of higher social class.

Yet in spite of this extensive empirical research tradition on the 'inequalities' in mental health services, these findings have limited impact on policy, since few have been able to relate differences in care to treatment outcomes. As Daniels (1982) states, 'it is at least arguable that only those utilisation rate variations are inequitable which reflect significant differences in the preventative, curing and caring functions of health care services'. Policy planners and professional groups have consistently been able to dismiss 'inequality' in treatment studies because of the lack of demonstrable differences in effectiveness between low-intensity treatment for low-income and minority groups, as compared to higher-intensity treatment for higher-income groups.

Quality of life for patients

Differences in the amenities afforded to different types of psychiatric patients represent a serious form of inequality which is observed when different types of hospitals are compared. These comparisons are most glaring when state mental hospitals are compared to private inpatient facilities. Few people need to be reminded of concentration camp-like images of the asylum inmates in the 1950s, yet in spite of dramatically smaller numbers of residents, many mental hospitals today are still poorly staffed and provide less than decent physical surroundings. Cochrane (1971), in reviewing this type of inequality, remarked that,

Here I'm not concerned with quality of treatment but with quality of living. There are many aspects of a hospital; the effectiveness of the treatment, the efficacy with which it is given by the staff and the basic standard of living of the place. Under the latter I included food, heating, lighting decoration and comfort. All doctors and many others have known for years of the growing gap between the standard of living in an acute general hospital on the one hand, and the psychiatric, geriatric, and mentally deficient institutes on the other.

Deinstitutionalisation, paradoxically, has contributed to the continued physical decline of many mental hospitals, as patients and financial resources are shifted to the community. In many states, the most debilitated patients are receiving care in delapidated state inpatient facilities which are reminiscent of the 1950s.

Lack of concern for quality of living can effect all psychiatric institutions, especially those caring for the poor and socially disabled such as CMHCs, half-way houses, etc. Societal acceptance of these different standards in quality of living for patients is widespread and the reasons for this acceptance complex, but the ability to transform these differences is apparently minimal.

CONCLUSIONS

Our journey through the major dimensions of mental health policy reveals the complex interactions within psychiatric care, both as an applied scientific discipline and as a social practice (Mollica 1987). The simplicity of the basic goal of mental health care — to make people better — is confounded by a bewildering range of social, historical, economic, and scientific constraints. Furthermore, national views of different societies and geographical regions make cross-national comparisons difficult. Modern mental health policy can be considered the summation of historically evolved approaches and scientifically based knowledge to the solution of mental health problems, through culturally and politically acceptable administrative and institutional methods. These methods reveal the 'moral' and 'scientific' orientation of the mental health system. This system is essentially moral in its orientation because it makes judgements which determine both the distribution of mental health care and the degree of equality of care. The mental health system is also fundamentally moral because it is concerned with the quality of an individual's social relationships — especially for those individuals afflicted with serious psychiatric disorder. Italian reformers, in particular, have recently sought to elucidate those political aspects of mental health which have not helped patients but have actually 'harmed' them, through the grim realities of severely under-funded custodially orientated mental hospitals during this century (Mollica 1985). The mental health system is also scientific because it uses scientifically derived knowledge to improve the effectiveness and efficiency of treatment. However, discoveries of new and better treatment approaches do not necessarily guarantee their introduction into the mental health system.

Does a model exist for an ideal mental health system in which every member of society receives access to equal and effective care? Within the United States, government controlled systems of all types are widely seen as increasing bureaucratisation, raising costs, and limiting technological innovation; they strive to maximise equity and equality, while compromising efficiency and excellence. On the other hand, price-competitive systems (e.g. the United States, more or less) promote effectiveness and efficiency and on occasion develop excellent innovative programmes, while simultaneously creating inequalities in the delivery and utilisation of services. Within every system, there are trade-offs and contradictions between its individual aspects. For Foucault (1965), these different national approaches revealed the historical foundations of their society, yet their origins are not easily understood. All the elements of psychiatric care reviewed in this chapter are part of a web of concrete practices, situated within a field of complex social forces. Foucault claimed that some the other factors which constitute the basis of any psychiatric system and which must also be considered include: professionalism, scientific orientation, commitment laws, and legal procedures. Of course, no policy planner or clinician can totally understand all the historical and social forces which influence the institutions in which he or she works. However, mental health policy can shift away from simplistic conceptualisations to multidimensional analyses which include the major dimensions of psychiatric care. It is to be hoped that a broader understanding of the meaning and relevance of the concepts of equity, effectiveness (efficiency) and equality can provide administrators with a systematic guide for assessing the relative advantages and/or disadvantages of a mental health system, as well as helping individual practitioners to achieve greater insights into the moral and scientific dimensions of their clinical practices.

REFERENCES

Action for Mental Health 1962 Final Report of the Joint Commission of Mental Illness and Health. Basic Books, New York

American Psychiatric Association 1983 Economic fact book for psychiatry. American Psychiatric Press, Washington DC.

Anderson R, Kravits T, Anderson O W 1975 Equity in health services: empirical analysis in social policy. Ballinger, Cambridge, Mass

Anthony W A, Jansen M A 1984 Predicting the vocational capacity of the chronically mentally ill: research and policy implications. American Psychologist 39: 537-544

Astrachan B M 1991 Economics of practice and inpatient care. General Hospital Psychiatry in press

Astrachan B M, Tischler G L 1984 Normality from a health systems perspective. In: Offer D, Sabshin M (eds) Normality and the life cycle. Basic Books, New York

Astrachan B M, Brauer L, Harrow M, Schwartz C 1974 Symptomatic outcome in schizophrenia. Archives of General Psychiatry 31: 155-160

Bollini P, Cotecchia S, DeBlase A, Romandini S, Tognoni G 1984 Drugs: guide and caveats to explanatory and descriptive approaches — II. Drugs in psychiatric research. Journal of Psychiatric Research 18: 391-400

Braun P, Kochansky G, Shapiro R, Greenberg S, Gudeman J E, Johnson S, Shore M F 1981 Overview: deinstitutionalization of psychiatric patients, a critical review of outcome studies. American Journal of Psychiatry 138: 736-749

Castel R, Castel F, Lovell A 1982 The Psychiatric Society. Translated by Goldhammer A. Columbia University Press, New York

Cochrane A L 1971 Effectiveness and efficiency. Burgess & Son (Abingdon) Ltd, London

Daniels N 1982 Equity of access to health care: some conceptual and ethical issues. Health & Society 60: 51-81

Dohrenwend B P, Dohrenwend B S 1969 Social status and psychological disorder: a casual inquiry. Wiley, New York

Dorwart R A, Schlesinger M, Pulice R T 1986 Competitive bidding and state's purchase of services: the case of mental health care in Massachusetts. Journal of Policy Analysis & Management 5: 245-263

Faris F E L, Dunham H W 1939 Mental disorders in urban areas: an ecological study of schizophrenia and other psychoses. University of Chicago Press, Chicago

Foucault M 1965 Madness and civilisation: a history of insanity in the age of reason. Trans. Howard R. Vintage/Random House, New York

Frank R G, Kamlet M S 1980 Unpublished Direct costs and expenditures for mental health in the United States — 1980. National Institute of Mental Health, Rockville, Maryland, 83M054337001D

Gostin L O 1983 The ideology of entitlement: the application of contemporary legal approaches to psychiatry. In: Bean P (ed) Mental illness: changes and trends. Wiley, New York: pp 27-54

Hollingshead A B, Redlich F C 1958. Social class and mentally ill. Wiley, New York

Holzer C E, Shea B M, Swanson J W et al 1986 The increased risk for specific psychiatric disorders among persons of low socioeconomic status. American Journal of Social Psychiatry 4: 259-271

Katz M B 1984 Poor houses and the origins of the public old age home. Health & Society 110-138

Katzper M, Manderscheid D W 1984 Applications of systems analysis to national data on the mental health service delivery system. Psychiatric Annals 14: 596-607

Kennedy J 1963 Message relative to mentally illness and mental retardation. February 5

Klerman G L 1984 Trends in utilisation of mental health services: perspectives for health services research. Medical Care 23: 584-596

Knepser D J 1978 Psychiatric manpower for state mental hospitals. Archives of General Psychiatry 35: 19-24

Kramer M J 1983 Perspectives on national health expenditures. Wall Street Journal Transcript, November 7

Langsley D G, Robinowitz C B 1979 Psychiatric manpower: an overview. Hospital & Community Psychiatry 30: 749-755

Lind J, O'Neil B, Wilson A, Bang A, Mahoney A 1984 The mental health system: where has it been and where should it go? Management and Policy Brief. Massachusetts Hospital Association 2: 1-8

Mazach N A, Lutterman T, Glover R 1985a Funding sources an expenditures of state mental health agencies: revenue/expenditure study results fiscal year 1983 (NIMH Contract, NIMH-DB-278-84-0020). Washington DC

Mazach N A, Lutterman T, Glover R 1985b Selected states and Federal Government agency mental health expenditures incurred on behalf of mentally ill persons. (NIMH Contract, NIMH-DB-278-84-0020). Washington DC

Mollica R F 1983 From asylum to community: the threatened disintegration of public psychiatry. New England Journal of Medicine 308: 367-373

Mollica R F (ed) 1985 The unfinished revolution in Italian psychiatry. In: International Journal of Mental Health Vol. 14. M E Sharpe, New York

Mollica R F (ed) 1986 Psychiatry in quest after orientation. In: Tymieniecka A-T (ed) The moral sense in the communal significance of life (Analecta Husserlina). D Reidel Publishing Company, Holland: 101-124

Mollica R F 1987 Upside down psychiatry: a genealogy of mental health. In: Levin D M (ed) Pathologies of the modern self: the social and cultural dimensions of psychiatric illness. University Press, New York

Mollica R F, Milic M 1986 Social class and psychiatric practice: a revision of the Hollingshead and Redlich model. American Journal of Psychiatry 143: 12-17:

Mollica R F, Redlich F 1980 Equity and changing patient characteristics — 1950 to 1975. Archives of General Psychiatry 37: 1257-1263

Musto D F 1975 Whatever happened to 'community mental health'? Public Interest 39: 53-79

National Institute of Mental Health 1971 Community mental health center program operating handbook. I. Policy and standards manual. United States Department of Health, Education, and Welfare, Washington DC

Pardes H 1979 Future needs for psychiatrists and other mental health personnel. Archives of General Psychiatry 36:1401-1408

President's Commission on Mental Health 1978 Report to the President from the President's Commission on Mental Health. Government Printing Office, Washington DC

Public Law 182 1955 84th Congress, 1st session, July 28

Public Law 88-164 1963 Approved October 31

Public Law 89-97 1965 Social Security Amendments of 1965, July 30

Public Law 89-749 1966 Comprehensive health planning and public health services amendments of 1966. United States Congress, 89th Congress, 2nd session, October 18

Redlich F C 1983 Medical rehabilitation and psychiatric rehabilitation. Psychiatric Annals 13: 564–511

Regier D A, Goldberg I D, Taube C A 1978 The de facto US mental health services system. Archives of General Psychiatry 35: 685-693

Rioch M J, Elkes C, Flint A A, Usdansky B S, Newman R G, Silber E 1963 National Institute of Mental Health pilot study in training mental health counsellors. American Journal of Orthopsychiatry 33: 678-689

Rose S M 1979 Deciphering deinstitutionalization: complexities in policy and program analysis. Milbank Memorial Fund Guar/Health & Society 57: 429-460

Schwartz C C, Myers J K, Astrachan B M 1973 The outcome study in psychiatric evaluation research: issues and methods. Archives of General Psychiatry 29: 98-102

Sharfstein S, Muszynski S, Myers E 1984 Health insurance and psychiatric care: update and appraisal. American Psychiatric Press, Washington DC

Sherlock D B 1984 The psychiatric hospital industry — industry overview. Salomon Brothers, 1-16

Stein L I, Test M A 1980 Alternative to mental hospital treatment. I. Conceptual model, treatment program and clinical evaluation. Archives of General Psychiatry 37: 392-397

Strauss J, Carpenter W 1972 The prediction of outcome in schizophrenia — I. Archives of General Psychiatry 27: 739-749

Strauss J, Carpenter W 1974 The prediction of outcome in schizophrenia — II. Archives of General Psychiatry 31: 37-42

Tsuang M T, Simpson J C 1985 Mortality studies in psychiatry. Archives of General Psychiatry 42: 98-103

Tudor-Hart J 1971 The inverse care law. Lancet i: 405-408

Weisbrod B A, Test M A, Stein L I 1980 Alternative to mental hospital treatment. II. Economic benefit-cost analysis. Archives of General Psychiatry 37: 400-405

Weissman G 1982 Foucault and the bag lady. Hospital Practice August: 28-29, 33-34, 39

Weissman M M 1975 The assessment of social adjustment: a review of techniques. Archives of General Psychiatry 32: 357-365

Williams D H, Bellis E C, Wellington S W 1980 Deinstitutionalisation and social policy: historical perspectives and present dilemmas. American Journal of Orthopsychiatry 50: 54-64

Witkin M J 1980 Trends in patient care episodes in mental health facilities, 1955-1977. National Institute of Mental Health (Statistical note 154) (DHHS publication # ADM80-158), Rockville, MD

Wolfe H L, Astrachan B M 1985 Community mental health services. In: Klerman G (ed) Psychiatry. Basic Books, New York

Wolfe H L, Astrachan B M, Scherl D J 1991 Psychiatric practice in organized health and proprietary care system. In: Prospective payment: implications for psychiatric patient care. American Psychiatric Press, Washington DC (in press)

21. Social policy and community psychiatry in the UK

J. Raftery

INTRODUCTION AND OVERVIEW

Mental health services comprise one of the oldest publicly financed services in the UK, as in most other industrialised countries. The form of services provided has been changing, though, over the past three decades in ways that increasingly minimise the use of inpatient care and treatment. In parallel, public policy has aimed at shifting existing long-stay patients from the old hospitals into the 'community'. The most recent plans of the UK government for health and social services open the way for rapid change towards these goals. This article reviews progress to date before considering the rationale for and implications of these major policy changes.

The distinction between treatment and care will be retained throughout, since, although it is not an absolute distinction, it usefully differentiates community orientated treatment of new referrals from the deinstitutionalisation of long-stay patients. Although some ex-inpatients may require treatment, they mainly require continuing care. Community psychiatry, then, concerns itself both with the community-orientated treatment of patients in general and with policies of deinstitutionalisation and care for existing long-stay patients.

The second section of this chapter provides data on levels of public spending, the numbers of people utilising services, progress towards meeting targets, and trends in manpower employed. At over £1.2 billion in 1986-1987, direct public spending on mental health services has never before taken so high a share of British national resources; over the last decade, though, institutional care has continued to absorb over 80% of direct public spending on mental illness services, despite the policy emphasis in favour of community-orientated services. Each year, around 1% of the British population receive treatment from the psychiatric sector of the NHS, half of them as new patients. The numbers of consultant psychiatrists and psychiatric nurses have risen over the past decade, both absolutely and in relation to population. However, up to now, progress toward official targets has been more rapid in the reduction of inpatient places and growth in outpatient attendances than in the expansion of day-places and hostels.

The meanings of both public and social policy are discussed in the next section, which also outlines the economic arguments in favour of public provision of mental health services and discusses the key concepts of policy analysis: effectiveness, efficiency, and equity. Psychiatric epidemology and mental health policy have, it is suggested, largely remained isolated from each other.

Similarly, too little attention has been given to *what* constitutes 'the community' or *who* will provide *what* type of care or treatment, and *where* it will be provided. Section 4 notes the complexities inherent in the term 'community', and reviews academic studies of community psychiatry against the criteria of effectiveness, efficiency, and equity. These studies include some relating to community-orientated treatments, as well as others on the effects of deinstitutionalisation; in general, they have been small-scale, short-term and methodologically deficient. While they suggest that community-orientated methods of treatment and care are as effective, and perhaps as efficient as institutionally-based treatment, equity considerations have received little attention in these comparisons.

Other factors which have influenced the development of a more community-orientated psychiatry in the UK are then considered. These include: the considerable costs of renovating the old institutions; wider entitlement to income maintenance arising out of developments in social security since World War II; new psychiatric treatments, particularly pharmacotherapies; legal redefinitions of the rights of the mentally ill; and finally, changes in the way mental health and illness are perceived.

Some of the barriers to successful implementation of the new community-orientated policies, particularly in relation to replacing institutional by community care, are outlined next. Relevant policy reviews in the mid to late 1980s are summarised, along with the two complementary White Papers in 1989 (HMSO 1989a,b) and the subsequent legislation in 1990.

Finally, different conclusions could be drawn, justifying either pessimistic or optimistic views depending on the framework one utilises. From the perspective of rational policy analysis, pessimism seems reasonable but such analysis perhaps tends towards pessimism about the practice of any policy. A more pragmatic view, though, of the limitations on policy-making and implementation in contemporary liberal-democratic societies would suggest a more optimistic judgement. The final section attempts to synthesise these two approaches.

THE SIZE OF THE SECTOR

Publicly provided health and personal social services for the mentally ill currently cost over £1 billion per annum in England, equivalent to almost 0.3% of the Gross National Product (GNP). By contrast, in 1954, when the number of psychiatric inpatients was more than double the present figure, direct public expenditure on mental health amounted to under 0.2% of the GNP (HMSO 1955). The growth in the share of national resources devoted to psychiatric illness has been due partly to the continuing cost of maintaining and improving the old mental hospitals, as well as to the extra costs of providing some new community-based services.

Measures such as the above, understate the level of public sector spending on mental health services to the extent that patients who have been discharged, or who would have been admitted in the past, also receive social security payments. Other public sector costs may be associated with housing subsidies, with the rest of the health services, and with the legal system. To date, then, changes in mental health policy have led, not to reductions in current public expenditure, but to increases.

Alongside public spending on mental health services, a private market caters not only for small numbers of people with psychiatric illness but also for those who seek 'personal enhancement' through a variety of methods traditionally associated with psychiatric treatment, ranging from psychoanalysis to a variety of self-help groups. Although the size of the personal enhancement sector remains unknown in the UK, casual observation suggests considerable growth, albeit from a small base compared with the United States, for instance. Only about 4% of acute psychiatric beds in the UK are private (Laing 1985).

Direct public expenditure changes

Direct NHS expenditure on mental health services in England and Wales, as shown below in Table 21.1, grew by just under 12% in constant prices (adjusted for inflation) between 1976–1977 and 1986–1987; despite the

Table 21.1 Public expenditure on mental health services by NHS, England (in 1986–1987 prices, deflated by health service prices)

	Mental illness inpatients £m	Mental illness outpatients £m	Psychiatric day patients £m	Total £m
1976/7	942.4	44.3	43.4	1030.1
1977/8	981.5	50.2	50.5	1080.2
1978/9	983.6	53.3	51.7	1088.6
1979/80	989.5	52.9	50.7	1093.1
1980/1	1004.7	53.1	58.3	1116.1
1981/2	1019.6	62.7	63.2	1145.5
1982/3	1013.7	67.6	63.7	1145.0
1983/4	1010.4	67.2	70.9	1148.5
1984/5	1013.5	69.9	73.8	1157.2
1985/6	1002.1	72.2	77.6	1151.9
1986/7	998.2	71.4	79.6	1149.2
% change	+5.9%	+61.2%	+83.5%	+11.6%

Source: HMSO 1988d

Table 21.2   Mental illness expenditure by local authorities and the NHS (all in 1986–1987 prices)

	Residential	Day care	Sub-total	NHS sub-total	Total
	£m	£m	£m	£m	£m
1976/7	15.9	9.60	25.5	1030.1	1055.6
1977/8	17.2	10.40	27.6	1082.2	1109.8
1978/9	19.1	12.19	31.2	1088.6	1119.8
1979/80	20.8	13.31	34.1	1093.1	1127.2
1980/1	22.0	13.87	35.8	1116.1	1151.9
1981/2	21.0	14.00	35.0	1145.5	1180.5
1982/3	21.9	16.51	38.4	1145.0	1183.4
1983/4	22.7	18.17	40.8	1148.5	1189.3
1984/5	23.0	19.60	42.6	1157.2	1199.8
1985/6	22.1	19.60	41.7	1151.9	1193.6
1986/7	21.8	22.10	43.9	1149.2	1193.1
% change	+37.1%	+130.2%	+72.2%	+11.6%	+13.0%

Source: HMSO 1988d.

commitment to non-institutional care, the hospital inpatient sector continued to absorb over 80% of this NHS spending. However, although outpatient and day-patient services accounted for only 10% of NHS spending in 1986–1987, expenditure on these services has been growing at high rates, though from a low base: 61% for outpatients and 84% for day-patients services, compared to 6% for inpatients, over the decade.

However, NHS expenditure accounts for only part of the picture, since the social services departments of Local Authorities also provide services for the mentally ill, though these absorbed relatively small amounts of money — around £43 million in 1986–1987, or 4% of NHS spending on the mentally ill. Trends in these expenditures are shown in Table 21.2; the two main headings being provision of residential and day care services, both of which expanded rapidly over the preceding decade. The combined total of NHS and Local Authority revenue spending came to £1193 million in 1986–1987, with the inpatient component continuing to dominate at 84% of this total, representing a fall from the 1976–1977 proportion of 89%. The continuing small size of the non-institutional sector and of the Local Authority component are problems that the most recent policy reviews aim to redress.

Numbers of persons in receipt of services

The significance of the public psychiatric sector in England and Wales can be gauged by the numbers of persons recorded as receiving treatment, which provide some measures of treated incidence and prevalence. Because of the difficulties associated with the concept of 'case', and the imprecision about when or if a patient is 'cured', prevalence in psychiatry arguably relates more to contact (or not) with a treatment agency, at least for the more serious disorders. Over a quarter of a million persons in England each year present as new patients — around 0.5% of the population: 80% of these receive outpatient or day-patient services with the remainder admitted as inpatients (HMSO 1986a).

Some 200 000 persons are admitted each year to psychiatric hospitals and units in England and Wales; three-quarters of these have been admitted at least once before. A rough estimate, then, would suggest that around half a million people, or about 1% of the population, are in receipt of services each year. Over the last 30 years, the total number of inpatient admissions has been rising slowly while the number of NHS psychiatric beds available has been declining — from over 3 beds to around 1 bed per 1000 population. Concomitantly, the average length of stay has fallen and the number of outpatient attendances has doubled from over one million in 1961 to just under two million in 1988.

The progress in meeting declared targets was reviewed by the National Audit Office (1987), showing that between 1975 and 1985, the ratio of NHS psychiatric beds to population fell by 24% and of residential places by 20%. Although day-hospital places per capita increased by 73% over the same period and the number of Local Authority day-places doubled, their combined provision remained only around one-third of the targets laid down in 'Better Services for the Mentally Ill' (HMSO 1975). The National Audit Office has also shown that according to the plans of Regional Health Authorities, the number of available beds is projected to decline further by 23% by 1993–1994, offset by increases in outpatient attendances of 15%, and in day-hospital attendances of 91%. In addition, many health authorities throughout the UK have developed community mental health centres, but without any agreement over objectives or potential achievements (Sayce 1987).

Judged in terms of activity, then, the shift in emphasis towards 'community care', in the sense of reduced inpatient and greatly increased outpatient provision, has been more significant than the expenditure data alone would suggest; however, this may result to some extent from those expenditure data failing to reflect the advent of new services. The substitution of outpatient for inpatient services still implies a hospital-centred service: more community-orientated modes of treatment involving community-based psychiatric teams have only developed slowly, as shown by the manpower data below.

Manpower changes

Despite the run-down in numbers of psychiatric beds and slow development of community-orientated programmes, the overall numbers

Table 21.3   Consultants and nurses in mental illness sector, England, 1976–1986 (all w.t.e)

	Consultants per 100 000 population	Nurses per 100 000 population	Total nurses	CPNs
1976	2.3	103.5	47347	(n.a.)
1986	3.1	122.3	57782	(2973)
% change	+35%	+18%	+22%	(+158%) (1979-1986)

Source: HMSO 1986a.
CPNs = Community Psychiatric Nurses.

employed in the NHS psychiatric sector have continued to grow over the last decade, as shown in Table 21.3.

The number of consultant psychiatric medical staff grew in England & Wales between 1976 and 1986 from 2.3 per 100 000 population to 3.1 (+35%), while the ratio of nurses grew from 103.5 to 122.3 (+18%) over the same period. In 1986, just over 1000 consultant psychiatrists were employed, out of around 3500 medical staff. The increase in nursing numbers resulted to some extent from reductions in the working week in 1980–1981. The NHS mental health services employed around 70 000 staff in England, of whom psychiatric nurses, at almost 58 000, made up the main group. Community Psychiatric Nurses numbered almost 3000 in 1986 — a rise of 158% from 1979, the earliest year for which data are available. Despite this growth, community-orientated nurses amount to only around 5% of all psychiatric nurses, indicating the degree to which labour resources remain centred on the psychiatric hospitals and units, where the remaining inpatients have a higher average degree of dependency than in the past. However, as with the financial data, the manpower data may be failing to reflect fully the newer, more community-orientated services, since a small proportion of the nursing staff are also involved in outpatient, day-patient, and community services.

Although community psychiatry in England and Wales provides the main focus for this article, the variation within the UK between England, Wales, and Scotland should be noted, not least for the diversity of policy formulation in each country. Hunter & Wistow (1987) showed that compared to England, Scotland had made relatively little progress towards community-orientated service targets, whereas Wales had moved furthest, particularly with the mentally handicapped (retarded). The same study suggested that the Welsh example indicated the influence that committed political leadership can have, though psychiatrists have serious reservations as to whether the mentally retarded there would continue to have the appropriate access to medical expertise.

The development of community care may be impeded by the transition difficulties faced by some key groups of staff. For instance, the policy shift towards community-based services has been seen as requiring a break by psychiatrists with the 'medical model', combined with un-learning and re-learning to prepare themselves for the task ahead (Sturt & Waters 1985).

SOCIAL POLICY AND PUBLIC POLICY

Questions about the role and appropriateness of public policy for the mental health services are necessarily prompted by the size of the sector, as measured by its costs, and the numbers of clients and staff employed. The macro question of why these services should be publicly provided has special relevance in view of the extension of 'privatisation' in several industrialised countries. Even if public sector involvement can be justified, micro questions arise as to how effectively particular services deal with individual illnesses, how efficiently these services are provided, and how equitably they are distributed.

History of public provision in mental illness

Any policy analysis of mental health services must note that these were among the first public services to be provided, along with defence, roads, and the police. In the UK, local authorities were empowered from 1828, and required from 1845, to build lunatic asylums (Jones 1972). Funding was from local property taxation until 1874, when the first central financing was introduced to help provide for pauper lunatics. The extent of direct central support remained limited to less than 25% of total spending, though, until the advent of the NHS in 1948. The fact that admission to a mental hospital generally involved formal certification and loss of legal rights meant that public financing was necessary, at least for the destitute who made up the overwhelming bulk of those admitted; compulsory treatment of those lacking resources could only be financed out of the public purse. However, the shift to informal admission after the 1959 Mental Health Act to some extent undermined the argument that the service should be publicly provided and financed.

Virtually all industrialised countries today provide mental illness services through the public sector, free of charge, regardless of whether confinement is voluntary or not. Why does the state remain involved, though? It will be argued here that the necessity for public provision arises primarily from the inevitable inadequacies of private market provision.

Theoretical reasons for public provision

Government intervention can be justified in economic theory on the grounds of market inefficiencies, which can result from violation of any of the following three conditions, often referred to as the standard assumptions (Barr 1987): (a) perfect information; (b) perfect competition; and (c) absence of public goods, economies of scale or externalities.

A private market for mental health care could not function adequately because of difficulties in meeting all these conditions. Were such a market to exist, the amounts of mental health services utilised would probably be sub-optimal from a social point of view.

Information deficiencies severely curtail the existence of a private market for most forms of health care. Typically, consumers have poor knowledge both of their illnesses and of the most suitable treatments, as well as of their future morbidity patterns. Applied to psychiatric illness, these problems are compounded by the possibility that the consumer may be no longer rational. Under a private market regime, much fewer mentally ill people would receive treatment than might be considered socially desirable.

A private market in mental health services would also be inhibited by the lack of competition in medicine, both because of its specialised nature and also because of legislation regulating practice. In addition, the medical profession, in conjunction with the education authorities, controls the numbers of entrants to the profession, and as with all professions, competition between practitioners is attenuated. The degree to which this lack of competition relates to the exigencies of professional specialisation or to the acquisition of monopoly power remains a matter for some debate (Green 1985). However, increasing freedom of movement of professionals within the European Community is tending to reduce the degree of control exercised by national bodies over these activities.

Of the factors making up the third standard assumption, only externalities might apply to psychiatric services. Externalities refer to the wider non-individual effects which may result from an individual's action. Psychiatric treatment may plausibly involve externalities because of the effects that non-treatment of the mentally disturbed may have on society generally.

Thus, economic theory would tend to favour public intervention in the provision of psychiatric services because of inadequate information about the services required, the lack of competition among suppliers, and the presence of wider social effects arising out of the treatment of mentally ill individuals. However, the weight given to each of these factors and the appropriate type of public intervention require more detailed investigation. The historical UK pattern of public finance plus public provision may be moving towards public finance of a range of providers, public, voluntary & private.

The argument that the private market could not adequately function for psychiatric disorder differs from the conventional social equity argument, which sees public provision as necessary because many people with low incomes might not be able to afford services (Frank 1981). The justification of public provision in terms of market failure need not detract from this equity-based argument, though; rather, it can strengthen the overall case for public provision by providing clear statements of both the efficiency and equity aspects.

Key concepts in policy analysis

Before proceeding to consider the justification for policies with a community rather than institutional slant, the terms 'social policy' and 'public policy' must be clarified. Social policy tends to be preoccupied with issues of fairness or equity, while much public policy analysis focuses on efficiency and effectiveness. Although any thorough policy analysis ought to deal with the three Es (efficiency, effectiveness, and equity), remarkably few do so, no doubt in part because of the difficulties involved; yet separation of these three aspects limits understanding. The issues raised by mental health policy and community psychiatry should be considered against the three dimensions of effectiveness, efficiency, and equity, but what do the terms mean?

Effectiveness has to do with how effectively particular services attain their goals. It can be measured by the amount of goal attainment in a particular time period, but studies of the effectiveness of medicine raise basic questions, since few procedures have been subjected to thorough evaluation of their effects on health status (Wing 1978, Drummond et al 1986). The most favoured evaluation is the randomised control trial or some variant. Such trials, which compare the effects of two or more treatments on several groups, with a random allocation of persons to each group, can be very powerful in comparing different treatment regimes and hence in judging effectiveness.

Efficiency deals with how productively resources are combined to achieve certain goals, and thus measures the cost in resources required to produce each unit of organisational or system output (Etzioni 1964). Efficiency fares less well from randomised control trial type studies because the small numbers employed can produce atypical economic results (Drummond et al 1986). Efficiency measures involve measuring, not only how much better one treatment was than another, but also how much better per unit of money spent. Complex measures of healthiness (Rosser 1983) are thus involved, as well as the costs of treatment. The quality of cost data in turn depends on the method of organisation of the health care system, with free-at-point-of-delivery systems like the NHS typically recording poor cost information.

Equity definitions range from the narrow to the broad. The narrow definition confines itself to the social characteristics of users of any service, e.g. by age, sex, social class, race, or area of residence. A somewhat wider view includes analysis of the funding of the service, asking for instance, whether the tax system is progressive, regressive, or neutral with respect to income levels. The widest approach looks at the effects of service use on life chances: by the fact of public intervention, the distribution not only of income but also of life chances will have been altered. Donnison (1975) has defined social policies widely as: 'those actions of Government which deliberately or accidentally affect the distribution of resources, status, opportunities and life chances among social groups and categories of people within the country, and thus help shape the general character and equity of its social relations'.

Equity in health service provision might also require knowledge of the degree of individual responsibility in contracting different ailments (LeGrand 1987). An evaluation of the mental health services, then, in terms of effectiveness, efficiency, and equity, would clearly require a considerable epidemiological understanding of psychiatric illness.

The epidemiology of psychiatric illness

The epidemiology of most illnesses, including psychiatric disorders, remains underdeveloped, particularly in relation to the formulation of policy; the assessment of effectiveness and efficiency would require information on the relative impact of alternative regimes and their costs. Epidemiological data on the prevalence and incidence of the various types of psychiatric illness, along with trends by time and variations by social group would be the prerequisites of an equitable health service policy. In practice, however, epidemiology and policy have generally remained uncontaminated by each other (Knox 1979).

Psychiatric illness, of course, comprises a variety of conditions. Unambiguous case definition being a prerequisite for epidemiology (Kendell 1975), the inadequacies of such definitions have posed considerable problems for psychiatry; these have only begun to be resolved in the past decade with progress towards standardised assessments and classification systems (Kreitman 1985).

The epidemiology of the psychoses, including schizophrenia, has received most attention, including cross-national studies by WHO (1973, 1979, Sartorius et al 1986) which suggest a fairly uniform incidence of schizophrenia on a worldwide basis. The controversy over the interpretation of the repeatedly demonstrated link between social class and schizophrenia remains unsettled, but recent reviews (Mechanic 1985, Cochrane 1983) see the disproportionate occurrence of schizophrenia as a consequence of genetic inheritance and social selection. Social selection could operate either through downward social mobility or through failure to move upwards as a result of the debilitating consequences of the disorder. Several studies (Goldberg & Morrison 1963, Wiersma et al 1983) reported that while new cases showed the expected class gradient, the class of their parents represented a typical occupational sample of the general population.

The epidemiology of the neuroses remains less developed, however, partly because of the ambiguity of definition and the uncertain boundaries of psychiatric disorder. Nevertheless, both a social class and a sexual gradient appear to operate (Mechanic 1985), and much research has focused on the specific factors which might account for these differences. Brown & Harris (1978), for example, suggest that the relatively higher prevalence of depression in lower-class urban women results from differential life events and greater vulnerability to such events because of life circumstances.

Historical data on prevalence and incidence have also been subject to controversy. Hare (1983), who has strongly argued, contrary to reigning orthodoxy, that insanity did increase in nineteenth century Britain, suggests — based on the age-related pattern of admissions — that this was primarily the case in respect of schizophrenia.

Klerman (1987), in one of the few articles examining the relationship between psychiatric epidemiology and policy, suggests four sub-populations which are potentially of interest to service planners: (a) an inner core group who are chronically mentally ill, amounting to around 1% of the population (all figures refer to the US); (b) an outer core group with diagnosable mental disorder, amounting to perhaps 15% of the population; (c) a large group who are each year exposed to the risk factors of stress and distress associated with life events and social adversity, amounting to perhaps 25% of the population; and (d) a new group using mental health facilities in the hope of realising their personal potential, estimated at 6–10% of the population.

Although the inner core group has traditionally been the focus of those providing services, Klerman argues for greater understanding of the factors which lead members of these other groups into contact with mental health services. Similarly, preventive policies would necessitate such information, which, however, remains so far noticeable by its absence.

POLICY ANALYSIS OF COMMUNITY PSYCHIATRY

The community

The concept of community is one of the more difficult in the whole field of public policy. An old term, it curiously does not seem to have had any negative connotations (Williams 1976) but encompasses a realm of vaguely positive sentiments. Community relates in complex ways to the concept of fraternity which, with liberty and equality, has been a key historical term in the evolution of modern liberal-democratic society, but whose contemporary application is soaked with nostalgia and utopianism (Ignatieff 1984). Although several commentators (HMSO 1985, Wilmott 1986) have acknowledged the desirability of adopting some alternative term, they have ruefully accepted the impossibility of change. 'Community care' has proved to be an extraordinarily seductive piece of alliteration, the origins of which remain open to some doubt. The phrase appears to have been first used by the Wood Committee Report on Mental Deficiency (HMSO 1929).

However, the ambiguities inherent in the concept of community have become apparent as attempts have been made to fashion a policy of 'community care'. Bulmer (1987) has defined four lacunae in relation to community care in Britain: (a) the lack of any consistent family policy; (b) the failure to develop any policy to support women acting as informal carers; (c) the failure to think through the implications for informal care of the deinstitutionalisation of the mentally ill and mentally handicapped; and (d) the lack of serious attention to the interweaving of formal and informal care. These shortcomings all apply to community-orientated psychiatry, which also involves assumptions about the nature of psychiatric illness, its course and treatment, the proper scope for psychiatry, and the efficacy of social work (Hawks 1975).

'Community psychiatry', as used here, includes both community-orientated treatment of the mentally ill and the deinstitutionalisation and care of long-stay patients. Treatment relates mainly to incidence, in the sense of 'new' patients, but may also involve treatment of 'old' patients. Patients who have been moved out of long-stay institutions may require the same or different treatment as others, but mainly require nursing, counselling, support, and shelter.

Central issues in community-orientated psychiatry include the questions of *who* provides *what* care or treatment and *where*. A useful distinction in policy terms separates care *in* and *by* the community (Bayley 1973). Receiving care by some member of the community, whether relative, friend, or neighbour, differs greatly from obtaining care from a professional carer, whether in the context of the community or of an institution.

The scope for care being provided by members of the community depends on many factors, including: (a) the availability of carers (traditionally women not in paid employment); (b) the provisions for income maintenance for both the cared and the carers; and (c) the types of treatment favoured.

All of these sets of variables have changed considerably during the past decades. The effects of changes in family structure, fertility, and the employment of married women have been extensively analysed (Ermisch 1985), showing that altered rates of births and of women's participation in the labour force result from deep-seated structural factors. The OECD (1986) has shown that the trends to smaller families, life-long involvement of women in the labour force, and the consequently reduced scope for informal caring, all apply internationally. Although the modern welfare state has evolved income-maintenance schemes which guarantee at least a minimum income to the sick, including the mentally ill, state support for carers remains one of the less developed aspects of policy.

Community psychiatry in Britain tends to involve treatment and care primarily 'in' rather than 'by' the community; it is necessarily carried out by psychiatrists or other members of community psychiatric teams. Similarly, care of those leaving long-stay hospitals tends to be mainly by professional staff, but a policy of treating new referrals in the community rather than in institutions might enable care to be provided mainly by that individual's personal network, at least for the less serious disorders. Care provided by the community, however, whether by family, friends, neighbours, or voluntary organisations, involves considerable burdens, with carers generally receiving little support, advice or information from official agencies (Fadden et al 1987).

Community-orientated psychiatric treatment can be characterised by the provision of the usual range of psychiatric interventions (diagnosis and treatment e.g. pharmacotherapy and psychotherapy) in the patient's home environment. While this may be as effective as hospital-centred treatment (see below), and provided at no greater financial cost, a number of other questions are raised including those relating to the privacy and autonomy of the client. For instance, Bulmer (1987) suggests that privacy, defined as the control over the way information about oneself is used, may be imperilled by community care. Treatment for psychiatric illness provided at home may be more difficult to conceal from family or neighbours, and may therefore stigmatise in the same way as institutional care. The problems of compulsory treatment in the community are discussed in the next section. The remainder of this section reviews studies of community-orientated treatment and of deinstitutionalisation.

Studies of community-orientated treatment

An 1981 review of the literature of studies of outcomes from different modes of treatment and care (Braun et al 1981) suggested that with few exceptions, these studies had been open to serious methodological objections, when examined against such criteria as: (a) randomised allocation; (b) well characterised patients; (c) detailed descriptions of experimental and control programmes; (d) outcomes measured with validated instruments; (e) follow-up for adequate period; and (f) large enough numbers for statistical inference.

Most of the treatment studies summarised in Table 21.4 covered young patients, used randomised allocation methods, and collected some economic data on costs. The numbers of patients included were generally small, though, and many studies were confined to schizophrenics. The report by Test & Stein (1980) has received least criticism, and has come to be seen as a prototype. Hoult & Reynold's study (1984), which was completed since the 1981 review, broadly replicated that of Test & Stein, in Australia as did Fenton (1982) in Canada and a number of more recent studies (see Olfson, 1990). Such a study has not yet been completed in the UK.

Table 21.4 Outcome studies of alternative treatments modes for new patients: a summary

	Country	Numbers studied	Follow-up (months)	Exclusions	Type of trial
Grad & Sainsbury (1968)	Eng	1408	24	none	Other
Pasamanick et al (1967)	US	152	6-30	Sch only	RCT
Langsley et al (1969)	US	300	1	Not stated	RCT
Goodacre et al (1975)	Can	212	12	Al/drugs	RCT
Polak & Kirby (1976)	US	85	?	Not stated	RCT
Mosher et al (1975)	US	57	12	Sch only	Other
Stein & Test (1980)	US	130	14	Al/Drugs/Br	RCT
Fenton et al (1982)	Can	162	24	Al/Drugs/Suic	RCT
Hoult & Reynolds (1984)	Aus	65	12	Sch only	RCT

Source: adapted from Fenton et al (1982) with Hoult added.
Notes: Sch = Schizophrenia, Al = Alcoholism, Br = Severe organic brain syndrome, Suic = High suicide risk, RCT = Randomised control trial.

Despite the shortcomings of some of these studies, particularly the small numbers involved and the groups excluded, they all agreed about the relative value of alternatives to hospital treatment:

(i) Effectiveness: in none of the studies did outcome measures favour hospital treatment, indicating that the effectiveness of community treatments was at least equal to that of hospital-based care. No comparison was made between different types of community-orientated treatments, however;

(ii) Efficiency: the relative efficiency of community-orientated treatments remains unclear. The Test & Stein study (Weisbrod et al 1980) showed that both benefits and costs were higher in the community-orientated programme, but as a common calculus to compare costs and benefits was lacking, relative efficiency could not be estimated. However, Hoult & Reynolds (1984) suggested that community-orientated treatment for schizophrenics was more efficient, in that it produced better outcomes at less cost;

(iii) Equity: the equity aspects of the different types of care was not explicitly considered, except insofar as the selection of control and trial groups adequately accounted for social differences. The small numbers involved in virtually all the studies would inhibit one from drawing conclusions about equity.

More generally, these studies took both 'hospital' and 'psychiatric' patients as unitary entities, whereas a more sophisticated approach would recognise the diversity of types included in both terms, and the possibility that some categories of hospital treatment were likely to be better for some groups of patients. Further, by setting hospital and community-orientated treatments as opposites, some studies precluded the possibility that combined hospital and community treatment may be the most appropriate in certain circumstances.

Studies of deinstitutionalisation

The main studies of alternatives to long-term hospital care, summarised in Table 21.5, also covered relatively few patients compared with the numbers who have been 'deinstitutionalised'. Only two of the studies reported were judged adequate on the methodological criteria noted above; those of Marx et al (1973) and of Weinman & Kleiner (1978). The lack of longer-term follow-up has also been stressed.

An important UK analysis of 28 pilot projects (Cambridge & Knapp 1988, HMSO 1990b) explored the effects of different models of care management in the deinstitutionalisation of 900 long-stay patients. Community care alternatives scored at least as well in measures of outcome and at no greater cost, but staff often experienced difficulties.

The conclusions from the studies of deinstitutionalisation were that: (a) Effectiveness seemed to be equal between those discharged more or less rapidly; (b) Efficiency also seemed equal, in that costs were no higher in the community; (c) Equity issues were hardly ever examined.

A later literature review (Avison & Speechley 1987) suggested that little theoretical or methodological progress has been made on these issues or in identifying factors conducive to the adjustment of discharged patients on their return to the community. Mosher (1983) has argued that despite the clear superiority of community-orientated services, as claimed to be shown by the above studies, only slow progress has been possible due to the reluctance of service providers to change. Against this, Tantam (1985) suggested that these studies had been insufficiently clear on the representativeness of the groups studied to warrant their generalisability, and that they had failed to demonstrate that seriously disturbed patients can be managed as well in the community as in hospital. The small numbers involved and the lack of clarity about the groups who were excluded lend weight to this argument.

The failure to consider equity issues in both sets of studies is also disturbing. Such an omission may be more serious in the case of deinstitutionalisation because of the evidence that many of those being discharged belong to the less advantaged social classes, regardless of which classes they originated in. Even if some patients ought not to have

Table 21.5 Summary of studies of deinstitutionalisation

	Country	Nos	Follow-up	Type of trial	Major exclusions
Brown et al (1966)	UK	339	5 years	Other	Hom/Suic
Wing (1960)	UK	30	12 months	RCT	Sev Dist
Marx et al (1973)	US	61	5 months	RCT	Chronic
Weinman & Kleiner (1978)	US	625	4 months	RCT	None
Linn et al (1977)	US	420	4 months	RCT	Sev Disabled
Cambridge & Knapp 1988	UK	900	36 months	Pilot projects	None

Source: Braun et al 1981

Notes: Hom/Suic = Homicidal, suicidal, Sev Dist = Too severely disturbed, Chronic = Too chronic, Sev Disabled = Too severely disabled.

become long-stay in the first place, once they have become so, the decision to discharge them often without adequate monitoring, let alone community support, can only be judged undesirable and likely to be inequitable.

OTHER FACTORS IN THE DEVELOPMENT OF MENTAL HEALTH POLICY

If the shift to community-orientated treatment and care was not driven by demonstrable advantages in terms of effectiveness, efficiency, and equity, what factors were involved? This section considers the influence of costs; of social security development; of new treatments; of legal changes; and of shifts in the perception of mental illness and health. In essence, the change to community-orientated policies was more a retreat from the institution than a positive move towards the community.

Costs

By the 1950s, the life-cycle of the original British mental hospital buildings was necessitating costly replacement or renovation. Many had been built shortly after the 1845 Lunacy Act, or during the second wave of asylum construction in the 1880s. After 1900, asylum building was on a much smaller scale so that by the 1950s, many of the structures were in a poor state. Although the costs of replacement were nowhere dealt with explicitly, they received fleeting mention in the main policy documents, such as *Better Services for the Mentally Ill* (HMSO 1975). An official study on underused and surplus property (HMSO 1982), however, estimated that one-third of mental hospitals were no longer viable and that some £2 billion would be required for full repair and maintenance of the rest.

Trends in other public policies

Treatment of the mentally ill was necessarily institutionally-orientated before the development of universal income maintenance schemes. Since such schemes emerged as a product of the post-World War II welfare state, the enthusiasm in the 1950s for community care policies is hardly surprising. The debate in the UK had earlier been dominated by the perceived inequity of the means-tested Poor Law, with the result that the distinction between insurance-based payments and public assistance was largely eroded. Similarly, payments to cover housing costs, which developed rapidly in the UK social security system during the 1970s and 1980s, can only have facilitated community care. Current plans for deinstitutionalisation depend critically on continuing social security payments to discharged patients, particularly in respect of housing costs, which can be three or four times greater than personal cash payments to claimants (National Audit Office 1987).

New treatments

New treatments, particularly pharmacotherapies, also favoured community-orientated care and treatment. While opinions have differed on the effects of the development of antipsychotic drugs, there can be little doubt that they at least played an enabling function in the shift to community care. Scull (1977) has scoffed at the claims that drugs played a leading role, mainly on account of timing; he has stated that deinstitutionalisation as a policy was adopted before such drugs were in common use. While community-orientated care may not have chronologically followed the development of new drugs directly, their promise almost certainly increased confidence in the newly emerging policy. Perhaps more importantly, the use of drugs enabled many of the more custodial aspects of mental hospitals to be removed.

The contemporary role played by new methods of drug delivery may be of greater importance; neuroleptic drugs can be administered by injection, with slow-release effects lasting for several weeks (depot drugs). Although there are obvious advantages, not least regarding compliance, the long-term effects of such therapy have been little studied. Freeman (1978), however, has argued that differences in the method of delivery of the same drug are pharmacologically irrelevant, although the practical and therapeutic advantages seem to have been considerable. Depot drug treatments, which greatly increase the scope for community-based treatment, also raise difficult issues about patients' rights, in particular whether treatment can be given in the community without their consent.

Legal rights

One of the effects of civil rights movements around the world in the 1960s and 1970s was the ever more widespread employment of the concept of 'rights' to cover new groups including psychiatric patients. The 1983 UK Mental Health Act fundamentally changed the law in their favour, thus reversing the trend away from legalism which was evident in the 1930 Mental Treatment Act and the 1959 Mental Health Act (Unsworth 1987). The 1983 Act resulted partly from the championing of patients' legal rights by the pressure group MIND, leading to the publication of a White Paper (HMSO 1978), a revised White Paper (1981a) following the change of government in 1979, and finally legislation in 1983 (HMSO 1983a). Much of the final legislation reflected MIND's detailed legal input to the policy-making process (Unsworth 1987).

The 1983 Act extended patient's rights through legal safeguards: further restrictions were placed on long-term compulsory detention; second opinions were required about the necessity for the more serious forms of treatment; legal immunities that service providers had hitherto enjoyed were reduced; the franchise was extended to informal patients; and the Mental Health Act Commission was established to monitor and report on patients' rights. However, the commitment in the Labour Government's White Paper (HMSO 1978) to a 'crisis intervention' service as a community-based alternative to formal emergency admission, was dropped on the grounds of cost. Similarly, the problem of compulsory treatment in the community was left unresolved, leading at times to the use of conditional leave as a means of ensuring treatment compliance after discharge (Unsworth 1987), until this was disallowed by the courts. the Mental Health Act Commission (1986) proposed a variety of options for discussion, and the Royal College of Psychiatrists (1987) called for a new legal power to allow compulsory medical treatment outside hospital. While psychiatrists have strongly supported such compulsory powers, almost unanimous opposition has come from community psychiatric nurses (Dyer 1987), social workers, and 'users' groups (Read 1988).

Anti-psychiatry, women's and gay movements

The move towards greater emphasis on patients' rights also drew on the anti-psychiatry movement, in turn based on the writings on Laing (1960, 1967), Laing and Esterson (1964), and Cooper (1970) in the UK, and Szasz (1972a, b) in the US. Although drawing on different political premises, these works represented an unprecedented assault on psychiatry by psychiatrists. Madness was seen by them less in terms of illness but rather as arising from problems in living (Szasz), or from contemporary capitalist society (Laing & Cooper), although there was no evidence that the level and morbidity in 'socialist' societies was any different.

A range of sociological studies lent support to the anti-psychiatry movement, including studies by Goffman (1962) and Scheff (1966), of deviancy by Matza (1969), Pearson (1975), and of psychiatric history by Rothman (1971), Foucault (1973), Scull (1979), and Castels (1976). In addition, the repeated scandals in long-stay hospitals (Martin 1984) contributed to the public disquiet about such institutions, which included mental handicap as well as psychiatric units.

The women's and gay movements drew on, and to some extent developed out of the assault on conventional psychiatry which queried the definition of normal behaviour and social roles. The initial inclusion of homosexuality as a psychiatric disorder in DSM II, before protests led to its discontinuation (Blashfield 1984), may have contributed to public malaise in the USA.

Inevitably, perhaps, this revolt found its literary and artistic accompaniment. The novel and film 'One Flew Over the Cuckoo's Nest', were the most popular and visible part of a sub-culture which eschewed the conventional view of madness, though novels on the theme of mental health services as evil conspiracies have a long tradition which the 1960s revived (Showalter 1987, Jones 1972).

BARRIERS TO POLICY IMPLEMENTATION AND PROPOSED SOLUTIONS

Following concern over lack of progress, the UK Government began the 1980s with a consultative document (HMSO 1981b) on ways that resources might be moved towards community care. Fragmentation of responsibility for the mentally ill was seen as providing incentives for the NHS to discharge patients, but not for Local Authorities to provide the necessary community-orientated facilities and care. The various policy documents reviewed below deepened understanding of these problems and led to the proposals for change. Following the 1981 consultative document, the DHSS (HMSO 1983b) announced support for two of the more modest options, the further facilitation of the joint finance arrangements which had existed since 1976, and allowing health authorities to make payments ('dowries') for long-stay patients discharged to other agencies. The more radical options, such as allocating administrative responsibility for the client group to a single authority, or of central transfer of funds to local government were rejected, only to re-surface in later reviews. While the changed joint finance arrangements have not been particularly successful, the dowry system has made possible the closure of some mental handicap hospitals (Korman & Glennerster 1985) and was being extended to the mental hospitals. Progress on deinstitutionalisation of the mentally ill was comprehensively reviewed and criticised in two official reports, one from a House of Commons Select Committee (HMSO 1985), the other from the Audit Commission (HMSO 1986c). Arising out of these trenchant critiques, the UK Government in December 1986, requested Sir Roy Griffiths 'to review the way in which public funds are used to support community care policy and to advise ... on the options for action that would improve the use of these funds as a contribution to more effective community care'. Griffiths reported in March 1988 (HMSO 1988a). In addition, two other official reports on residential care were published: the Firth (HMSO 1987a) and the Wagner Report (HMSO 1988b&c). The Government responded favourably to the Griffiths Report and published a White Paper, *Caring in the Community* (HMSO 1989a) which, in conjunction with other NHS reforms (HMSO 1989b), will fundamentally affect the development of services for the mentally ill.

The Short Committee Report

The House of Commons Select Committee Report (or Short Report, after the name of its Chair, Mrs Short) noted that theirs was the first inquiry of this scope to be carried out by elected representatives. Despite misgivings, the Committee decided to continue to use the term 'community care'. After reviewing a wide range of submissions, it considered that the 'cart had been put before the horse', in that the removal of hospital facilities had far out-run the provision of services in the community to replace them. 'Any fool can close a long term hospital: it takes time and trouble to do it properly and compassionately'. More positively, the Short Report recommended improved planning, increased involvement of patients and their families, and better take-up by patients of social security benefits. The Committee advocated increased funding — 'the proposition that community care could be cost-neutral is untenable'. Real increases in expenditure on services for mentally ill and mentally retarded people were seen as essential if community care policies were to be achieved. The Committee, however, did not attempt to quantify the extra finances needed.

The Audit Commission Report

The necessity for extra finance was challenged in a report from the Audit Commission (1986), which argued strongly that much more could be achieved within existing budgets. Community care, it claimed, had been successfully implemented in some areas, but national policies were in disarray due to agencies pulling in different directions; health and social services, in particular, were poorly co-ordinated. The methods for transferring funds were judged to have been inadequate in a number of ways. Dowry payments which took no account of the degree of disability had led to some agencies accepting and making a profit on the fitter ex-patients, while the inability to transfer all long-stay patients had meant that some hospitals had to remain open, thus preventing the full transfer of resources. Further, dowries have been confined to discharged patients, thus ignoring those in need of care who had not managed to be admitted.

The Audit Commission Report also detailed the problems of bridging finance, suggesting that strategies have been developed in ad hoc ways, sometimes leading to perverse incentives and cost shifting from one public authority to another. Local authorities faced particular problems in that funds for community care had to compete with many other claims, at a time of severely constrained budgets, and when social services were being drastically reduced in some areas.

However, the Commission argued strongly that the success of some authorities indicated that much could be achieved with committed local leadership and a preparedness to bend the rules where necessary. Other identified ingredients for success included: the delegation of budgets for providing services to small localities, the development of multidisciplinary care teams, and partnership between statutory and voluntary organisations.

The Audit Commission, concluding that radical change was necessary, suggested the nomination of 'lead authorities' for the mentally ill, the elderly, and the mentally and physically handicapped, respectively. Such authorities would have separate budgets, to be used to purchase services from other agencies, if and as appropriate. A proposal of this kind was raised but rejected by UK policy makers in the early 1980s, and also by Griffiths in 1988.

Griffiths' review

The Government, in March 1988, published the review of community care prepared under Sir Roy Griffiths, whose earlier report has led to fundamental restructuring of NHS financial practices (HMSO 1983c). Rejecting the Audit Commission's proposal for lead authorities in favour of strengthening the role of local authorities, the report proposed the radical option for the public sector 'to spell out responsibilities, insist on performance and accountability and to evidence that action is being taken; and even more radical, to match policy with appropriate resources and agreed timescales'. The mentally ill, the mentally handicapped and the elderly would all become the responsibility of the Local Authorities, but Griffiths avoided the issue of whether extra funding was required by stressing that regardless of the level of funding, improved structures were required.

Under Griffiths' proposals, responsibilities for community care would be clarified at both national and local levels. He proposed that a new central focus should be provided by a new Minister for Community Care responsible for approving and, in part, funding programmes produced by the local authorities. The social services authorities within the local authorities should be responsible for ensuring that the needs of individuals within specified groups were identified, packages of care devised and services co-ordinated, and, where appropriate, a specific care manager assigned.

Funding of programmes at local authority level should, according to Griffiths, be made up from a variety of sources and in such a way as to remove the short-term variability which had hitherto inhibited planning. Between 40% and 50% of funding should be from central government, the rest to be made up from charges and the new 'community charge' (poll tax). The main component of central funds should be that part of the current rate support grant which is provided to social services authorities from central government for community care responsibilities but which is not at present earmarked for this purpose. Rather than proposing new funding mechanisms, then, Griffiths recommended defining the responsibilities inherent in the present system and building control mechanisms into them. Existing entitlements would be preserved whilst putting the social services authorities in a position of 'financial neutrality' in deciding what form of care would be in the best interests of the individual.

GPs, who potentially play a critical role in community-orientated psychiatry, also received attention from Griffiths. In the UK, some 60%

to 70% of the population see their GP annually and between one-quarter and one-third of all illnesses treated by family doctors are thought to be psychiatric in origin. To the extent that early rather than late diagnosis and treatment are to be preferred, GPs could provide that intervention. However, GPs have little time for assessment and treatment, and their recognition of psychiatric disorder depends largely on their own attitudes and training (Goldberg 1981). Despite an enthusiasm for extending the role of GPs in treating psychiatric illness in the 1970s, such interest appears to have waned more recently: the White Paper on primary care (HMSO 1987b) paid minimal attention to this question. Griffiths, however, suggested that the full potential of the family doctor services had not been realised, and recommended amending GP's contracts to specify that they should inform the social services authority of possible community care needs of their patients.

With regard to the specific problems of deinstitutionalisation, Griffiths recommended that special funds be made available for large-scale projects such as closing a long-stay hospital and developing alternative community services. Such projects should take the form of a joint plan by the health and social services authorities, including the nomination of a 'care manager' for each long-stay patient who was to be discharged.

The Firth Report

An important influence on Griffiths was the Report of a Joint Central and Local Government Working Party on Public Support for Residential Care (HMSO 1987a), under Mrs Firth, which provided a detailed account of the perverse financial incentives affecting local authorities' decisions concerning choice of residential or domiciliary care. These incentives resulted from the complex interactions of national social security entitlements and Local Authority resources. The Firth Report recommended, on the basis of a detailed appraisal of options, in favour of giving local authorities responsibility for financing all public sector residential care. 'Financial neutrality' (a phrase picked up by Griffiths) should be achieved by harmonisation of the social security and local government financing systems, involving the transfer of National Social Security funds to the local authority. Local authorities would also be responsible for the assessment of care needs, but with an obligation to provide a reasonable degree of choice to clients. Although confined to residential care, which is mainly provided for the elderly, these proposals also affect the mentally ill and bear a close resemblance to those put forward by Griffiths.

The Wagner Report

The Report of the Independent Review of Residential Care (HMSO 1988b,c), referred to as the Wagner Report after its Chair, Lady Wagner, provided a considered review of the subject, along with useful background surveys of recent research. Recommendations were made concerning residential care in statutory, voluntary, and private establishments. Perhaps of most importance, Wagner agreed with Griffiths (and Firth) on the central role of local authorities, recommending that they should be responsible for the strategic planning of accommodation and support services for community care. Wagner also stressed, with Griffiths, the desirability of consumer choice. On the particular needs of the mentally ill, increased investment was recommended to extend the range of services in the community for people with or recovering from psychiatric illness. Recommendations were also made regarding individual rights, the setting and maintaining of standards, and staffing and training. This report provided a detailed account of residential care, which in turn made up part of Griffiths' brief. The similarity of the Firth, Wagner, and Griffiths findings regarding the enhanced role of the local authorities and of consumer choice was striking.

Griffiths' proposals classed the mentally ill with the elderly and the mentally handicapped, and proposed giving responsibility to the local authorities for them all; since the NHS currently provides the bulk of services for the mentally ill, this would have involved a major change. Doubts were expressed about the ability of the social service authorities to manage the complex mix of services necessary for community care for the mentally ill (Day & Klein 1988).

The Government's response

In late 1989, the government published the White Paper 'Caring for People' (HMSO 1989a) which accepted much of the Griffiths report and proceeded to legislate accordingly in the NHS & Community Care Act of 1990. The long-standing commitment to community care was reiterated and the main changes announced concerned ways of ending the perverse incentives resulting from the unplanned interaction of social security and residential accommodation. In future, a single budget would cover the costs of care, regardless of where provided. All claimants would be equally entitled, whether living in their own homes, independent residences or nursing homes. Local authorities were to be given responsibility for the use of public funds for new applicants for residential accommodation. A Minister for Community Care would not, however, be appointed.

Proper management of the care of the severely mentally ill was stressed, and hospital discharges were to be allowed only when adequate medical and social care was available; individual care plans for patients would be a prerequisite for the closure of mental hospitals. Perhaps most importantly, a new specific grant to local authorities would be channelled through the Regional Health Authorities who would thus be empowered to ensure that Local Authorities met their obligations to the mentally ill.

In addition, a number of other initiatives specific to the mentally ill were announced, including: (a) Guidance to Health Authorities on the development of individual care programmes for psychiatric patients discharged from hospitals with the Royal College of Psychiatrists assisting in drawing up a code of good practice. (b) Guidance on compulsory admissions, with a code of practice on admitting and treating patients compulsorily detained under the 1983 Mental Health Act. (c) Health service resources would be eased by allowing greater flexibility in disposing of mental hospital sites before closure, by means of bridging loans and deals with private developers. (d) Quality of services would be monitored by the Health Advisory Service, which itself would be reviewed for effectiveness, and (e) The role of the voluntary sector would be reviewed, in particular the £2.5 million funding currently provided to it; (f) Closer links between GPs and social service departments would be fostered.

Although virtually all the White Paper proposals were included in the NHS and Community Care Act of 1990, the implementation of many was postponed to 1993 due to fears of their impact on the Community Charge (Poll Tax). Several reforms affecting mental health services will, however, become operational from April 1991, including the new grant to local authorities and a capital loans fund. Mental illness services funded by local authorities will receive a £30m injection in 1991 made up 70/30 from central & local funding. A £50m three-year rolling programme will loan funds to facilitate the transition between closing mental hospitals and opening non-hospital facilities.

Other reforms of the National Health Service, as outlined in the White Paper 'Working for Patients' (1989b) will also change the way health services are provided for the mentally ill. Two reforms stand out in particular: the separation of purchaser and provider roles; and the introduction of capital charges. Health authorities will become purchasers of services from other agencies. As contracting agencies, they will have the power to ensure that services are provided appropriately. To the extent that those supplying the mental health services have been responsible for the slow development of community-orientated policies, the advent of service contracts will facilitate progress. If community-orientated treatments can be shown to be cost effective, they may well become the norm.

Perhaps of equal importance in encouraging the closure of the old mental hospitals will be the introduction of capital charges on all NHS hospitals from 1991. These capital charges, to be made up of depreciation and interest on the capital assets of each hospital, are likely to increase significantly the average revenue cost per mental hospital patient for several reasons: firstly many mental hospitals now occupy valuable sites; secondly, the amount of space per inpatient has increased as numbers have fallen; and thirdly, the relatively low revenue cost per mental hospital bed, compared with acute hospital beds, means that the capital charge will amount to a relatively higher proportion of the revenue cost per bed.

Thus, at the end of the 1980s, and after 30 years of slow progress with community-orientated mental health policies, some of the major organisational barriers are to be swept away. The combination of a single budget for the mentally ill, combined with service contracts specifying modes of treatment and increased costs for inpatient treatment may mark a policy conjuncture which will lead to fundamental changes. The monolithic pattern of provision centred on the former lunatic asylums looks like being replaced by a network of smaller, community-orientated facilities, publicly financed but provided by a mix of voluntary and private agencies.

CONCLUSIONS

The above discussion has suggested that the major changes in mental health policy over the past three decades in Britain have been reactive, owing as much to developments in social security, law and wider social perceptions as to any demonstrated advantages of the more community-orientated services. Partly as a consequence of this broad support, but particularly due to policy changes implemented in 1990, the shift towards community-orientated care and treatment will almost certainly continue and accelerate. However, as the number of inpatient places declines further, greater concern may emerge over the amount of 'asylum' care available (Kings Fund 1987).

While the analysis of public policy must concern itself with the criteria of effectiveness, efficiency, and equity, the practice of policy, both in its making and implementation, results from the interplay of competing forces. Consequently, policy in practice resembles a mosaic, parts of which make sense to different groups but whose overall message may be less than completely coherent. The conclusions to be drawn from any review of policy, then, depend on the framework within which one is operating — whether that of rational policy analysis or of practical policy formation and implementation.

What can reasonably be expected from public policy in practice in a liberal-democratic society? Lindblom (1980) suggests that those who expect reality to conform to the rational model tend to become disillusioned and cynical, as policies in practice are made by settlements, reconciliations, adjustments and agreements. Lindblom's preferred criteria for evaluation of policy include acceptability, openness to reconsideration, responsiveness to a variety of interests, and equity. In a similar vein, Rein (1983) has pointed to the limits of comprehensive policy analysis and has warned against the fallacy of promoting co-ordination as anything more than a useful but limited remedy, when multiple participants continue to press competing claims. Co-ordination, he suggests, will not allow difficult choices to be avoided.

Depending on whether one operates in the rationalist-analytical mode or follows the more pragmatic approach, either pessimistic or optimistic conclusions can be drawn about mental health policy. A synthesis between the two might see the role of analysis as continually attempting to make the practice of policy more rational, more effective, efficient, and equitable, while at the same time accepting that in contemporary society, policy will in practice remain a complex resultant of many forces. Sisyphus may thus provide the most appropriate role-model for policy analysts.

A judgement on mental health policy within the framework of rational policy analysis would tend toward a pessimistic conclusion. Pessimism could be justified on the basis of lack of clarity about objectives; slow progress in closing the old mental hospitals; difficulties in establishing new community-based facilities; and insufficient resources. Alternative policies have not been thoroughly evaluated in terms of effectiveness, efficiency, and equity. Inadequate epidemiological knowledge about psychiatric illness casts doubts over possible causes and cures, as well as about the 'needs' of different groups. The fragmentation of services between health, social security, and local authorities persists. The concept of 'community', when examined, dissolves into a multiplicity of possible meanings, and the latest set of proposals for improved planning will invariably run up against these barriers.

Within such a perspective, critics often go on to apportion blame for this sorry state of affairs to one or several groups: the government; the various agencies; psychiatrists and nurses; local communities; even the mentally ill themselves. Once blame has been allocated, it usually follows that the solution lies with reforming the guilty party or parties. At this point, the analysis clearly becomes partisan and unfortunately, much commentary on policies for dealing with psychiatric illness has taken such an approach.

However, more optimistic conclusion could be based on the continued growth in resources devoted to mental health services, and the apparent acceptability of the services to the large numbers who use them each year. Policy has been flexible, with no less that five major Acts of Parliament in the UK over the last century — roughly one every generation. Custodial care has been replaced by informal regimes, often outside hospital. The run-down of institutional care in the UK, particularly in Scotland, has been slower and more cautious than in the US or Italy. Various academic studies have indicated, however roughly, the relative merits of alternative policies, broadly favouring the community-orientated stance of current policy. Epidemiological understanding has advanced, notably in mental retardation, in preventing GPI, in developing pharmacopotherapies, and in greater knowledge about schizophrenia. The official publication in Britain of no less than five reviews of community care by various agencies in the period 1986–1989, culminating in the 1990 NHS and Community Care Act, signals a preparedness to change policies as required. The fragmentation of responsibilities and associated policy inertia may be coming to an end. Within the pragmatic framework that is arguably appropriate to modern, pluralistic, Western society, then, mental health policy performs fairly well.

A balanced overall conclusion might incorporate both rational and pragmatic perspectives. Although mental health policy remains somewhat incoherent in terms of its objectives and methods of care and treatment, the sector has maintained and expanded the resources devoted to it and remains broadly acceptable to its users. Policy has developed cautiously but, in future, health authorities look like being free to purchase a variety of types of care and treatment. With constrained budgets, they will also have incentives to pursue the most cost-effective packages.

Several common grounds for concern can be discerned and grouped under the headings of service provision, finance, manpower, and research. Much of the information which is routinely collected emphasises the first of these, to the detriment of the others. Much more remains to be known about the effectiveness, efficiency, and equity of current services before they can be improved. While some progress has begun to be made in evaluation of procedures carried out on the acutely physically ill, hardly a start has been made in the mental illness sector.

The financial information available remains crude and possibly fails to reflect the diversity of types of treatment and care provided. Only direct public spending on mental health services can be ascertained, despite the certainty that other public sector programmes are also providing support. Thus, the total size of the public psychiatric sector, let alone the private one, remains unknown. The cost data that are available tend to be hospital-centred, but within this, fail to differentiate between service users, e.g. by diagnosis or severity or type of treatment. Many of the organisational difficulties have hitherto related to finance, particularly those to do with moving resources together with patients as they transfer to the newer community-orientated services. The attribution of financial responsibility to health authorities should involve improvements in the range and quality of financial data collected.

The role of professionals, despite its importance both financially and in changing the emphasis in service provision towards the community, remains under-researched, and again the focus remains on measuring inputs rather than outputs. Little is known, for example, about what psychiatric doctors and nurses actually do and how effective and efficient their actions might be. Much remains to be known about the degree to which different professions can be substituted for one another, and which combinations provide the best service. The literature on community-orientated mental health services contains remarkably little on the attitudes of existing service providers to the proposed changes, yet their support would seem to be essential if services are to change in content as well as form.

The priority in mental health services research must be to remedy these information deficiencies. There are some encouraging signs that such research is being commissioned, both officially (Renshaw & Knapp 1987) and independently (Sayce 1987). Much of this work, however, focuses on the monitoring of pilot schemes in community living, on the run-down of particular hospitals, and on broad evaluations of alternative modes of treatment. Much more detailed work would appear to be required on the evaluation of the effectiveness, efficiency, and equity aspects of particular treatments for specific ailments, as well as on their financial and manpower aspects.

No matter what changes are made in the organisation, financing, and staffing of the mental health sector, however, its long history and size, as well as society's fascination with the subject will ensure that interest and controversy continue. Because they attempt to provide for some of the more fundamental, demanding, and complex needs which individuals can have, the mental health services deserve our continuing attention.

REFERENCES

Avison W R, Speechley K N 1987 The discharged psychiatric patient: a review of the social, social-psychological and psychiatric correlates of outcome. American Journal of Psychiatry 144:1
Barr N 1987 The economics of the welfare state, London
Bayley M J 1973 Mental handicap and community care. RKP, London
Blashfield R K 1984 The classification of psychopathology: neo-kraepelinian and quantitative approaches. Plenum Press, New York
Braun P, Kochansky G, Shapiro R et al 1981 Overview: deinstitutionalisation of psychiatric patients, a critical review of outcome studies. American Journal of Psychiatry 136: 736-749
Brown G W, Harris T 1978 Social Origins of depression: a study of psychiatric disorder in women. Tavistock, London
Brown G W, Bone M, Dalison B et al 1966 Schizophrenia and social care: a comparative follow-up of 339 schizophrenic patients. OUP, London
Bulmer M 1987 The social basis of community care. Allen & Unwin, London
Cambridge P, Knapp M 1988 Demonstrating successful care in the community. Canterbury. PSSU, University of Canterbury
Castels R 1976 L'ordre psychiatrique: l'age d'or de l'alalienisme, Paris
Cochrane R 1983 The social creation of mental illness. Longman, London
Cooper D 1970 The death of the family. Pantheon, New York
Day P, Klein R 1988 Creating a revolution in community care. Health Services Journal 24 March: 326-327
Donnison D 1975 An approach to social policy. NESC, Dublin: 30
Drummond M, Ludbrook A, Lowson K, Steele A 1986 Studies in economic evaluation in health care. Vol. 2 Oxford University Press, Oxford
Dyer C 1987 Compulsory treatment in the community for the mentally ill? British Medical Journal 295: 991-992
Ermisch J 1985 The political economy of demographic change. HEB, London
Etzioni A 1964 Modern organisations. Englewood Cliffs, New Jersey, Prentice Hall
Fadden G, Bebbington P, Kuipers L 1987 The burden of care: the impact of functional psychiatric illness on the patient's family. British Journal of Psychiatry 150: 285-292
Fenton F R, Tessier L, Struvening E L, Smith F A, Benoit C 1982 Home and hospital psychiatric treatment. Croom Helm, London
Foucault M 1973 Madness and civilisation. Vintage Books, New York
Frank R 1981 Cost benefit analysis in mental health services: a review of the literature.

Administration in Mental Health 8: 164

Freeman H 1978 Pharmacological treatment and management. In: Wing J K (ed) Schizophrenia: towards a new synthesis. Academic Press, London

Goffman I 1962 Asylums: essays on the social situation of mental illness patient and other inmates. Aldine, Chicago

Goldberg D 1981 Recognition of psychological illness by general practitioners, In: Edwards G (ed) Psychiatry and general practice. University of Southampton

Goldberg E M, Morrison S L 1963 Schizophrenia and social class. British Journal of Psychiatry 209: 785-802

Goodacre R H, Coles E M, MaCurdy E A, Coates D B, Kendall LM 1975 Hospitalisation and hospital bed replacement. Canadian Psychiatric Association's Journal 20: 7-14

Grad J, Sainsbury P 1968 The effects that patients have on their families in a community and a control psychiatric service. British Journal of Psychiatry 114: 265-278

Green D 1985 Which doctor? Research Monograph 40. Institute of Economic Affairs, London

HMSO 1929 Report of the mental deficiency committee, Part III. The Audit Defective. London

HMSO 1955 Ministry of Health, Report of the Ministry of Health for the Year Ending 31 December 1954. London

HMSO 1975 Better services for the mentally ill, Cmnd. 6233. London

HMSO 1976 Priorities for personal health and social services in England: a consultative document. London

HMSO 1978 A review of the Mental Health Act 1959 Cmnd 7320. London

HMSO 1981a Reform of mental health legislation Cmnd 8405. London

HMSO 1981b Care in the community: a consultative document on moving resources for care in England. London

HMSO 1982 Report on under-utilised and surplus property in the NHS. London

HMSO 1983a Mental Health Act. London

HMSO 1983b Health service development: care in the community and joint finance. Circular HC (83)6/LAC(83)5. London

HMSO 1983c NHS management inquiry by Sir Roy Griffiths

HMSO 1985 Second Report from the Social Service Committee Session 1984/5 on Community Care. London

HMSO 1986a Statistics of mental illness and mental handicap hospitals in England, various years, and subsequent booklet series. DHSS, London

HMSO 1986b Fourth Report of the Social Services Committee, Vol II. House of Commons, 387-II. London

HMSO 1986c Making a reality of community care. Audit Commission, London

HMSO 1987a Public support for residential care: report of a joint central and local government working party. Chaired by Mrs Firth. DHSS, London

HMSO 1987b Primary health care: an agenda for discussion. London

HMSO 1988a Community care: agenda for action, a report to the Secretary of State for Social Services by Sir Roy Griffiths. London

HMSO 1988b Residential care: a positive choice, report of the independent review of residential care. Chaired by Gillian Wagner. London

HMSO 1988c Residential care: the research reviewed. Literature surveys commissioned by the independent review of residential care. Chaired by Gillian Wagner London

HMSO 1988d Public expenditure on the social services. Social Services Committee. 548. House of Commons, London

HMSO 1989a Caring for People: community care in the next decade and beyond. Secretaries of State for Health, Social Security, Wales and Scotland, London

HMSO 1989b Working for patients. Presented to the Parliament by the Secretaries of State for Health, Wales, Northern Ireland and Scotland by Command of Her Majesty. London

HMSO 1990 NHS and Community Care Act. House of Commons, London

HMSO 1990b Care in the community: making it happen. Department of Health and Central Information Office, London

Hare E 1983 Was insanity on the increase? British Journal of Psychiatry 142: 439-455

Hawks 1975 Community care: an analysis of assumptions. British Journal of Psychiatry 127: 276-85

Hoult R, Reynolds I 1984 Schizophrenia: a comparative trial of community oriented and hospital oriented psychiatric care. Acta Psychiatrica Scandinavica. 69: 359-372

Hunter D J, Wistow G 1987 Community care in Britain: variations on a theme. King's Fund, London

Ignatieff M 1984 The needs of strangers. Chatto, London: 138

Jones K 1972 A history of the mental health services. RKP, London

Kendell R E 1975 The concept of disease and its implications for psychiatry. British Journal of Psychiatry 127: 305-315

King's Fund 1987 The need for asylum in society for the mentally ill of infirm: consensus statement from the third King's Fund Forum, London

Klerman G L 1987 Psychiatric epidemiology and mental health policy. In: Levine S, Lilienfeld A (eds) Epidemiology and health policy. Tavistock London

Knox E G 1979 Epidemiology and health care planning. Oxford University Press, Oxford

Korman N, Glennerster H 1985 Closing a hospital: the Darenth Park Project. Bedford Press, London

Kreitman N 1985 Epidemiology in relation to psychiatry. In: Shepherd M (ed) The Scientific Foundations of Psychiatry. Psychiatric Handbook 5, London

Laing R D 1960 The divided self. Tavistock, London

Laing R D 1967 The politics of experience and the bird of paradise. Penguin, London

Laing R D, Esterson A 1964 Sanity madness and the family: families of schizophrenics. Tavistock, London

Laing W 1985 Private health care. Studies of current health problems No. 79. Office of Health Economics, London

Langsley D G Fromenhaft K, Mackhota P 1969 Follow up evaluation of family crisis therapy. American Journal of Orthopsychiatry 39: 735-759

LeGrand J 1987 Three essays on equity. STICERD, LSE, London

Lindblom C E 1980 The policy making process. Prentice Hall, New Jersey

Linn M W, Caffey E M Jr, Klett C J et al 1977 Hospital vs community (foster) care for psychiatric patients. Archives of general psychiatry 34: 78-83

Martin J 1984 Hospitals in trouble. Blackwell, Oxford

Marx A J, Test M A Stein L I 1973 Extrahospital management of severe mental illness: feasibility and effects of social functioning. General Archives of psychiatry 29: 505-511

Matza D 1969 Becoming deviant. Prentice Hall, New Jersey

Mechanic D 1969 Mental health and social policy. Prentice Hall, New Jersey

Mechanic D 1985 Social science in relation to psychiatry. In: Shepherd M (ed) The scientific foundations of psychiatry. Psychiatry Handbook 5, London

Mechanic D 1987 Correcting misconceptions in mental health policy: strategies for improved care of the seriously mentally ill. In: The Millbank Quarterly, 65: 2

Mental Health Act Commission 1986 Compulsory treatment in the community, a discussion paper. HMSO, London

Mosher L R 1983 Why has research failed to be translated into practice? New England Journal of Medicine 309: 1579–1580

Mosher L R, Menn A, Matthews S M 1975 Soteria: evaluation of a home-based treatment for schizophrenia. American Journal of Orthopsychiatry 45: 455-467

National Audit Office 1987 Community care developments. HMSO London

OECD 1986 The integration of women into the economy. Paris

Olfson M 1990 Assertive community treatment: an evaluation of the experimental evidence. Hospital and Community Psychiatry June 1990, Vol 41, 634-641.

Pasamanick B, Scarpitti F R, Lefton M, Dinitz S, Wernert J J, McPheeters H 1967 Schizophrenics in the community: an experimental study in the prevention of hospitalisation. Appleton Century, Crofts, New York

Pearson G 1975 The deviant imagination, psychiatry, social work and change. Macmillan, London

Polak P R, Kirby M W 1976 A model to replace psychiatric hospitals. Journal of Nervous & Mental Diseases 162: 132-52

Read J 1988 Asylums with long arms. New Society 83: 36-37

Rein M 1983 From policy to practice. Macmillan, London

Renshaw J, Knapp M 1987 Measuring out the real costs of caring. Health Services Journal 13 August, London: 934-935

Rosser R 1983 Issues of measurement in the design of health indicators: a review. In: Culyer A L (ed) Health indicators. Marin Robertson, Oxford: 39

Rothman D 1971 The discovery of the asylum, social order and disorder in the new republic. Little Brown, Boston

Royal College of Psychiatrists 1987 Community treatment orders: a discussion document. London

Sartorius N, Jablensky A, Korten A et al 1986 Early manifestations and first-contact incidence of schizophrenia in different cultures. Psychological Medicine 16: 909-928

Sayce L 1987 Revolution under review. Health Services Journal 97: 1378-1379

Scheff T J 1966 Becoming mentally ill: a sociological study. Aldine, Chicago

Scull A T 1977 Decarceration: community treatment and the deviant: a radical view. Prentice Hall, New Jersey

Scull A T 1979 Museums of madness: lunacy in Britain, 1800-1860. Penguin, London

Showalter E 1987 The female malady. Virago, London

Stein L I, Test M A 1980 Alternative to mental hospital I: conceptual model, treatment program, and clinical evaluation. Archives of General Psychiatry 37: 392-397

Sturt J, Waters H 1985 Role of the psychiatrist in community-based mental health care. Lancet i: 507-508

Szasz T S 1972a The manufacture of madness. Paladin, London

Szasz T S 1972b The myth of mental illness. Paladin, London

Tantam D 1985 Alternatives to hospitalisation. British Journal of Psychiatry 146: 1-4

Test M A, Stein L I 1980 Alternative to hospital treatment II: Social cost. Archives of General Psychiatry 37: 409-412

Unsworth C 1987 The politics of mental health legislation. Clarendon Press, Oxford

WHO 1973 Report of the international pilot study of schizophrenia. Vol 1. WHO, Geneva

Weinman B, Kleiner R J 1978 The impact of community living and community member intervention on the adjustment of the chronic psychotic patient. In: Stein L I, Test M A (eds) Alternatives to mental hospital treatment. Plenum Press, New York

Weisbrod B A, Test M A, Stein L I 1980 Alternative to mental hospital III: economic cost-benefit analysis. Archives of General Psychiatry 37: 400-405

WHO 1979 Schizophrenia: an international follow-up study. Wiley, Chichester

Wiersma D, Giel R, De Jong A, Sloof C J 1983 Social class and schizophrenia in a Dutch cohort. Psychological Medicine 13: 141-150

Williams R 1976 Keywords. London

Wilmott P 1986 The debate about community. Policy Studies Institute, London

Wing J K 1960 Pilot experiment in the rehabilitation of long stay hospitalised male schizophrenic patients. British Journal of Preventive and Social Medicine 14: 173-180

Wing J K 1978 Reasoning about Madness. Blackwell, Oxford

22. The international perspective

D.H. Bennett

Those who have sought to make international comparisons of mental health services find that this involves difficulties which stem not only from differences in the definition of a 'patient' or a 'bed', but from fundamental disparities in the recording of data. May (1976) noted that the process is further hampered by the absence of standardised criteria and terminology in relation to both the organisation and operation of facilities, as well as to the training and qualification of staff. More surprisingly, there are gaps in the information available to governments themselves, while an account simply of overall national profiles can also mislead, since in all countries, there are serious regional inequalities in the distribution of services. The most reliable data are still those referring to mental hospitals and to the services which they provide; the more services are decentralised among a variety of facilities, the more difficult it becomes to collect consistently reliable information about their activities.

Assumptions tend to be made about the achievements of some other country which stress its ideals, rather than giving examples of its failure to meet them. Though Jones (1979), a widely respected commentator on social policy, could claim that the United States 'had made a much better job of the business of deinstitutionalisation' than Britain, Mollica (1980) and Scull (1984) thought that this seemed to indicate an intimate knowledge of British policies but too ready an acceptance of American claims. Who is right? There have also been many over-enthusiastic but superficial accounts of developments in Italy. So the value of such international discussion might well be questioned, since it is unlikely to offer solutions to pressing domestic problems by providing any country with a system which could be transplanted there wholesale. Nevertheless, some comparisons can challenge current national assumptions and can add extra dimension to the perception of any country's problems, as well as providing clues for possible new approaches to their resolution. They might also indicate pitfalls which others could try to avoid (Mangen 1985), though it must be recognised that differences between services in different countries may owe as much to broad social policy and to economic change as to alterations in psychiatric outlook and treatment. For instance, current mental health developments and plans in Britain are highly dependent on the social security system, so that any loss of support from that side would throw the whole development into jeopardy. But whatever the organisational pattern, each system has positive and negative features: highly centralised administrations can plan comprehensively and allocate staff where they are most needed, while decentralised, loosely organised systems may result in excellent local or community services, which cannot then be reproduced on a national scale (May 1976).

A working group of WHO (1980) reaffirmed the value of comprehensive community mental health care, but concluded that it was 'not properly applied because of prejudice and professional ignorance, lack of staff and material resources, poor co-ordination and administration, political vacillation, and outdated legislation'. Because of these influences of both professional and non-professional factors on changes in the pattern of care, WHO decided that instead of examining national trends in Europe, it would look at a number of selected local experiments in different countries that might serve as demonstration models — the 'Pilot Study Areas' (WHO 1987) (vide infra). Similarly, while this chapter makes no claims to undertake a comparative analysis of national differences, it does seek to highlight variations within the general framework of mainstream European and North American assumptions about psychiatric services — that their aim is improvement in the mental health of populations and the reduction of psychiatric morbidity, by making a better quality of care available to all those who are at risk.

In the late 1960s, May believed that in spite of national differences, each European country faced similar problems in providing for the care and management of the mentally ill, and that they had developed broadly similar services for dealing with most serious forms of psychiatric illness. To test this assumption, he circulated a questionnaire to the governments in all countries of the European region of WHO. In spite of the surprising fact that many countries lacked the most basic details of their services, it was hoped that the exercise would not only improve the subsequent collection of data in each country, but that it would prove to be repeatable. In view of the changes that had occurred since the end of World War II, it was expected that the study would show a shift from hospital to community care — that patients were being treated to a large extent only on an outpatient basis and receiving medical and social support in their normal environments. In *Mental Health Services in Europe* (May 1976), shortcomings in the data were acknowledged, but the study did provide a useful baseline and did in fact stimulate some countries to collect more adequate data. May emphasised that in public health, the main emphasis was no longer on acute and communicable diseases, but on chronic, relapsing illness and that 'this had been responsible for more state direction of mental health services in most countries'.

A review of progress in Europe, 10 years after May's study, showed that information on mental health services was still seriously deficient (Freeman et al 1985). For example, though outpatient services had been widely developed, half the countries could not provide any list of their outpatient resources, while the rest could give only incomplete details. Full data on day patient facilities were not available in 7 countries and no information at all could be given about them in another 6; only 17 countries were able to report on the number of day places available, and 8 on the number of patients attending. A certain degree of movement was seen to have taken place away from dependence on largely custodial care in remote institutions, and these facilities were no longer seen as a central point for the psychiatric service. Instead, sectorised, diversified, and multidisciplinary services were being provided in many European countries. Nevertheless, progress had not generally been very impressive and in most areas, services alternative to the hospital remained so limited as to have little or no influence on inpatient care. Perhaps this relative lack of change should not be so surprising, though; forward-looking psychiatrists in Britain have been trying for at least a hundred years to implement changes in a pattern of care dominated by the mental hospital. Therefore, perhaps the evidence that the number of mental hospitals in Europe with over a thousand beds have been reduced in this period by 50% should be seen as fairly satisfactory evidence of some progress, on the assumption that very large institutions will tend to have generally lower standards of care.

The Pilot Study Areas initiative eventually involved 21 areas in 16 European member states (WHO 1987). One lesson learned from it was that any patient progresses through a series of service elements, and that his/her use of the particular elements of that service is determined more by the nature of the service than by his/her characteristics as a patient; this particularly applies to readmission (Freeman & Fryers 1987). Another important lesson was that 'a shift in the emphasis of care cannot be achieved simply by providing a new alternative; other action is necessary, e.g. closure of the less desirable type of service' (Giel et al 1987). The importance emerged of social and demographic determinants in both the provision of services and their use: for services depend on inter-relationships between the environment, the experience of illness, the community's resources, professional traditions, and demographic history. This perhaps explains why there are no ideal services; while most psychiatric services have some or many of the features needed in a good network, none has them all, and those that do may be exceptions to the general run of that particular nation's provision.

In the subsequent discussion here, emphasis will be given to the divergent views, different methods of administration, and variable funding services revealed by the WHO studies, as well as to the difficulties which these cause for the implementation of community care. In the European region, the aims of WHO have gathered sophistication since the 1970s, and now include a reduction of the psychiatric morbidity of the member states' population 'by making services of better quality available to everyone at risk' (Freeman et al 1985). It is hoped that progress towards this objective may be achieved by moving the system of care from mental hospitals under medical direction to comprehensive community-orientated services, staffed by multidisciplinary teams, though there are, of course, subsidiary objectives, including recruitment and training of staff, liaison with primary care, co-ordination and specialisation of services, etc. While health services obviously differ enormously between various countries, the innovations made by pioneers have shown a remarkable similarity to each other. Does this mean that as international travel and communications improve, pioneering advances will tend to follow a common pattern? Perhaps so, since these innovations often bear little relation to the current provision of services in any country, but are more closely related to each other.

FRANCE

In spite of geographical closeness, there is surprisingly little contact between British and French psychiatry; the account given here owes much to the views of Mangen & Castel (1985). The French Lunacy Act of 1838 required that each *département* build a public asylum or else make suitable arrangements with another local authority. Special training was developed for psychiatrists, but the centralised organisation and administration, together with the forms of certification, remained unchanged until the 1960s. While the old law of 1838 is still largely operative, its lack of concern with individual patients' rights is an obstacle to progress (Demay 1987). Psychiatry was isolated from the beginning, with the patients housed mostly in remote asylums, and although resources could be allocated to extramural activities as early as 1851, only a fraction of the budget was ever spent in that way.

During the Second World War, the French mental hospital population fell from 115 000 to 65 000, much of this being due to death from mass starvation. An experimental service was created at Saint-Alban by two doctors, Bonaffé and Tosquelles. Assisted by resistance workers, they placed their patients in the closely-knit local community, where survival was not only better than that of patients who remained in hospital, but also contributed to the survival of the village and did something to change public attitudes (Mangen & Castel 1985). Therapeutic communities were established after the war and in 1945, voluntary treatment became possible. The Saint-Alban psychiatrists were Lacanian, but a group of anti-Lacanians in the thirteenth arondissement of Paris, led by Paumelle, formed a private association which offered day care and outpatient services which were widely admired (Chick 1967). None of these services had much effect on the general picture, but a small group of hospital directors were able to influence national policy, and a Ministerial Circular, issued in 1960, emphasised the importance of local community-based services, as well as promulgating plans for the conversion of old mental hospitals and even for building new 'community' type hospitals. However, the closure of mental hospitals, which then housed a total of 120 000 patients, was not envisaged; the hospitals were generally large and 44% had over 1000 beds — this was the highest proportion of large hospitals in Europe (May 1976), one hospital having over 4000 beds (Mangen & Castel 1985). On the other hand, there were only minimal numbers of patients in general hospital units.

The Ministerial Circular also outlined a comprehensive plan in which France would be divided into 750 sectors — the 'politique du secteur'. Each sector was to be of about 70 000 population, be the responsibility of a multidisciplinary team, and have a day hospital, night hospital, sheltered workshop, and *dispensaire*. The subsequent realisation of these plans owed much to the work of Henri Ey, whose discussions with a diverse group of psychiatrists were published in the *Livres Blancs de la Psychiatrie Française* (1965, 1966, 1967). In 1968, the 1838 law was amended, giving patients more rights over property and finance, but with little other reforming effect. Psychiatric hospitals were given administrative autonomy, psychiatrists received improved status and salaries and new posts were created for junior psychiatrists, while psychiatry and neurology were formally separated. Unfortunately, these changes were made by ordinances or guidelines, which carried little weight with the financial authorities, so that no funds were allocated for the creation of extramural services, and the future of the hospitals was never seriously considered (Demay 1987). Since then, in spite of aspirations to community-based services, the mental hospitals have not only remained in being, but have actually expanded their role, though a government report of 1982 advocated the replacement of mental hospitals by 'public residences', related to sectors.

A considerable amount of fully private office psychiatry continues, while private hospitals provide 10% of the psychiatric beds — on the basis of profitability rather than need. Hospital and community organisations have contrary aims; there are too many hospital beds, which attract continued finance through admissions of patients, and so hospital staff resist discharges which would lead to a reduction in their budget. Largely as a result of this situation, extramural services have done nothing to reduce hospital admission rates. Though the financial arrangements are complex, much health service expenditure is met by insurance funds; global budgeting has been introduced since 1984 and state financial subsidies have been raised, in the hope of reducing the need for costly inpatient care. But local authorities still show little interest in providing alternative services: there is still a triple system of finance, with the sickness funds responsible for hospital costs, the State for extra-hospital expenditure, and the local authorities for long-term care and rehabilitation. Sectorisation has always been hospital-based, but the sector team lacks responsibility for the psychiatric establishments in its area and there is little continuity of care or co-ordination between community and hospital-based services. With these varied forms of reimbursement and administration, the sector is so far little more than a geographical entity, without responsibility or an integrated budget. In 1981, 50% of sectors offered only an outpatient service and some home visiting, in addition to inpatient care, while 90% had no sheltered accommodation. Sectors were finally put on a legally established basis in 1985.

While the status of psychiatrists has been improved, that of nurses has not, and only a minority of them work in the community at all; training of staff is based on inpatient experience, community work being narrowly interpreted as the provision of after-care. Finally, under the Handicapped Persons Act (1975), chronic patients are being moved into long-stay homes, some with as many as 400 beds, yet with few staff, little medical attention, and a failure to appreciate that some disabilities may have the capacity to improve.

WEST GERMANY

The development of German psychiatry was interrupted by the Nazis, who formulated their own policy of mental health care, resulting in between 70 000 and 120 000 victims of euthanasia and between 200 000 and 350 000 cases of compulsory sterilisation (Dörner et al 1980).

Psychoanalysis was banned, extramural services diminished, and Jewish psychiatrists were dismissed or forced to flee abroad, while the cultural and political atmosphere paralysed developments in psychiatry. After the Second World War, the innovations in psychiatric care which were taking place in Anglo-Saxon and Scandinavian countries took time to establish themselves in West Germany. There was little interest in community psychiatry, the university departments and mental hospitals going their separate ways (Mangen 1985). By the 1960s, however, signs of change were appearing and in 1968, as in France, neurology and psychiatry were formally separated. The West German psychiatric system was reorganised, as the country itself had been earlier, to operate as a federation of 11 Länder (States) of varying size. It is a system in which 'care' and 'treatment' are funded at different rates: hospitals are paid on the basis of a daily fee, while psychiatrists in private practice are paid a 'fee for service'. Such policies have the negative effect of maintaining high bed occupancy rates, and are said to encourage doctors to undertake unnecessary interventions. About a half of the hospitals containing 8 out of every 10 beds, are administered by the Federal States, the remainder being operated by voluntary or private bodies, although there are wide differences between the provision made by individual states. The separation persists between university clinics, which have no catchment area and which select acute patients for treatment, and hospitals, which cannot do so. *Niedergelassene Aerzte* (specialist psychiatrists in private practice) have what is almost a monopoly of outpatient treatment and until 1976, only university clinics could see their own outpatients. This restriction was then lifted, but to establish an outpatient department outside a state hospital, a shortage of private practitioners has to be demonstrated in any locality.

In 1970, a Commission of Enquiry (the *Psychiatrische Enquête*) was appointed by the Federal Government, with all-party support: all but 2 of its 26 members were medically qualified, but only 4 worked in mental hospitals, and there was only 1 private practitioner. It was expected to report on the 'standards of psychiatric, psychotherapeutic and psychosomatic care of the population'; tackling the problem with typical German thoroughness, it took four years to complete this task. The Bundestag Report and the accompanying statements of policy published in 1975 run to 3700 pages (Deutscher Bundestag 1975), and are said by Mangen (1985) to make 'depressing reading' with accounts of how patients were living in impoverished and inhumane conditions. The mental hospitals had large catchment areas and were remote from the populations which they served, over half the patients were on locked wards, while only 42% of the nurses had a training recognised by the state, in which in any case psychiatry played little part, so that only 6% had specific qualifications in psychiatric nursing. The Commission found that day care and hostels were non-existent in some areas. The outpatient specialists were not distributed in a way which allowed them to fulfill their contracts, so that only one-third of those patients advised to consult them when they were discharged from hospital actually did so. In fact, these specialist psychiatrists were isolated from hospital practice and only a few of their patients were ever referred to hospital by them (Dilling et al 1975).

The Commission proposed equality of status for the mentally and physically ill, and endorsed community-based mental health care; prevention was to take precedence over cure, and counselling and crisis intervention services were to be established. Together with rehabilitation, it was hoped that those services would help to transfer the care of patients away from the mental hospital. Measures of sectorisation were proposed, as well as strong support for psychiatric units in general hospitals. The report was, however, reticent about the future of mental hospitals, only recommending that they should have a maximum size of 600 beds and that chronic patients were to be transferred to residential or nursing home care.

Criticisms of the Enquête have been directed at what some see as a narrow medical approach, in which the major objective was the integration of psychiatry into medicine and the devaluing of social problems, so that they were seen as problems of the individual. Other critics wanted lay help and self-help to be encouraged. Some of these criticisms were justified, but the fundamental problem was that the Commission proposed to reform mental health in an unreformed health care system. Both the Federal Government and the States were critical in their response to the Commission's report, tending to feel the existing services had not been sufficiently appreciated, or that the whole strategic plan was too expensive. Individual States reacted in different ways, however, according to their political stance, those with Christian Democratic majorities being probably less co-operative than those governed by the Social Democrats. Future plans continue to see the inpatient mental hospital services as the pivot of the new system, and money is still directed towards upgrading of hospitals, rather than to the provision of alternative, sector-based services.

Nevertheless, there has been a decline in the number of occupied beds and a rise in the number of hospital admissions, especially of alcoholic patients. Hospital directors have complained about the budgetary effect of reduced bed capacity which, of course, increases the cost per case of inpatient care. The development of day hospitals has been hindered by an insurance system which reimburses the cost of inpatient care more liberally than that of day or outpatient treatment. Some 50 000 to 60 000 patients — a number similar to that of patients in the chronic wards of mental hospitals have been placed in residential and nursing homes but there is a lack of occupation during the day in those homes, and Kunze (1985) has described their inadequate conditions, with no professional input from hospital staff. Compulsory detention of patients cannot be expressed as a national figure, as each State tends to calculate the data differently: in some, 40% of current inpatients are compulsorily detained, but in others the figure would be much lower. In the current situation though, cost containment seems to be the dominating consideration (Mangen 1983). The German system of payment is almost as complicated as the French: 1300 different health insurance schemes bear the cost of inpatient treatment, and compete by offering slightly different benefits, while there are also state subsidies and a tendency to look to the nursing homes and to private provision for the care of long-stay patients. Since nurses cannot be guaranteed posts in community care, jobs are threatened by these economic pressures, which also hinder co-operation between different parts of the service. Community care is only one of the many objectives proposed and, in a country where psychiatrists have received a strong neuropsychiatric training, it has often been viewed with suspicion as a means of undermining medical expertise.

Haerlin (1985) has drawn attention to the 14 pilot projects which, under the leadership of Kulenkampff (1981), sought to show how community psychiatric services might be developed. These projects produced statistics useful for monitoring change, but not sufficiently detailed for evaluative purposes, since there are no before-and-after comparisons (Cooper & Bauer 1987). In Solingen (a town in the Ruhr), there is an innovative programme which developed out of the mental hospital at Langenfeld; it includes crisis and hostel beds, sheltered accommodation, places in staffed community houses and group homes, as well as a day centre, social clubs, and a co-operative workshop. A most important development is the 24-hour, 7-day-a-week emergency team, which offers immediate service to patients, their relatives, and the public at large when they telephone or call. Of equal importance is the involvement of volunteers from families in the policy development and running of the service (Nouvartné 1987). In Mannheim, a network of extramural services includes 5 hostels, 7 group homes, 2 sheltered workshops, and a number of voluntary initiatives, co-ordinated by the Central Institute for Mental Health (Haefner 1987).

BELGIUM

In Belgium, the present situation does not seem to be conducive to the development of community psychiatry. The majority of patients are still cared for in large asylums, many of which are administered by religious orders; general hospital units have only been developed in the past 14 years. Until 1974, Belgium had one of the highest psychiatric bed ratios in North-West Europe, and two-thirds of the hospital patients were treated in closed services, governed by archaic legislation passed between 1850 and 1873. Since then, the number of detained patients has been significantly reduced, but there are still gaps in the legal protection of detained patients; yet legislative reform is stalled, since the upper and lower houses of Parliament cannot agree whether patients should be admitted by a magistrate or a doctor.

Nationally, the system of psychiatric care is fragmented between the regions of Wallonia, Flanders and Brussels. More seriously perhaps for community care, the acute treatment facilities are classed as 'A' services, whilst there are separate 'T' services for long-term patients. Private neuropsychiatrists see themselves as being threatened by multidisciplinary teams and outpatient *dispensaires,* which provide counselling, crisis intervention, and work with parents and children; their origins go back to the 1930s and it seems that they were set up as part of the mental hygiene movement, with a preventive hope, so that they can be described as part of a 'community mental health' rather than a 'community psychiatric' movement.

Thus, Belgian services are fragmented between hospitals, 'A' and 'T' services, open and closed facilities, *dispensaires,* local authorities, voluntary bodies, and private neuropsychiatrists. Since most services operate on a 'fee-for-service' basis, patients' care is further fragmented by conflicting financial and professional interests, with collective respon-sibility 'increasingly replaced by private liability' (Baro et al 1985).

THE NETHERLANDS

Giel (1987) refers to a jigsaw puzzle of mental health care in Holland: those who are unable to say what AGGZ, APZ, AWBZ, BOPZ, CAD, and a large number of similar abbreviations mean, are unlikely to be able to grasp the complexities of Dutch mental health care. Certainly, the situation is complicated by former confessional divisions between Roman Catholic, Protestant, Jewish, the Humanist services, while there is a plethora of financial regulations in this confusing care network. The outcome, according to van der Grinten (1985), is an inefficient, patchy service with duplication in some sectors co-existing with a total absence of services in others. The government has attempted to create some order in the system, but as in France, this has been done by memoranda, which have been widely ignored and have so far done little to affect patterns of service. There is a separation between community (social psychiatric) and inpatient services, because hospitals do not draw their patients from catchment areas, nor undertake functions on that basis.

Dutch social psychiatry is often associated in Britain with the name of Querido, who was the Medical Officer for Health of Amsterdam and since 1934, had organised a domiciliary, 24-hour emergency service mainly to prevent admission to mental hospitals, which had to be paid for by the city and was expensive (Querido 1954). Later the plan was copied nationally, but provided neither the 24-hour service nor the regulation of admission, so that in practice, 'social psychiatry' became simply counselling and psychotherapy for the less severely ill. (See also Chs. 1 and 12).

With the denominational divisions that exist in Holland, the attempt to co-ordinate services had been made no easier by the financial arrangements of 'fee-for-service' and daily payments for the number of residents in hospitals. However, since 1980, with fixed budgets for the mental hospitals, for outpatients, and for extramural services, (but excluding outpatient services by the mental hospitals), the need for more alternatives to hospital care has been generally accepted: it is intended to provide a community mental health centre for each 90 000–100 000 people. There is still conflict, however, since the major problem is the lack of a comprehensive organisational framework within which to co-ordinate new innovations (van der Grinten 1985, Giel 1987). Changes have, of course, taken place, but as elsewhere, there has been no evaluation of the psychiatric care that is now offered. Little is done for the community care of chronic patients, doctors and other staff being more interested in counselling the less ill than in treating severe disorders, and

Giel (1987) believes that a critical situation is therefore developing in the care of this group of patients. Psychiatric hospitals now concentrate on intensive psychotherapy, using a therapeutic community model; their outpatient services do not provide continuity of care for discharged patients with chronic disabilities. It is strange that with the great variety and wealth of services provided in the Netherlands, these still maintain their traditional independence from national and local health authorities and from each other (Giel & ten Horn 1982).

SCANDINAVIA

Finland

Finland is a country with great space and a limited population. The law requiring local authorities not only to provide care for the poor but to establish departments for chronic mental patients in connection with work-houses, was passed in 1889, and many psychiatric institutions were built in the 1900s. While in English hospitals inpatient rates were declining, in Finland the rates increased from 235 per 100 000 population in 1954 to 425 in 1972, but then decreased to 362 in 1980 (Salokangas et al 1985); 50% of those residents are still involuntary patients (Lehtinen 1987). However, there is now a two-tier system: following the Mental Health Act of 1952, local authorities were encouraged to build new hospitals for chronic psychiatric patients — 'B' hospitals. Community mental health centres have also been established, but have not led to any reduction of the inpatient population; they are staffed by different specialists from the hospitals so that the outpatient and inpatient services really operate separately, and continuity of care is largely lacking. Instead, the centre staff tend to look after people who in England would be cared for by general practitioners. In addition, the attitudes of the public to psychiatric disorder may be more authoritarian or paternalistic than in Britain, as evidenced by the higher rate of involuntary admission. Sectorisation of services is recommended, but will present difficulties, since the local authorities have considerable autonomy and fear the loss of power from giving up their established admission 'territories' (Lehtinen 1987). State services are supplemented by a private organisation (Sopimusvuori) which operates six rehabilitation homes for handicapped schizophrenic patients (Ojanen 1984); it has some similarities to the Richmond Fellowship in Britain.

Denmark

Denmark is different; it has had health insurance for many years and from 1933 this was compulsory (Strømgren 1985); but since 1976, the 14 counties and city of Copenhagen have taken responsibility through taxation for the funding and administration of health services. These authorities have to submit their plans for ministerial approval, to ensure that they remain in line with national policy. Services for the mentally retarded have been separated from services for the psychiatrically ill for more than 100 years. Today, Danes can choose from two compulsory health insurance schemes, but hospital treatment is free, as is care for long-stay patients and those in nursing homes who surrender their welfare pension and are given a small amount of pocket money. There is some competition between local authorities and the central government (but not between hospitals and private practitioners), which may lead to changes in policy.

From 1921 to 1976, state mental hospitals were administered on a centralised basis by a special national directorate. During the 1930s and 1940s, a feeling of the need for reorganisation grew, and in 1952, a government commission was set up. Its report, published in 1956, recommended that psychiatry should be integrated with the rest of medicine, since mental hospitals were too far from the population they served, old large and overcrowded. All psychiatric hospitals should instead be adjacent to or part of a general hospital, and their size should not exceed 300 to 400 beds; the differentiation between acute and chronic hospitals was rejected and outpatient services were to be extended. Glostrup Hospital in Copenhagen, which opened in 1960 as a joint general and psychiatric hospital, provided a model for these developments; where lack of space made such developments impossible, smaller psychiatric units were to be established (Strømgren 1985). In fact, though, only 4 of the planned hospitals were operating after 15 years. A number of small psychiatric units were established in general hospitals, but since admissions to mental hospitals did not decrease, these units seem to have been catering for patients who had not formerly been admitted. During the 1960s, plans for the administration of mental hospitals to be decentralised to the counties were gathering impetus, since the counties were already managing the general hospitals. However, following a change of government, nothing happened until the Danish Psychiatric Association established a commission, which reported in 1970. Agreement was then reached on plans for 60-bed units, also accommodating day patients and having extensive outpatient facilities; up to 4 of these units, each serving a sector of 30 000 people, could be grouped together. A community mental health project, undertaken on the island of Samsø, was used as a guideline for planning.

This report had considerable influence, and a law to effect these changes was passed in 1975. Though it was intended then that all counties should become self-sufficient, their situations differ; some have a large old hospital, others a new unit, while others have no facilities at all. When the ratio of psychiatric beds to population was determined, it was discovered that while the national average was 2.3 per 1000 inhabitants, Ringkøping in Jutland had 1.3, and Copenhagen 7. Subsequently, this difference was found to be partly due to different levels of nursing home provision, as well as to local demographic factors. The different counties, therefore, had to decide how to combine the various elements of psychiatric care, before submitting their plans to the Ministry of Health. While these plans differ, they all emphasise sectorisation, although the sizes of the sectors vary, and all also emphasise outpatient services, but only a few intend to build new psychiatric inpatient units; most intend to reduce their number of beds. Total inpatients had fallen from 10 312 in 1977 to 8524 in 1982, while day patients had increased; in 1982, 40% of admissions were to general hospital psychiatric units, but mental hospitals still provided the long-term beds.

Strømgen (1985) describes the present position in Denmark as confused; counties vary in their plans, but he sees this as a hopeful period of experimentation. In fact, the outlook of the mental health services and of psychiatry as practised in Denmark, corresponds closely to the British view, as does that of Norway, where primary health facilities have always treated patients with psychiatric disorders. The ratio of patients in mental hospitals there, has declined from 2.28 per 1000 population in 1965 to 1.0 in 1982. In the recent reorganisation of services, there has been emphasis on non-institutional care and comprehensive community provision (Lavik 1987). Paradoxically, the introduction of a sectorised service in Bergen was reported to have resulted in a large increase of hospital multiple readmissions (Holsten & d'Elia 1985).

Sweden

Sweden, on the other hand, has not participated in the last two world wars and has had a stable social-democratic government for most of the last 40 years; health services are funded by a national insurance system, and the Swedes were proud of having a large number of psychiatric beds as indicating a high standard of care. In 1963, it was proposed by the government that responsibility for psychiatric care should shift from the state to the counties. The number of beds subsequently dropped from 24 328 in 1970 to 15 455 in 1984; less than 20% of these are in general hospitals (Holmberg 1988). The main debate, however, has been between the biological and psychotherapeutic outlooks; legislation is said to have followed the Italian Law 180, although 30% of the patients are still compulsorily detained and changes in Sweden seem to have followed a very uneven course (Freeman et al 1985). Great disparities remain between cities and rural areas in the number of practising psychiatrists per 100 000 population, and the development of extramural facilities has not kept pace with the run-down of mental hospitals. Sectorisation has been strongly criticised, e.g. for causing deterioration in existing resources, and the need has been acknowledged for specialised milieu therapy units for chronically handicapped schizophrenics, serving a wider area of population. A study of the introduction of a community-based service to a suburb of Stockholm (Stefansson & Cullberg 1986) showed that after two years, this had resulted in a large increase in the number of people receiving psychiatric care, with a fall in hospital admissions; primary medical care and social services in the area were rather poorly developed at the time. However, a sophisticated study of the effects of a nearby sectorised service on former mental hospital patients was unable to find any additional benefit, compared with the traditional service (Lindholm 1983).

ITALY

In recent years, the Italian experience has conformed to many of the European trends (Bennett 1985). However, in its rhetoric, its attack on the asylum, its attempts to restructure the organisation of services, and in the criticisms of those who note the failure of its dispersion countrywide it has become the 'outlier' of European psychiatry (Mangen 1985). What has been happening in Italy has certainly attracted more attention, more argument, more admirers, and more detractors than any other European service (Perris & Kemali 1985, Pirella 1987, Paparo & Bacigalupi 1985). Unfortunately, due to a lack of careful evaluative studies, there is much that can still be argued about, especially since in Italy, the debate begins from the 'ideological assumptions of Right or Left' (Robb 1986). This situation contrasts sharply with that of Germany, where totalitarianism was also defeated, but political changes did not filter through to the psychiatric services in Italy for many years, and the number of inpatients increased until 1963. When the republic was promulgated in 1947, the principle of decentralisation was accepted, but it was not until 1973 that a system of regional government was actually in operation. Medical practice remained mostly private and there was no elaborate system of health insurance in the hands of an army of national and local organisations, the south is still a dependent, peripheral economy, exporting workers and cheap food to the north, and dominated by corrupt political machines, used to deliver votes to northern-based politicians (Robb 1986). Mental health reform (Law 180) was enacted in 1978, seven months before Law 833, establishing the National Health Service. Both were drafted by the Communists, and their enactment involved complicated political manoeuvres by the Christian Democrats, to avoid a possibly embarrassing defeat in a referendum, such as they had previously experienced in the cases of divorce and abortion.

Franco Basaglia, the founder of the reform movement, was concerned by the excessive use of mental hospitals in Italy in the 1960s, when conditions were extremely poor and the patients 'utterly abandoned'. All doors were locked, nurses had no psychiatric training, ECT was used extensively and perhaps indiscriminately, so that Basaglia concluded that rather than meeting the needs of the patients, the mental hospital was an end in itself. He looked towards the British therapeutic community as a model for reform, but felt it overlooked the political dimension. The anti-institutional movement began in 1968 in Gorizia, but three years later, Basaglia moved to Trieste (Bennett 1985). Humanitarian sentiments in relation to this antiquated system of asylums led to Law 180; Basaglia's philosophy, which underlies the Act, was that mental illness was due to a distortion in the communication network linking a person to his family, his work environment, and society in general. Mental disorders were said to be caused by social inhumanity and repression, the large mental institutions being the major sources of these forces (Cassano et al 1985). The goal of Law 180 was the abolition of the asylum, which was seen as the place where the displaced poor were segregated and punished. The other aim was to enable the mentally ill to re-enter society fully and be integrated into it, but social welfare also was said to make people dependent on the asylum.

The second 'disease' according to Basaglia, was chronicity caused through institutionalisation, though he overlooked the primary illness and never defined it. Staff were also said to be institutionalised, and had to be 'liberated' from the asylum, so that there had to be the elimination of locked wards, demedicalisation of treatment, elimination of psycho-therapy, unionisation of patients, and the transformation of their status, so that they became 'guests' of the institution (Mollica 1985). Further aims were the creation of a decentralised service in which mental illness could be prevented and patients treated and rehabilitated, giving priority to voluntary treatment and eliminating all concepts of dangerousness. Unfortunately, the problems of creating the alternative services and facilities such as day hospitals, foster homes, hostels, group homes, homes for the elderly, and sheltered workshops were not discussed in practical details (Cassano et al 1985). Further problems in implementation were caused by political and economic instability, the shift of mental health professionals from public to the private sector, and the fact that chronicity has a clinical as well as a social dimension. There was also a failure to appreciate that there is a tendency for even the most idealistic practitioners to avoid treating psychotic patients (Mollica 1985). The new law reflected a social climate in Italy that was generally liberal and anti-institutional, but it was not adequately thought through or prepared (Freeman et al 1985). Bennett, studying services in Trieste, detailed profound changes following Basaglia's appointment as director of the mental hospital in 1971 (Bennett 1985). However, in spite of the democratic ideology, power seemed to remain largely in the hands of the doctors, there was little or no emphasis on diagnosis, and an untested belief prevailed that if the impositions of a repressive mental hospital were removed, improvement in patients' mental health could be confidently expected. There were no treatment programmes: group therapy was considered a sophisticated form of staff manipulation and even certain forms of occupational therapy were seen as oppressive. The combination of ideological pressures and uncritical humanitarian convictions seemed to have pushed scientific knowledge into the background (Bennett 1985).

The type and extent of change which has developed in practice from the psychiatric reform varies greatly from one geographical area of Italy to another (Robb 1986). Local enthusiasm has been curbed everywhere by financial constraints and by cultural pressure in the South, as well as by the shortage of well qualified professional personnel, whose training at present does not fit them for their new tasks. Robb believes that reform of the education system is essential for the completion of health and psychiatry reforms; both reliable sociological information and systematic evaluation of the services are so far lacking. He does not accept Mosher's (1982) enthusiastic view and suggests that this depends on experience limited to Trieste, where the developments have been relatively successful. Tansella (1986) admits that there are many places, especially in the South, where the reform has not been implemented and where community services are obviously not functioning. As Sarteschi et al (1983) point out, in Italy there are very few hard facts. Freeman et al (1985) also emphasise that there is no reliable information on whether or not certain categories of mentally disordered people in Italy are failing to receive treatment or care because of the effects of the new legislation. The old order cannot be reformed just by pointing out its faults; the new order cannot be created simply through ideology.

A more realistic view of the situation in Italy, based on data from the National Statistical Institute, is given by Crepet (1988). Another account, which gives data on what has actually happened in Turin and Piedmont, is rarely quoted; Becker (1985), a German psychiatrist who worked there for over a year, provides a careful review of the changes. Of 1500 patients discharged from Turin's psychiatric hospitals, 12% could not be accounted for; Becker believed there were more than 100 homeless patients in the Turin area, 650 had found accommodation in old peoples' homes and nursing homes, and 600 were accommodated in the 28 community-type facilities *within* the mental hospital as 'guests'. There were 76 community psychiatric centres in Piedmont and 44 in Turin; the multidisciplinary teams were led by doctors, whose numbers had increased from 4.5% of the hospital staff to 18% of the community staff. Becker concluded that Italy's mental health legislation cannot be seen as a blueprint for a comprehensive psychiatric system, though in Piedmont, it had been pragmatically implemented, with both beneficial results and unresolved problems.

Jones & Poletti (1984, 1985) strongly criticised the practical consequences of the reform, especially as they saw it in Southern Italy;

their visits were to Milan, Pavia, Pisa, Lucca, Florence, Salerno and Reggio di Calabria — none of them centres of *Psychiatrica Democratica*, as the group of psychiatrists committed to these changes are known. Later, in response to criticisms of their earlier views, they visited Trieste (Jones & Poletti 1986), concluding that the system, can work and that there at least, it is impressive in practice; however, they did not refer in detail to the excellent shared apartments in Trieste or to the continuity of care, comprehensiveness, and integration of services that Bennett noted there — if not throughout the country (1985). Jones (1988b) may have performed a useful function in pointing out that this is no model for British or American society. Large numbers of former patients are still living in mental hospitals as 'guests'; their conditions are worse than ever, while they lack structured work or activities in the mental health centres. But for Italy it may be much more humane than some university or private clinics, where patients in pyjamas receive medication through the almost universal *Flebo* or intravenous drip (Muscettole et al 1987). Certainly, feelings on both sides are eloquently proclaimed; Basaglia was a constructive iconoclast, who relished paradox and did not shun publicity. He practised what he preached, helping patients both in and outside hospital to live their lives in their own territory, rather than that of the professionals. As Peter Nichols, one-time Times correspondent in Italy, said (1975): 'it is not that Italians are basically untruthful, but their flair is dramatisation, not simple exposition. They are not much concerned about facts. They find rhetorical complications and confusion preferable to a well ordered system of public life; it is perhaps the best they can expect in an imperfect world'.

OTHER EUROPEAN COUNTRIES

It is impossible to give accounts here of all the European countries. In Vienna, a psychosocial service was established in 1980 to operate all outpatient and community services for the population of 1.53 million, which was divided into eight catchment areas. Between 1978 and 1982, the two mental hospitals serving the city reduced their occupied beds from 3750 to 2261. In addition to the services being developed in each sector, an emergency visiting team is available for nights and weekends (Rudas 1986). Switzerland, which is conservative in outlook, but sound in practice, is described by Müller (1987). Greek services are still rudimentary, although some advances are being made; half the psychiatric beds are located in the two largest cities and 60% of the psychiatrists practice in Athens. Yugoslavia has, among other things, an unusually well developed but almost unknown community service at Modrica on the river Bosna. Some interesting developments have been started in Spain, but ambitious plans have been drastically curtailed by economic constraints.

AFRICA

Describing the African scene, German (1987) drew attention to the fact that international policies 'have increasingly urged the development of health services based on village health workers and other primary health care workers' (WHO 1978). Such primary health services also help to redress social evils, and offer support to their victims through education and community resources. German shows that mental ill-health extends throughout black Africa and is not the prerogative of advanced societies. He believes that there is a need to resist the wishes of politicians to establish hospitals and medical schools in an attempt to foster their chances of re-election. Giel (1985), discussing Ethiopia, thought that chronic psychotics in Africa generally resist hospital admission; they live scattered about towns, but are not altogether homeless or vagrant. 'In their own queer way they were self-reliant, albeit in a precarious balance with regard to their physical health.' Asuni (1986) felt that Nigerian psychotics lacked the apathy, slowness, and utter disinterest seen in Western institutionalised patients. They were more concerned about what they were going to eat, and psychotics in Addis Ababa also combined serious mental disability with a capacity for survival. Referring to West Africa, Harding (1973) said that, in spite of the mechanical restraints often employed, traditional healing should be encouraged; these healers should be given advice about psychotropic drugs and also about the detection of organic psychiatric disorder. In the Sudan, collaboration between religious healers and mental health services has been reported to be very helpful (Workneh & Giel 1975). While the universal extent and nature of mental ill-health does not seem to suggest that psychiatric disorders are strongly culture-bound, purely medical approaches are insufficient in themselves to contain or reduce these problems.

JAPAN

In Japan, a mental health act was enacted in 1950 and this was amended in 1965; before then, there were 32 beds per 100 000 population, and most mentally ill people were cared for by their families or by the community. Subsequently, prevailing attitudes were strongly in favour of hospital admission and the number of inpatients reached its maximum in 1984, when there were 283 per 100 000 population. Unlike most other countries, 81% of psychiatric hospitals are private, while 89% of inpatients are in private beds. Okagami & Wada (1985) say that this 'could be part of the reason that Community Residence Programs, such as, halfway houses and halfway hostels have not fully progressed'. Few psychiatrists want to involve themselves in community psychiatry services, which are supported by taxes, while hospital care is paid by four types of health insurance. However, there are only two mental health centres in the Tokyo area, and the *mean* number of staff for all mental health centres in Japan is only nine. An interesting account of Japanese attitudes to the mentally ill up to 1958 is given by Totsuka (1990) together with a study of the events leading to the Mental Health Act of 1987.

CHINA

Generally, China represents a huge gap in international knowledge of psychiatric services, and it seems strange to Western thought that such an ancient culture and such pragmatic and resourceful people should have accorded mental disorders such little concern (Brown 1980). During the Great Leap Forward and the Cultural Revolution, care is said to have been given by barefoot doctors and Red Guards, the treatment was politicised, as was everything else in the society (Sidel 1973). Since Mao's death in 1976, the Chinese have apparently selected what they think they need from Western culture. However, when Jones (1988a) says that they are now manufacturing pharmacotherapeutic drugs and Lin (1985) says that services 'especially in rural areas may be said to be non-existent', it is difficult to balance such advances with such overall backwardness. It appears that in cities at least, only the severely disturbed patients are admitted to hospital, as an attempt to focus services on those most likely to benefit from them (Parry-Jones 1986). Chinese culture stresses self-control and conformity, together with loyalty to the family unit and service to the state. But as Jones (1988a) concludes, there is simply not enough evidence to enable Western observers to judge what is really happening.

SOVIET UNION

The Soviet Union is such a diverse collection of countries that again, it is difficult to generalise about its services and, in any case, there is little information available. Communication with psychiatrists there is difficult, and has been bedevilied by the misuse of psychiatric treatment for political dissidents (Koryagin 1989), and also by a diagnostic system which is different from the International Classification of Disease. Wing (1974), who warned that he had no deep knowledge of Russian life or language, said that social or community psychiatry has a long history in Russia. During the 1920s and 1930s, a system of extramural psychiatry is said to have been established which was based on a network of dispensaries, day hospitals and workshops, while services for the social and industrial resettlement of patients were apparently well developed — at least in large cities. Polyclinics are staffed by surgeons, physicians, pediatricians, and gynaecologists, so that a patient with psychiatric disorder will at first be seen by a general physician and then referred to a 'neuropathologist' who works in a dispensary. Psychiatrists also do home visits. If the patient is admitted to hospital, he/she will have a different doctor, but liaison with the dispensaries is said to be close and patients discharged from hospital are expected to attend the dispensary again within five days. Other psychiatric specialists in dispensaries deal with alcohol addiction. Each dispensary has a day hospital, but the figures for the number of day hospitals or the number of their patients were not made available for inclusion in the WHO data (May 1976, Freeman et al 1985). Sheltered workshops may be well developed, as they were in Poland and East Germany. Wing said there were no hostels in the British sense, and that patients without families had to live in long-stay hospitals; Isaev, in an account of mental health services in Leningrad, did not add anything which could enable the situation to be assessed more fully (WHO 1980). The WHO figure show considerable differences in European countries of the Eastern bloc, although with the exception of Czechoslovakia, they tend to have fewer beds than West European countries. Wing believed, however, that British services could profitably learn from some aspects of the experiences of Moscow and Leningrad.

OTHER COUNTRIES

The North American outlook is dealt with in Chapters 19 and 20, while pioneering Australian services in Sydney are mentioned in Chapter 1. South American countries vary considerably in the availability of care, except to those members of the population who can afford to pay for it. Elsewhere, many countries have populations with idiosyncratic ways of communicating distress (Leff 1988), languages poorly understood by European psychiatrists, fundamentalist religious beliefs, or widespread reliance on traditional healing practices. Some comparisons of psycho-geriatric services are given in Chapter 9.

CONCLUSION

It is obviously difficult to draw lessons from the often inadequate accounts of services in countries with very different histories and traditions. In Europe, sectorisation of services in some form seems to be being pursued very widely (May 1976, Mangen 1985, Freeman et al 1985, Breemer Ter Stege & Gittelman 1987). Most countries have inherited over-large and sometimes decaying mental hospitals, often remote from the populations they serve. Though there is a general loss of faith in traditional institutional care, it is difficult for these institutions to be abolished, but almost everywhere, living conditions in them are being improved and beds reduced in number. In the Netherlands, however, a major hospital construction programme is said to be still going ahead. France, West Germany, the Netherlands, and Belgium all have insurance-based health systems which are willing to pay for inpatient but not for day patient treatment. They also offer 'fees-for-service', which encourage private neuropsychiatric practice. 'Treatment' in hospital or private practice is paid for at higher rates than 'care' in social-psychiatric services and dispensaries, with the result of under-funding community services. This handicaps the development of community psychiatry, which seeks to consider not only the patient, but his influence on his social milieu, as well as its influence on him and his disordered condition. It also makes hospitals reluctant to discharge patients on whose daily fees they rely. The paradox in both France, Germany, and elsewhere in Europe is that 'sickness insurance authorities are prepared to pay for more expensive hospital treatment but refuse to accept responsibility for less costly community interventions' (Mangen 1983). It seems clear that the provision of private hospitals in Japan is related to their rising occupancy, which is also mainly a result of the payment system.

Even as smaller and more locally based services are being developed, it has been shown that mental health centres tend to treat a new population of patients, rather than reduce hospital admissions. Psychiatric units in general hospitals are being developed almost everywhere; new psychiatric legislation is being enacted to offer legal safeguards against arbitrary admission; lay and self-help groups are developing, while multi-disciplinary teamwork is increasingly praised but less often implemented, as is the continuity of care. May (1976) stressed the fact that in general, outpatient services had developed to a greater extent in the Eastern than the Western European countries. There are perhaps overall differences in Europe between those countries following the Anglo-Saxon/Scandinavian tradition, the Roman tradition, as in Spain and Portugal, and the Eastern tradition. Even so, Italy is currently the exception: severely restricting admission to hospital, attempting (at least in theory) to mobilise the mentally impaired as a political force and, above all, threatening the social hegemony which embodies the meanings and values which society assigns to the mentally ill and to asylums. However, there must be doubts as to whether this experiment can or will succeed. More moderate attempts at reform have considered the advantages of either centralised or more localised systems of government, but when the advantages and disadvantages of the system in the Netherlands are compared with West Germany's federal one, it seems that whatever the circumstances, development will be slow (WHO 1987). So there is a varying emphasis from country to country, modified by local necessities, which has an important influence on the development of a community psychiatry; both economic conditions and political changes influence these innovations more or sometimes less directly. There is, however, a general if slow movement towards sectorisation and the run-down of hospitals, within widely different systems of psychiatric care, and these processes seem to offer at least some prospect of change.

REFERENCES

Asuni T 1986 Vagrant psychotics in Abeokuta. Procédés du Deuxième Coloque Africaine de Psychiatrie. Audecam, Paris

Baro F, Prims A, De Schouwer P 1985 Belgium: psychiatric care in a pluralist system. In: Mangen S P (ed) Mental health care and the European community. Croom Helm, London

Becker T 1985 Psychiatric reform in Italy — how does it work in Piedmont? British Journal of Psychiatry 147: 254-260

Bennett D H 1985 The changing pattern of mental health care in Trieste. International Journal of Mental Health 14: 70-92

Breemer Ter Stege C, Gittelman M (eds) 1987 Trends in mental health care in Europe in the past 25 years. International Journal of Mental Health 16: 6-20

Brown L B 1980 A psychiatrist's perspective on psychiatry in China. Australian & New Zealand Journal of Psychiatry 14: 21-35

Cassano G B, Mauri M, Petracca A 1985 The current status of psychiatric care in Italy. International Journal of Mental Health 14: 174-183

Chick J D 1967 Community mental health services in the thirteenth arrondissement of Paris. In: Freeman H, Farndale J (eds) New aspects of the mental health services. Pergamon, Oxford

Cooper B, Bauer M 1987 Developments in mental health care and services in the Federal Republic of Germany. International Journal of Mental Health 16: 78-93

Crepet P 1988 The Italian mental health reform nine years on. Acta Psychiatrica Scandinavica 77: 515-523

Demay J 1987 The past and future of French psychiatry. International Journal of Mental Health 16: 69-77

Deutscher Bundestag 1975 Bericht über die lage der psychiatrie in der Bundesrepublik Deutschland (Psychiatrie Enquête). Drucksache 7/4200. Heger, Bonn

Dilling H, Weyerer S, Lisson H 1975 Zur ambulanten psychiatrischen Versorgung durch niedergelassene nervenärzte. Social Psychiatry 10: 111-131

Dörner K, Härlin C, Rall V, Schernus R, Schwendy A 1980 Der krieg gegen die psychisch kranken. Psychiatrie Verlag: Rehburg-Loccum

Freeman H L, Fryers T 1987 The pilot areas study and the context of mental health care. In: Mental Health Services in Pilot Study Areas. WHO, Copenhagen

Freeman H L, Fryers T, Henderson J H 1985 Mental health services in Europe: 10 years on. Public Health in Europe: No 25 WHO, Copenhagen

German G A 1987 Mental health in Africa: II The nature or mental disorders in Africa today: some clinical observations. British Journal of Psychiatry 151: 440-446

Giel R 1985 Chronic psychosis and vagrancy in contrasting cultural settings. In: Sluss-Radebaugh T, Gruenberg E M, Kramer M, Cooper B (eds) The chronic mentally ill: an international perspective. Johns Hopkins University, Baltimore

Giel R 1987 The jigsaw puzzle of Dutch mental health care. International Journal of Mental Health 16: 152-163

Giel R, Ten Horn G H M M 1982 Patterns of mental health care in a Dutch register area. Social Psychiatry 117: 117-123

Giel R, Ten Horn G H M M, Hermann P, Tricot L 1987 Patterns of care and service utilization. In: Mental health services in pilot study areas: report on a European study. WHO Regional Office for Europe, Copenhagen

Haefner H 1987 Do we still need beds for psychiatric patients? Acta Psychiatrica Scandinavica 75: 113-126

Haerlin C 1985 Community care in West Germany: concept and reality. Mimeo paper. Mental health care in the European community. Institute of Psychiatry 2-3 May 1985

Harding T W 1973 Psychoses in a rural West African community. Social Psychiatry 8: 198-203

Holmberg G 1988 Treatment, care and rehabilitation of the chronic mentally ill in Sweden. Hospital & Community Psychiatry 39: 190-194

Holsten F, d'Elia G 1985 Patients with multiple admissions in a community mental health service in Western Norway. Social Psychiatry 20: 55-59

Jones K 1979 Integration or disintegration in the mental health services. Journal of the Royal Society of Medicine 72: 640-648

Jones K 1988a A note on China. In: Experience in mental health. Sage, London
Jones K 1988b Experience in mental health: community care and social policy. Sage, London
Jones K, Poletti A 1984 The mirage of a reform. New Society 70: No 1137
Jones K, Poletti A 1985 Understanding the Italian experience. British Journal of Psychiatry 146: 341-347
Jones K, Poletti A 1986 The 'Italian experience' reconsidered. British Journal of Psychiatry 148: 144-150
Koryagin A 1989 The involvement of Soviet psychiatry in the prosecution of dissenters. British Journal of Psychiatry 154: 336-340
Kulenkampff C 1981 Modellprogramme des Bundes und der Länder in der Psychiatrie: kritische ubersicht. Rheinland Verlag, Cologne
Kunze H 1985 Rehabilitation and Institutionalisation in community care in West Germany. British Journal of Psychiatry 147: 261-264
Lavik N J 1987 Trends in the organisation of mental health services in Norway. International Journal of Mental Health 16: 164-169
Leff J 1988 Psychiatry around the globe: a transcultural view. Gaskell, London
Lehtinen V 1987 The development of mental health services in Finland. International Journal of Mental Health 16: 58-68
Lin Tsung-yi 1985 The shaping of Chinese psychiatry. In: Lin Tsung-yi, Eisenberg L (eds) Mental health for one billion people: a Chinese perspective. University of British Columbia Press, Vancouver
Lindholm H 1983 Sectorised psychiatry. Acta Psychiatrica Scandinavica Supplementum 67: 304-312
Mangen S P 1983 French and German lessons in community care. Mimeo B S A Sociology Conference. University of York September 24th 1983
Mangen S P 1985 (ed) Mental health care in the European community. Croom Helm, London
Mangen S P, Castel F 1985 France: the 'psychiatrie de secteur'. In: Mangen S P (ed) Mental health care in the European community. Croom Helm, London
May A R 1976 Mental health services in Europe. WHO offset publication: No 23. WHO, Geneva
Mollica R 1980 Community mental health centres: an American response to Kathleen Jones. Journal of the Royal Society of Medicine 73: 863-870
Mollica R F (ed) 1985 The unfinished revolution in Italian psychiatry: an international perspective. International Journal of Mental Health 14: 1-2
Mosher L 1982 Italy's revolutionary mental health law: an assessment. American Journal of Psychiatry 139: 199-203
Müller C 1987 The organisation of mental health services in Switzerland. International Journal of Mental Health 16: 225-235
Muscettole G, Casiello M, Bollini P, Sebastioni G, Pampallona S, Tognori G 1987 Pattern of intervention and role of psychiatric settings: a survey of two regions of Italy. Acta Psychiatrica Scandinavica 75: 55-61
Nichols P 1975 Italia, Italia. Fontana, London
Nouvartné K 1987 Zur bedeutung von tagesangeboten für langzeitkranke zum überleben in der gemeinde. Mimeographed report. Psychosozialer Träger Verein, Solingen
Ojanen M 1984 The Sopimusvuori Society: an integrated system of rehabilitation. International Journal of Therapeutic Communities 5: 193-207
Okagami K, Wada S 1985 Community mental health services in Japan: the roles of public health centres and the national institute of mental health. International Journal of Mental Health 32: 141-146
Paparo F, Bacigalupi M 1985 The Italian experience: further considerations. International Journal of Mental Health 14: 93-104
Parry-Jones W L 1986 Psychiatry in the Peoples Republic of China. British Journal of Psychiatry 148: 632-641
Perris C, Kemali D (eds) 1985 Focus on the Italian psychiatric reform. Acta Psychiatrica Scandinavica Supplement 316
Pirella A 1987 Institutional psychiatry between transformation and rationalisation. International Journal of Mental Health 16: 118-141
Querido A 1954 Experiment in mental health. Bulletin of World Federation of Mental

Health 6: No 4

Robb J H 1986 The Italian health services: slow revolution or permanent crisis? Social Science & Medicine 22: 619-627

Rudas S 1986 Comprehensive mental health services. Acta Psychiatrica Belgica 86: 630-635

Salokangas R K R, Der G, Wing J K 1985 Community psychiatric services in England and Finland. Social Psychiatry 20: 23-29

Sarteschi P, Cassano G B, Mauri M, Petracca A 1983 The social effects of the new mental health laws in Italy. In: Roth M, Bluglass R (eds). Psychiatry, human rights and the law. Cambridge University Press, Cambridge

Scull A 1984 Decarceration, community treatment and the deviant: a radical view. 2nd edn. Polity Press, Cambridge

Sidel V W 1973 Discussant (pp72-74) The greater medical profession. Josiah Macy Jr. Foundation, New York

Stefansson G G, Cullberg 1986 Introducing community mental health services. Acta Psychiatrica Scandinavica 74: 368-378

Strømgren T 1985 Devolution and reform of psychiatric services in Denmark. In: Mangen S P (ed) Mental health care in the European community. Croom Helm, London

Tansella M 1986 Community psychiatry without mental hospitals — the Italian experience: a review. Journal of the Royal Society of Medicine 79: 664-669

van der Grinten 1985 Mental health care in the Netherlands. In: Mangen S P (ed) Mental health care in the European community. Croom Helm, London

Totsuka E 1990 The history of Japanese psychiatry and the rights of mental patients. Psychiatric Bulletin 14: 193-200

Wing J K 1974 Psychiatry in the Soviet Union. British Medical Journal i: 433-436

Workneh F, Giel R 1975 Medical dilemma: a survey of the treating practice of a Coptic priest and an Ethiopian sheik. Tropical & Geographical Medicine 27: 431-439

WHO 1978 The WHO medium-term mental health programme 1975-1982 interim report. Division of Mental Health, WHO, Geneva

WHO Regional Office for Europe 1980 Changing patterns in mental health care. Report on a working group. Euro Reports and Studies No 25, Copenhagen

WHO Regional Office for Europe 1987 Mental health services in pilot study areas. Report on a European study. WHO, Copenhagen

Index